Essentials of

ANATOMY

for Dental Students

(With Colour Atlas)

Essentials of ANATOMY for Dental Students (With Colour Atlas)

Inderbir Singh

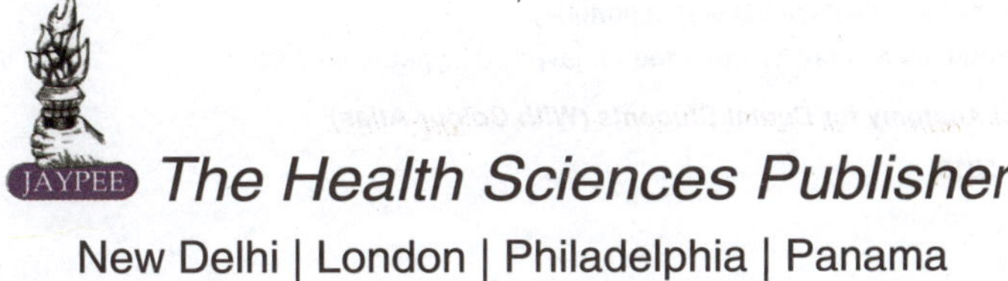

The Health Sciences Publisher
New Delhi | London | Philadelphia | Panama

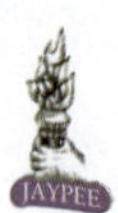

Jaypee Brothers Medical Publishers (P) Ltd

Headquarters

Jaypee Brothers Medical Publishers (P) Ltd
4838/24, Ansari Road, Daryaganj
New Delhi 110 002, India
Phone: +91-11-43574357
Fax: +91-11-43574314
Email: jaypee@jaypeebrothers.com

Overseas Offices

J.P. Medical Ltd
83 Victoria Street, London
SW1H 0HW (UK)
Phone: +44 20 3170 8910
Fax: +44 (0)20 3008 6180
Email: info@jpmedpub.com

Jaypee Medical Inc
The Bourse
111 South Independence Mall East
Suite 835, Philadelphia, PA 19106, USA
Phone: +1 267-519-9789
Email: jpmed.us@gmail.com

Jaypee Brothers Medical Publishers (P) Ltd
Bhotahity, Kathmandu, Nepal
Phone: +977-9741283608
Email: kathmandu@jaypeebrothers.com

Jaypee-Highlights Medical Publishers Inc
City of Knowledge, Bld. 237, Clayton
Panama City, Panama
Phone: +1 507-301-0496
Fax: +1 507-301-0499
Email: cservice@jphmedical.com

Jaypee Brothers Medical Publishers (P) Ltd
17/1-B Babar Road, Block-B, Shaymali
Mohammadpur, Dhaka-1207
Bangladesh
Mobile: +08801912003485
Email: jaypeedhaka@gmail.com

Website: www.jaypeebrothers.com
Website: www.jaypeedigital.com

Inquiries for bulk sales may be solicited at: jaypee@jaypeebrothers.com

Essentials of Anatomy for Dental Students (With Colour Atlas)

First Edition: **2015**

ISBN 978-93-5152-591-2

Printed at Sanat Printers, Kundli.

Preface

Essentials of Anatomy for Dental Students (With Colour Atlas) emphasises throughout the book on a picture memory rather than a verbal one. It is with this objective that the book incorporates a colour atlas. The atlas is realistic to the extent that normal contours and relationships are maintained in the illustrations; but it is schematic in that some structures present in the field of dissection are omitted, or are delineated more clearly than is possible to see in actual dissections. In describing any part of the body, the region is first reviewed using the atlas figures as a guide. This is followed by detailed consideration of individual structures.

For the dental student, the study of anatomy is not an end in itself. It is a necessary beginning to the study of physiology, pathology, and the signs and symptoms of disease. The subject acquires interest if the student is made aware of the clinical importance of what he/she studies in the anatomy class room. This is why there has always been emphasis on what has been called 'applied anatomy.' In this book emphasis is on providing students some examples of clinical correlations of anatomical structures. Instead of spreading out this information in small bits throughout the book, a separate chapter is devoted to clinical correlations at the end of each major part.

The text has been graded into three levels:

1. The descriptions of essential features, which every student must know, are printed on a white background.
2. Details that a good undergraduate student should know are printed on a light green background.
3. Further details that will interest bright students and postgraduates are printed on a light red background.

However, to preserve continuity of narration, matter belonging to all the three categories is given in appropriate sequence.

It is hoped that students as well as teachers will find the book complete and useful.

Inderbir Singh

Contents

PART 1: HEAD AND NECK

PART 2: CENTRAL NERVOUS SYSTEM

PART ONE

Head and Neck

CHAPTER

1

Colour Atlas of the Head and Neck

This chapter consists of a colour atlas of the head and neck. The atlas should be used while reading the text presented from Chapter 52 onwards. In studying any region it will be useful to begin by looking carefully at the figures in the atlas depicting the structures present, their layout, and mutual relationships.

As the drawings are realistic, and in full colour, it will be like seeing the structures in a dissection (but much more clearly!). Thereafter, the descriptions of individual structures will be easy to understand. For quick location of the figures of any region consult the table below. The last three plates are devoted to radiographs.

Arteries, of orbit	24
Artery, common carotid	12, 14 to 17
Artery, external carotid	9 to 17
Artery, internal carotid	9, 10, 14 to 17
Artery, subclavian	14 to 18
Artery, vertebral	18, 19
Cervical fascia	25
Cervical pleura	18
Cervical plexus	14, 15, 18
Cranial fossae	20
Face, deep structures	8, 10
Face, lateral view	6, 8 to 10
Face, muscles of, anterior view	5
Falx cerebri	21
Infratemporal region	10 to 12
Intracranial sinuses	20, 21
Larynx	12, 16, 17, 22
Nasal cavity	22
Neck, anterior triangle	13, 14, 16
Neck, anterior view	16, 17
Neck, deep structures	15, 17

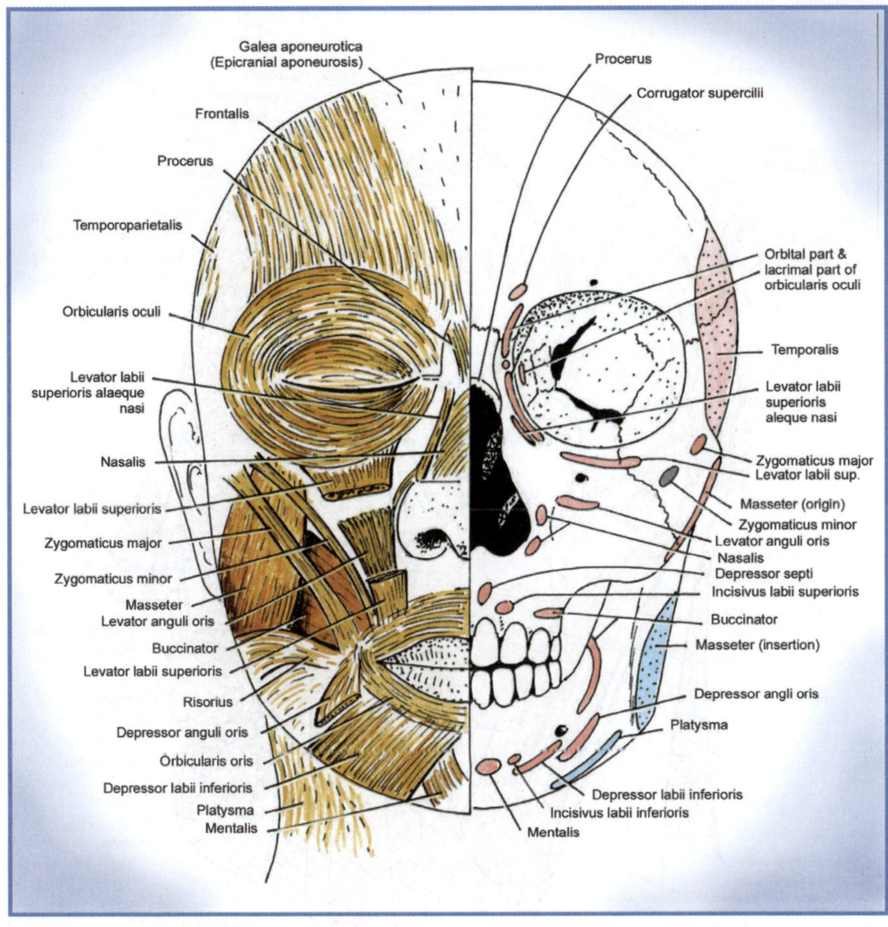

Fig. 1.1 Muscles of the face as seen from the front.

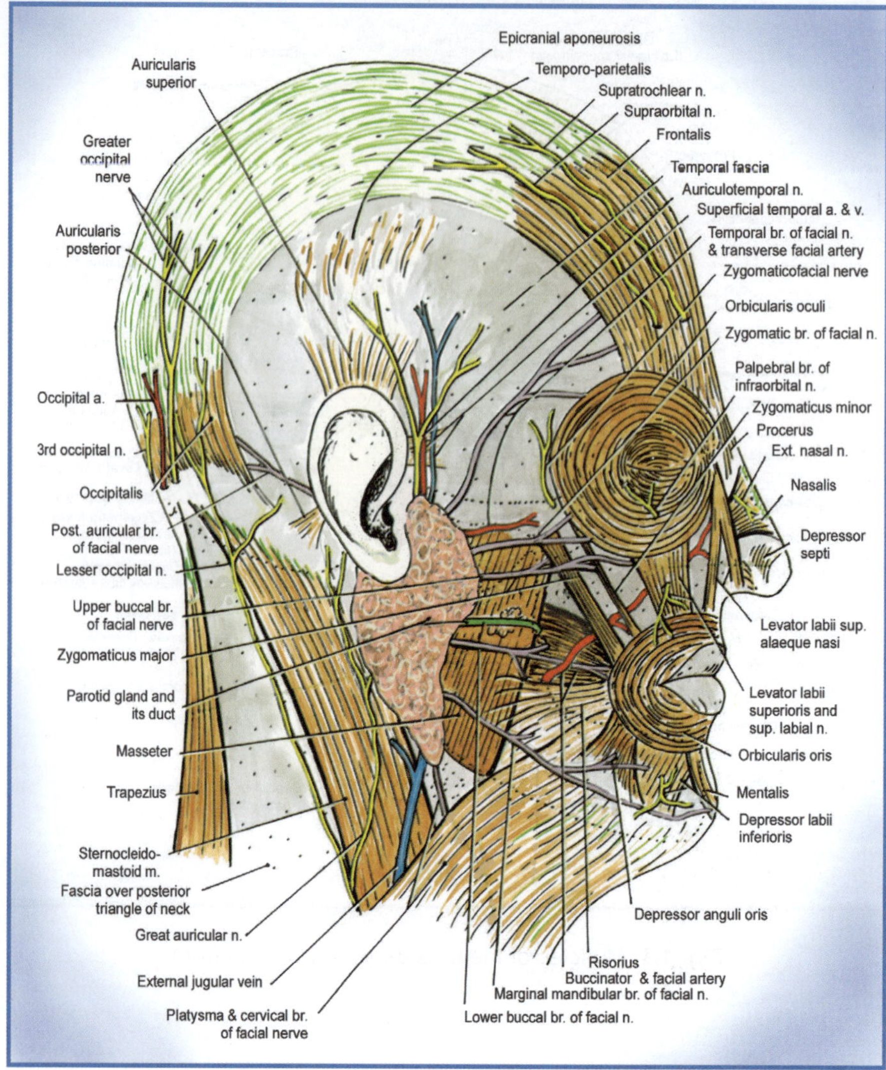

Fig. 1.2 Superficial dissection of the face, scalp, parotid region and temporal region. Branches of the facial nerve are shown in violet.

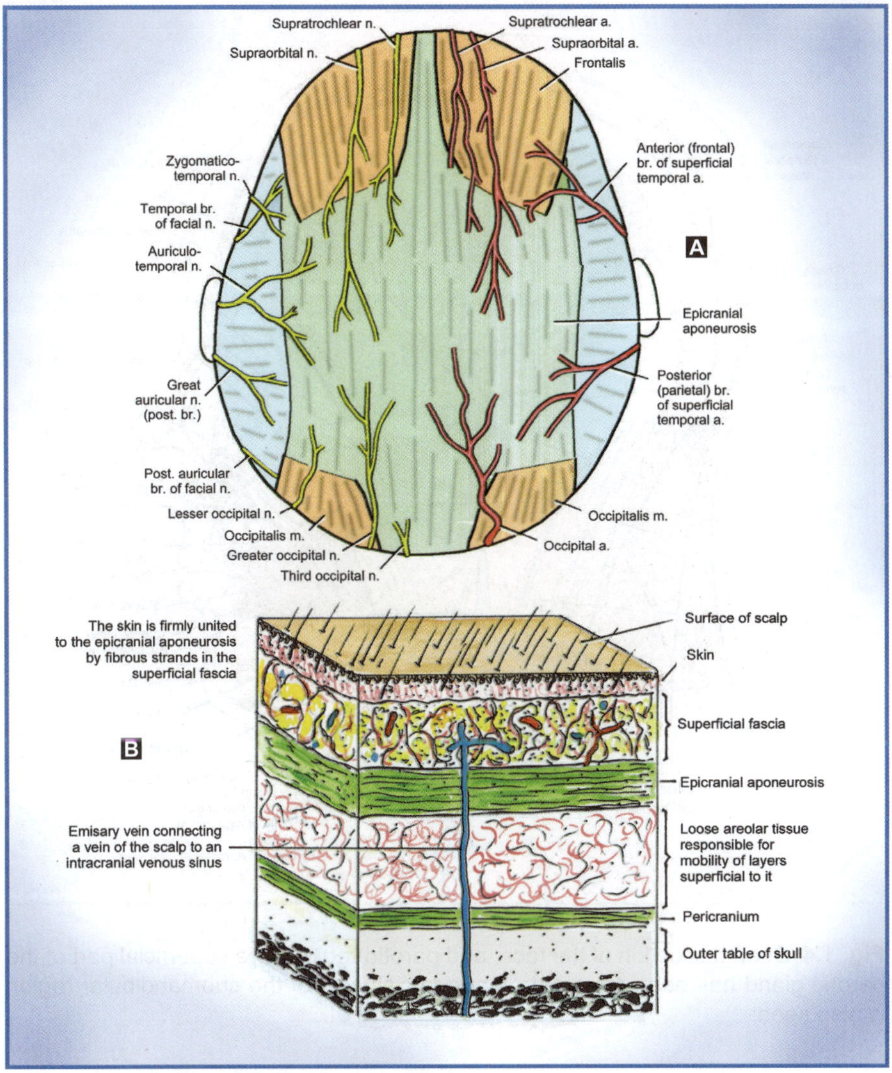

Figs. 1.3A and B A. Nerves and arteries of scalp seen from above. B. Scheme to show the layers of the scalp.

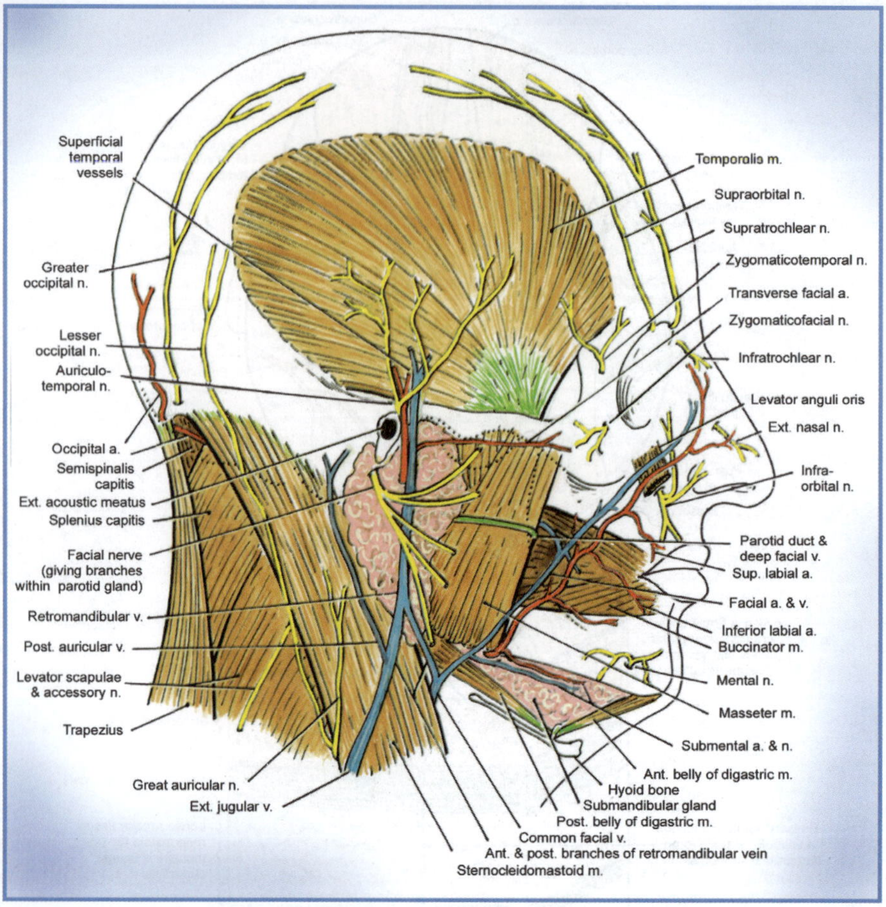

Fig. 1.4 Deep dissection of the face, and parotid region. The superficial part of the parotid gland has been removed. A superficial view of the submandibular region is also seen.

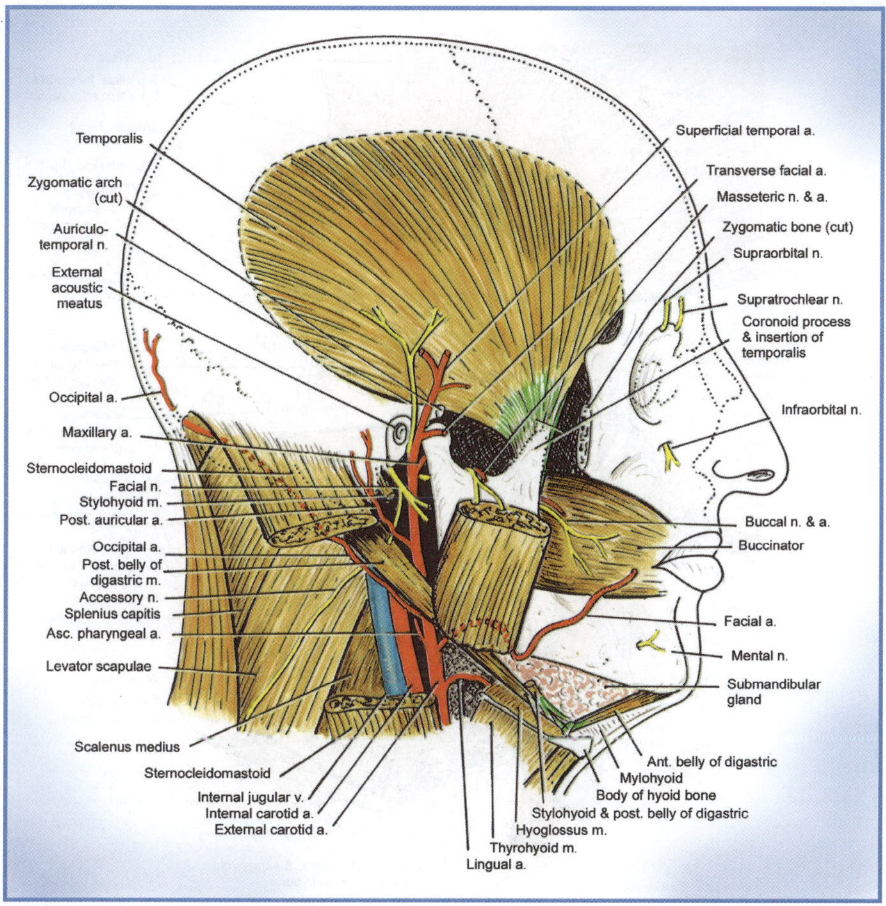

Fig. 1.5 Dissection of side of the head at a deeper plane than shown in Fig. 1.4. The parotid gland, the zygomatic arch, a segment of the sternocleidomastoid, and a segment of the masseter have been removed. The entire temporalis muscle is now seen.

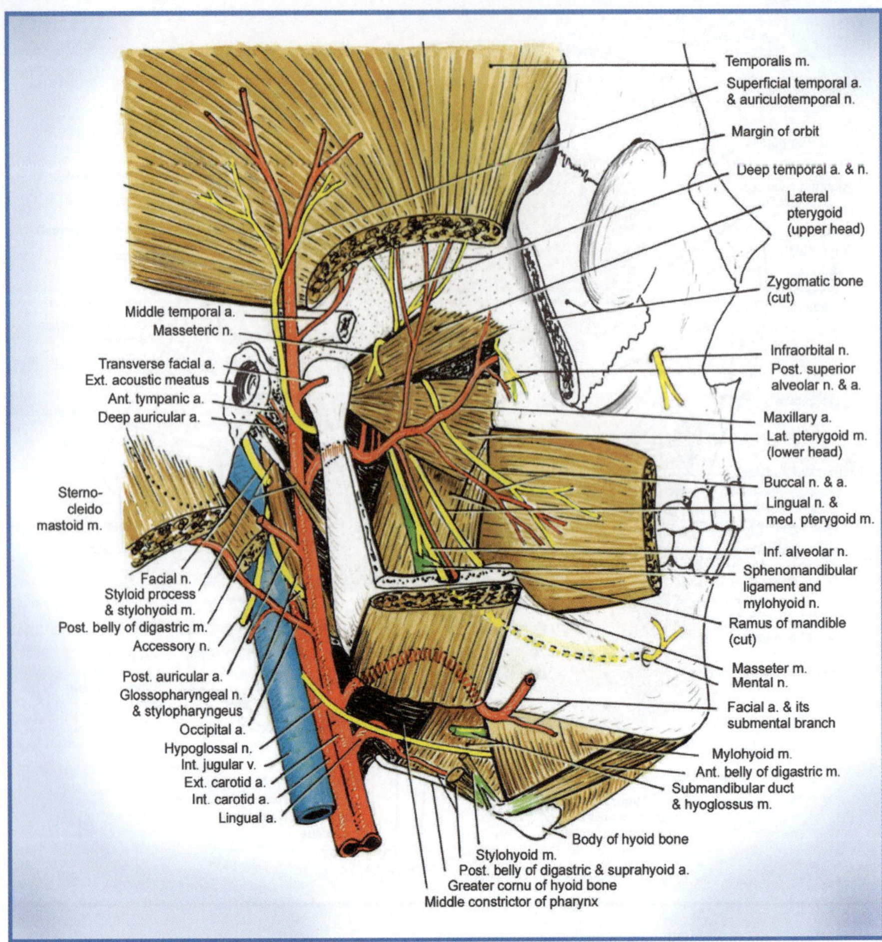

Fig. 1.6 Dissection of the side of the head at a deeper plane than shown in Fig. 1.5. The infratemporal, temporal and submandibular regions are seen. Removal of the sternocleidomastoid brings the internal and external carotid arteries, and the internal jugular vein into view. Note the various branches of the external carotid artery.

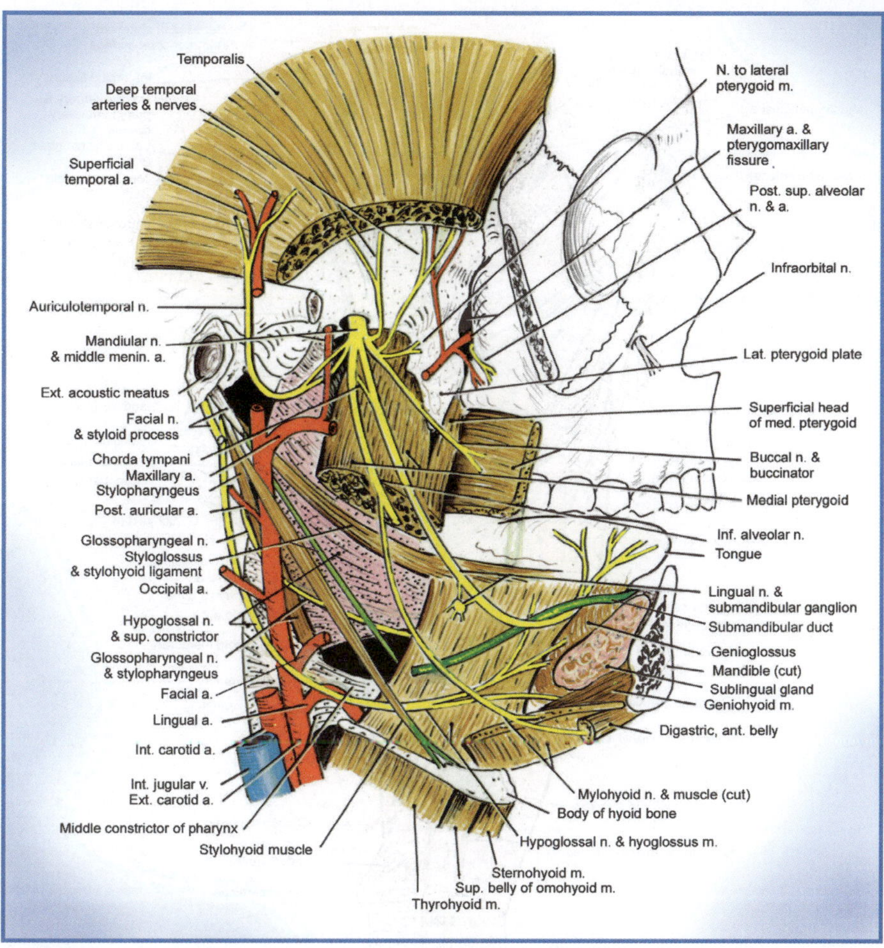

Fig. 1.7 Dissection of the side of the head at a deeper plane than shown in Fig. 1.6. Deep structures in the temporal, infratemporal and submandibular regions are exposed. Note the mandibular nerve and its branches, the structures lying superficial to the hyoglossus muscle, the superior and middle constrictors of the pharynx and the structures related to them.

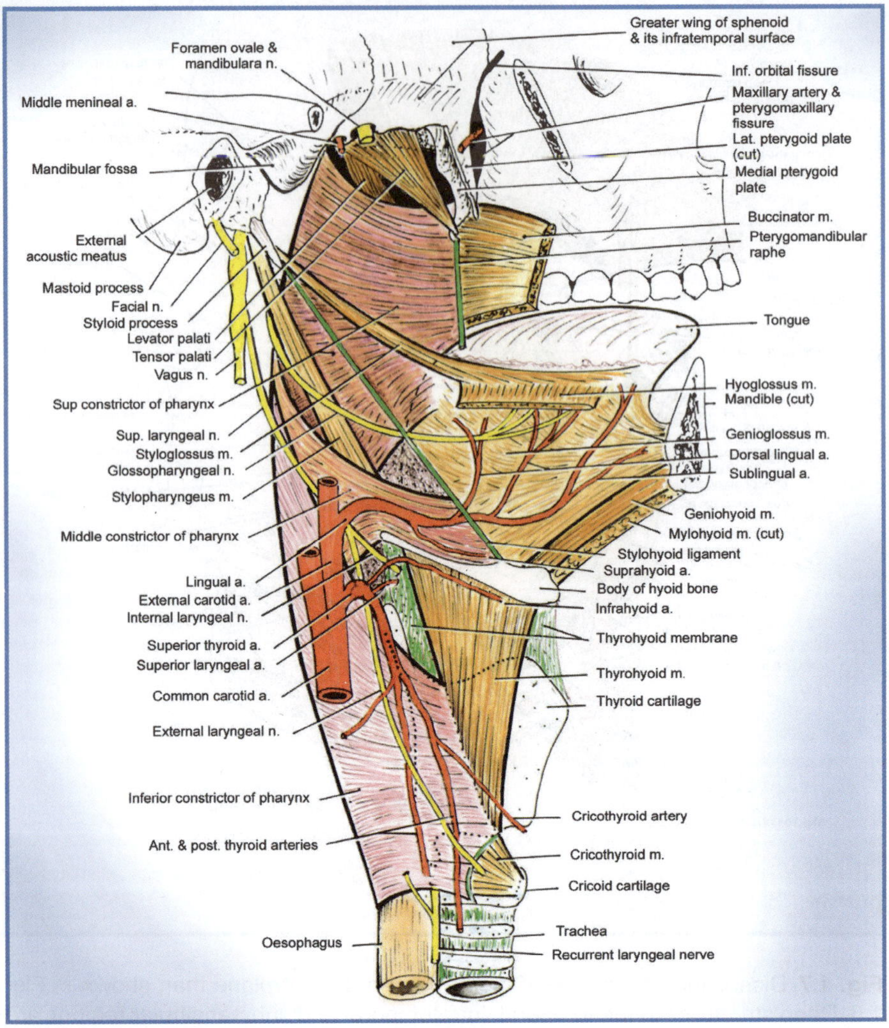

Fig. 1.8 Dissections to show the superior, middle and inferior constrictors of the pharynx and structures related to them. In the submandibular region structures deep to the hyoglossus muscle are seen. Note the course of the glossopharyngeal and superior laryngeal nerves.

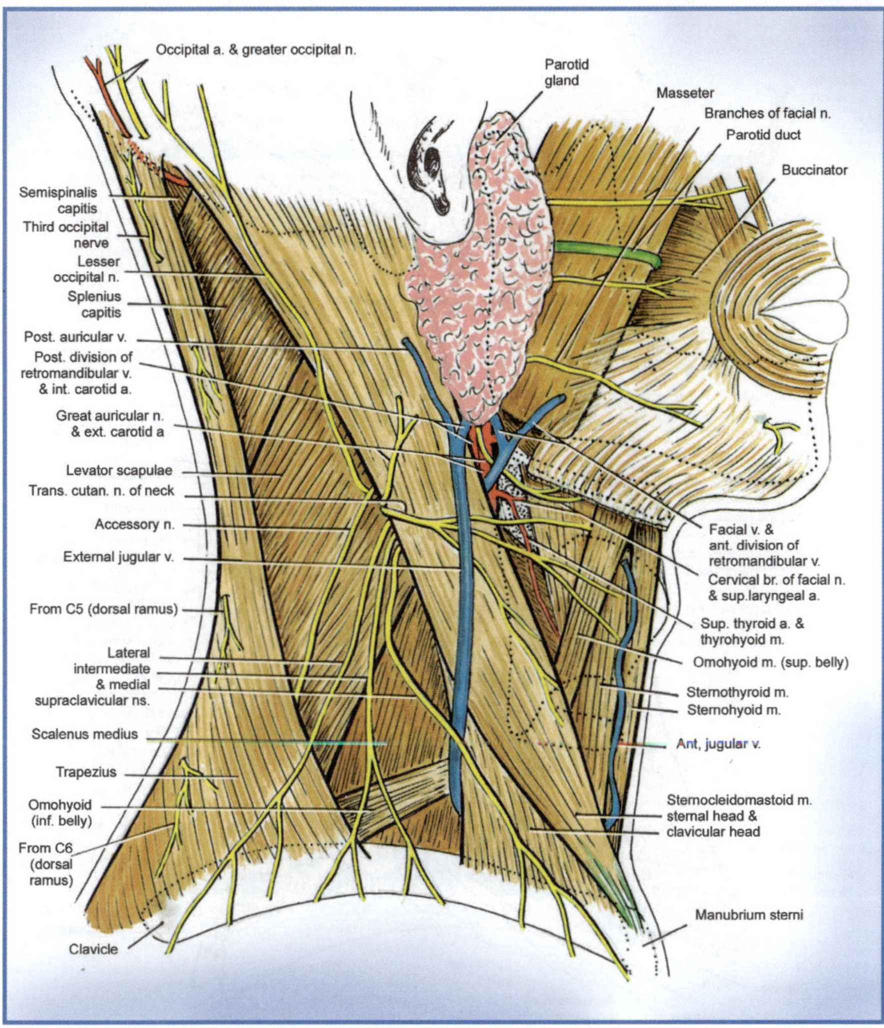

Fig. 1.9 Lateral side of the neck. The fascia covering the muscles has been removed, but superficial nerves and veins are retained. Note the sternocleidomastoid muscle dividing the side of the neck into anterior and posterior triangles, and the various muscles present in these triangles. Some structures of the parotid region and face are also seen.

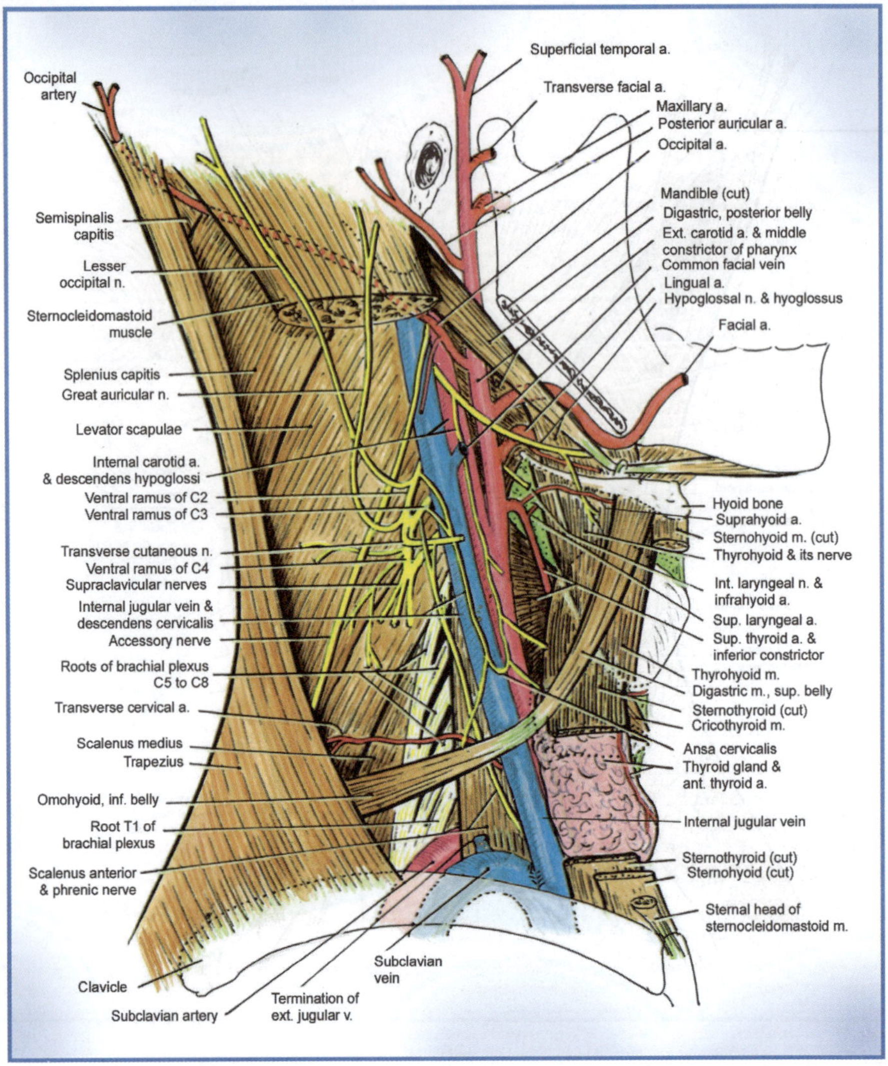

Fig. 1.10 Dissection of lateral side of neck in a deeper plane than in Fig. 1.9. The greater part of the sternocleidomastoid has been removed to reveal deeper structures. Note the cervical and brachial plexuses, the accessory nerve, the carotid arteries, the internal jugular vein and the subclavian vessels. Part of the thyroid gland is also seen.

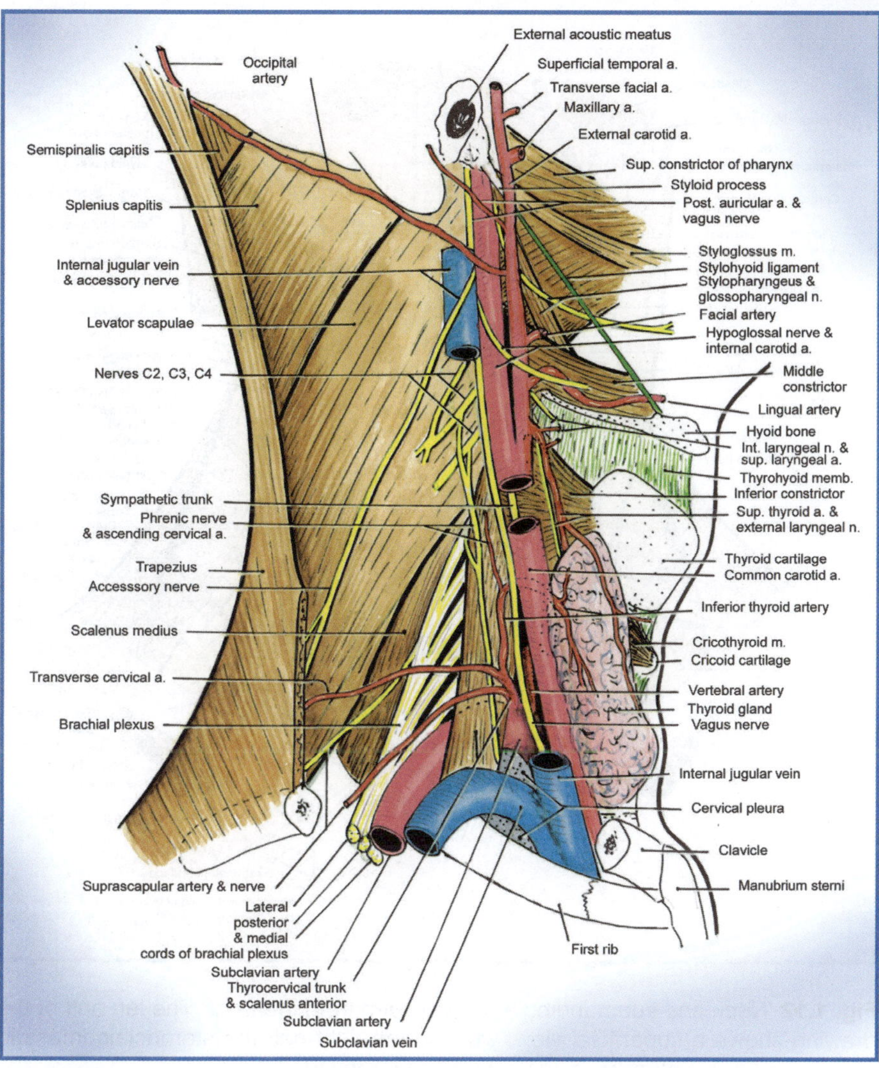

Fig. 1.11 Dissection of lateral side of neck in a deeper plane than in Fig. 1.10. Note the thyroid gland and its arteries, the subclavian vessels and the carotid arteries. Also observe the vagus, phrenic and accessory nerves.

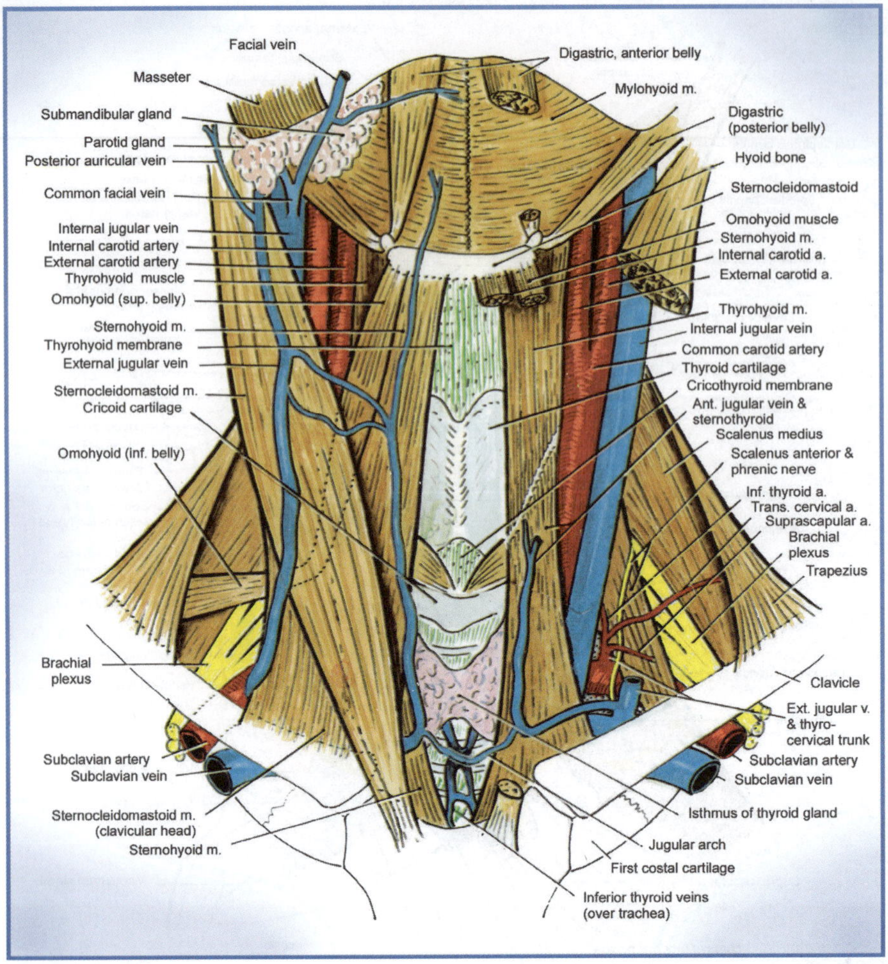

Fig. 1.12 Neck and submandibular region seen from the front. The left half of the drawing shows a superficial view, while in the right half the sternocleidomastoid muscle and some other muscles have been removed.

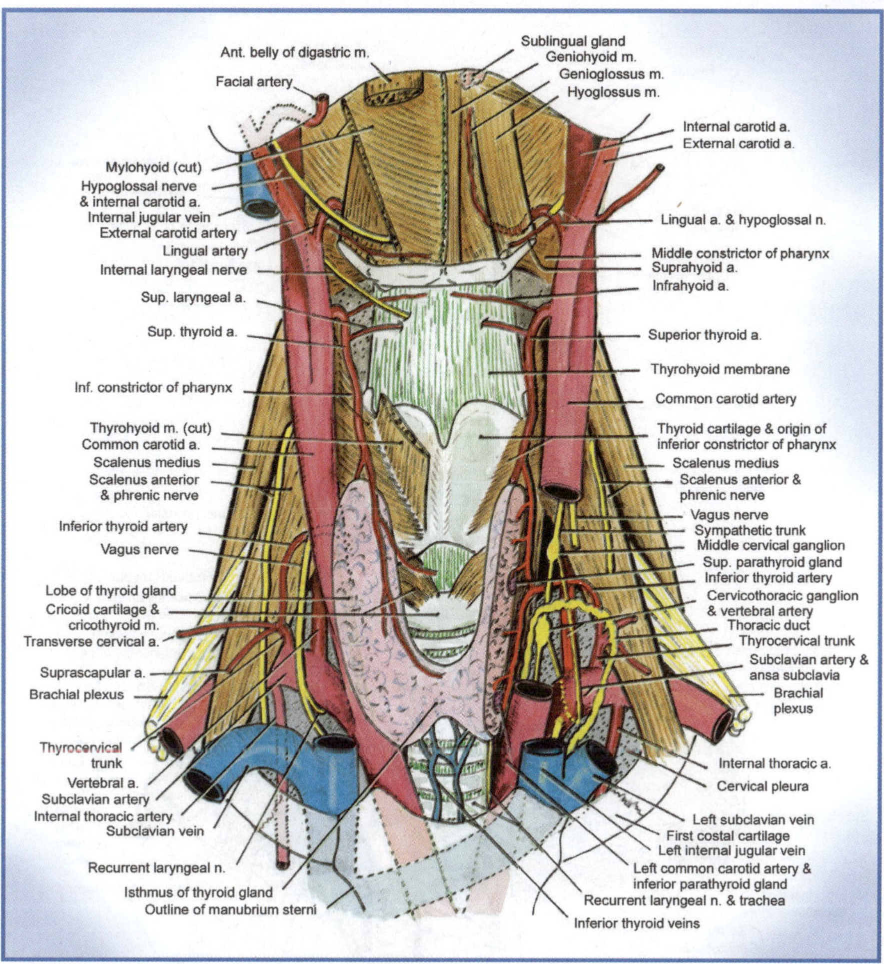

Fig. 1.13 Neck and submandibular region seen from the front at a deeper plane than in Fig. 1.12. Note the thyroid gland and its relations, the branches of the subclavian artery, the thoracic duct and the sympathetic trunk and ganglia.

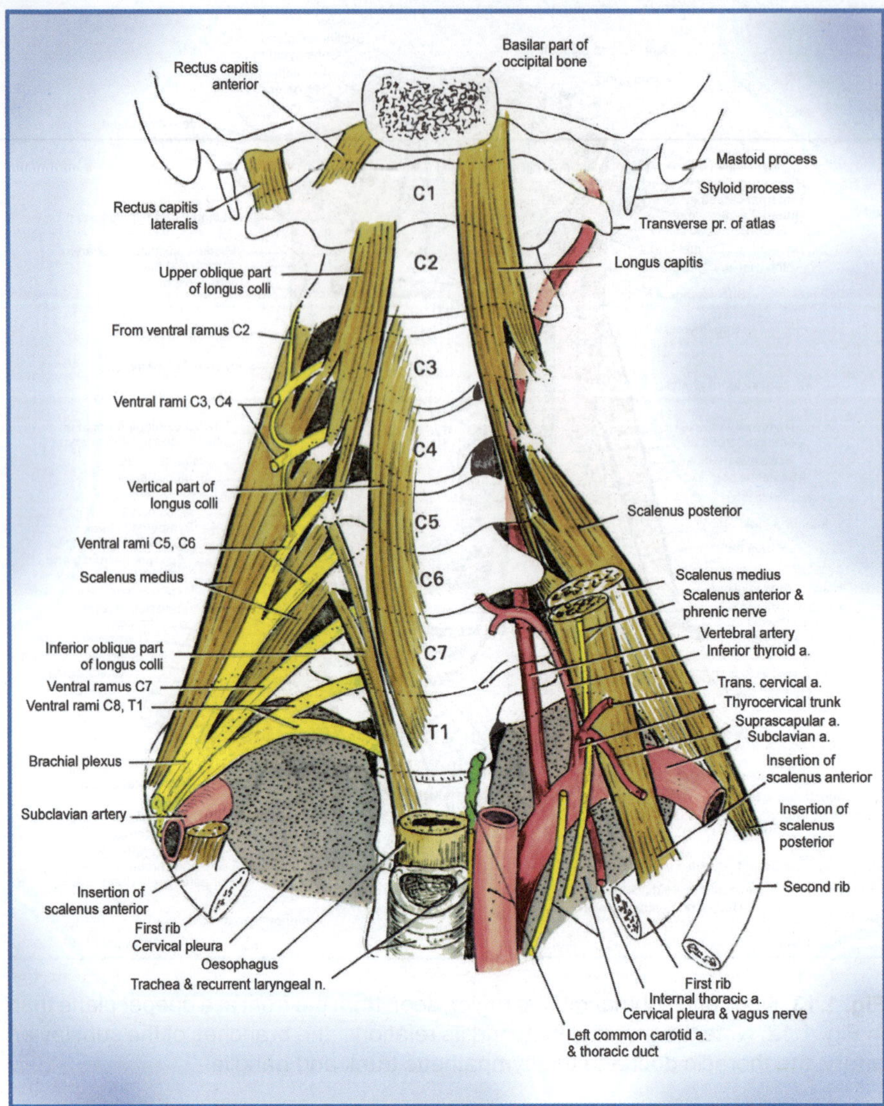

Fig. 1.14 Dissection to show the prevertebral muscles. The brachial and cervical plexuses, the cervical pleura, and the branches of the subclavian artery are seen.

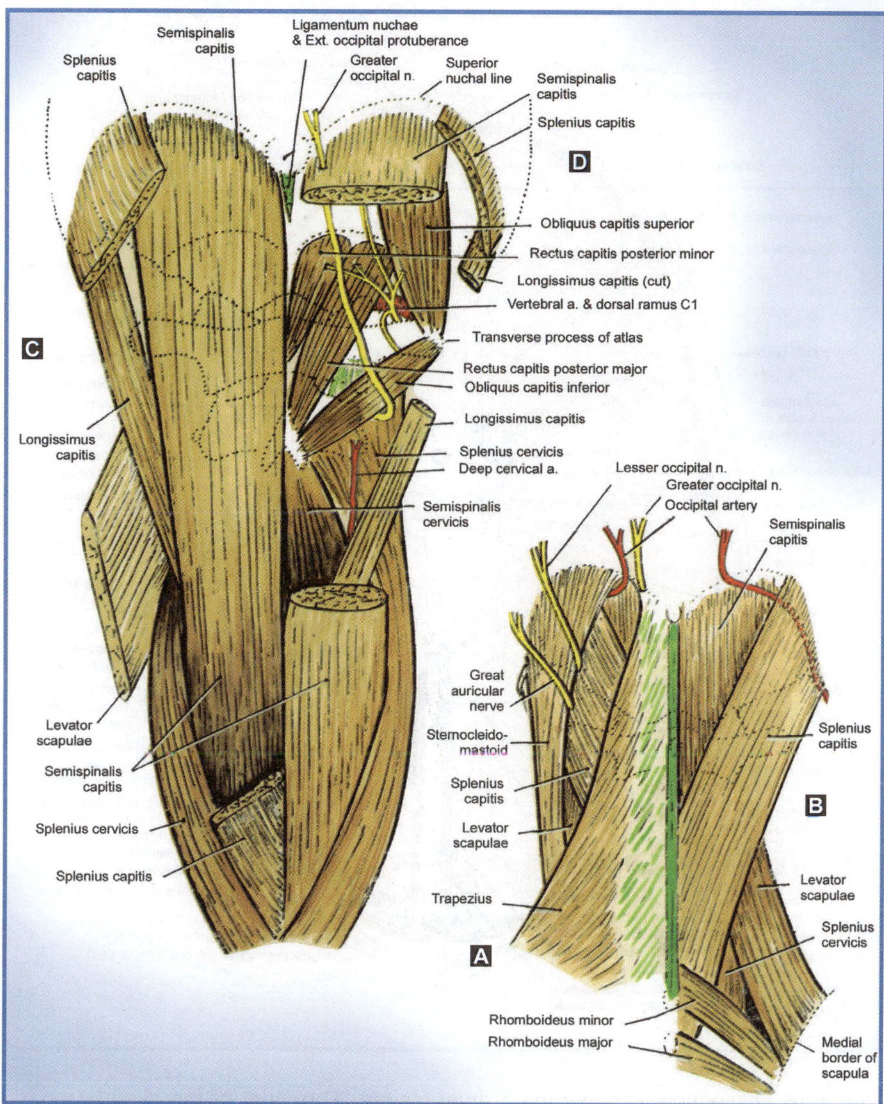

Figs. 1.15A to D A to D. Successive stages in displaying the muscles of the back of the neck. In 'D' note the boundaries and contents of the suboccipital triangle.

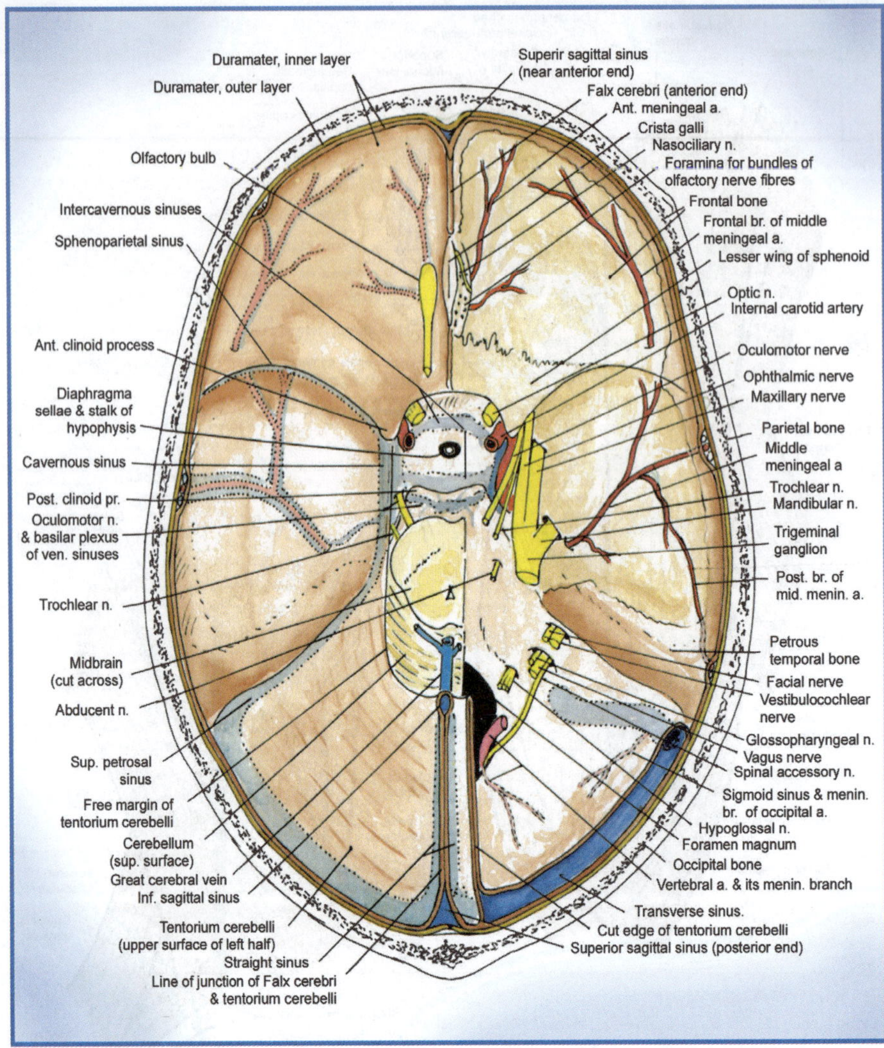

Fig. 1.16 Dissection to show the cranial fossae. The vault of the skull has been removed. In the right half of the drawing the tentorium cerebelli and the cerebellum have been removed.

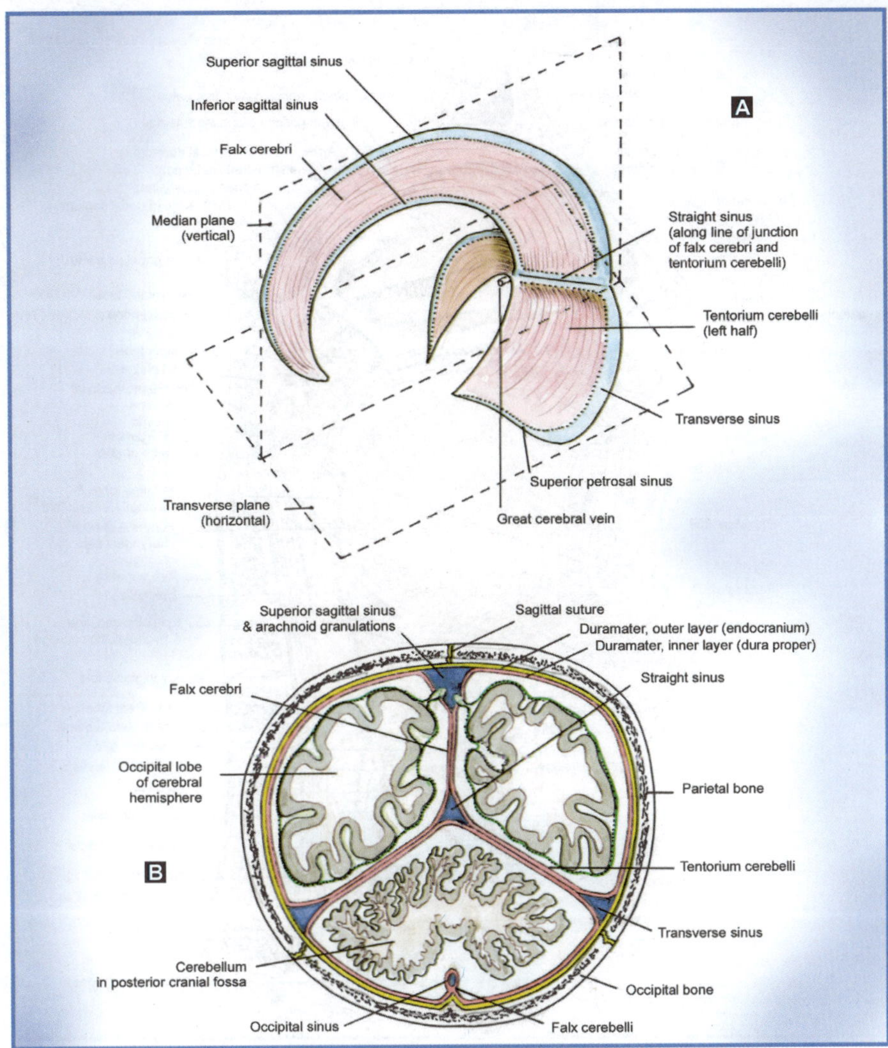

Figs. 1.17A and B A. Scheme to show the orientation of the falx cerebri and tentorium cerebelli. Note the related venous sinuses. B. Coronal section through posterior part of skull to show the relationship of the falx cerebri and tentorium cerebelli to each other and to the venous sinuses of the region.

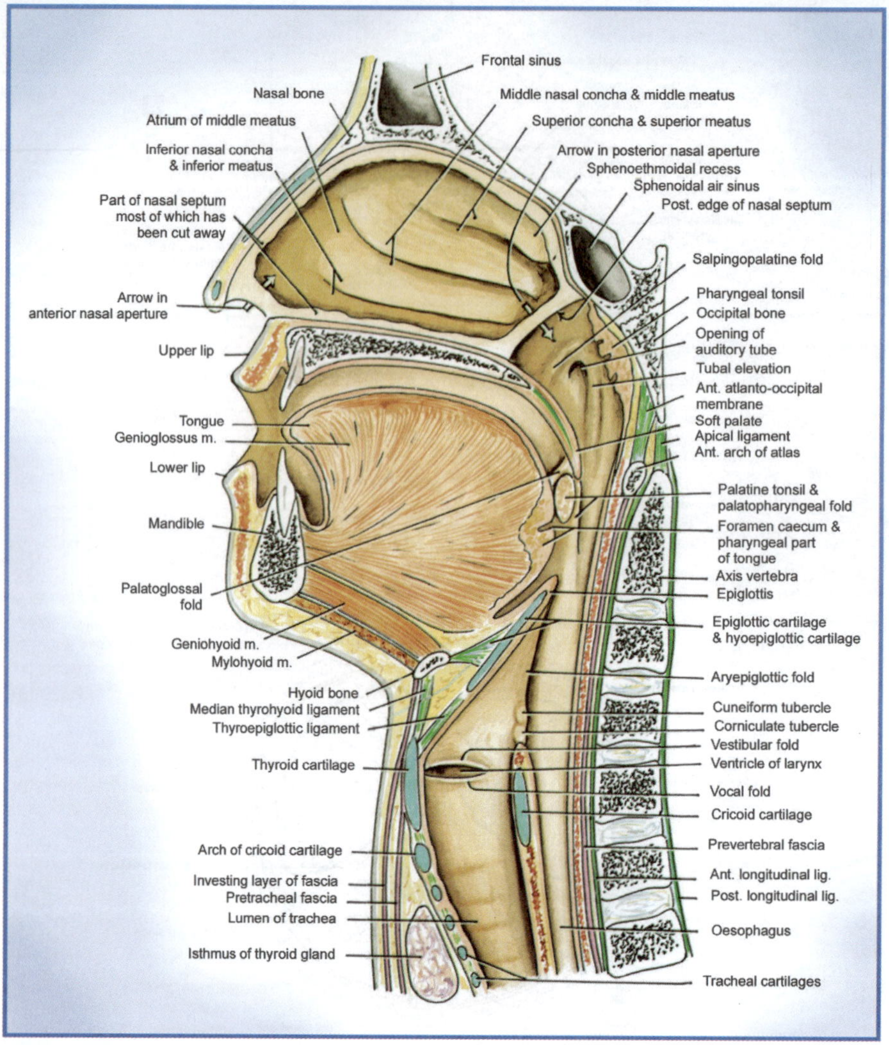

Fig. 1.18 Median section through the neck and anterior part of the head to show the interior of the nose, the mouth, the pharynx and the larynx.

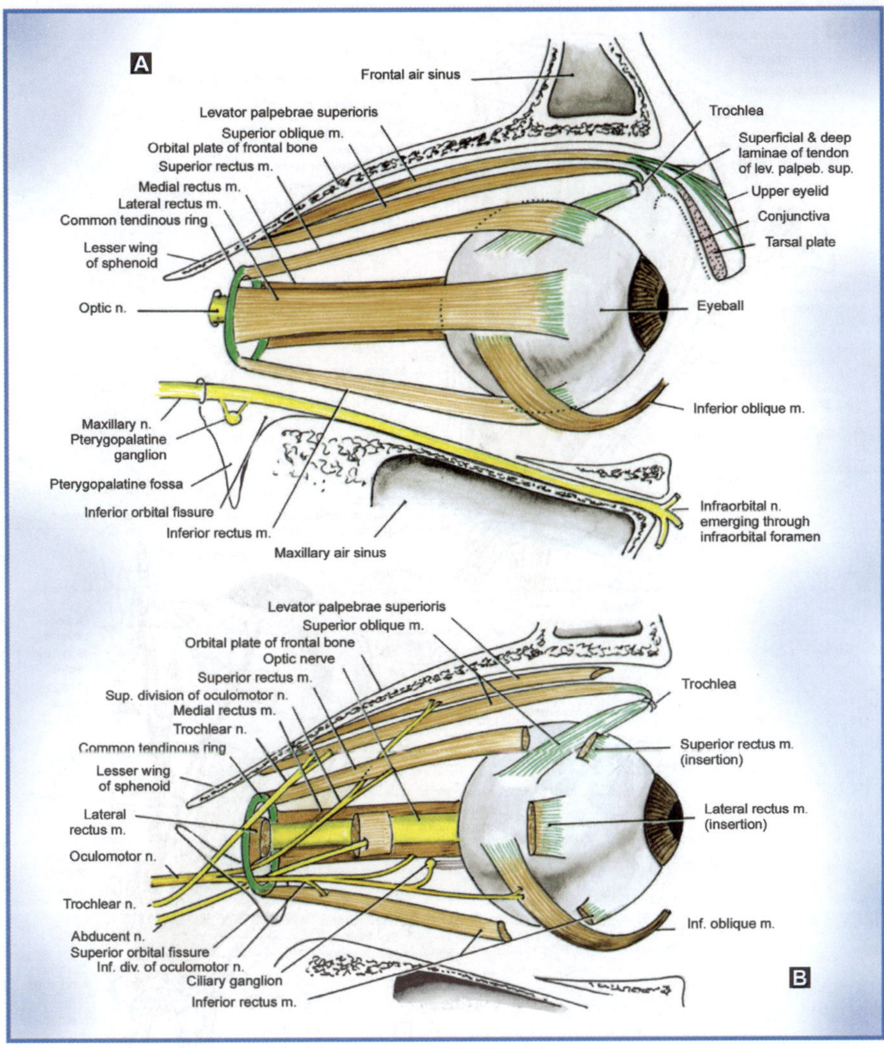

Figs. 1.19A and B A. Scheme to show extraocular muscles as seen from the lateral side. B. Scheme to show the arrangement of nerves supplying the extraocular muscles. The optic nerve is also shown.

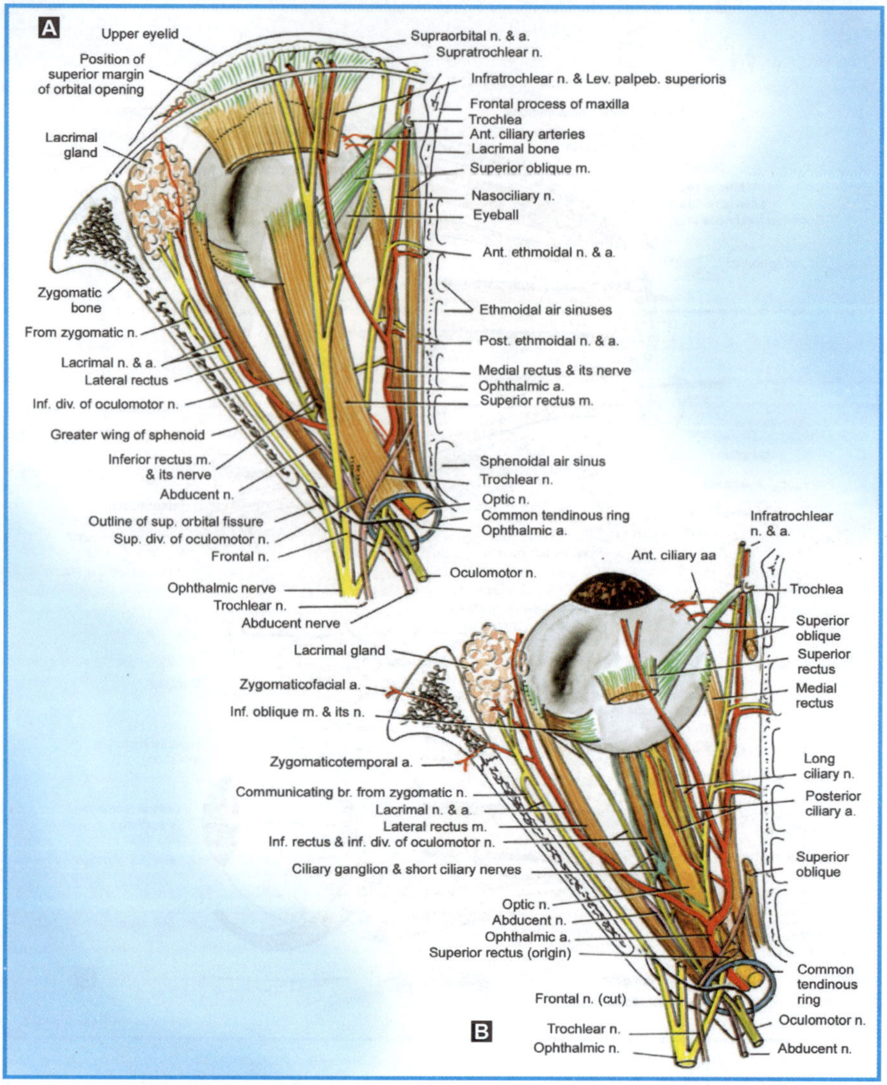

Figs. 1.20A and B Dissections of the orbit seen from above.

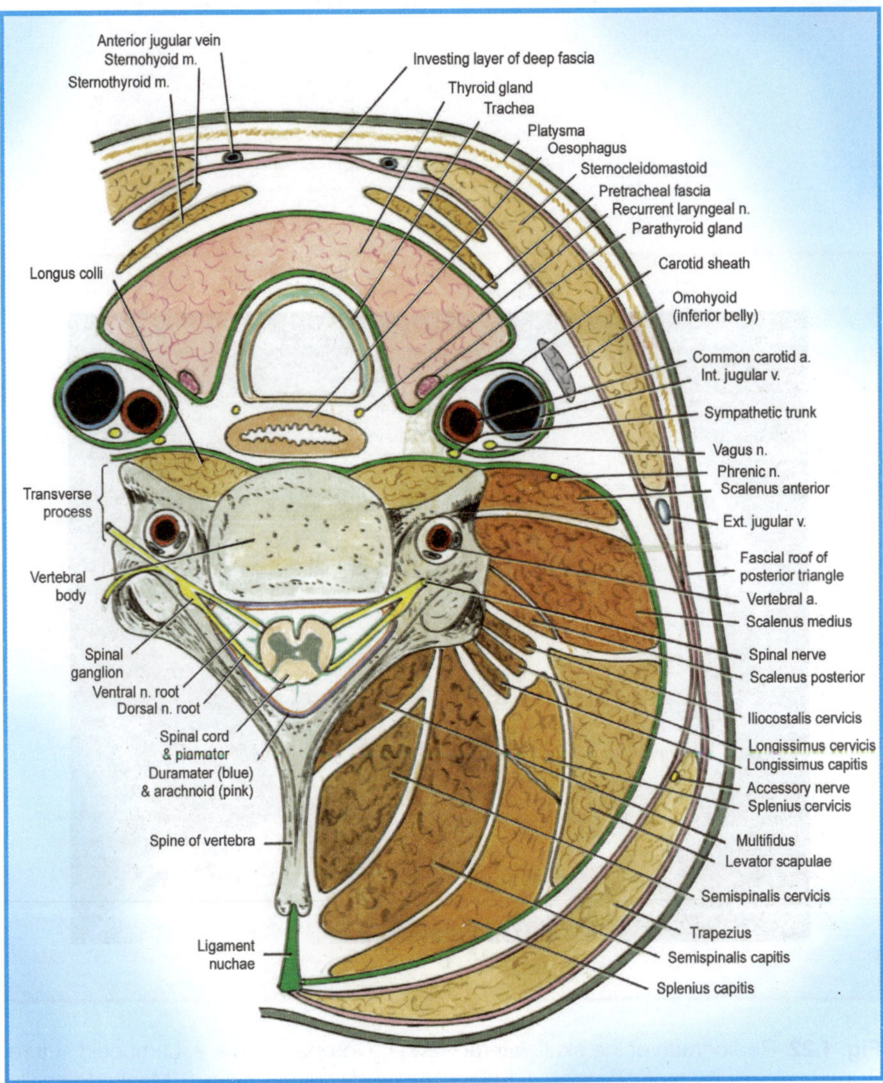

Fig. 1.21 Transverse section through lower part of neck. Note the various groups of muscles, the trachea and oesophagus, the thyroid gland, the carotid sheath, and the layers of cervical fascia.

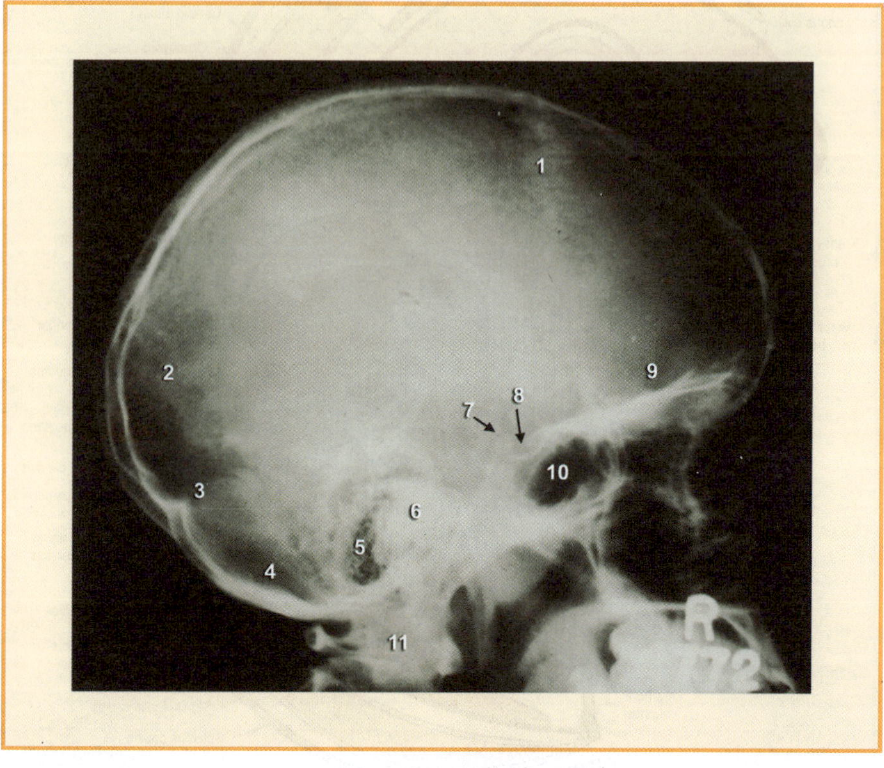

Fig. 1.22 Radiograph of the skull, lateral view. 1. Coronal suture. 2. Lambdoid suture. 3. Internal occipital protuberance. 4. Floor of posterior cranial fossa. 5. Mastoid air cells. 6. Petrous temporal bone. 7. Dorsum sellae. 8. Hypophyseal fossa. 9. Floor of anterior cranial fossa. 10. Sphenoidal sinus. 11. Cervical vertebrae.

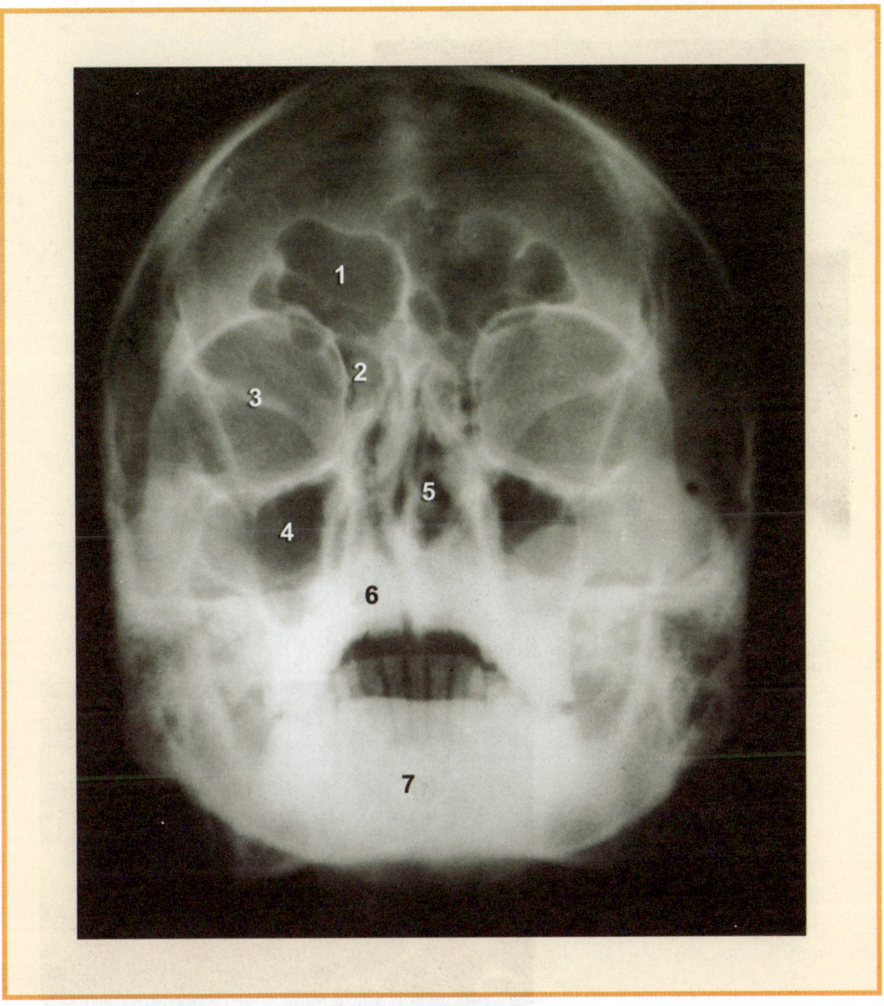

Fig. 1.23 Radiograph of the skull to show paranasal sinuses (PNS) view. 1. Frontal sinus. 2. Ethmoidal sinuses. 3. Orbit. 4. Maxillary sinus. 5. Nasal cavity. 6. Maxilla. 7. Mandible.

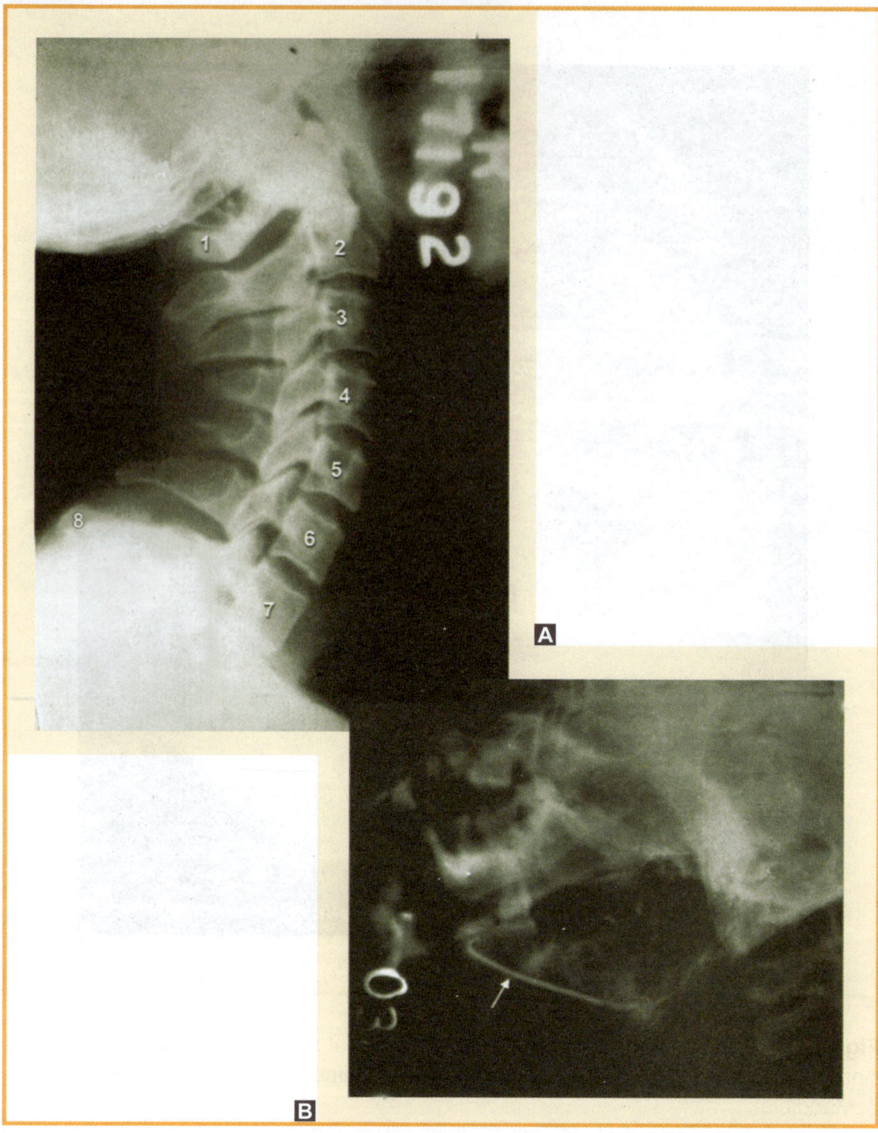

Figs. 1.24A and B A. Radiograph to show the cervical spine (lateral view). 1. Posterior arch of atlas. 2 to 7. Bodies of second to seventh cervical vertebrae. 8. Tip of spine of C7; B. Radiograph after injecting contrast medium into the submandibular duct (Sialography). The arrow points to the duct.

CHAPTER

2

Introduction to the Head and Neck

The head and neck are very important regions of the body. The brain, which is the seat of intelligence, of memory, and of all our emotions, is lodged here. The eyes through which we see, the ears which enable us to hear, the mouth tongue and larynx which help us in speech are all located here. The neck is the great pathway through which the head is connected to the rest of the body. Large blood vessels passing through the neck keep the brain alive by constantly supplying it with blood. Other structures of vital importance lying in the neck are the spinal cord, the pharynx, the larynx, the trachea and the oesophagus. Some endocrine glands that exert a profound influence on tissues throughout the body are located in the head and neck. These are the hypophysis cerebri, the pineal gland, the thyroid gland and the parathyroid glands.

Because of the presence of all these organs, along with numerous muscles, blood vessels and nerves, the head and neck is a challenge to any student of anatomy. Many important structures are small and difficult to see in dissections. As a large number of structures are packed into a relatively small space the relationships to be studied become complex. It is for this reason that the study of the head and neck is usually regarded as difficult and time consuming. However, a student who tries to develop an overall mental picture (rather than mugging up details) will find the study of this region most interesting and rewarding.

In almost all medical institutions in India, dissection of cadavers remains the standard method for the study of gross anatomy including that of the head and neck. In doing so superficial structures have, of necessity, to be studied first, before going on to deeper ones. However, this is far from being the best approach for obtaining a good mental picture of the layout of structures. In particular it is neither interesting nor useful to study nerves and blood vessels in small bits (in the process of which many students fail to acquire a clear picture of their overall distribution). In this book an attempt has, therefore, been made to present the anatomy of different regions in a sequence that will, hopefully, lead to good overall comprehension.

Skeleton of the head and neck

The skeletal basis of the head is formed by the skull and the mandible. These have been described in Chapter 8. Students are strongly advised to read this chapter as a knowledge of the skull is fundamental to understanding the anatomy of the head.

The skeletal basis of the neck is formed by the seven cervical vertebrae. These are described in Chapter 6. Several structures in the neck have attachments on the clavicle, the scapula, the sternum and the upper two ribs. The features of these bones should be revised as and when references are made to them.

Demarcation of the head from the neck

For convenience of description the head and neck are subdivided into several regions. Before considering these subdivisions it is necessary to clearly understand exactly where the head joins the neck, because this is not as obvious as it may appear.

The first point to understand is that the neck is longer posteriorly than it is anteriorly. Anteriorly, in the middle line, the lower limit of the neck lies at the

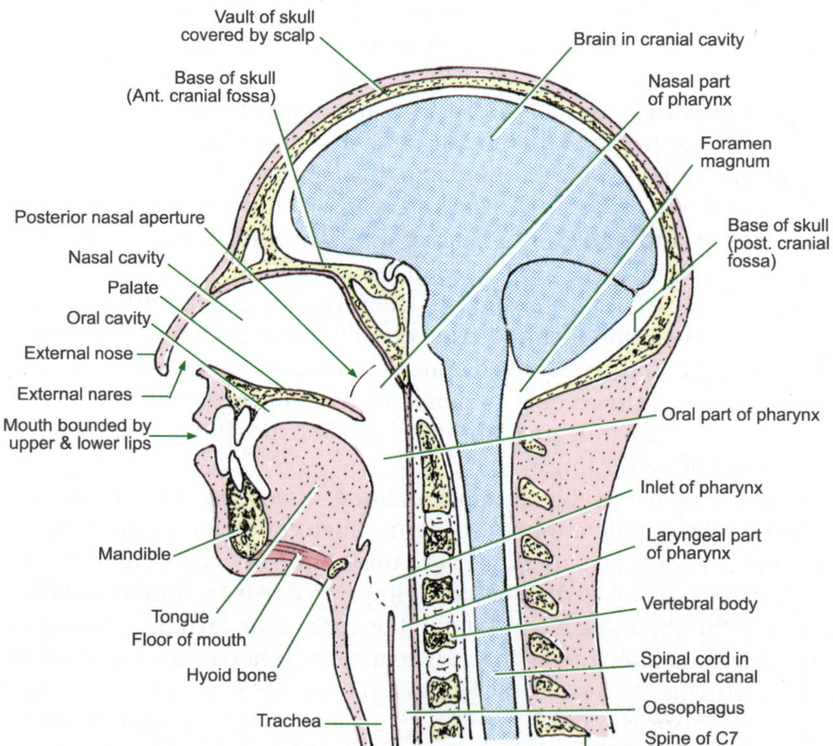

Fig. 2.1 Schematic and highly simplified presentation of some structures to be seen in a median section through the head and neck.

upper border of the manubrium sterni. If gentle backward pressure is applied here with a finger the trachea can be felt. If the finger is passed upwards for about an inch we can feel a thick bar of cartilage lying transversely. This is the cricoid cartilage (a part of the larynx). Passing further upwards we can feel a median cartilaginous projection. This is the thyroid cartilage (again a part of the larynx). A short distance above the thyroid cartilage we can feel the hyoid bone. For all practical purposes we can regard the level of the hyoid bone as the upper limit of the neck in front.

Between the hyoid bone behind, and the chin in front, we have the floor of the mouth. It is bounded on each side by the lower border of the body of the mandible. Most of the structures here belong to the head, but some superficial muscles lying in the region are included amongst muscles of the neck.

Lateral to the manubrium sterni the lower end of the neck extends to the clavicles. Traced upwards it extends up to the mandible. Behind the mandible the neck extends upwards to reach the mastoid process.

The back of the neck is covered by a thick muscle mass. In the middle line the muscles extend up to the external occipital protuberance; and more laterally their upper limit lies along a line passing from the external occipital protuberance to the mastoid process. The spines of the upper six cervical vertebrae cannot be palpated as they are short and covered by soft tissues. However, the spine of the seventh cervical vertebra is prominent and can be taken as the lower limit of the neck on the back.

Finally it has to be stressed that the lower limit of the neck is not horizontal but slopes downwards and forwards. It corresponds to the plane of the superior thoracic aperture.

AN OVERVIEW OF THE LAYOUT OF STRUCTURES IN THE HEAD AND NECK

CRANIAL CAVITY AND VERTEBRAL CANAL

The skull is divisible into a large upper and posterior part occupied by the ***cranial cavity***; and the ***facial skeleton*** forming the anterior and inferior part.

The cranial cavity is occupied by the brain which is surrounded by three membranes (meninges) called the ***duramater*** (outermost), the ***arachnoidmater*** and the ***piamater*** (innermost). Between the arachnoidmater and the piamater there is the ***subarachnoid space*** which is filled by ***cerebrospinal fluid*** (usually abbreviated to CSF). In addition to the brain, meninges and CSF the cranial cavity contains twelve pairs of cranial nerves that emerge from the brain and leave the cranial cavity through foramina in its walls. The cranial cavity also contains arteries that enter it from the neck to supply the brain and meninges. Venous blood drains into a series of ***intracranial venous sinuses***.

The roof and side walls of the cranial cavity are formed by the vault of the skull. The skin and other soft tissues that cover the vault of the skull constitute the ***scalp***. The floor of the cranial cavity is in the form of three large depressions. These are the ***anterior, middle and posterior cranial fossae***. Apart from the

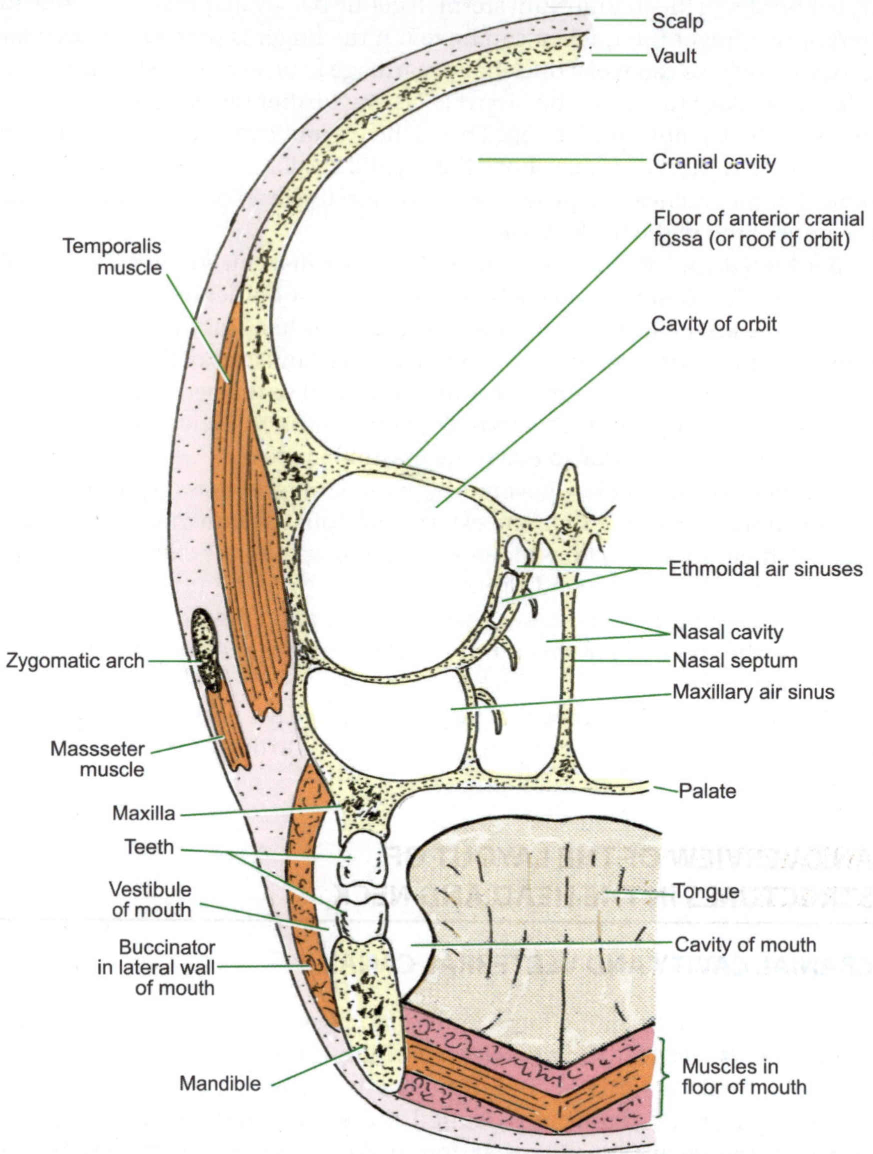

Fig. 2.2 Schematic coronal section through the anterior part of the head to show its main features.

brain the cranial cavity contains two important endocrine glands. These are the hypophysis cerebri and the pineal gland.

Inferiorly, the cranial cavity has a large opening the ***foramen magnum***, through which it communicates with the ***vertebral canal***. The vertebral canal contains the spinal cord which is continuous with the lower end of the brain. Like the brain the spinal cord is surrounded by duramater, arachnoidmater and piamater. The subarachnoid space and CSF extend into it. The vertebral canal also contains blood vessels and roots of a series of spinal nerves that emerge from the spinal cord. The vertebral canal descends through the length of the vertebral column and reaches up to the sacrum. However, the spinal cord extends only up to the lower border of the first lumbar vertebra.

The cranial cavity and vertebral canal may be regarded as one unit housing the central nervous system (brain and spinal cord) (Fig. 2.1). It is appropriate that they be studied together. [Even though the greater part of the vertebral canal lies outside the confines of the head and neck, it is traditional to study the contents of the canal along with the head and neck].

THE BACK

The soft tissues that cover the vertebral column from behind are referred to simply as ***the back***. The region contains a number of muscles, the most conspicuous of which is the erector spinae (Fig. 2.4). Even though the back extends right down to the sacral region, the muscles here are traditionally studied along with the head and neck.

Superficially, muscles of the back are overlapped by muscles of the extremities that gain attachment to the vertebral column (e.g., the trapezius and latissimus dorsi). These muscles have already been studied in the section on the upper extremity.

FACIAL REGION AND NECK

It has been mentioned above that the cranial cavity and the cervical part of the vertebral column can be regarded as one unit of the head and neck. Similarly, the facial region (of the head) and the tissues of the neck lying in front of the vertebrae can be regarded as a unit that contains structures belonging to the alimentary and respiratory systems. The region also contains the eyes and orbits; numerous muscles that move the head and the neck; large blood vessels and nerves. In addition it contains the thyroid and parathyroid glands (which are important endocrine glands).

To understand the layout of structures in the facial region and in the neck we will begin by examining a highly simplified sagittal section through the head and neck (Fig. 2.1). Note again the broad division of the head and neck into an upper and posterior subdivision including the cranial cavity, the vertebral column, the vertebral canal, and structures on the back; and a second division lying below the anterior part of the cranial cavity, and in front of the cervical vertebrae.

Note the following structures lying in the facial region and in the front of the neck.

a. The ***nasal cavity*** is the first part of the respiratory passages. Anteriorly, it opens on the face through the nostrils (or external nares). Posteriorly, it opens into the upper part of the pharynx (see below). Note that superiorly the nasal cavity is separated only by a thin plate of bone from the anterior cranial fossa. Inferiorly, the nasal cavity is bounded by the palate which separates it from the oral cavity. The anterior part of the palate is made up of bone covered by mucosa (***hard palate***), but the posterior part is made up only of soft tissues (***soft palate***).

b. Immediately below the nasal cavity there is the oral cavity. Anteriorly, the oral cavity opens to the outside through the mouth. Posteriorly, it opens into the pharynx (see below). The roof of the oral cavity is formed by the palate. The greater part of the palate is formed by the right and left maxillae. The upper teeth are attached to the alveolar process of the maxilla. The floor of the mouth is predominantly muscular. Anteriorly, and on the sides these muscles gain attachment to the body of the mandible. Posteriorly they are attached to the hyoid bone. The mandible and hyoid bone thus maintain the shape of the floor of the mouth and give strength to it. The lower teeth are attached to the alveolar process of the mandible. The tongue is attached to the floor of the mouth.

The Pharynx and Larynx

In Fig. 2.1 note the presence of a long passage lying in front of the cervical vertebrae. Its upper end reaches the base of the skull, and inferiorly it extends to the level of the 6th cervical vertebra. This passage is the pharynx. It is divisible into three parts.

The uppermost part of the pharynx communicates anteriorly with the nasal cavity. It is, therefore, called the ***nasal part of the pharynx*** (or nasopharynx). The middle part communicates anteriorly with the oral cavity. It is, therefore, called the ***oral part of the pharynx*** (or oropharynx). The lower part of the pharynx is the ***laryngeal part***. Near its upper end the laryngeal part opens anteriorly into the larynx. Lower down the laryngeal part of the pharynx lies behind the larynx.

The pharynx and larynx extend downwards up to the level of the lower part of the sixth cervical vertebra. Below this level the pharynx becomes continuous with the oesophagus and the larynx becomes continuous with the trachea.

The pharynx is a passage common to the alimentary and respiratory systems. Food passes from the mouth into the oral part of the pharynx, down into the laryngeal part, and into the oesophagus. Air breathed in through the nose passes through the nasal, oral and laryngeal parts of the pharynx to enter the larynx and the trachea. The soft palate acts as a flap that can shut off the nasopharynx from the oropharynx during swallowing. The palate also plays an important role in speech by preventing leakage of air through the nose.

The walls of the pharynx are predominantly muscular. As seen in Fig. 2.1 the anterior wall is mostly deficient because of the presence of openings into the nasal cavity, the oral cavity and the larynx.

The ***larynx*** is placed anteriorly in the neck. It has a dual function. Firstly, it is a respiratory passage and is continuous inferiorly with the trachea. Secondly it is responsible for production of voice. Its walls have a cartilaginous basis covered by some muscles and mucosa.

The ***trachea*** and ***oesophagus*** lie in front of the 7th cervical vertebra and pass into the thorax through the superior thoracic aperture.

In the above paragraphs we have studied the placing of the nasal cavity, the oral cavity, the pharynx and larynx as seen in a sagittal section. Some additional facts can be appreciated by studying a coronal section through the anterior part of the head (Fig. 2.2).

The upper part of Fig. 2.2 shows the anterior part of the cranial cavity. Note that its roof and lateral wall are formed by bones in the vault of the skull. The floor (anterior cranial fossa) is formed by a thin plate of bone. Near the median plane the region just below the anterior cranial fossa is occupied by the ***nasal cavity***. This cavity is divided into right and left halves by a median ***nasal septum***. The roof of the nasal cavity is narrow and is separated from the anterior cranial fossa only by a thin plate of bone. The floor of the nasal cavity is formed by the palate, and is much broader than the roof.

In Fig. 2.2 note some important relationships of the maxilla. We can see that the maxilla helps to form the wall of the orbit, the wall of the nasal cavity and the palate. Also note its alveolar process jutting down into the oral cavity and bearing the upper teeth.

Oral Cavity

The oral cavity is seen in the lower part of the Fig. 2.2. Note the roof formed by the palate, and the muscular floor and lateral walls. The tongue and teeth lie within the cavity. When the mouth is closed the upper and lower teeth come into apposition. The cavity is then seen to be divided into a main part containing the tongue, and a part between the teeth and the cheeks. The latter part of the oral cavity is called the vestibule.

SOME REGIONS OF THE HEAD

In the above paragraphs we have seen that the core of the head and neck is formed by a series of cavities and passages. The remaining space in the head and neck is filled in by muscles, along with large blood vessels and nerves. Some glands are also present. For convenience of description we can consider these structures in groups as follows.

Face

A view of the face seen after removal of skin is shown in Figs. 1.1 and 1.2. Note the presence of numerous small superficial muscles. (Don't worry about their names yet). These muscles of the face are responsible for facial expression. [In these figures note that some superficial muscles are also present in the scalp and in the upper part of the neck].

In the region of the cheek we see some deep structures in the face. Identify the ***buccinator*** muscle (that forms the substance of the cheek), and behind it the ***masseter***. The masseter is one of several muscles of mastication that are responsible for movements of the jaw while eating. The masseter and buccinator are better seen in Fig. 1.4 in which the facial artery and vein are also seen.

Also note the presence of numerous nerves in the face. The nerves shown in white in Fig. 1.2 are branches of the facial nerve. They supply muscles of the face. Other nerves seen in the face are terminal ramifications of the trigeminal nerve. They are sensory and supply the skin of the face.

Parotid Region

Lying just below the ear we see the parotid gland (Fig. 1.2). This is one of the salivary glands that produce ***saliva*** which keeps the mouth moist. The area occupied by the parotid gland is the ***parotid region***. The gland extends deep into the space behind the mandible. In Fig. 1.4. the superficial part of the parotid gland has been removed. We now see that the gland is traversed by blood vessels and by the facial nerve. The nerve is seen dividing into a number of branches within the gland substance. In Fig. 1.5 the entire parotid gland has been removed and we see that deep to the gland there are several nerves and blood vessels.

Temporal Region

In Fig. 1.4. we see a large muscle over the lateral aspect of the vault of the skull. This muscle is the ***temporalis***. It is one of the muscles of mastication. The region occupied by the temporalis is called the ***temporal fossa***. In Fig. 1. 4 note some superficial vessels and the nerves ascending over the temporalis. In Fig. 1.5 (in which the zygomatic arch has been removed) we see the temporalis muscle in its entire extent. In Fig. 1.6 the lower part of the temporalis has been removed. We now see that some nerves and vessels ascend deep to the muscle.

Infratemporal Fossa

In Fig. 1.6. the lower part of the temporalis and part of the mandible have been removed revealing a region called the infratemporal fossa. In it we see muscles, vessels and nerves. This fossa lies deep under cover of the base of the skull.

The main muscles seen in the infra-temporal region are the lateral pterygoid and medial pterygoid muscles. Like the temporalis and masseter (also seen in this diagram) the lateral and medial pterygoids are muscles of mastication. The main artery of the region is the maxillary artery. A deeper dissection of the region is seen in Fig. 1.7 in which we see that the main nerve of the region is the mandibular nerve.

Submandibular Region

In Fig. 1.5. observe the region below the body of the mandible. Here we see the submandibular gland which (like the parotid) is a salivary gland. Just below the gland we see the digastric muscle arranged like the letter 'V'. The muscle has a posterior belly and an anterior belly. In Fig. 1.6 the submandibular gland has been removed. We see that deep to the gland there are several muscles,

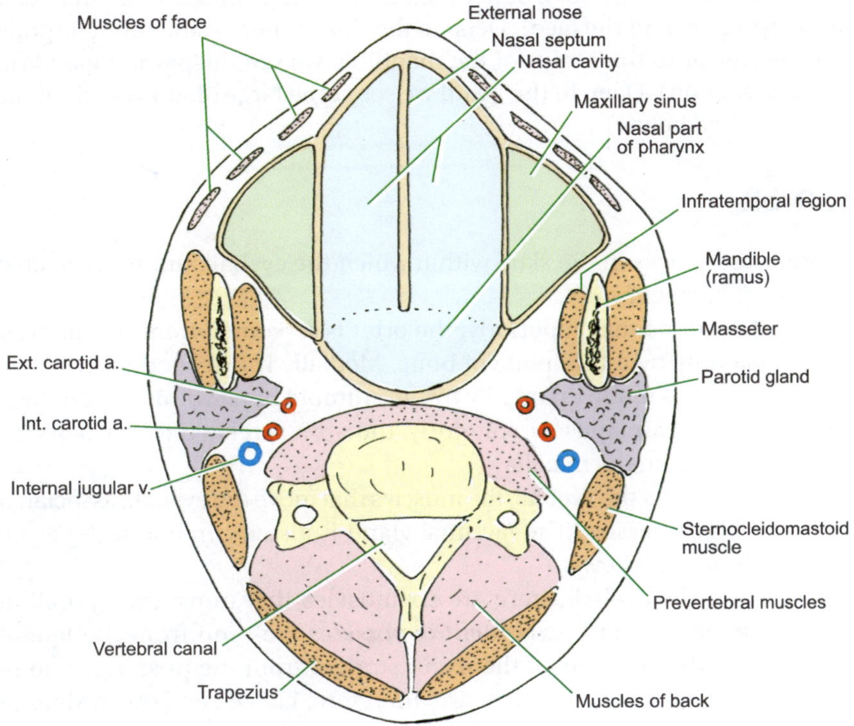

Fig. 2.3 Highly schematic horizontal section through the head at the level of the nasal part of the pharynx. Note the relative position of the various groups of muscles. Many additional structures present are omitted for sake of clarity.

nerves and vessels. Identify the mylohyoid muscle, and behind it the hyoglossus muscle. The mylohyoid muscle forms the floor of the mouth. The hyoglossus is a muscle of the tongue. A still deeper level of the submandibular region is seen in Fig. 1.7. The greater part of the mylohyoid muscle has been removed exposing the hyoglossus fully. Several nerves are seen superficial to the muscle (and will be identified later). Anterior to the hyoglossus note the ***sublingual gland***, which is yet another salivary gland.

In Fig. 1.7 we can see that the continuity between the infratemporal and submandibular regions. The structures see behind the infratemporal and submandibular regions belong to the upper part of the neck.

In the preceding paragraphs we have tried to identify some regions of the head (as seen from the lateral side). The relative depth at which some of these regions lie is better appreciated by studying a horizontal section through the head (Fig. 2.3). In this figure note the right and left halves of the nasal cavity, flanked by the maxillary air sinuses. The nasal cavity opens posteriorly into the nasal part of the pharynx. The region between the pharynx and the vertebral column is the ***prevertebral region***.

On either side of the drawing note the triangular interval bounded anteriorly by the maxilla, and posteriorly by the prevertebral region. In it note the ramus of the mandible (cut across). Superficial to the ramus observe the masseter muscle (lying deep in the face). Deep to the ramus there is the infratemporal region. Posterior to the ramus of the mandible we see the parotid gland (in transverse section). Deep to the gland we see some large blood vessels of the neck (described below).

The Orbit

The orbits are spaces in the skull within which the eyeball and some related structures are present.

In Fig. 2.2 we see that superiorly, the orbit is separated from the anterior cranial fossa only by a thin plate of bone. Medially it is related to the nasal cavity. (This wall is made up mainly by the ethmoid bone within which there are the ethmoidal air sinuses). Inferiorly, the orbit is related to maxillary air sinus, present within the maxilla.

The orbit contains the eyeball, the muscles that move the eyeball, associated nerves and blood vessels. The lacrimal gland is also a content of the orbit. Some details are as follows.

Attached to the eyeball there are six muscles that move the eyeball in various directions. These ***extraocular muscles*** are seen from the lateral side in Figs. 1.19 A,B. Four of them run straight from the posterior end of the orbit to the eyeball, and they are, therefore, called recti. According to their position relative to the eyeball they are termed the ***superior rectus***, the ***inferior rectus***, the ***medial rectus*** and the ***lateral rectus***. The two remaining muscles follow an oblique course. The ***superior oblique muscle*** (Figs. 1.19 A,B) runs forwards along the angle between the upper and medial walls of the orbit. It ends in a tendon that passes through a pulley (trochlea) to turn backwards and laterally to reach the eyeball. The ***inferior oblique*** muscle arises from the anterior and medial part of the floor of the orbit. It runs a curved course first lying below the eyeball and then lateral to it (Fig. 1.19B). Running forwards just below the roof of the orbit there is another muscle the ***levator palpebrae superioris***. This muscle ends in the upper eyelid. It is not attached to eyeball.

Several nerves are seen in the orbit (Fig. 1.19B). The most important of these is the ***optic nerve*** which is attached to the posterior pole of the eyeball. Also identify the oculomotor, trochlear and abducent nerves. These three nerves supply the extraocular muscles. In Fig. 1.20A we see the ophthalmic division of the trigeminal nerve dividing into the lacrimal, frontal and nasociliary nerves. These three nerves enter the orbit and provide sensory innervation to structures in the orbit and to some adjoining regions.

The main artery of the orbit is the ophthalmic branch of the internal carotid artery (Fig. 1.20B). It gives numerous branches to structure in the orbit. In Fig. 1.20 note the lacrimal gland lying in the anterior part of the orbit at the junction of the upper and lateral walls. Note also that the lacrimal nerve and artery supply the lacrimal gland.

Eyelids, Conjunctiva and Lacrimal Apparatus

The front of the eyeball is protected by the upper and lower eyelids. The deep surface of each eyelid is lined by a thin membrane called the ***conjunctiva***. Conjunctiva also lines the anterior part of the eyeball (excluding the cornea). When the eyelids are closed they are separated from the front of the eyeball by a capillary space. This space is called the ***conjunctival sac***. The conjunctiva and cornea are kept moist by lacrimal fluid secreted by the lacrimal gland into the conjunctival sac. After flowing across the front of the eyeball lacrimal fluid enters the ***lacrimal canaliculi*** through which it reaches the ***lacrimal sac***. The lacrimal sac lies in close relation to the medial wall of the orbit. Inferiorly, it becomes continuous with the nasolacrimal duct which opens into the nose. The secretion of lacrimal fluid is greatly increased during emotional stress and flows out as tears. Some of this fluid reaches the nose. [That is why a person in tears needs to blow his/her nose].

LAYOUT OF STRUCTURES IN THE NECK

In Fig. 2.4 we see a highly simplified view of structures to be seen in a horizontal section through the lower part of the neck. Such a section enables us to form a good picture of the arrangement of various structures present in the neck.

Approximately in the centre of the drawing we see a cervical vertebra. Immediately in front of the vertebra there is the prevertebral region occupied by prevertebral muscles. The prevertebral region extends upwards right up to the base of the skull. (In Fig. 2.3 we have seen it lying behind the pharynx).

In front of the prevertebral region, in the middle line, we see the oesophagus, the trachea and the thyroid gland. (In a section at a higher level in the neck the oesophagus is replaced by the pharynx, and the trachea by the larynx). Comparison of Fig. 2.4 with 2.3 will show that throughout the length of the neck the median region in front of the vertebral column (and prevertebral muscles) is occupied by viscera.

In Fig. 2.4 now observe the angular interval between the prevertebral region (posteriorly) and the oesophagus and trachea (medially). This angle is occupied by large blood vessels and nerves running up or down the neck. At the level shown in Fig. 2.4 the large vessels are the ***common carotid artery*** and the ***internal jugular vein***. They are enclosed in a common fibrous covering called the ***carotid sheath***.

Superficial to the foregoing visceral structures (oesophagus, trachea, thyroid gland, carotid sheath) we see a number of flat ribbon like muscles. These are collectively referred to as the ***infrahyoid muscles***. The infrahyoid muscles are in turn overlapped by a large muscle the ***sternocleidomastoid***.

We will now turn our attention to structures behind the vertebra. In the angle between the spine and transverse process of the vertebra we see a mass formed by deep muscles of the back. (The upper part of the same mass is seen in Fig. 2.3). The deep muscles of the back are overlapped by two muscles already studied in the upper extremity. These are the levator scapulae (Fig. 2.4), and the trapezius (Figs. 2.3, 2.4).

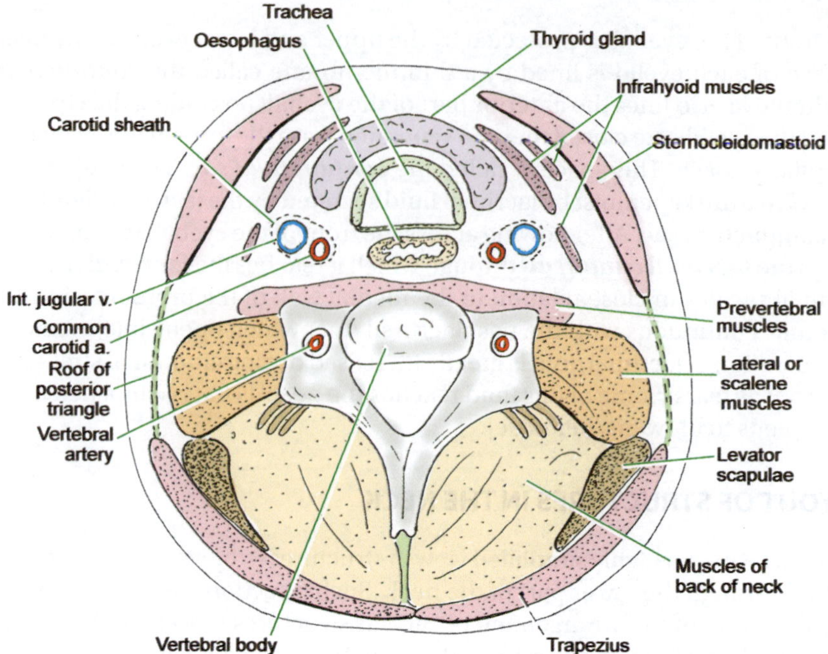

Fig. 2.4 Schematic transverse section through the lower part of the neck to show the relative position of various groups of muscles present. For more detail see Fig. 1.21.

With this introduction we are now in a position to understand some further details. Turn over to Fig. 1.21 (atlas section) in which we see a section very similar to that in Fig. 2.4, but with much more detail. We will begin by identifying some muscles.

1. In the infrahyoid group of muscles identify the ***sternohyoid*** (superficial) and the ***thyrohyoid*** (deep). [At a higher level in the neck the sternothyroid is replaced by a muscle called the ***thyrohyoid***]. Superficial to the carotid sheath note the ***omohyoid*** muscle.
2. At this level in the neck the prevertebral muscles are represented by the ***longus colli.***
3. Just behind the carotid sheath there are the ***lateral (or scalene) group*** of muscles attached to the transverse process. These are the ***scalenus anterior***, the ***scalenus medius*** and the ***scalenus posterior***.
4. The ***deep muscles of the back*** are arranged in four groups. They lie deep to the trapezius and the levator scapulae.
   a. The splenius group is most superficial. It consists of the ***splenius capitis*** and the ***splenius cervicis.***
   b. Over the back of the thoracic part of the vertebral column we have a large muscle the ***erector spinae*** which lies deep to the splenius group. In the neck the erector spinae is represented only by three narrow slips called the ***iliocostalis cervicis***, the ***longissimus cervicis***, and the ***longissimus***

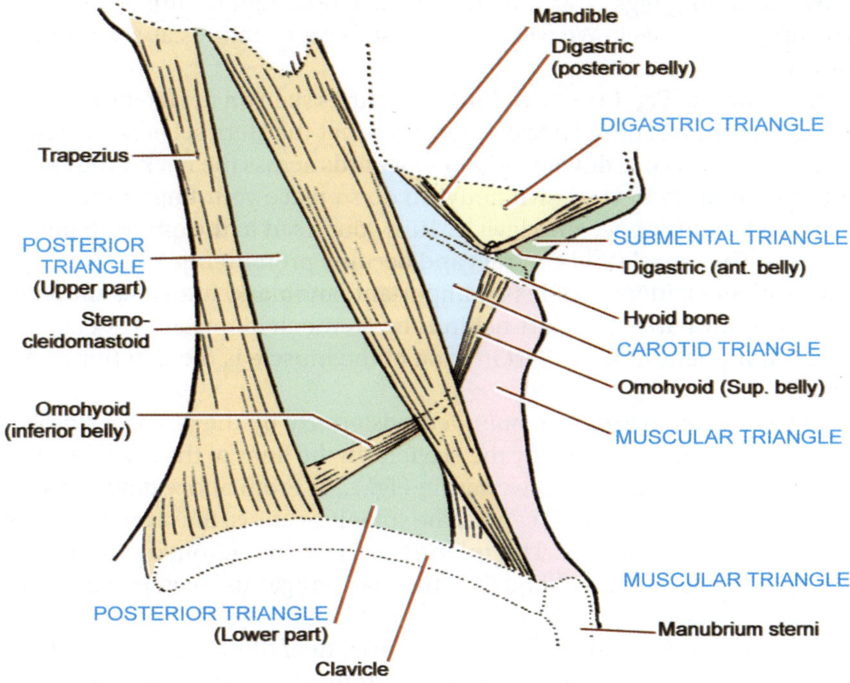

Fig. 2.5 Triangles of the neck (lateral view).

capitis. The three slips are seen lateral to the posterior part of the transverse process.

c. Immediately deep to the splenius muscles (Fig. 1.21) we see the semispinalis group consisting of the ***semispinalis capitis*** and the ***semispinalis cervicis***. (On the back of the thorax this group is deep to the erector spinae).

d. The deepest group of muscles of the back is represented at this level by the ***multifidus*** (lying in the angle between the vertebral spine and the transverse process). Other members of this group are seen lower down in the back.

After identifying the muscles (in Fig. 1.21) note that in the neck the deep fascia (or cervical fascia) is arranged in several layers as follows.

a. The outermost or ***investing layer*** of fascia consists of two layers that go right round the neck. The two layers split to enclose the sternocleidomastoid and the trapezius muscles. Some superficial veins (anterior jugular, external jugular) also lie between the two layers.
b. The pretracheal fascia forms an investment for the thyroid gland.
c. The prevertebral fascia covers the prevertebral muscles and passes backwards over the scalene muscles and the levator scapulae.

Finally, in Fig. 1.21 note the presence of the spinal cord in the vertebral canal. Observe the ventral and dorsal roots that join to form a spinal nerve. The vertebral artery is seen in the foramen transversarium.

By examining Figs. 1.21 and 2.4 we have obtained a 'birds eye view' of structures in the neck. We will now look at these structures as seen from the surface

Please turn to Fig. 1.9 which shows structures seen on the lateral side of the neck after removal of deep fascia. Observe that the sternocleidomastoid is a long muscle that runs downwards and forwards across the neck. [You can feel this muscle easily in your own body. To do so place your fingers on the side of the neck a little above the clavicle. Turn your head to the opposite side and upwards. The muscle will contract and become prominent].

The sternocleidomastoid is an important landmark. It divides the side of neck into two parts. The part behind the sternocleidomastoid is called the posterior triangle, and the part in front of the muscle is the anterior triangle (Fig. 2.5).

The ***posterior triangle*** is bounded posteriorly by the anterior border of the trapezius, and inferiorly by the clavicle. In the floor of the triangle we can identify several muscles that we saw in Fig. 1.21. From above downwards we see parts of the semispinalis capitis, the splenius capitis, the levator scapulae, and the scalenus medius. The inferior belly of the omohyoid (one of the infrahyoid muscles) runs obliquely across the triangle and divides it into upper and lower parts.

The ***anterior triangle*** of the neck lies in front of the sternocleidomastoid. Medially it is bounded by the anterior midline of the neck. Its third (upper) boundary is formed by the lower border of the mandible. In Fig. 1.10 identify the superior belly of the omohyoid that runs upwards and forwards across the triangle. Also identify the digastric muscle. These muscles are used to divide the anterior triangle of the neck into four smaller triangles (Fig. 2.5) as follows.

a. The space between the anterior bellies of the right and left digastric muscles is called the ***submental triangle***. This triangle lies just below the floor of the mouth which is formed here by the mylohyoid muscle (Fig. 1.12).
b. The ***digastric triangle*** is bounded above by the lower border of the body of the mandible, behind by the posterior belly of the digastric, and in front by the anterior belly of the same muscle. The triangle is better seen in Fig. 1.5 in which we see that the triangle is covered by the submandibular gland.
c. The ***carotid triangle*** is bounded posteriorly by the anterior border of the sternocleidomastoid, above and in front by the posterior belly of the digastric muscle, and below and in front by the superior belly of the omohyoid muscle. The reason why this is called the carotid triangle is obvious from Fig. 1.12 in which we see that the carotid arteries are most superficial here.
d. The ***muscular triangle*** is bounded medially (and anteriorly) by the anterior middle line of the neck, posterosuperiorly by the omohyoid, and posteroinferiorly by the sternocleidomastoid. In the floor of the muscular triangle (Fig. 1.12) we see the infrahyoid muscles (already identified in Fig. 1.21). These are the sternohyoid (and the omohyoid itself) superficially, and thyrohyoid and sternothyroid muscles lying in a deeper plane. In the

anterior median region of the neck we see part of the larynx, part of the thyroid gland, the trachea, and some superficial veins.

Other Muscles in the Neck

In Fig. 1.9 we have viewed the muscles on the lateral side of the neck after removal of deep fascia. In Fig. 1.10 we see a view after the greater part of the sternocleidomastoid has been removed. The position of the omohyoid muscle is now better seen. The two bellies of the muscle are united by a intermediate tendon.

Removal of the sternocleidomastoid also brings the scalenus anterior into view (Also see Figs. 1.13 and 1.14). The muscle is crossed by the phrenic nerve (which runs downwards and forwards across it) and by the subclavian vein which lies in front of the lower part of the muscle. The subclavian artery crosses behind the muscle which intervenes between the artery and the vein. Observe that the brachial plexus emerges from under the lateral margin of the muscle (Fig. 1.13).

In Fig. 1.14 we see the neck from the front after the pharynx, larynx and the anterior part of the skull have been removed. This brings the prevertebral muscles into view. Running more or less vertically over the vertebral column we see the longus coli (in three parts), and the longus capitis. Two short muscles connecting the base of the skull to the atlas are the rectus capitis anterior and the rectus capitis lateralis. In Fig. 1.14 we also see a good display of the scalene muscles (scalenus anterior, scalenus medius and scalenus posterior). Note that the roots of the cervical and brachial plexuses lie anterior to the scalenus medius, and deep to the scalenus anterior.

To round off our review of muscles of the neck turn to Fig. 1.15 which illustrates the muscles of the back (already seen in Fig. 1.21 in section). In Fig. 1.15A we see the region of the posterior triangle of the neck from behind. In Fig. 1.15B the trapezius has been removed revealing the ***splenius capitis*** in its full extent. Removal of the trapezius also brings the lower part of the levator scapulae into view. In Fig. 1.15C the greater part of the splenius capitis has been cut away to expose the ***semispinalis capitis***. In Fig. 1.15D a segment of the semispinalis capitis has been cut away revealing four short muscles in the suboccipital region. Identify the rectus capitis posterior minor, the rectus capitis posterior major, the obliquus capitis superior, and the obliquus capitis inferior. The triangular interval enclosed by these muscles is the ***suboccipital triangle***.

Finally identify the splenius cervicis (Figs. 1.15 B,C,D), the semispinalis cervicis (Fig. 1.15D), and the longissimus capitis (Fig. 1.15D) reaching the mastoid process.

MAIN ARTERIES OF HEAD AND NECK

The main arteries supplying the head and neck are the common carotid arteries (Fig. 1.11), and the subclavian arteries. On the right side the ***common carotid***

artery is a branch of the brachiocephalic trunk, while on the left side it is a direct branch of the arch of the aorta. The artery ascends into the neck and divides into the internal and external carotid arteries.

The ***internal carotid artery*** continues upwards to reach the base of the skull. Here it has a complicated course through the base of the skull and finally enters the cranial cavity. In the cranial cavity it gives off the ophthalmic artery to the eye and orbit, and then divides into the anterior cerebral and middle cerebral arteries that supply the brain. (Some other small branches are also given off).

Structures in the head and neck lying outside the cranial cavity are supplied mainly by branches of the ***external carotid artery***. These branches are the ***superior thyroid artery*** to the thyroid gland (Figs. 1.11, 1.13); the ***lingual artery*** to the tongue (Figs. 1.8, 1.13); the ***facial artery*** to the face (Figs. 1.4, 1.5); the ***occipital artery*** to the scalp and back (Figs. 1.3, 1.10, 1.11); the ***posterior auricular artery*** to the auricle (of the ear) and scalp (Figs. 1.10, 1.11); the ***maxillary artery*** to the infratemporal and temporal regions (Fig. 1.6); and the ***superficial temporal artery*** to the auricle, the temporal region and the scalp (Figs. 1.3, 1.4, 1.6).

The right ***subclavian artery*** is a branch of the brachiocephalic trunk. The left subclavian artery is a direct branch of the arch of the aorta and runs part of its course in the thorax. On each side the ***subclavian artery*** passes through the lower part of the neck on its way to the upper limb. The artery gives some important branches to the head and neck. For descriptive purposes the artery is divided into three parts by the scalenus anterior muscle. The part medial to the muscle is the first part, the part deep to the muscle is the second part, and the part lateral to the muscle is the third part.

The branches given off by the subclavian artery in the neck are shown in Figs. 1.11, 1.13 and 1.14. They are as follows.

a. The ***vertebral artery*** arises from the first part of the subclavian artery. It passes through the foramina transversaria in the transverse processes (of the upper six cervical vertebrae) (Fig. 1.14) to reach the suboccipital region (Fig. 1.15). Finally it enters the vertebral canal and passes through it to reach the cranial cavity (Fig. 1.16). The right and left vertebral arteries unite to form the basilar artery. The vertebral and basilar arteries take part in supplying the brain.
b. The ***internal thoracic artery*** arises from the first part of the subclavian artery and descends into the thorax.
c. The ***thyrocervical trunk*** is a short vessel arising from the subclavian artery near the medial edge of the scalenus anterior (Fig. 1.13). It divides into the **inferior thyroid**, ***suprascapular*** and ***transverse cervical*** arteries. The last two arteries send branches into the upper limb and take part in the anastomosis around the scapula.
d. The ***costocervical trunk*** divides into the ***deep cervical artery*** (to muscles in the neck) and the ***superior intercostal artery***.

All other arteries to be seen in the head and neck are branches of one or other of the arteries described above.

MAIN VEINS OF HEAD AND NECK

The chief veins of the head and neck are the right and left ***internal jugular veins***. Each vein begins at the base of the skull and descends alongside the internal and common carotid arteries. It ends by joining the corresponding subclavian vein to form the brachiocephalic vein. (Recall that the right and left brachiocephalic veins join to form the superior vena cava which ends in the right atrium).

The internal jugular vein receives the common facial, lingual and superior thyroid veins which accompany the corresponding arteries. It also receives a middle thyroid vein. The ***thoracic duct*** opens into the junction of the left internal jugular and subclavian veins, while the right lymphatic duct has a similar termination on the right side.

Superficial Veins of Head and Neck

Several superficial veins to be seen in the neck correspond to branches of the external carotid artery. In Fig. 1.4 observe the ***superficial temporal vein***. Within the substance of the parotid gland it is joined by the ***maxillary vein*** (from the infratemporal fossa) to form the ***retromandibular vein***. Inferiorly, the retromandibular vein divides into anterior and posterior branches. The anterior branch joins the ***facial vein*** to form the ***common facial vein***. This vein ends by joining the internal jugular vein. The posterior branch of the retromandibular vein is joined by the ***posterior auricular vein*** to form the external jugular vein.

The ***external jugular vein*** is the most prominent superficial vein of the neck. It runs downwards over the sternocleidomastoid muscle to reach the lower part of the posterior triangle (Fig. 1.9). Here it ends by joining the subclavian vein (Fig. 1.12). Veins accompanying the transverse cervical artery and the suprascapular artery drain into the external jugular vein. The external jugular vein is also joined by the anterior jugular vein (see below). Therefore, the external jugular vein can be regarded as the main channel of drainage of superficial veins of the neck.

The ***anterior jugular vein*** runs down the front of the neck a short distance from the middle line. At its lower end it turns laterally and ends by joining the external jugular vein.

Some veins from the neck (vertebral, inferior thyroid) descend into the upper part of the thorax and terminate in the brachiocephalic veins.

LYMPH NODES OF HEAD AND NECK

Numerous groups of lymph nodes are present in the head and neck. Some of them are placed superficially in the occipital region (***occipital nodes***); behind the auricle (***retroauricular nodes***); in relation to the parotid gland (***superficial and deep parotid nodes***); in relation to the submandibular gland (***submandibular nodes***); and below the chin (***submental nodes***). Lymph nodes are also present along some veins. The ***buccal nodes*** lie along the facial vein; the ***superficial cervical nodes*** along the external jugular vein; and the ***anterior cervical nodes*** along the anterior jugular vein. Lymph from all these nodes ultimately drains into the ***deep cervical lymph nodes*** that lie along the internal jugular vein. The deep cervical nodes drain into a jugular lymph trunk which joins the thoracic duct (on the left side), or the right lymphatic duct (on the right side).

MAIN NERVES OF THE HEAD AND NECK

The nerves of the head and neck are the twelve pairs of cranial nerves (arising from the brain) and the eight pairs of cervical nerves (arising from the spinal cord). The upper part of the sympathetic trunk lies in the neck.

THE CRANIAL NERVES

The first cranial nerve or ***olfactory nerve*** is the nerve of smell. Each nerve is made up of several bundles that begin in the mucosa lining the upper part of the nasal cavity. The bundles pass through numerous foramina (in the cribriform plate of the ethmoid bone) and end by joining the olfactory bulb (Fig. 1.16).

The second cranial nerve or ***optic nerve*** is the nerve of vision. It is attached to the back of the eyeball and runs backwards through the orbit (Figs. 1.19B, 1.20B). It passes into the cranial cavity through the optic canal (Fig. 1.16).

The third (***oculomotor***), fourth (***trochlear***) and sixth (***abducent***) nerves arise from the brainstem and pass forwards through the middle cranial fossa (Fig. 1.16). They enter the orbit through the superior orbital fissure and supply muscles that move the eyeball (Fig. 1.19).

The fifth or ***trigeminal nerve*** arises from the brainstem. Its initial part lies in the floor of the middle cranial fossa (Fig. 1.16). This part is marked by an enlargement called the ***trigeminal ganglion***. Distal to the ganglion the nerve divides into three branches (hence the name trigeminal). The branches (often called divisions) are as follows.

a. The ***ophthalmic division*** of the trigeminal nerve divides into three branches (***lacrimal***, ***frontal*** and ***nasociliary***) that pass through the superior orbital fissure (Fig. 1.20A) to provide a sensory supply to structures in the orbit and neighbouring regions. The lacrimal nerve also supplies the lacrimal gland. The frontal nerve divides into the ***supraorbital*** and ***supratrochlear*** nerves that supply the anterior part of the scalp (Figs. 1.3, 1.4).
   Other nerves derived from the ophthalmic division that take part in supplying the skin of the face are the infratrochlear and external nasal nerves (Fig. 1.4). The area of skin of the face supplied by the ophthalmic division of the trigeminal nerve includes the forehead, the upper eyelid and the greater part of the nose. The ophthalmic division does not supply any muscle.
b. The ***maxillary division*** of the trigeminal nerve has a complicated course through parts of the base of the skull (Fig. 1.19), but ultimately it enters the

orbit as the infraorbital nerve. This nerve emerges on the face just below the inferior orbital margin (Fig. 1.4) and takes part in supply of the skin of the face. Branches of the maxillary division take part in supplying the nasal mucosa and the palate, the upper jaw and upper teeth. In addition to the infraorbital branch, the zygomaticofacial and zygomaticotemporal nerves seen in Fig. 1.4 are also terminal ramifications of the maxillary nerve that supply the skin of the face. Cutaneous branches of the maxillary division supply the upper part of the cheek, the lower eyelid and the upper lip. The maxillary division does not supply any muscle.

c. The ***mandibular division*** of the trigeminal nerve provides a motor supply to the muscles of mastication (and some other muscles), and also takes part in supplying the skin of the face and the mucous membrane of the mouth including that of the tongue. The branches of this nerve are shown in Fig. 1.7.

The motor branches supply the temporalis (***deep temporal nerves***, Fig. 1.7); the medial and lateral pterygoid muscles, and the masseter (Fig. 1.5). Branches are also given to the anterior belly of the digastric muscle and to the mylohyoid muscle (Fig. 1.7).

The sensory branches include the ***auriculotemporal nerve*** (that accompanies the superficial temporal vessels), the ***buccal nerve*** that supplies the skin over the cheek (Fig. 1.7), the ***lingual nerve*** to the tongue, and the ***inferior alveolar nerve*** that supplies the lower jaw and teeth. The terminal part of this nerve emerges on the face as the ***mental nerve*** (Figs. 1.4, 1.8). The mandibular division supplies skin over the temple, the lower part of the cheek, and the lower lip.

The seventh cranial nerve is the ***facial nerve***. After a complicated course through the skull it emerges in the parotid region and divides into branches within the substance of the parotid gland (Fig. 1.4). These branches emerge from under the anterior border of the gland and supply the muscles of the face (Fig. 1.2) They also supply the buccinator muscle. Fibres of taste for the anterior two thirds of the tongue travel part of their course in the facial nerve, and through its ***chorda tympani*** branch which joins the lingual nerve (Fig. 1.7). Secretomotor nerve fibres for the submandibular and sublingual gland also travel through the facial nerve, the chorda tympani and the lingual nerve.

The eighth cranial nerve or ***vestibulocochlear nerve*** consists of two functional parts. The cochlear nerve is the nerve of hearing. The vestibular nerve supplies end organs in the internal ear that are responsible for equilibrium. The course and distribution of the vestibulocochlear nerve is too complex to be considered here.

The ninth cranial nerve or ***glossopharyngeal nerve*** is predominantly sensory. As its name implies it is distributed to the tongue and pharynx. Fibres for taste from the posterior one third of the tongue travel through this nerve. Secretomotor fibres for the parotid gland travel part of their course through this nerve and partly through the auriculotemporal branch of the mandibular nerve.

The tenth cranial nerve (or vagus nerve) has a wide distribution. Its distribution in the thorax and abdomen has already been considered. In the neck this nerve runs downwards alongside the internal and common carotid arteries (Fig. 1.11). The nerve lies within the carotid sheath (Fig. 1.21). It gives branches to the pharynx and larynx. The fibres to the larynx travel through the ***superior laryngeal nerve*** which divides into the ***internal laryngeal*** and ***external laryngeal*** nerves. Fibres to the larynx also travel through the ***recurrent laryngeal nerve***. On the right side this branch arises from the vagus in the lower part of the neck (Fig. 1.13) and winds round the right subclavian artery. Finally it runs upwards to the larynx. On the left side the recurrent laryngeal nerve is given off in the thorax and has been described on page 499. The vagus nerve also gives off cardiac branches that descend into the thorax to supply the heart.

The eleventh or ***accessory nerve*** consists of cranial and spinal parts. The cranial part joins the vagus nerve and is distributed along with it to the palate, the pharynx and the larynx. The spinal branch runs downwards and backwards over the floor of the posterior triangle of the neck (Fig. 1.11). It supplies the sternocleidomastoid and the trapezius muscles.

The twelfth or ***hypoglossal nerve*** enters the neck and runs down along the internal carotid artery and internal jugular vein. The nerve then runs forwards to enter the submandibular region (Figs. 1.7 and 1.11). It supplies the muscles of the tongue).

The account of the cranial nerves given above should be regarded as a brief summary of their main features. Numerous details will be considered later.

CERVICAL NERVES

There are eight cervical nerves in the neck. Like other spinal nerves, each cervical nerve is formed by union of dorsal and ventral roots (Fig. 1.21). The dorsal roots bears a ganglion. After a very short course the nerve divides into a dorsal ramus and a ventral ramus. As a rule dorsal rami are much smaller than ventral rami. However, the dorsal rami of the first and second cervical nerves are larger than the ventral rami.

1. The ***dorsal ramus of the first cervical nerve*** is seen in the suboccipital region (Fig. 1.15) where it divides into branches that supply muscles around the suboccipital triangle.
2. The dorsal ramus of the second cervical nerve is large. Its main continuation is the ***greater occipital nerve*** which supplies the scalp (Figs. 1.2, 1.3, 1.15).
3. The dorsal ramus of the third cervical nerve is smaller than the ventral ramus. Its main continuation is the ***third occipital nerve*** (Figs. 1.2, 1.3).
4. The ventral rami of the 1st, 2nd, 3rd and 4th spinal nerves unite with one another to form the ***cervical plexus*** (Figs. 1.10, 1.11). The plexus gives off several branches to muscles of the neck. It also gives off a number of cutaneous branches which are as follows.
   a. The ***lesser occipital nerve*** runs upwards along the posterior border of the sternocleidomastoid. It takes part in supply of the auricle, and part of the scalp in that region (Figs. 1.3, 1.9).
   b. The ***greater auricular nerve*** runs upwards over the surface of the sternocleidomastoid to supply the auricle and some skin around it (Figs. 1.9, 1.10).

c. The ***transverse cutaneous nerve*** of the neck runs forwards across the sternocleidomastoid to supply skin of the front of the neck (Fig. 1.9).
d. The ***supraclavicular nerves*** (medial, intermediate, and lateral) run downwards over the posterior triangle. They run across the clavicle to reach the pectoral region and shoulder (Fig. 1.9).

In addition to the cutaneous branches mentioned above the cervical plexus gives off the ***phrenic nerve***. In Fig. 1.11 the nerve is seen descending over the surface of the scalenus anterior muscle. It also crosses the subclavian artery (Figs. 1.13, 1.14) to descend into the thorax where it has been described on.

The ventral rami of the 5th, 6th, 7th and 8th cervical nerves take part in forming the brachial plexus. From Figs. 1.11 and 1.13 note that the upper part of the brachial plexus lies in the neck. The roots of the plexus pass laterally in the plane between the scalenus medius and the scalenus anterior. The plexus crosses the first rib to enter the axilla.

SYMPATHETIC TRUNK

The sympathetic trunk runs down the entire length of the neck, the thorax and the abdomen. In the neck the sympathetic trunk lies posterior to the internal and common carotid arteries lying outside the carotid sheath (Figs. 1.11, 1.13, 1.21). In the neck the sympathetic bears three ganglia, superior, middle and cervicothoracic (Fig. 1.13). The cervical sympathetic ganglia give branches to various structures in the head and neck. The fibres travel along blood vessels. The cervical part of the sympathetic trunk also gives cardiac branches that take part in forming the cardiac plexuses.

ENDOCRINE GLANDS OF HEAD AND NECK

The endocrine glands present in the head and neck are as follows.

1. The ***hypophysis cerebri*** (or pituitary gland) lies within the cranial cavity in the floor of the middle cranial fossa. It is attached to the base of the brain by a stalk (Fig. 1.16)
2. The ***pineal gland*** (or pineal body) is also attached to the brain. Its importance as an endocrine gland has been recognised only recently.
3. The ***thyroid gland*** is present in front of the larynx and trachea (Figs. 1.11, 1.13). It consists of right and left lobes that are united across the midline by the ***isthmus*** of the gland.
4. The ***parathyroid glands*** are four in number (two on each side). They lie in relation to the posterior border of the corresponding lobe of the thyroid gland (Fig. 1.13)

These endocrine glands produce hormones that have a wide influence on tissues throughout the body.

CHAPTER

3

Scalp, Face, Parotid Region and Lacrimal Apparatus

In this chapter we will consider some structures that are placed at a relatively superficial level in the head. The regions to be considered will include the scalp, the face and parotid region, and some parts of the lacrimal apparatus. References will be made to blood vessels, lymphatics and nerves to be seen in the region but these will be considered in detail (and in proper continuity) in Chapters 8, 9 and 13.

Many of the structures in these regions have been briefly reviewed in Chapter 2. Beginners must read Chapter 2 before reading this chapter.

THE SCALP

The term scalp is applied to the soft tissues covering the vault of the skull. This region extends anteriorly up to the eyebrows (and, therefore, includes the forehead), posteriorly up to the superior nuchal lines, and laterally up to the superior temporal lines.

Layers of the Scalp

These are shown in Fig. 1.3B and are as follows.

1. The most superficial layer is ***skin***. Being hairy it contains numerous sebaceous glands. The skin is closely adherent to underlying tissues.
2. The ***superficial fascia*** is represented by dense connective tissue that is firmly united to the skin and to the underlying epicranial aponeurosis. Fibrous strands divide the superficial fascia into numerous small pockets.
3. The third layer of the scalp is partly muscular and partly fibrous. It corresponds to deep fascia. The greater part of this layer is formed by the ***epicranial aponeurosis*** (or galea aponeurotica). The muscular part is formed by a muscle called the ***occipitofrontalis*** (see below).
4. The three layers of the scalp described above are firmly united to one another. All the three layers move together over the fourth layer which is made up of ***loose areolar tissue***. The extent of the layer of loose

connective tissue corresponds to the extent of the scalp itself. This layer is traversed by emissary veins passing from the scalp to intracranial venous sinuses.

5. The deepest layer of the scalp is the ***pericranium*** (which is the periosteum over the bones of the vault of the skull). It is important to note that at the edge of each bone of the skull the pericranium is fixed because it is attached to sutural ligaments that are present in sutures of the skull.

Occipitofrontalis

The occipito-frontalis covers the upper curved roof of the skull. (Figs. 1.2, 1.3) It consists of a posterior ***occipital part*** (or ***occipitalis***), and an anterior ***frontal part*** (or ***frontalis***). Each of these is divided into a right half and a left half. These four parts are continuous with each other through the epicranial aponeurosis.

Each ***occipital part*** arises from the occipital bone (lateral two thirds of the highest nuchal line). Laterally, the line of origin extends on to the mastoid part of the temporal bone. The fibres of the occipitalis run upwards and forwards to end in the epicranial aponeurosis. The occipital parts of the two sides are separated from each other by a part of the epicranial aponeurosis that gains attachment to the external occipital protuberance, and to the medial parts of the highest nuchal lines.

The ***frontal parts*** are attached posteriorly to the epicranial aponeurosis. Anteriorly, the fibres have no bony attachment. The medial-most fibres merge with the procerus, which is a small muscle overlying the upper part of the nose (Fig. 1.1). More laterally, the deeper fibres merge with the corrugator supercilii, which is a small muscle underlying the medial part of the eyebrow. The majority of the fibres of the frontalis merge with the upper edge of the orbicularis oculi. (The procerus, the corrugator supercilii and the orbicularis oculi are considered later in this chapter under muscles of the face).

Nerve Supply

The occipital part is supplied by the posterior auricular branch of the facial nerve, and the frontal part by the temporal branches of the same nerve.

Actions

Acting alternatively, the frontal and occipital parts can move the scalp forwards and backwards over the vault of the skull. The frontal parts raise the eyebrows (as in surprise): acting from below they produce transverse wrinkles of the forehead.

Blood Vessels and Nerves of the Scalp

The ***arteries*** that supply the scalp are seen in Fig. 1.3. These are the supratrochlear and supraorbital branches of the ophthalmic artery in front,

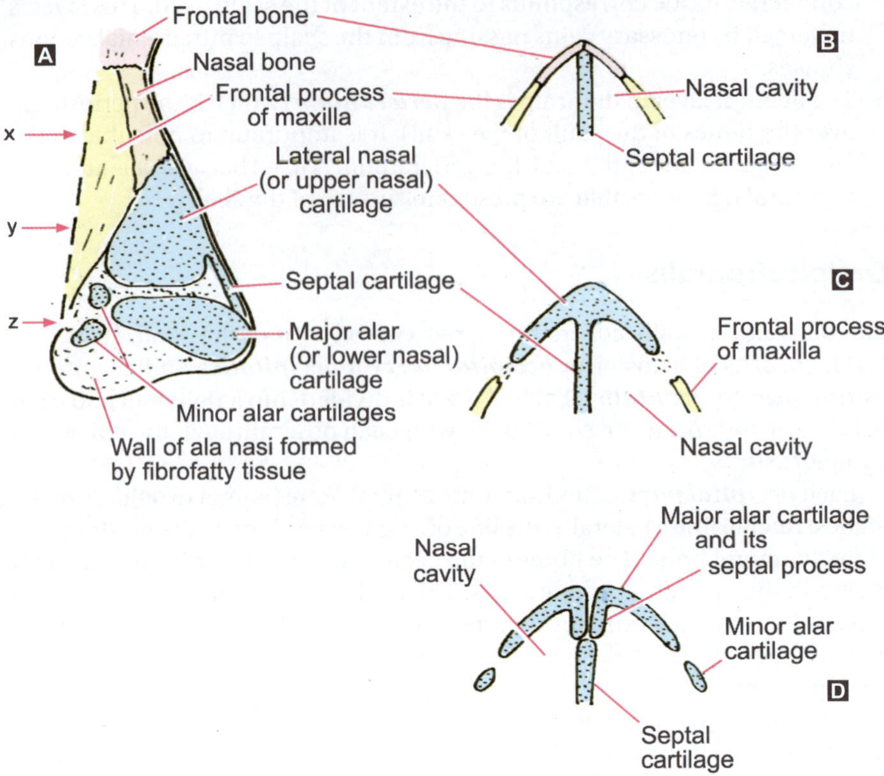

Fig. 3.1 A. Structures forming the skeleton of the external nose (lateral view). B, C, D. Transverse sections through the nose at levels x, y and z shown in Fig. A.

the anterior and posterior branches of the superficial temporal artery laterally, and the occipital artery posteriorly. The ***veins*** of the scalp accompany the corresponding arteries.

The ***nerves*** of the scalp may be divided into motor nerves that supply the occipito frontalis and sensory nerves that supply skin and other tissues of the scalp (Figs. 1.2 to 1.4).

As stated above the motor nerves are the temporal and posterior auricular branches of the facial nerve.

The sensory nerves are as follows:

1. In front there are the supratrochlear and supraorbital nerves, which are branches of the frontal nerve (which is itself derived from the ophthalmic division of the trigeminal nerve).
2. Laterally there are the zygomatico-temporal, the auriculo-temporal, and great auricular nerves.
3. Posteriorly, there are the greater occipital, lesser occipital, and third occipital nerves.

The ***lymphatic drainage*** of the scalp is described in Chapter 3.

Important ***clinical correlations*** are discussed in Chapter 5.

THE FACE

A brief introduction to the layout of structures in the face has been given on page 734. Here we will consider some features seen on the surface of the face, and the muscles of the face. The blood vessels and nerves of the region will be considered along with those of the parotid region.

It is common knowledge that when we think of the face we visualize the forehead, the eyes, the nose, the mouth and the cheeks. The forehead is really a part of the scalp. We will begin by noting some facts about the nose, the mouth the cheeks and the eyes.

THE EXTERNAL NOSE

The prominence on the face that the layman refers to as the nose is strictly speaking the external nose. (The nasal cavities constitute the internal nose.) Certain descriptive terms applied to parts of the external nose are as follows. The upper end (where the nose becomes continuous with the forehead) is called the ***angle.*** The ridge-like free border passing downwards from the angle is called the ***dorsum nasi.*** The dorsum nasi ends below in a rounded prominence which forms the tip, or ***apex***, of the nose. On either side the external nose has lateral surfaces that are continuous behind with the cheeks. The lowest parts of the lateral surfaces are rounded and mobile: these are called the ***alae nasi.*** The upper parts of both lateral surfaces (just below the angle) together form the ***bridge*** of the nose.

The shape of the nose is maintained by the presence of a skeleton made up partly of bone and partly of cartilage. Some details of the elements forming the skeleton are shown in Fig. 3.1.

The ***external nares*** (or anterior nares) are the external openings of the nasal cavities. They are located on the inferior aspect of the nose. They are bounded laterally by the alae nasi and medially by the lowest part of the nasal septum.

LIPS AND CHEEKS

Some facts worth noting about the lips and cheeks are as follows.

The ***lips***, upper and lower, are lined on the outside by skin and on the inside by mucous membrane. The junction between the two forms the 'edge' of each lip. The substance of the lip is formed by the orbicularis oris muscle and by numerous smaller muscles that blend with it (See below under muscles of face). The points, on either side, where the upper and lower lips meet are called the ***angles of the mouth.*** The deep surface of each lip is connected to the gum by a median fold of mucous membrane called the ***frenulum***.

The ***cheeks*** are, like the lips, made up of an outer layer of skin, an inner layer of mucous membrane and an intervening layer of muscle, connective tissue and fat. The muscle layer is formed chiefly by the buccinator (Fig. 1.5). The fat is specially prominent in infants and is responsible for the rounded appearance of the cheeks. Numerous glands are present in relationship to the lips and cheeks. They open into the vestibule of the mouth.

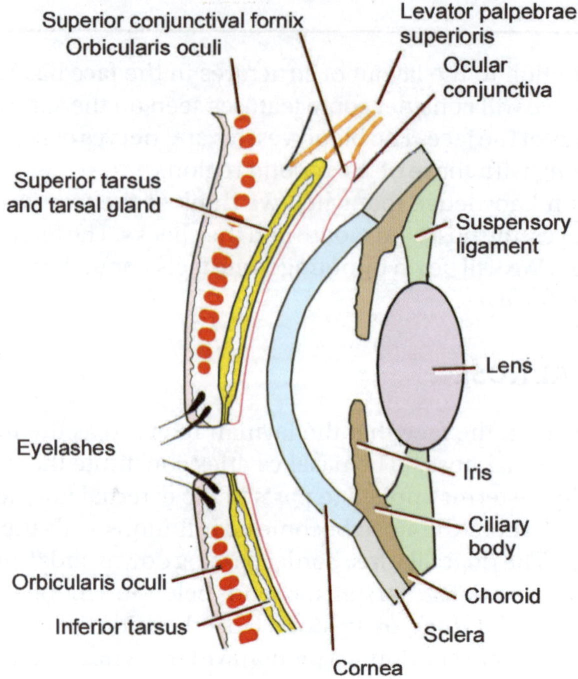

Fig. 3.2 Schematic sagittal section through the eyelids and anterior part of the eyeball.

THE EYELIDS AND CONJUNCTIVA

The basic parts of the eyeball are probably already known to you. They will be studied in detail later. The part of the eye seen on the face consists of a part that is white, and a circular area in front that looks dark. The 'white of the eye' is formed by the outermost coat of the eyeball which is called the ***sclera***. The sclera is lined by a thin transparent membrane the ***ocular conjunctiva***. The circular dark part in the centre is the ***iris*** which we see through a transparent disc like structure the ***cornea*** which covers it. At the centre of the iris there is an aperture called the ***pupil***. The pupil appears black because the interior of the eye (which we see through the pupil) is dark. When we view the 'eyes' we see only a small part of the eyeball in the interval between the upper and lower eyelids. This interval is called the ***palpebral fissure*** (Fig. 3.3).

The upper and lower eyelids (or palpebrae) protect the eyeball, specially the cornea, from injury in several ways.

Firstly, they provide protection against mechanical injury by reflex closure when any object suddenly approaches the eye. The same happens when the cornea is touched (***corneal reflex***).

Secondly, they help to keep the cornea moist as follows: When the eyelids are closed (i.e., when the upper and lower eyelids meet) a capillary space separates the posterior surfaces of the lids from the cornea and the anterior part of the

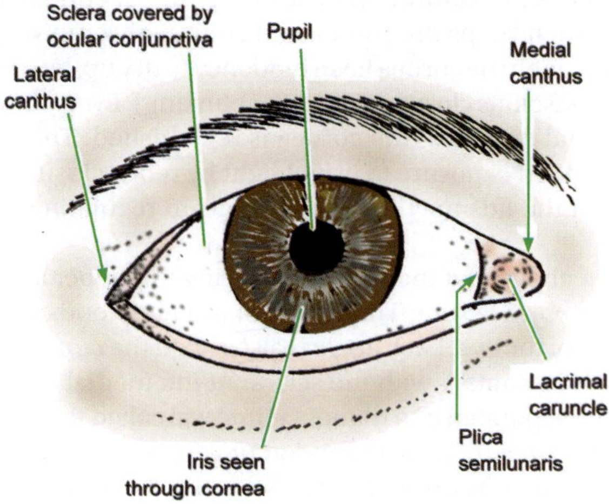

Fig. 3.3 Some features of the eye as seen on the face. The eyelashes are omitted. The interval between the two eyelids is the palpebral fissure.

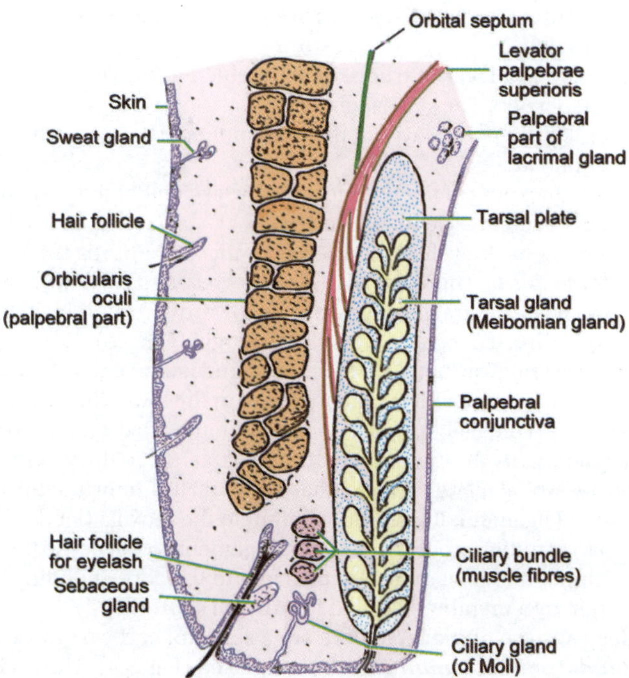

Fig. 3.4 Schematic sagittal section through the upper eyelid.

sclera. This space is the ***conjunctival sac*** (Fig. 3.2). It contains a thin film of lacrimal fluid, which keeps the cornea and conjunctiva moist.

With the 'eyes' open the cornea has a tendency to dry up, but this is prevented by periodic, unconscious closure of the lids (blinking). Every time this happens the film of lacrimal fluid over the cornea is replenished. Thirdly, lids protect the eyes from sudden exposure to bright light by reflex closure. In bright light partial closure of the lids may assist the pupils in regulating the light falling on the retina.

We have seen above that the space separating the upper and lower eyelids is called the palpebral fissure. The medial and lateral ends of the fissure are called the ***angles*** of the eye. Each angle is also called the ***canthus*** (Fig. 3.3). The lateral canthus is in contact with the sclera. At the medial canthus the upper and lower lids are separated by a triangular interval called the ***lacus lacrimalis***. In the floor of this area there is a rounded pink elevation called the ***lacrimal caruncle***. Just lateral to the caruncle there is a fold of conjunctiva called the ***plica semilunaris*** which represents the third eyelid present in some lower animals (in whom it is called the ***nictitating membrane*)**. Each eyelid has a free edge to which eyelashes are attached. Just lateral to the lacrimal caruncle each lid margin has a slight elevation called the ***lacrimal papilla***. On the summit of the papilla there is a small aperture called the ***lacrimal punctum***. It is important to note that the punctum is normally in direct contact with the ocular conjunctiva.

The basic structure of an eyelid is shown in Fig. 3.4. The various structures forming the eyelid are as follows:

1. Anteriorly there is a layer of true skin with which a few small hair and sweat glands are associated. The skin is thin.
2. Deep to the skin there is a layer of delicate connective tissue, which normally does not contain fat.
3. Considerable thickness of the lid is formed by fasciculi of the palpebral part of the orbicularis oculi muscle (described below).
4. The 'skeleton' of each eyelid is formed by a mass of fibrous tissue called the ***tarsus***, or ***tarsal plate***. The shape of the tarsi corresponds to that of the lids: they are semi-oval having a straight edge directed towards the margin of the lid and a convex margin directed towards the orbital margin (Fig. 3.5). The 'height' of the tarsus is greatest midway between the medial and lateral ends of the tarsus. It is about 10 mm in the upper lid and about 5 mm in the lower lid. The tarsi narrow down laterally and medially and become continuous with the ***lateral and medial palpebral ligaments*** through which they are attached to the walls of the orbit, just inside the orbital margin. The medial palpebral ligament is better developed than the lateral ligament. It gains attachment to the maxilla (lacrimal crest and adjoining part of frontal process). The lateral ligament is attached to the zygomatic bone. The upper and lower tarsi are attached to the corresponding part of the orbital margin by a membrane called the **orbital septum.**
5. On the deep surface of the tarsi there are a series of vertical grooves in which ***tarsal glands*** (or ***Meibomian glands***) are placed (Fig. 3.4). These glands may occasionally be embedded within the tarsal plates. Each gland has a duct that opens on the free margin of the lid. The tarsal glands are modified sebaceous glands. They produce an oily secretion a thin film of which spreads over the lacrimal fluid and delays its evaporation.

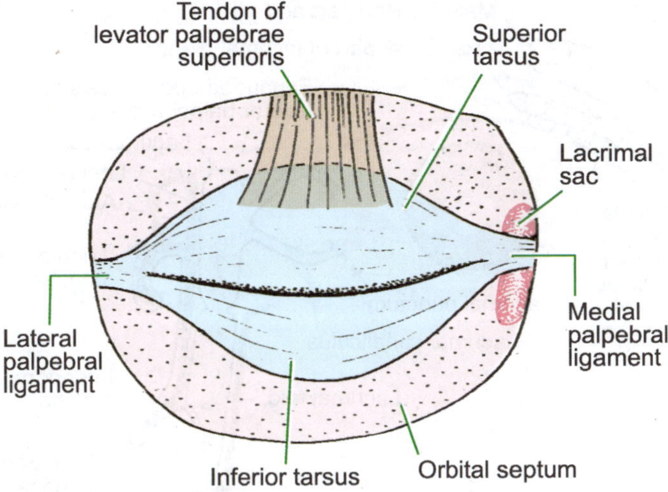

Fig. 3.5 Scheme to show the tarsal plate and the palpebral ligament as seen from the front.

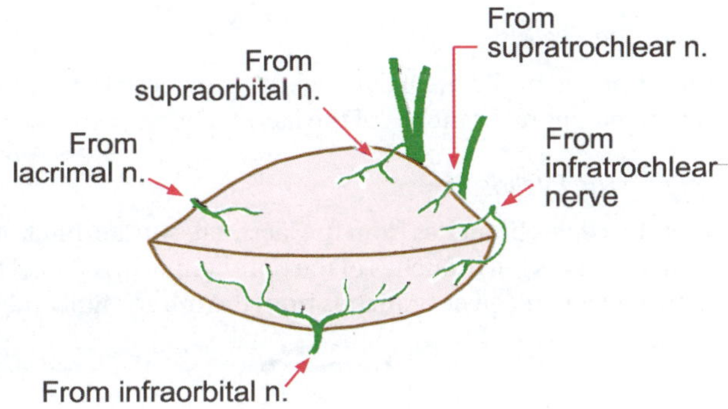

Fig. 3.6 Nerves supplying the eyelids.

In addition to tarsal glands, modified sweat glands called ***ciliary glands***, are present in the lids near their free edge.

6. The inner surface of the eyelid is lined by ***palpebral conjunctiva***. This is a thin transparent membrane continuous with the ***ocular conjunctiva*** lining the anterior part of the sclera. The sharp line of reflection (of the conjunctiva) from the lid to the sclera is called the ***conjunctival fornix*** (superior or inferior) (Fig. 3.2).

The levator palpebrae superioris extends into the upper eyelid anterior to the tarsal plate to gain insertion into it. This muscle elevates the upper eyelid, in opening the palpebral fissure. Some fibres of the muscle, which are inserted into the superior conjunctival fornix, pull the fornix up during this movement (Figs. 3.2, 3.4). The palpebral fissure is closed by contraction of the orbicularis oculi.

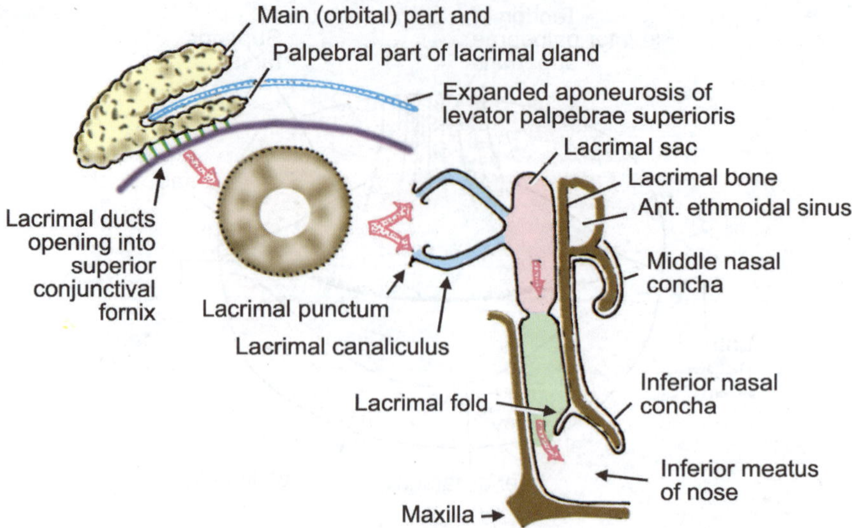

Fig. 3.7 Scheme to show the parts of the lacrimal apparatus. The pink arrows indicate the direction of flow of lacrimal fluid.

Blood Vessels of the Eyelids

The eyelids are supplied by the medial palpebral branches of the ophthalmic artery and by the lateral palpebral branches of the lacrimal artery.

Nerves Supplying the Eyelids

The upper eyelid receives branches from the lacrimal, supraorbital, supratrochlear and infratrochlear nerves (all branches of the ophthalmic division of the trigeminal nerve). The lower eyelid receives branches from the infraorbital and infratrochlear nerves (Fig. 3.6).

THE LACRIMAL APPARATUS

We have seen that the cornea is kept moist by the lacrimal fluid. The lacrimal apparatus consists of the organs concerned with the secretion and drainage of this fluid. Lacrimal fluid is secreted by the ***lacrimal gland*** and is poured into the conjunctival sac at the superior conjunctival fornix. The fluid passes downwards and medially to reach the lacus lacrimalis. Here it passes through the lacrimal puncta into narrow tubes called the ***lacrimal canaliculi***. These canaliculi open into the ***lacrimal sac.*** The lacrimal sac drains into the inferior meatus of the nasal cavity through the ***nasolacrimal duct***.

The lacrimal gland is seen in Figs. 1.20A,B. It will be described in detail when we study the orbit. For the time being note that the lacrimal gland lies in relation to the upper lateral part of the wall of the orbit. An extension of the gland, that passes into the upper eyelid, is called its ***palpebral part*** (Figs. 3.4, 3.7). The lacrimal gland drains into the superior conjunctival fornix through about twelve ducts.

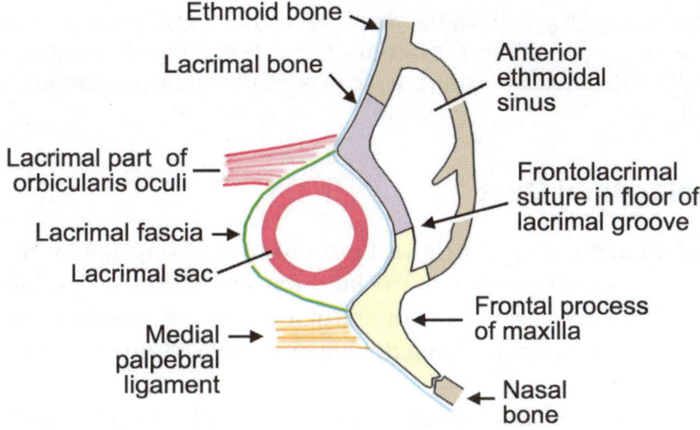

Fig. 3.8 Transverse section through lacrimal sac and some surrounding structures.

The other parts of the lacrimal apparatus are described below. To understand some of the details you will need to know some features of the bony orbit and the bony nasal cavity.

The Lacrimal Canaliculi

There are two lacrimal canaliculi, upper and lower, in relation to each eye. Each canaliculus is about 10 mm long. It is a narrow tube that starts at the lacrimal punctum and ends by joining the lacrimal sac. Note the direction of each canaliculus as shown in Fig. 3.7.

The Lacrimal Sac

The lacrimal sac lies in the lacrimal groove on the medial wall of the orbit (Figs. 3.5, 3.7).

The floor of this groove is formed by the lacrimal bone (posteriorly) and the frontal process of the maxilla (anteriorly). The groove is bounded anteriorly by the anterior lacrimal crest, and behind by the crest of the lacrimal bone.

The lacrimal sac is blind at its upper end. Inferiorly, the sac is continuous with the nasolacrimal duct. Laterally, it receives the lacrimal canaliculi near its upper end.

Some relationship of the lacrimal sac can be seen in Fig. 3.8 which is a schematic transverse section across the sac. Note the bones forming the floor of the lacrimal groove. Medially the sac is separated by a thin partition of bone from the anterior ethmoidal sinus; and lower down from the middle meatus of the nasal cavity (Fig. 3.7). Laterally the lacrimal sac is covered by lacrimal fascia which is attached to the anterior and posterior margins of the lacrimal groove. The medial palpebral ligament is placed in front of the lacrimal sac and is separated from it only by the lacrimal fascia (Figs. 3.4, 3.7). The lacrimal part of the orbicularis oculi muscle (see above) takes origin partly from the lacrimal fascia. Every time the muscle contracts there is pull on this fascia causing the sac to expand and helping to suck lacrimal fluid into the sac.

The Nasolacrimal Duct

The nasolacrimal duct (Fig. 3.6) is a tube about 18 mm long. It may be regarded as the downward continuation of the lacrimal sac. It is closely related to the lateral wall of the nasal cavity, and opens below into the inferior meatus of the nose. The wall of the nasolacrimal duct is made up of bone lined by mucous membrane.

The lower end of the nasolacrimal duct is separated from the inferior meatus of the nose by a fold of mucous membrane called the ***lacrimal fold***.

The bones helping to form the wall of the duct are the maxilla (laterally); and the lacrimal bone and the inferior nasal concha (medially).

MUSCLES OF THE FACE

Deep to the skin of the face there are several muscles that produce varying facial expressions (Figs. 1.1, 1.2). Many of them converge upon the mouth. These are also concerned with speech and with feeding.

The ***orbicularis oculi*** is made up of fasciculi that run concentrically round the palpebral aperture (This muscle is described in detail below). Its upper margin merges with the fibres of the ***frontalis*** (described above under the scalp). The oral aperture is also surrounded by concentrically arranged muscle bundles that constitute the ***orbicularis oris*** (This muscle is described in detail below). Underlying the eyebrows there are two muscles. The ***corrugator supercilii*** runs obliquely deep to the frontalis while the ***depressor supercilii*** consists of some muscle fibres continuous with the upper medial part of the orbicularis oculi. Over the upper part of the nose we have some vertically running fibres which constitute the ***procerus***. Lower down on the nose we have the ***nasalis*** which has a transverse (constrictor) and an alar (dilator) part. Just below the nasal septum we have the ***depressor septi***. As many as nine muscles converge on the orbicularis oris. The ***levator labii superioris alaeque nasi*** arises from the frontal process of the maxilla (Fig. 1.1). Below it divides into two slips, one for the ala of the nose, and the other to the upper lip.

As many as nine muscles converge on the orbicularis oris. The ***levator labii superioris alaeque nasi*** arises from the frontal process of the maxilla (Fig. 1.1). Below it divides into two slips, one for the ala of the nose, and the other to the upper lip. The ***levator labii superioris*** arises from the lower margin of the orbit (partly from the maxilla and partly from the zygomatic bone) and merges below with the orbicularis oris. The ***levator anguli oris*** lies deep to the foregoing muscle. It arises from the maxilla below the infraorbital foramen and

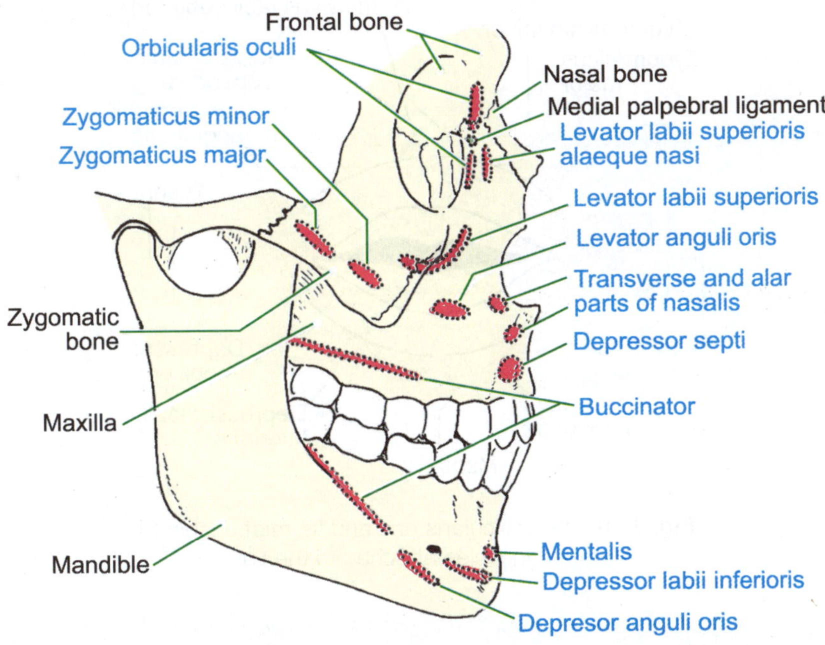

Fig. 3.9 Facial skeleton seen from the side to show some muscle attachments.

is inserted into the angle of the mouth. The ***zygomaticus major and minor*** arise from the zygomatic bone and converge on the angle of the mouth. The ***risorius*** arises from fascia overlying the parotid gland and is inserted into the angle of the mouth. It is continuous below with the ***platysma*** which extends into the neck (Fig. 1.2). The ***depressor anguli oris*** arises from the mandible and reaches the angle of the mouth. The ***depressor labii inferioris*** also arises from the mandible deep to the foregoing muscle and merges with the lower part of the orbicularis oris. The ***mentalis*** arises from the mandible just below the incisor teeth: its fibres run downwards to gain insertion into the skin of the chin.

All the muscles of the face are supplied by the facial nerve. They are derivatives of the second pharyngeal arch. The actions of most of them are indicated by their names. The corrugator supercilii produces vertical wrinkles on the forehead. The procerus produces transverse wrinkles on the bridge of the nose. The depressor septi assists the alar part of the nasalis in widening the external nares. The zygomaticus minor elevates the upper lip while the zygomaticus major draws it upwards and laterally as in laughing.

The mentalis produces wrinkles on the chin. The risorius retracts the angle of the mouth.

The areas of bony attachment of some of the muscles considered above are shown in Figs. 1.1 and 3.9.

Some further details of the orbicularis oris, the orbicularis oculi, and the buccinator are given below.

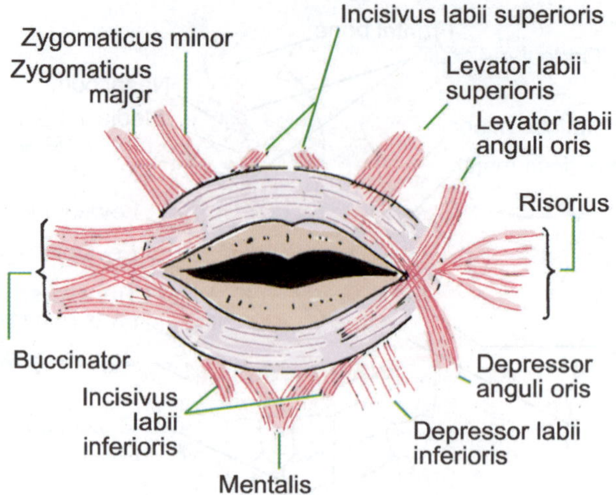

Fig. 3.10 The orbicularis oris and its relationship to vaious muscles attached to the lips.

Orbicularis Oris

The fibres of the orbicularis oris surround the opening of the mouth. They make up the muscular basis of the lips. The muscle contains three types of fibres.

a. Many of the fibres are derived from other facial muscles as shown in Fig. 3.10. At the angle of the mouth many of the fibres cross, those from above entering the lower lip, and vice versa. The middle fibres of the buccinator cross in this manner while the upper and lower fibres go into the corresponding lips.
b. The intrinsic fibres of the lips run obliquely from the skin to the mucous membrane.
c. Some fibres connect the orbicularis oris to the maxilla (opposite the lateral incisors) These fibres constitute the incisivus labii superioris. Similar fibres in the lower lip constitute the incisivus labii inferioris; they arise from the mandible just below the incisor teeth and run laterally to the angle of the mouth.

The orbicularis oris is supplied by the lower buccal and mandibular marginal branches of facial nerve. The orbicularis oris closes the lips. It is responsible for complex movements of the lips associated with speech, eating and drinking.

Orbicularis Oculi

The orbicularis oculi consists of muscle fasciculi arranged concentrically around the palpebral fissure (Fig. 1.1). The innermost rings lie within the eyelids and form the ***palpebral part*** of the muscle (Fig. 3.4). Succeeding rings surround the margin of the orbit and extend on to the temple and cheek: they constitute the ***orbital part.*** Some fibres closely related to the lacrimal sac form the ***lacrimal part.***

The orbital part consists of fasciculi that are attached to the nasal part of the frontal bone (Fig. 3.11). From here they wind above, lateral to, and then below the orbital margin to be attached to the frontal process of the maxilla. Some fibres are also attached to the medial palpebral ligament which intervenes between the two

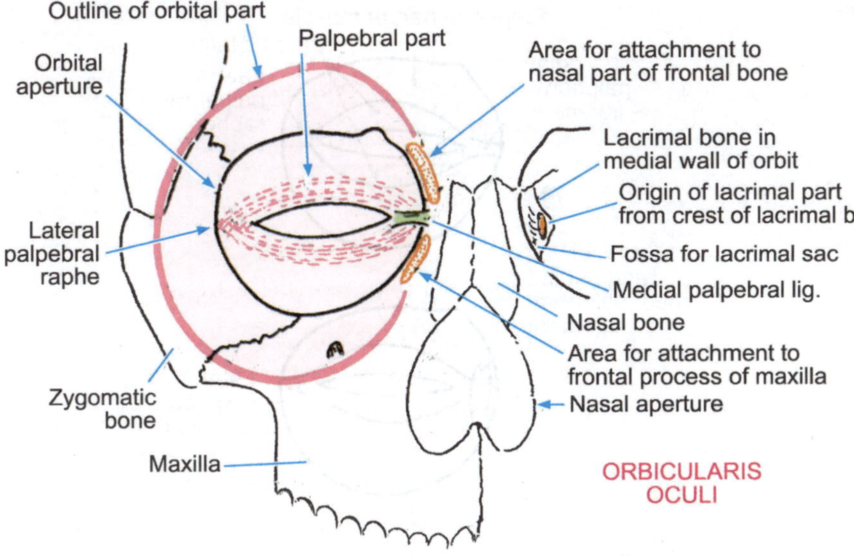

Fig. 3.11 Scheme to show the attachments of the orbicularis oculi muscle.

body attachments. The fibres of the palpebral part arise from the medial palpebral ligament (Fig. 3.11). They pass laterally through the eyelids; the upper and lower fibres then decussate to form the lateral palpebral raphe (Figs. 3.11, 3.12C). A group of fibres close to the margins of the lids form the ciliary bundle.

The lacrimal part of the muscle is attached to the lacrimal bone behind the lacrimal sac (3.12C). Some fibres are also attached to fascia covering the sac. The fibres pass laterally to join the palpebral part.

The orbicularis oculi muscle closes the palpebral fissure. The lacrimal part draws the eyelids medially. It dilates the lacrimal sac thus helping to suck lacrimal fluid into it.

The muscle is supplied by the temporal and zygomatic branches of the facial nerve.

Buccinator

Origin: The buccinator has a 'C' shaped line of origin (Fig. 3.13) from :

a. the outer aspect of the maxilla just above the three molar teeth;
b. a tendinous arch connecting the maxillary tuberosity to the pterygoid hamulus;
c. the pterygo-mandibular raphe (see below); and
d. the outer surface of the body of the mandible just below the molar teeth. At its posterior end the line of origin from the mandible passes behind the 3rd molar tooth to reach the medial side.

The pterygomandibular raphe is made up of interlacing tendinous fibres. It is attached above to the pterygoid hamulus (at the lower end of the medial pterygoid plate), and below to the posterior end of the mylohyoid line of the mandible. The raphe gives attachment anteriorly to fibres of the buccinator, and posteriorly to fibres of the superior constrictor of the pharynx.

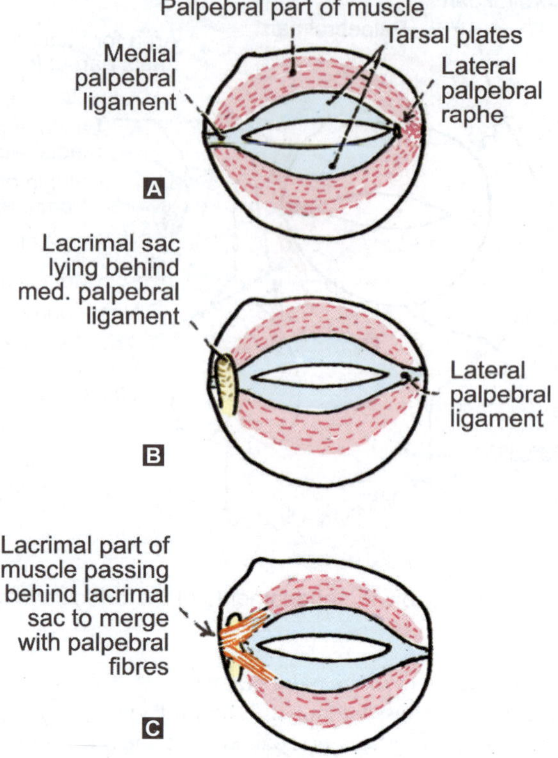

Figs. 3.12A to C Scheme to show the relationship of the lacrimal part of the orbicularis oculi to the lacrimal sac and to the medial palpebral ligament as seen from behind. A. Tarsal plates, medial palpebral ligament, and palpebral part of orbicularis oculi. The lateral palpebral ligament has been cut away to show the lateral palpebral raphe. B. Lacrimal sac lying behind the medial palpebral ligament. The lateral palpebral ligament is seen behind the lateral palpebral raphe. C. Lacrimal part of orbicularis oculi lying behind the lacrimal sac and passing laterally to blend with the palpebral part.

Insertion: The fibres of the buccinator run forwards where they are continuous with the orbicularis oris (Fig. 3.10).

Nerve Supply: The muscle is supplied by the lower buccal branches of the facial nerve.

Actions: The buccinator aids mastication by pushing food between the teeth. The muscle increases air pressure within the mouth as in blowing. (Laterally, the word buccinator means one who blows a trumpet).

Important Relations: The muscle is lined on the inside by the mucous membrane of the mouth. It is related on its outer aspect to the parotid duct which pierces it opposite the third upper molar tooth; to the superficial muscles inserted into the angle of the mouth; to the facial artery and vein; and to branches of the facial and buccal nerves (Figs. 1.2, 1.4 to 1.6).

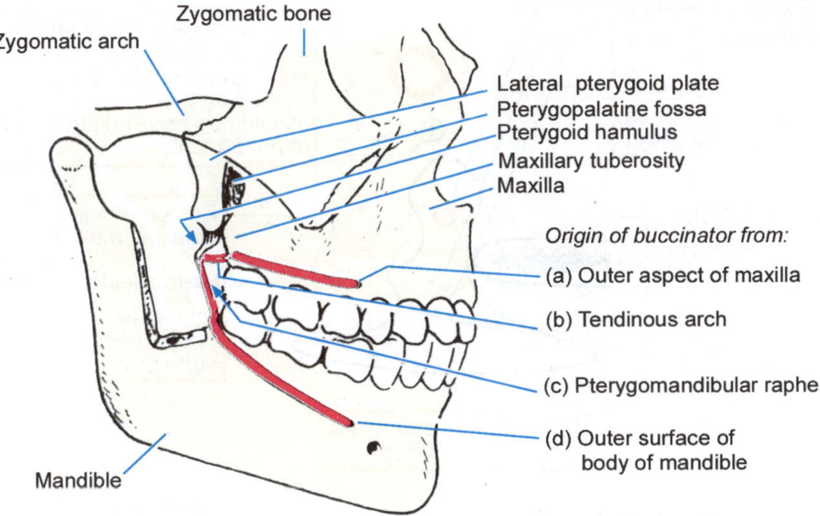

Fig. 3.13 Origin of the buccinator muscle. For insertion see Fig. 3.10.

PAROTID GLAND

The parotid gland lies on the lateral side of the face in a depression below the external acoustic meatus, behind the mandible, and in front of the sternocleidomastoid muscle (Fig. 1.2). It is roughly triangular on cross section. It has a lateral or superficial surface, an anteromedial surface, and a posteromedial surface (Fig. 3.14). At its upper end it has a small superior surface. Its lower end is rounded and is called the apex.

The superficial surface of the parotid gland extends upwards to the zygomatic arch. Its lower end (apex) lies behind and below the angle of the mandible. Anteriorly, it is prolonged forwards superficial to the masseter. Posteriorly, it overlaps the anterior margin of the sternocleidomastoid (Fig. 1.2). This surface is covered by skin and fascia. Lymph nodes of the superficial parotid group lie over it.

The superior surface of the parotid is concave and fits under the external acoustic meatus. It is also in contact with the posterior surface of the temporomandibular joint (Fig. 3.15).

The anteromedial surface is in contact with the posterior border of the ramus of the mandible (Fig. 3.14). It will be recalled that lateral to the ramus there is the masseter muscle, and deep to it there is the medial pterygoid. The anteromedial surface is related to all these structures.

The posteromedial surface is in contact, in its upper part with the mastoid process, and lower down with the sternocleidomastoid (superficially) and the posterior belly of the digastric (deep). The deepest part of the gland reaches the styloid process and the structures attached to it. These separate the gland from the internal carotid artery and the internal jugular vein (Figs. 3.14, 3.15).

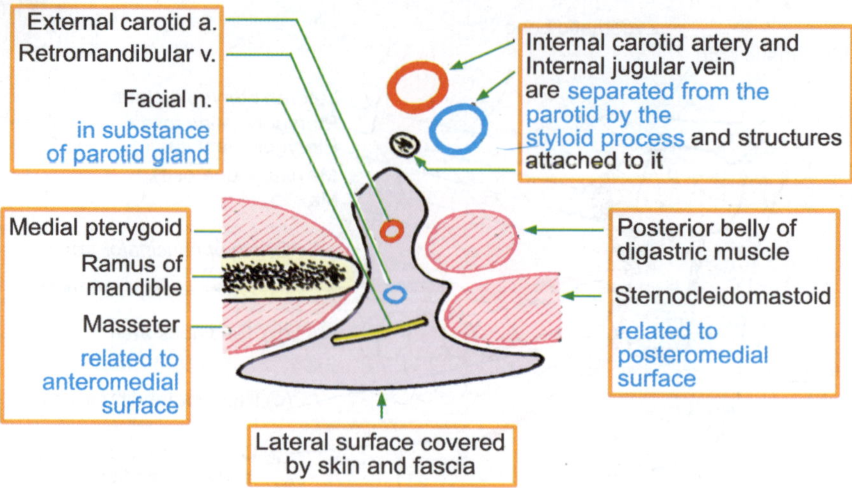

Fig. 3.14 Schematic transverse section through parotid gland to show its relations.

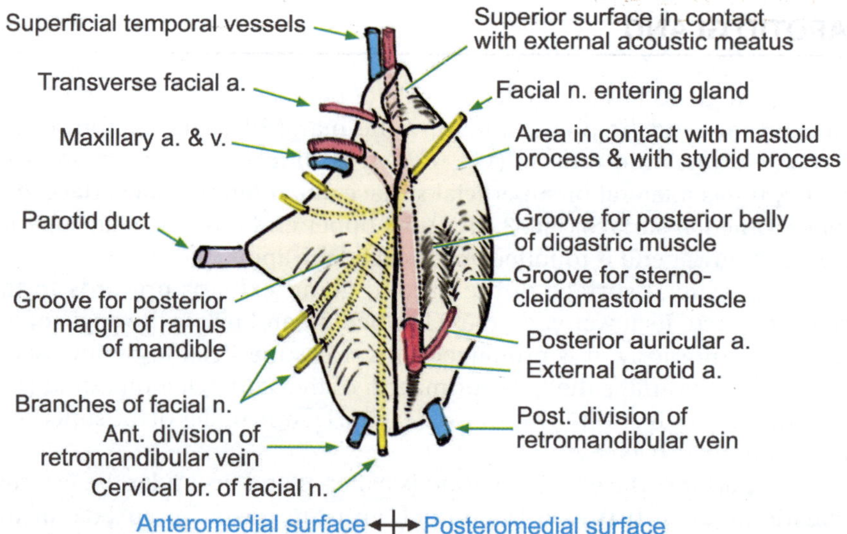

Fig. 3.15 Schematic view of parotid gland as seen from the medial side. Note the structures entering or leaving the gland.

The parotid gland is related to several nerves and vessels as follows.

1. The external carotid artery enters the lower part of the posteromedial surface (Fig. 3.13). Ascending within the substance of the gland it divides into its terminal branches (superficial temporal and maxillary) which emerge on the anteromedial surface of the gland. The posterior auricular branch of the external carotid artery arises just before the latter enters the gland. Sometimes it arises within the

substance of the gland and emerges on the posteromedial surface. The transverse facial branch of the superficial temporal artery may arise within the substance of the gland.
2. The retromandibular vein lies in the substance of the parotid superficial to the external carotid artery (Fig. 1.4) (See below).
3. The trunk of the facial nerve enters the upper part of the posteromedial surface. Within the gland it divides into its terminal branches which emerge from the anteromedial surface near its anterior margin (Figs. 1.4, 3.15). The cervical branch of the nerve emerges from the lower end of the gland (Fig. 1.2). The facial nerve is often described as dividing the parotid gland into superficial and deep parts.
4. The auriculotemporal nerve passes laterally between the neck of the mandible and the superior surface of the gland. It gives branches to the gland. (The nerve is seen in the region of the parotid gland in Fig. 1.5. The gland has been removed).
5. The anterior (facial) branch of the great auricular nerve passes forwards over the superficial surface of the gland and supplies the overlying skin.

Secretions of the parotid gland are collected by a system of ducts which unite to form the ***parotid duct.*** This duct emerges at the anterior margin of the gland and runs forwards across the masseter (Fig. 1.2). At the anterior border of the masseter the duct turns medially and pierces the buccinator. The terminal part of the duct runs forwards deep to the mucous membrane of the cheek. It opens into the vestibule of the mouth opposite the crown of the upper second molar tooth.

A detached part of the parotid gland present just above the parotid duct is called the ***accessory part*** of the parotid gland (Fig. 1.2).

The parotid gland is enclosed in a fibrous capsule derived from the deep cervical fascia as follows. At the lower end of the gland the investing layer of the deep cervical fascia splits into two layers. One layer ascends superficial to the parotid gland to reach the zygomatic arch to which it is attached. This fascia is thick and strong and is called the ***parotid fascia.*** The other layer ascends deep to the gland. Part of this layer forms a thickened band extending from the posterior margin of the ramus of the mandible to the styloid process. This band is the ***stylomandibular ligament.*** It separates the parotid gland from the submandibular gland.

The parotid gland is supplied by small branches of the external carotid artery or of its terminal divisions. The veins drain into the retromandibular and external jugular veins. The lymph vessels from the gland drain into the deep cervical nodes after passing through the superficial parotid nodes (lying on the lateral surface of the gland) and the deep parotid nodes (lying in the substance of the gland).

Secretomotor nerves reach the gland through branches from the auriculotemporal nerve. The gland also receives sympathetic nerves.

VESSELS OF THE FACE AND PAROTID REGION

Arteries

The arteries to be seen in the face are the facial artery and the transverse facial branch of the superficial temporal artery (Figs. 1.2, 1.4). The arteries to be seen in relation to the parotid gland have been mentioned above.

Facial artery

The facial artery runs part of its course in the neck, and in the submandibular region. It then enters the face by passing round the lower border of the body of the mandible just in front of the masseter muscle. it then runs upwards and forwards across the body of the mandible and the buccinator to reach the angle of the mouth. Finally it ascends along the side of the nose to reach the medial angle of the eye. In the face the artery gives off branches to the lower lip (inferior labial artery), the upper lip (superior labial artery), and to the nose (lateral nasal artery). The terminal part of the facial artery is called the angular artery.

The ***superficial temporal artery*** arises from the external carotid artery within the parotid gland. It runs upwards behind the temporomandibular joint and ends by dividing into frontal and parietal branches that supply the scalp. It also gives off the ***transverse facial artery*** which runs forwards across the masseter muscle.

We have seen that the external carotid artery runs through the parotid gland and gives off a number of branches in the region.

Veins

The veins to be seen in the face and parotid region are the facial vein, the superficial temporal vein, the retromandibular vein.

The retromandibular vein is formed within the upper part of the parotid gland by the union of the superficial temporal and maxillary veins. Its lower end divides, within the gland, into anterior and posterior divisions which emerge from the gland near its lower end. The posterior division, which is the main continuation of the retromandibular vein, joins the posterior auricular vein to form the external jugular vein. The anterior division joins the facial vein to form the common facial vein.

The facial vein runs downwards and backwards just behind the facial artery, and receives tributaries corresponding to branches of the artery. It end by joining the anterior division of the retromandibular vein to form the common facial vein. The common facial vein ends in the internal jugular vein.

Lymphatics

A brief introduction to the lymph nodes of the head and neck has been given on page 45.

The lymphatics of the face drain into the superficial and deep parotid lymph nodes, into the submental nodes, and also into the submandibular lymph nodes. As mentioned above the parotid gland drains into the superficial and deep parotid nodes.

NERVES OF THE FACE

The nerves seen on the face are motor and sensory. The motor nerves are terminal branches of the facial nerve. We have seen that after emerging from

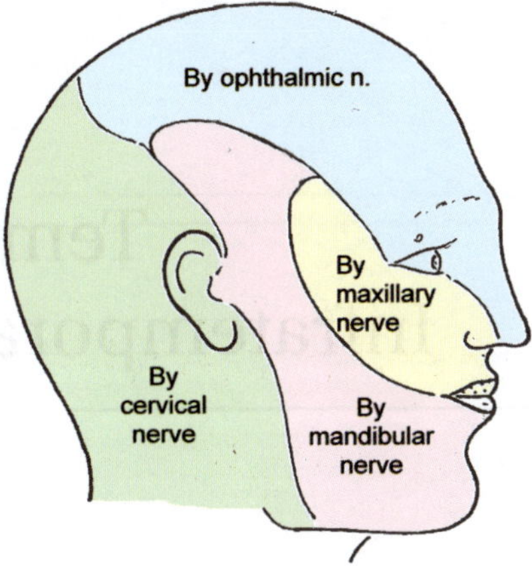

Fig. 3.16 Areas of skin supplied by the ophthalmic, maxillary and mandibular divisions of the trigeminal nerve.

the skull, the facial nerve enters the parotid gland and divides within it into several branches that emerge along the borders of the gland (Fig. 1.4).

In Fig. 1.2 note that the facial nerve gives off a temporal branch, a zygomatic branch, upper and lower buccal branches, a marginal mandibular branch, and a cervical branch. These branches supply the various muscles of the face.

The sensory nerves seen on the face are terminal ramifications of the trigeminal nerve (Fig. 1.4). Branches arising from the ophthalmic division are the supratrochlear, supraorbital, infratrochlear and external nasal nerves. Some branches are also given off to the upper eyelid.

Branches of the maxillary division of the trigeminal nerve to be seen on the face are the infraorbital nerve, the zygomaticofacial and zygomatico-temporal nerves (Fig. 1.5). Branches of the mandibular division seen on the face are the auriculotemporal, buccal (Fig. 1.5) and mental nerves. The area of skin of the face supplied by the three divisions of the trigeminal nerve are showing in Fig. 3.16.

Clinical Correlations

Clinical correlations of the scalp, of the face, and of the parotid gland are given in Chapter 15.

CHAPTER

4

Temporal and Infratemporal Regions

TEMPORAL REGION

Review of Structures to be Seen in the Temporal Region

The temporal region overlies the ***temporal fossa*** present on the lateral aspect of the skull. The fossa is bounded above by the temporal line and inferiorly by the zygomatic arch. Its floor is formed by parts of the frontal and parietal bones, part of the squamous temporal bone, and part of the greater wing of the sphenoid bone. The wall has an anterior wall made up mainly by the temporal surface of the zygomatic bone with contributions from the greater wing of the sphenoid and from the frontal bone.

A superficial view of the temporal region is seen in Fig. 1.2. The lower part of the region is overlapped by the auricle. A thick fibrous membrane, the ***temporal fascia*** covers the region. This fascia is attached superiorly to the temporal lines, and inferiorly to the zygomatic arch. Attached to the superficial aspect of the temporal fascia there are some subcutaneous muscles attached to the auricle. These are the ***auricularis superior***, the ***auricularis posterior*** and the ***auricularis anterior***. A few scattered muscle fibres that run vertically over the upper part of the region are given the name ***temporoparietalis***. [These are all vestigial muscles of no functional importance. We will, therefore, not go into any further details about them].

In Fig. 1.2 we also see a number of nerves and vessels. Immediately in front of the external acoustic meatus we see the ***auriculotemporal nerve*** emerging from under cover of the upper end of the parotid gland. The nerve ascends into the temporal region and scalp and divides into branches that supply them.

Just in front of the auriculotemporal nerve we see the superficial temporal vessels. The ***superficial temporal artery*** is a terminal branch of the external carotid artery. It divides into branches that supply the temporal region and scalp.

The ***superficial temporal vein*** is a tributary of the retromandibular vein.

Some other nerves seen in the region are as follows. The ***temporal branch of the facial nerve*** is seen running upwards and forwards to reach the frontalis muscle which it supplies. It also helps to supply the orbicularis oculi and the auricular muscles. The ***posterior auricular branch of the facial nerve*** is seen behind the auricle in the lower part of the temporal region. It runs backwards to reach and supply the occipitalis muscle. It also helps to supply the auricular muscles. The ***zygomatico-facial nerve*** (Fig. 1.2) and the ***zygomatico-temporal nerve*** (Fig. 1.4) are derived from the zygomatic branch of the maxillary division of the trigeminal nerve, They help to supply the skin of the region.

In the above paragraphs we have considered structures seen superficially in the temporal region. Removal of the temporal fascia brings the ***temporalis muscle*** into view (Fig. 1.4). This is the main content of the temporal fossa. It can seen that the muscle has a broad origin form the floor of the temporal fossa. The lower part of the muscle is obscured from view by the zygomatic arch. Removal of the arch (Fig. 1.5) brings the entire muscle into view. We can now see that the muscle is inserted into the coronoid process of the mandible. The temporalis is one of the muscles that is responsible for chewing movements (mastication). In Figs. 1.6 and 1.7 the lower part of the temporalis muscle has been removed. We now see that deep to the muscle there are the (anterior, middle and posterior) ***deep temporal nerves*** and vessels. The arteries are branches of the maxillary artery (Fig. 1.6), while the nerves arise from the anterior division of the mandibular nerve (Fig. 1.7, 9.48).

The deep temporal nerves supply the temporalis muscle.

This completes our review of the temporal region. The only structure that needs further consideration is the temporalis muscle which is described along with other muscles of mastication (below).

INFRATEMPORAL FOSSA

Relationship to the Skull

The term infratemporal fossa is applied to an irregular space lying below the lateral part of the base of the skull. The roof of the fossa is formed mainly by the greater wing of the sphenoid bone, with a small contribution from the squamous temporal bone. Superiorly, the lateral part of the fossa communicates with the temporal fossa through the gap between the zygomatic arch and the rest of the skull.

The fossa is bounded medially by the pterygoid process (of the sphenoid bone), the medial and lateral pterygoid plates being intimately related to structures in the fossa.

The anterior wall of the infratemporal fossa is formed by the posterior surface of the maxilla. The infratemporal fossa communicates with the pterygopalatine fossa through the pterygomaxillary fissure. Anteriorly, the infratemporal fossa communicates with the orbit through the inferior orbital fissure. These boundaries and communications should be confirmed in a skull. This will help in understanding the relationships of various structures to be seen in the region.

Structures to be Seen in the Infratemporal Fossa

Begin by examining Fig. 1.4 in which the head is viewed from the lateral aspect. We see the structures of the parotid region and some deep structures of the face. In particular note the masseter muscle the posterior part of which is overlapped by the parotid gland. Also identify the buccinator muscle already studied in the face.

Now turn to Fig. 1.5 in which the parotid gland has been removed. The zygomatic arch and the upper part of the masseter (which is attached to the arch) have also been removed. Identify the external carotid artery ascending a short distance behind the ramus of the mandible and terminating by dividing into the superficial temporal and maxillary arteries. Next observe the auriculotemporal nerve which is seen passing backwards deep to the neck of the mandible and then turning upwards to enter the temporal region. Also note that a nerve passes laterally through the mandibular notch to enter the masseter muscle. This is the masseteric branch of the mandibular nerve. Finally observe the buccal nerve and artery emerging from under the anterior margin of the ramus of the mandible to run forwards on the buccinator muscle.

In Fig. 1.6 dissection has been carried to a deeper level by removing a segment of the ramus of the mandible, and the lower part of the temporalis muscle. We now see the superficial contents of the infratemporal fossa. First identify the ***lateral pterygoid muscle***. The muscle has two heads, upper and lower. Their fibres run more or less horizontally and converge posteriorly to reach the neck of the mandible. Anteriorly, the two heads diverge and an interval can be seen between them. Inferior to the lateral pterygoid muscle we see the ***medial pterygoid muscle***. The fibres of this muscle run downwards and backwards. Anteriorly, some fibres of the muscle lie superficial to the lower head of the lateral pterygoid muscle. These fibres constitute the superficial head of the medial pterygoid muscle (which is better seen in Fig. 1.7). Note that the medial and lateral pterygoid muscles lie deep to the ramus of the mandible; and that the ramus separates the medial pterygoid muscle from the masseter. Finally note that the medial pterygoid muscle overlaps the posterior part of the buccinator muscle. The medial and lateral pterygoid muscles, the masseter, and the temporalis are muscles of mastication and are described below.

Now pay attention to the arteries of the region (Fig. 1.6). Note that the ***maxillary artery*** arises from the external carotid artery just behind the ramus of the mandible. The artery runs forwards deep to the neck of the mandible to enter the infratemporal fossa. It first runs forwards along the lower border of the lateral pterygoid muscle (first part) and then runs upwards and forwards across the lower head of the muscle (second part). Finally, it enters the interval between the two heads and disappears into the pterygomaxillary fissure. Note some branches of the artery that can be seen in Fig. 1.6. While still posterior to the mandible the maxillary artery gives off the ***anterior tympanic*** and ***deep auricular*** arteries. Within the infratemporal fossa it gives off the ***middle***

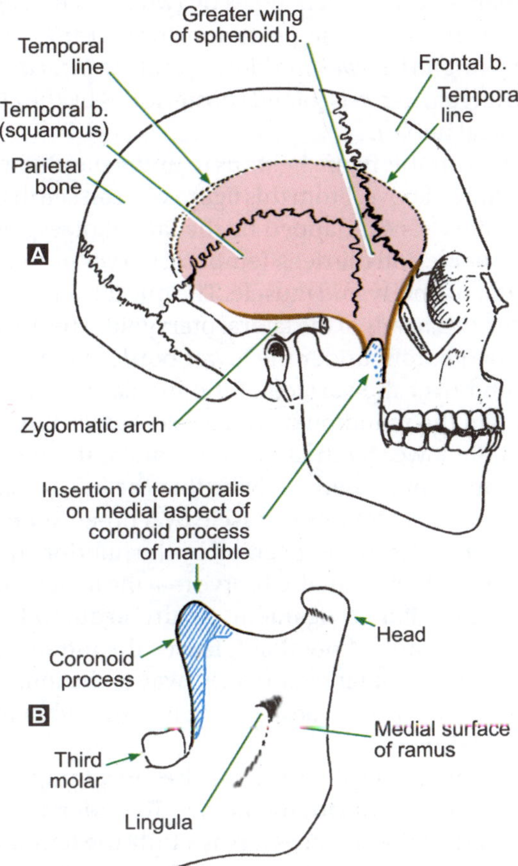

Fig. 4.1 A. Lateral view of the skull showing the origin of the temporalis muscle from the temporal fossa. Note the bones involved. B. Ramus of mandible seen from the medial side to show the insertion of the temporalis.

meningeal artery (shown in Fig. 1.6, but not labelled. It is better seen in Fig. 1.7). It also gives off the ***inferior alveolar artery***, the ***buccal artery***, and the ***deep temporal arteries.*** Just before entering the pterygomaxillary fissure it gives off the ***posterior superior alveolar artery***. From Fig. 8.24 it will be seen that the artery has a very wide distribution and gives off several branches not seen in the infratemporal region.

The main nerve of the infratemporal fossa is the ***mandibular nerve*** (Fig. 1.7). In this figure the nerve is seen entering the fossa through the foramen ovale. After a very short course the trunk of the nerve divides into a thin anterior division and a much thicker posterior division.

In Fig. 1.7 note that the anterior division gives off the ***deep temporal nerves.*** It also gives branches to the masseter (Fig. 1.6) and to the lateral pterygoid. Finally the anterior division continues on to the surface of the buccinator muscle as the ***buccal nerve.*** The thick posterior division gives off the ***auriculotemporal nerve*** which arises by two roots that are separated by the middle meningeal artery. The posterior division then divides into two main branches, the ***lingual nerve*** (anteriorly), and the ***inferior alveolar nerve*** (posteriorly). The lingual nerve is joined (posteriorly) by the ***chorda tympani*** (a branch of the facial nerve).

Now turn to Fig. 1.6 as this figure helps us to understand some relationships of the nerves mentioned above. From this figure you can see that the upper part of the mandibular nerve is overlapped by the lateral pterygoid muscle. Note that the masseteric nerve and the deep temporal nerves become superficial by passing above the lateral pterygoid muscle. The buccal nerve emerges through the gap between the two heads of the lateral pterygoid. The lingual and inferior alveolar nerves emerge from under the lower border of the lateral pterygoid muscle and descend over the surface of the medial pterygoid. The inferior alveolar nerve enters the mandibular canal and passes through it to supply the mandible and the lower teeth. It gives a branch, the ***mental nerve***, that emerges through the mental foramen. Note that the inferior alveolar nerve is separated from the medial pterygoid muscle by a broad ***sphenomandibular ligament***. The ***mylohyoid nerve*** is given off by the inferior alveolar nerve just before it enters the mandibular canal. Observe that the mylohyoid nerve pierces through the sphenomandibular ligament. Return again to Fig. 1.7 and trace the lingual nerve downwards. Note that it leaves the infratemporal region to pass through the submandibular region on its way to the tongue. In this figure also observe the mylohyoid nerve descending into the submandibular region to reach some muscles there.

This completes our general review of the infratemporal region. The muscles of mastication are considered below. To understand the actions of these muscles properly it is also necessary to study the temporo-mandibular joint.

MUSCLES OF MASTICATION

TEMPORALIS

Origin:

The temporalis arises from the temporal fossa on the lateral aspect of the skull (Fig. 4.1A). The area is bounded above by the temporal line, and below by the zygomatic arch. It includes parts of the frontal, parietal, and squamous temporal and of the greater wing of the sphenoid bone.

The anterior fibres of the muscle run vertically downwards; the posterior fibres run horizontally forwards; while the intermediate fibres run obliquely to converge in a tendon (Fig. 1.5). The tendon passes deep to the zygomatic arch.

Insertion:

The muscle is inserted into the coronoid process of the mandible. The region of insertion covers the entire medial aspect of the coronoid process (including its apex, anterior and posterior borders). Some fibres are inserted into the anterior border of the ramus (Fig. 4.1B).

Nerve Supply:

The temporalis is supplied by the deep temporal branches of the mandibular nerve.

Actions:

The temporalis helps to close the mouth by elevating the mandible.

The movements of elevation and depression of the mandible have two components. Firstly, there is a hinge like movement between the condyle of the mandible and the inferior surface of the articular disc of the temporomandibular joint. The second component is a gliding movement of the disc (along with the head of the mandible). In wide opening of the mouth the disc glides forwards so that the head of the mandible comes to lie below the articular eminence.

In closing the mouth the posterior horizontal fibres of the temporalis pull the mandible backwards (along with the intra-articular disc), whereas the anterior vertical fibres produce the angular hinge like movement.

Temporal Fascia:

The temporalis is covered by a thick temporal fascia. The fascia is attached above to the (superior) temporal line, and below to the zygomatic arch.

MASSETER

The masseter is a quadrilateral muscle placed superficial to the ramus of the mandible ((Figs. 1.4, 1.5).

Origin:

The muscle arises from the zygomatic arch (Fig. 4.2).

The more superficial muscle fibres arise from the anterior two thirds of the lower border of the arch; whereas the deeper fibres arise from its deep surface, and from the posterior one third of its lower border. The most anterior fibres arise from the zygomatic process of the maxilla.

Insertion:

The muscle is inserted into the lateral surface of the ramus and angle of the mandible.

Nerve Supply:

The masseter is supplied by a branch of the anterior division of the mandibular nerve. The nerve reaches the muscle by passing through the notch between the coronoid process and neck of the mandible (Fig. 1.5).

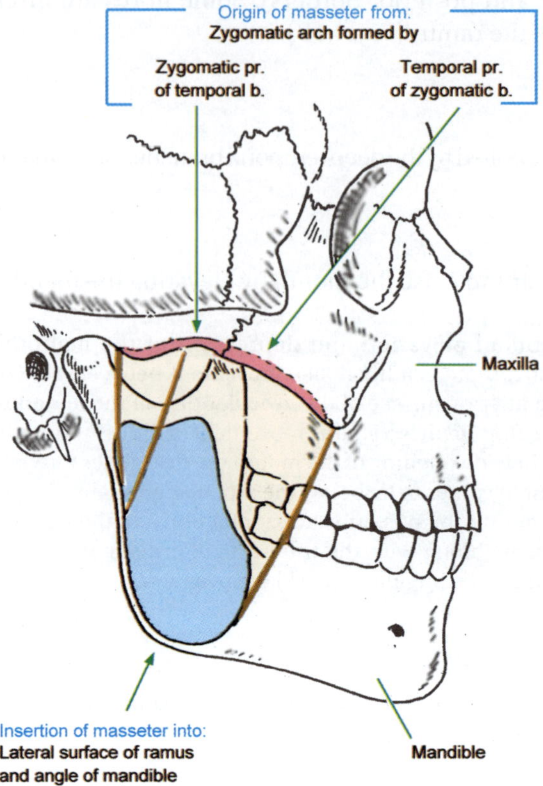

Fig. 4.2 Attachments of the masseter muscle.

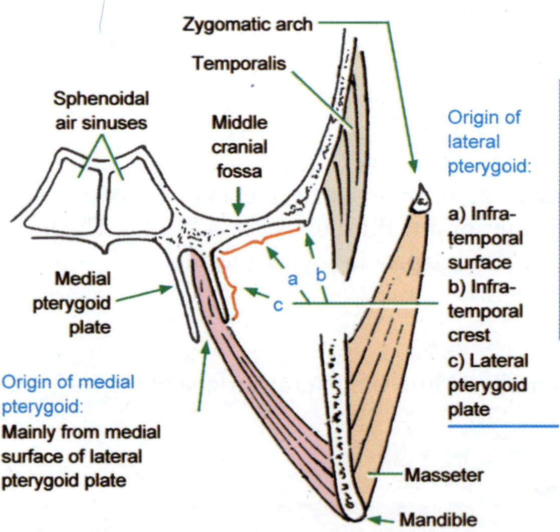

Fig. 4.3 Schematic coronal section across the base of the skull, in the region of the infratemporal fossa, to show the area of origin of the lateral pterygoid muscle. The medial pterygoid, the masseter, and part of the temporalis are also shown.

Actions:

The masseter elevates the mandible to close the mouth. Its anterior fibres help in protraction (forward movement) of the jaw.

Important Relations:

Apart from the skin and some superficial muscles of the face the masseter is overlapped by the anterior part of the parotid gland, the parotid duct, the branches of the facial nerve and the transverse facial vessels. Deep to the masseter there are the ramus of the mandible, the lower part of the temporalis and the posterior part of the buccinator (Fig. 1.2).

LATERAL PTERYGOID

The position and general appearance of the muscle are shown in Fig. 1.6. It is seen that the muscle has two heads of origin, upper and lower.

Origin:

The ***upper head*** arises from:

(i) the infratemporal surface, and (ii) the infratemporal crest, of the greater wing of the sphenoid bone (Fig. 4.3).

The ***lower head*** arises from the lateral surface of the lateral pterygoid plate.

Insertion:

The fibres of both heads run backwards and laterally to be inserted into a depression (pterygoid fovea) on the anterior aspect of the neck of the mandible (Fig. 4.5). Some fibres are inserted into the intra-articular disc and some into the capsule of the temporo-mandibular joint.

Nerve Supply:

Mandibular nerve (anterior division).

Actions:

These are considered along with those of the medial pterygoid below.

MEDIAL PTERYGOID

Origin:

The medial pterygoid muscle takes origin from:

a. the medial surface of the lateral pterygoid plate and
b. the adjoining part of the palatine bone (pyramidal process) (Figs 4.3, 4.4).
c. A superficial slip arises from the lateral aspect of the pyramidal process of the palatine bone and from the maxillary tuberosity. (This slip is seen in Fig. 1.6 superficial to the lower head of the lateral pterygoid muscle).

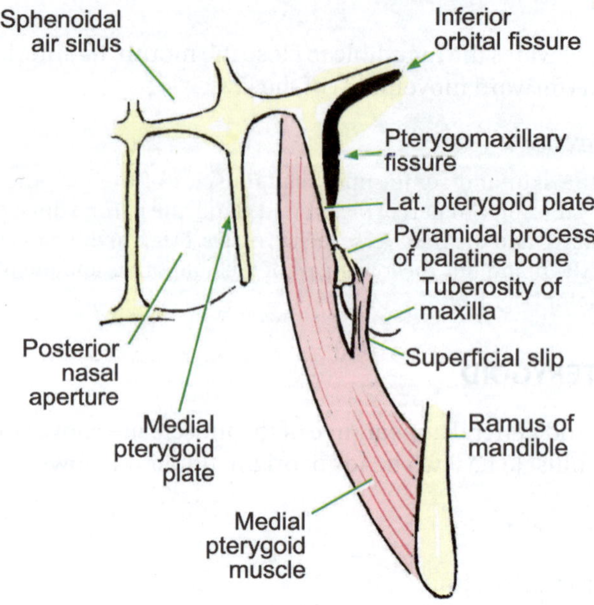

Fig. 4.4 Scheme to show the arrangement of the medial pterygoid muscle.

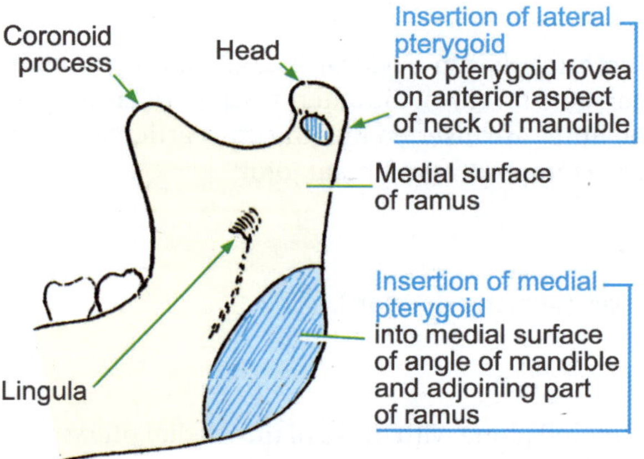

Fig. 4.5 Medial aspect of the ramus of the mandible showing areas for insertion of the lateral and medial pterygoid muscles.

Insertion:

The fibres of the muscle pass downwards, backwards and laterally (Figs. 1.6, 4.3, 4.4) to be inserted into the medial surface of the angle of the mandible and the adjoining part of its ramus (Fig. 4.5).

Nerve Supply:

Mandibular nerve.

Actions of Pterygoid Muscles:

In analysing the actions of these muscles it may be remembered that the pull of a muscle is opposite to the direction of its fibres. The fibres of the lateral pterygoid pass backwards and laterally. They can, therefore, pull the mandible forwards (protraction) and medially. The effect of the medial pull is that the chin moves to the opposite side. The fibres of the medial pterygoid also pass backward and laterally. This muscle can therefore, perform the same actions as described for the lateral pterygoid. However, its fibres also pass downwards: hence the muscle can elevate the mandible. Now note the following corollaries:

a. The medial and lateral pterygoids of both sides acting together protract the mandible.
b. The medial and lateral pterygoids of one side acting together pull the mandibular condyle of that side forwards (and medially). As a result the chin moves forwards and ***to the opposite side***. This movement is facilitated by slight rotation of the head of the mandible of the opposite side. Alternate action of the muscles of the two sides results in side to side chewing movements.
c. The two pterygoid muscles have opposite actions as far as opening and closing of the mouth is concerned. The medial pterygoid elevates the jaw. The lateral pterygoid helps in opening the mouth by pulling the head of the mandible forwards along with the intra-articular disc (as explained above under actions of temporalis).

Relations of Pterygoid Muscles

In considering the relations we will deal with the deepest structures first and move on to more superficial ones.

A. Deep relations of medial pterygoid

There are many structures deep to the medial pterygoid muscle. These can be visualised by examining 1.8. In this figure one half of the mandible has been removed (along with muscles attached to it) exposing structures lying in relation to the upper part of the wall of the pharynx. Note the following:

1. In this region the wall of the pharynx is formed by the ***superior constrictor*** muscle. Anteriorly, the muscle is attached to a tendinous band called the ***pterygomandibular raphe***. This raphe also gives attachment to the ***buccinator muscle***. Parts of all these lie deep to the medial pterygoid muscle (This can be appreciated by comparing Figs. 1.7 and 1.8).
2. The lower part of the superior constrictor of the pharynx is crossed by the ***styloglossus muscle*** (a muscle of the tongue), the ***stylopharyngeus*** (a muscle of the pharynx), and by the ***stylohyoid ligament***. It is also crossed by the ***glossopharyngeal nerve***. Parts of these structures are also deep to the medial pterygoid muscle.
3. Note that the upper border of the superior constrictor of the pharynx is curved, and that there is a gap between it and the base of the skull. In this gap we see a muscle of the palate, the ***tensor palati***. A little anterior to the tensor palati we see the ***medial pterygoid plate***. These are additional medial relations of the medial pterygoid muscle.

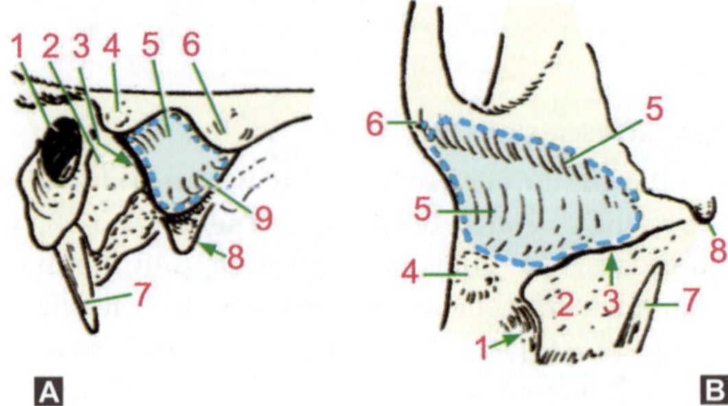

Fig. 4.6 Superior articular surface of the temporomandibular joint as seen (A) from the lateral side, and (B) from below. 1. Ext. acoustic meatus. 2. Tympanic plate. 3. Squamo-tympanic fissure. 4. Postglenoid tubercle. 5. Articular fossa. 6. Tubercle of root of zygoma. 7. Styloid process. 8. Spine of sphenoid. 9. Articular tubercle.

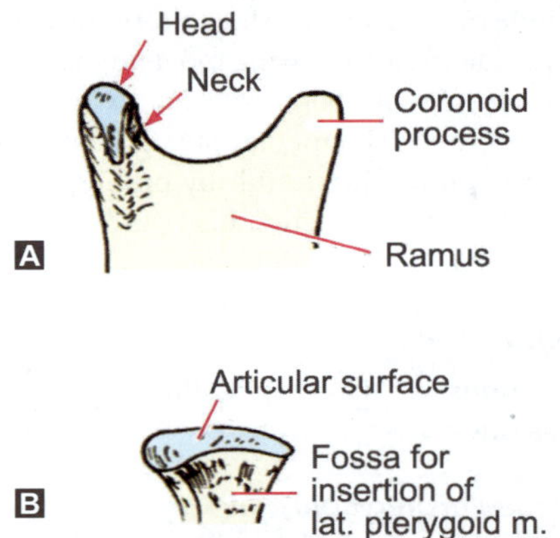

Fig. 4.7 Inferior articular surface of the temporomandibular joint (head of mandible). A. Seen from lateral side. B. Seen from the front.

B. Superficial relations of medial pterygoid:

These are as follows. The upper part of the muscle is separated from the lateral pterygoid muscle by the ***lateral pterygoid plate***, and by the upper parts of the ***lingual and inferior alveolar nerves*** (Fig. 1.7). Lower down the muscle is separated from the ramus of the mandible by the same nerves (Fig. 1.6), the ***maxillary artery*** and by the ***spheno-mandibular ligament***. The lower part of the ***ramus of the mandible*** separates the medial pterygoid muscle from the masseter (Also see Fig. 4.3).

C. Deep relations of lateral pterygoid:

These can be appreciated by comparing Figs. 1.6 and 1.7. The structures deep to the lateral pterygoid muscle are the ***auriculotemporal nerve***, the ***sphenomandibular ligament***, the ***middle meningeal artery***, the trunk of the ***mandibular nerve***, the upper parts of the ***lingual and inferior alveolar nerves***, the ***chorda tympani***, the ***lateral pterygoid plate*** and the upper part of the ***medial pterygoid muscle***.

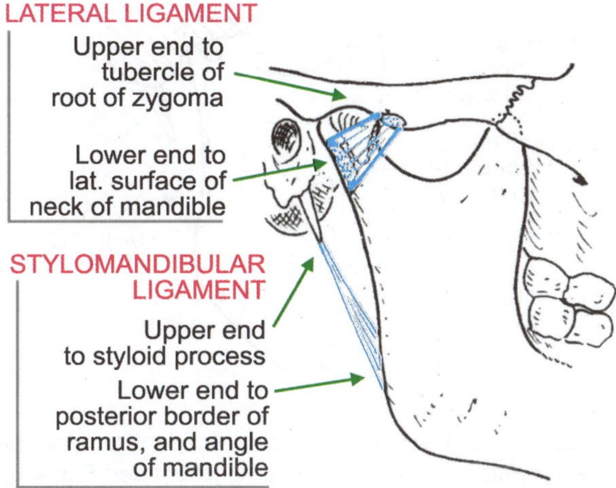

Fig. 4.8 Ligaments of the temporomandibular joint as seen from the lateral side.

D. Superficial relations of lateral pterygoid:

These are seen in Fig. 1.6. They are the tendon of the ***temporalis***, the ***maxillary artery***, the **buccal nerve** and the ***ramus of the mandible***. The upper border of the lateral pterygoid is related to the deep temporal and masseteric nerves.

THE TEMPOROMANDIBULAR JOINT

This is a synovial joint of the condylar variety. It is a complex joint as its cavity is divided into upper and lower parts by an intra-articular disc.

The ***upper articular surface*** of the joint is formed by the mandibular fossa of the temporal bone (Figs. 4.6 A,B). Anteriorly, the surface extends onto the articular tubercle. The posterior part of the surface is, therefore, concave downwards; and the anterior part is convex.

The ***inferior articular surface*** is formed by the head of the mandible which is markedly convex anteroposteriorly (Fig. 4.7A), and more gently convex from side to side (Fig. 4.7B). The articular surfaces are covered with white fibrocartilage (and not hyaline cartilage as in most other synovial joints; this is because the bones concerned ossify in membrane).

The ***articular disc*** is also made of fibrocartilage (Fig. 4.10A). Its upper surface is concavoconvex to fit the upper articular surface of the joint. Its lower surface is concave, the head of the mandible fitting into the concavity.

The ***capsule*** of the joint is attached to the margins of the articular surfaces. It is shown in interrupted line in Figs. 4.6 and 4.7. The inside of the capsule is lined by synovial membrane. The lateral part of the capsule is strengthened by the ***lateral temporomandibular ligament*** (Fig. 4.8). The upper end of this ligament is attached to the tubercle of the root of the zygoma and its lower end

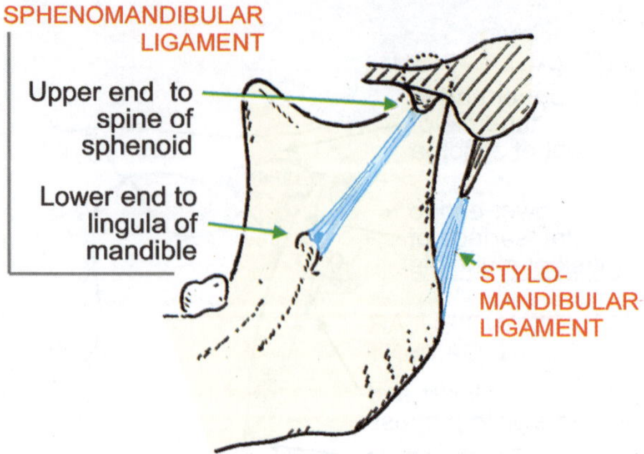

Fig. 4.9 Ligaments of temporomandibular joint as seen from the medial side. For attachments of stylomandibular ligament see Fig. 4.8.

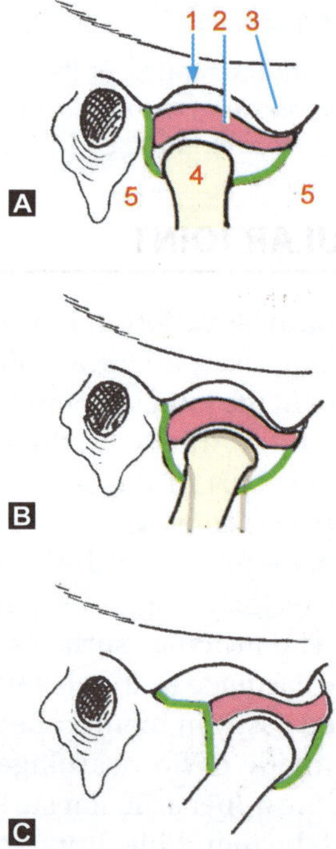

Fig. 4.10 Scheme to show phases in movements at the temporomandibular joint. A. Mouth closed. B. Mouth opened slightly. C. Mouth widely open. 1. Articular fossa. 2. Articular disc. 3. Articular tubercle. 4. Head of mandible. 5. Joint capsule

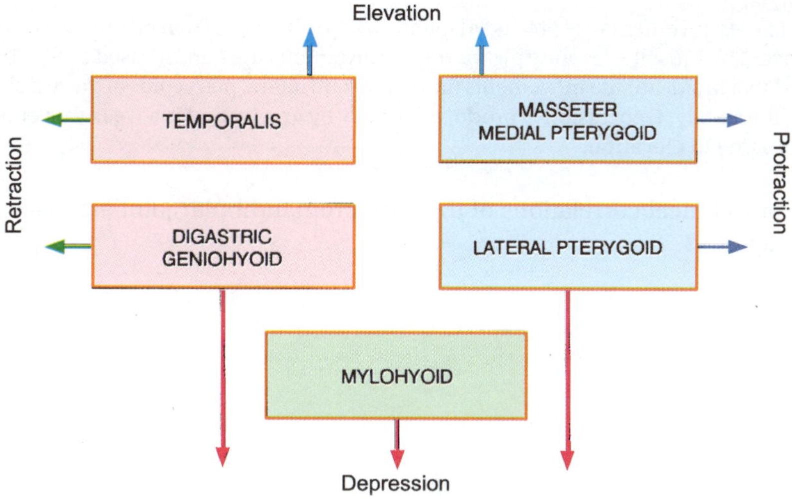

Fig. 4.11 Scheme to show the muscles responsible for movements at the temporomandibular joint.

to the lateral aspect of the neck of the mandible. In addition the joint has two accessory ligaments (that are independent of the capsule and lie some distance away from it). The ***sphenomandibular ligament*** (Fig. 4.9) is attached above to the spine of the sphenoid, and below to the lingula of the mandible. The ***stylomandibular ligament*** (Figs. 4.8, 4.9) extends from the apex of the styloid process to the angle and posterior border of the ramus of the mandible. It is formed by a thickening of the deep fascia of the region.

Movements at the temporomandibular joint

The movements at the joint can be divided into those between the upper articular surface and the articular disc, and those between the disc and the head of the mandible. Most movements occur simultaneously at the right and left temporomandibular joints. In forward movement or ***protraction*** of the mandible the articular disc glides forwards over the upper articular surface, the head of the mandible moving with it. The reversal of this movement is called ***retraction***. In slight opening of the mouth (depression of the mandible) the head of the mandible moves on the under-surface of the disc like a hinge (Compare Figs. 4.10 A and B). In wide opening of the mouth, this hinge like movement is followed by a forward gliding of the disc and the head of the mandible, as in protraction (Fig. 4.10C). At the end of this movement the head comes to lie under the articular tubercle. These movements are reversed in closing the mouth (or ***elevation*** of the mandible).

Chewing movements involve side to side movements of the mandible. In these movements, the head of one side glides forwards along with disc (as in protraction) but the head of the opposite side merely rotates on a vertical axis. As result of this the chin moves forwards and to one side (the side on which no gliding has occurred). Alternate movements of this kind on the two sides result in side to side movements of the lower jaw.

These movements are produced mainly by the muscles of mastication described above. The muscles responsible for these movements are summarised in Fig. 4.11. Note that in side to side movements the medial and lateral pterygoids of the two sides act alternately. Depression is produced mainly by gravity and is a weak movement compared to elevation.

Some clinical correlations of the temporomandibular joint are discussed in Chapter 15.

CHAPTER

5

Submandibular Region and Tongue

In this Chapter we will consider the submandibular region. We will see that muscles, blood vessels and nerves that supply the tongue lie in this region. It is, therefore, logical to combine the study of the submandibular region with that of the tongue.

SUBMANDIBULAR REGION

We will begin the study of this region by identifying the various structures to be seen here, and their layout, using figures in the atlas section.

The submandibular region lies between the mandible and the hyoid bone. Many structures that we will encounter will gain attachment to one or both of these bones or will be related to them.

A superficial view of the submandibular region is seen in Fig. 1.2. We see that apart from skin and fascia, the region is covered superficially by the platysma. A view after removal of skin, fascia, and platysma, is seen in Fig. 1.4. Observe the V-shaped ***digastric muscle***, consisting of anterior and posterior bellies united by an intermediate tendon. The tendon passes through a fibrous pulley attached to the hyoid bone. The region bounded by the two bellies of the digastric muscle, and by the lower border of the mandible is the ***digastric triangle***. It is occupied by the ***submandibular salivary gland***. Observe the submental branch of the facial artery (and accompanying vein) running across the gland just below the lower border of the mandible.

In Fig. 1.5 note some further details. The region between the anterior belly of the digastric and the anterior middle line is occupied by the ***mylohyoid muscle***. (For a much better view of this muscle see Fig. 1.12). In the interval between the hyoid bone and the posterior belly of the digastric muscle we see a small part of the ***hyoglossus muscle***. The ***lingual artery*** (a branch of the external carotid artery) is seen passing deep into the submandibular region under cover of the posterior margin of the hyoglossus. Just above the digastric tendon we see a small part of the ***stylohyoid muscle***, gaining attachment to the hyoid bone. (This muscle is seen fully in Fig. 1.7). Finally, in Fig. 1.5 note that the posterior belly of the digastric muscle passes backwards deep to the angle of the mandible. Further back it lies deep to the sternocleidomastoid muscle and reaches the mastoid process. (Observe the carotid arteries and the internal jugular vein deep to the posterior belly, in the neck, behind the submandibular region).

We will now turn to Fig. 1.6 in which the submandibular region is seen after removal of the submandibular gland. We now see that the 'bed' for the gland is formed anteriorly by the mylohyoid muscle, and posteriorly by the hyoglossus. Observe the ***submandibular duct***, and lower down the ***hypoglossal nerve***, running across the hyoglossus and disappearing deep to the posterior edge of the mylohyoid muscle. Observe again, the lingual artery passing deep to the hyoglossus. It gives a suprahyoid branch that runs across the hyoglossus near its lower end.

Now we will go on to Fig. 1.7. This figure shows a dissection in which one half of the mandible has been removed so that we can now see the tongue lying in the oral cavity. The greater part of the mylohyoid muscle has been cut away exposing the hyoglossus in almost its full extent. Note that the muscle is attached inferiorly to the hyoid bone. Its fibres pass upwards and forwards to enter the substance of the tongue. (As the suffix 'glossus' in its name implies it is a muscle of the tongue). Also observe the styloglossus muscle, another muscle of the tongue, passing from the styloid process to the tongue. Its fibres merge with those of the hyoglossus muscle near the upper end of the muscle.

Several structures are seen over the hyoglossus muscle. These are as follows (Fig. 1.7).

1. The ***lingual nerve*** is seen passing from the infratemporal fossa to the submandibular region. It runs across the hyoglossus, winds below the submandibular duct (see below), and enters the tongue.
2. The ***submandibular ganglion*** is seen hanging from the lingual nerve by two roots.
3. The ***submandibular duct*** (which drains the submandibular gland) runs upwards and forwards to reach the oral cavity inferior to the anterior part of the tongue.
4. The ***mylohyoid nerve*** (branch of the inferior alveolar nerve) is seen crossing the hyoglossus muscle, the submandibular duct and the hypoglossal nerve to reach the mylohyoid muscle which it supplies. It also gives a branch to the anterior belly of the digastric muscle.
5. The ***hypoglossal nerve*** is seen running downwards and forwards across the external carotid artery, and the (upward) loop formed by the lingual artery, to reach the hyoglossus muscle. The nerve then turns upwards over the muscle and divides into branches that supply muscles of the tongue (including the hyoglossus).
6. In Fig. 1.7 we see the ***stylohyoid muscle*** in its full extent. Observe that it is attached above to the styloid process, and below to the hyoid bone. Its tendon divides into two parts that embrace the digastric tendon (Fig. 1.6).

In the paragraphs above we have listed the various structures lying over the hyoglossus muscle. Next observe (Fig. 1.7) some structures that pass deep to the posterior edge of the muscle. From above downwards these are the ***glossopharyngeal nerve***, the ***stylohyoid ligament***, and the ***lingual artery***.

To end the examination of Fig. 1.7, observe the region anterior to the hyoglossus muscle. Just above the mylohyoid muscle we see a part of the ***geniohyoid muscle***. Above the geniohyoid muscle we see the ***sublingual salivary gland***.

Finally, turn to Fig. 1.8. The hyoglossus has been removed, and the mylohyoid cut near the middle line. The ***geniohyoid muscle*** is now seen fully. Note that it passes from the mandible (near the symphysis menti) to the hyoid bone. Just above the geniohyoid muscle we see the ***genioglossus muscle***. The fibres of this muscle begin from the posterior aspect of the symphysis menti and fan out to reach the tongue. The glossopharyngeal nerve and the lingual artery run across this muscle to reach the tongue. Observe the ***stylohyoid ligament*** stretching between the styloid process and the hyoid bone.

This completes our general review of the layout of structures in the submandibular region. We will now consider the following topics in detail in the sequence listed.

1. Submandibular salivary gland.
2. Sublingual salivary gland.
3. Suprahyoid muscles: digastric, stylohyoid, mylohyoid and genioglossus. Along with them we will also consider the stylohyoid ligament.
4. Tongue and its muscles.

The blood vessels to be seen in the region are the lingual artery and lingual vein (Chapter 8). Nerve supply involves the lingual nerve, the submandibular ganglion, the glossopharyngeal nerve and the hypoglossal nerve (Chapter 9). These will be considered in detail in the Chapters stated.

THE SUBMANDIBULAR GLAND

The submandibular gland is located partly below, and partly deep to the body of the mandible. The part below the mandible lies in the digastric triangle. The gland has three surfaces, inferior, lateral and medial, which are best appreciated in a coronal section through the gland (Fig. 5.1).

The ***inferior surface*** is superficial, and is the one seen in the digastric triangle. It is directed downwards and some what laterally.

The ***lateral surface*** is hidden from view by the body of the mandible. It lies in contact with the medial surface of the body of the mandible, below the attachment of the mylohyoid muscle (Fig. 5.5). The posterior part of the lateral surface is separated from the mandible by the medial pterygoid muscle (Fig. 5.2).

The ***medial surface*** rests on several structures (Fig. 5.3). The most important of these are the mylohyoid muscle (in front), the hyoglossus (in the middle) and the wall of the pharynx (posteriorly). At the posterior margin of the mylohyoid muscle a prolongation of the submandibular gland called the ***deep part*** passes forward in the interval between the mylohyoid (laterally) and the hyoglossus (medially) (Fig. 5.2).

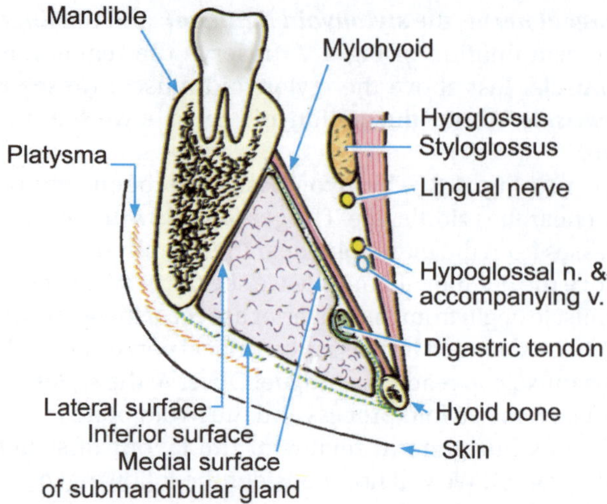

Fig. 5.1 Coronal section through the submandibular region to show the surfaces of the submandibular gland and their relations.

The following additional relationships may now be noted.

1. The submandibular gland is enclosed by two layers of fascia formed by splitting of the investing layer of deep cervical fascia. The superficial layer covers the inferior surface of the gland and is attached to the lower border of the mandible. The deeper layer covers the medial surface and is attached above to the mylohyoid line of the mandible.
2. Apart from skin and fascia the inferior surface is overlapped by the platysma. It is crossed by the facial vein, and the cervical branch of the facial nerve. The submandibular lymph nodes lie over it. Some of the nodes may be embedded within the gland.
3. The relationship of the facial artery to the gland is worthy of note. The artery first runs upwards along the posterior end of the gland (grooving it). It then runs downwards and forwards between the lateral surface of the gland (deep to the artery) and the medial pterygoid muscle (superficial to it) (Fig. 8.17).
4. The posterior end of the gland reaches as far as the stylomandibular ligament which separates it from the parotid gland (Fig. 5.2).
5. The following additional relations of the medial surface may be noted (Fig. 5.3).
   a. The anterior part of this surface is separated from the mylohyoid muscle by the mylohyoid nerve and vessels and by the submental vessels.
   b. The intermediate part of the medial surface is separated from the hyoglossus by the styloglossus, the lingual nerve, the submandibular ganglion, the hypoglossal nerve and the deep lingual vein.
   c. Behind the posterior margin of the hyoglossus the gland is related to the styloglossus, the stylohyoid ligament and the glossopharyngeal nerve.

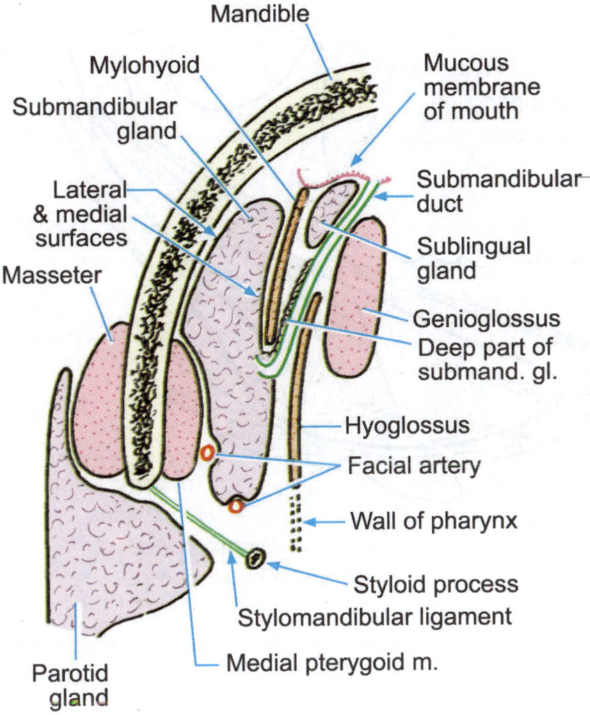

Fig. 5.2 Schematic transverse section through the body of the mandible, to show some relationships of the salivary glands.

The Submandibular Duct

The submandibular duct emerges from the medial surface of the submandibular gland near the posterior margin of the mylohyoid. In company with the deep part of the submandibular gland it runs forwards in the interval between the mylohyoid (laterally) and the hyoglossus (medially) (Fig. 5.2). Its anterior part lies between the sublingual gland (laterally) and the genioglossus (medially). The duct opens into the oral cavity on the sublingual papilla (located below the anterior part of the tongue, Fig. 5.12).

Blood Vessels, Nerves, Lymphatics

The arteries supplying the submandibular gland are branches of the facial and lingual arteries. The veins accompany the arteries.

The secretomotor (parasympathetic) nerve supply of the gland follows a complex pathway that is described in Chapter 9. The gland also receives sympathetic fibres.

Lymphatics from the submandibular gland drain into the submandibular lymph nodes and through them into the deep cervical nodes, particularly the jugulo-omohyoid node.

For histology of the submandibular gland see the author's HUMAN HISTOLOGY. For development see the author's HUMAN EMBRYOLOGY.

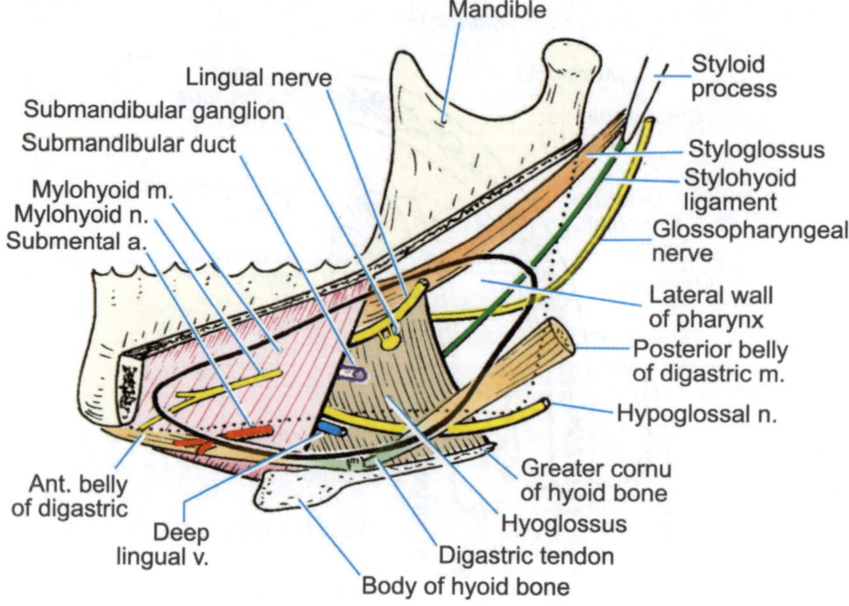

Fig. 5.3 Scheme to show structures deep to the submandibular gland. The outline of the area covered by the gland is shown in bold line.

THE SUBLINGUAL GLAND

The sublingual gland is present in relation to the floor of the anterior part of the oral cavity. It is placed just deep to the oral mucous membrane and is responsible for raising up the sublingual fold (Fig. 5.12). Inferiorly, the gland rests on the mylohyoid muscle. Laterally it is in contact with the anterior part of the mandible above the mylohyoid line (Fig. 5.5). These relationships are best appreciated in a coronal section through the gland (Fig. 5.4). In Fig. 5.2 note that the anterior end of the gland lies near the midline, close to the gland of the opposite side. The same figure shows that posteriorly the gland is near the deep part of the submandibular gland; and that the submandibular duct intervenes between the sublingual gland and the genioglossus.

Secretions of the sublingual gland leave it through a number of small ducts which open into the oral cavity on the sublingual fold (Fig. 5.12).

The secretomotor nerve supply (parasympathetic) of the gland is described in Chapter 9. The gland receives its blood supply through the sublingual branch of the lingual artery and the submental branch of the facial artery.

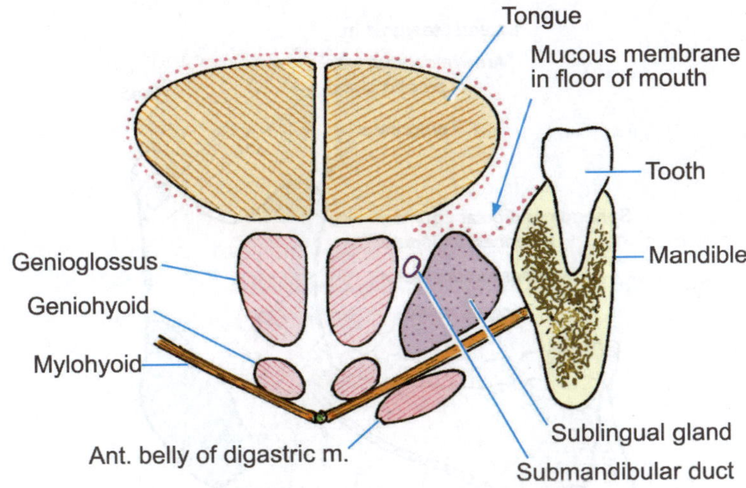

Fig. 5.4 Schematic coronal section through anterior part of tongue and mouth to show relationships of the sublingual salivary gland, and the oral diaphragm.

SUPRAHYOID MUSCLES

These are the digastric, stylohyoid, mylohyoid and geniohyoid muscles.

Digastric Muscle

The digastric muscle has two bellies, anterior and posterior, united by an intermediate tendon (Fig. 1.5). The posterior belly arises from the base of the skull just deep to the mastoid process. The anterior belly is attached to the anterior part of the base of the mandible near the midline (Figs. 5.5, 5.6). The intermediate tendon passes through a fibrous pulley that is attached to the hyoid bone (at the junction of body and greater cornu (Figs. 5.8, 5.9). The deep surface of the anterior belly rests on the mylohyoid (Fig. 5.15A: part of the belly is cut away to expose the mylohyoid).

Nerve Supply

The nerve supply of the anterior belly is by the mylohyoid branch of the inferior alveolar nerve; and that of the posterior belly by the facial nerve.

Actions

The digastric can elevate the hyoid bone. Acting along with other muscles attached to the hyoid bone it can fix the bone.

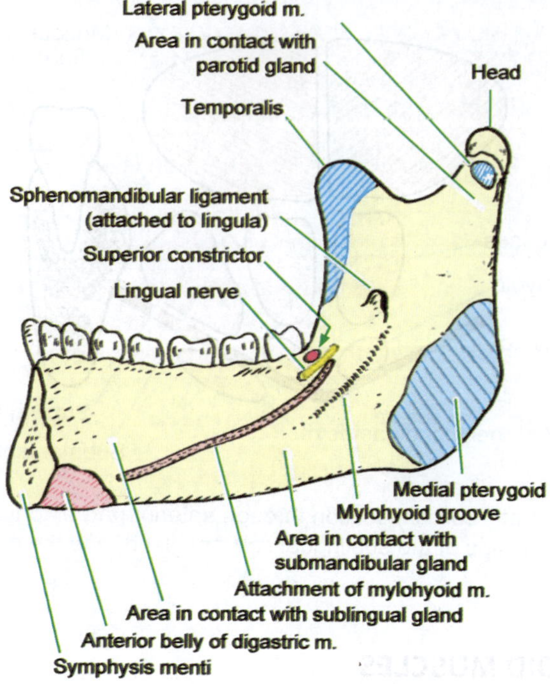

Fig. 5.5 Attachments on one half of the mandible seen from the medial side.

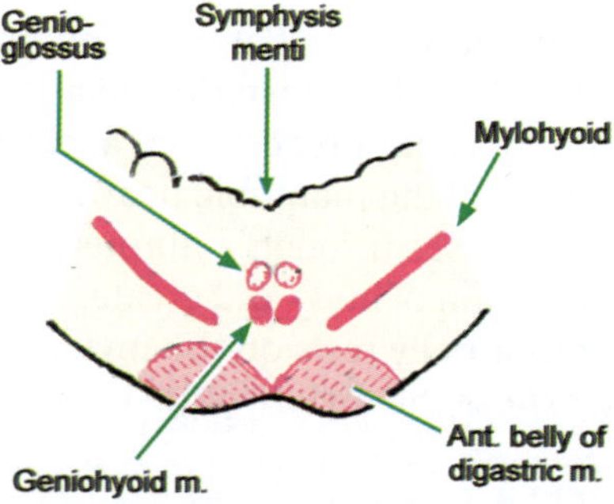

Fig. 5.6 Median part of mandible (region of symphysis menti) seen from behind to show attachments.

Stylohyoid Muscle

The stylohyoid muscle (Fig. 5.15A) arises from the posterior aspect of the styloid process (Fig. 5.7). It runs downwards and forwards to end in a tendon which splits into two to enclose the intermediate tendon of the digastric muscle. The

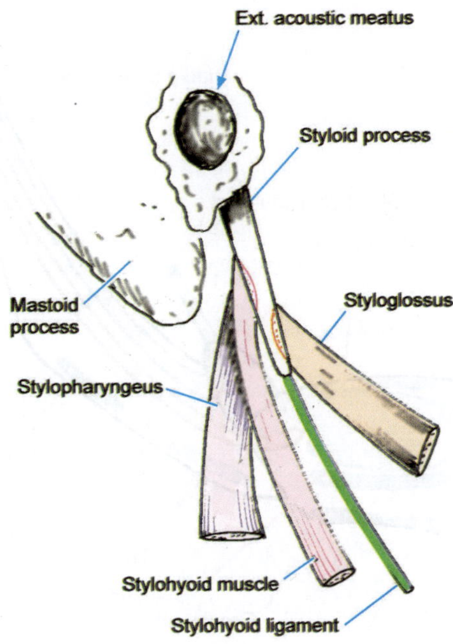

Fig. 5.7 Structures attached to the styloid process. The stylohyoid ligament is attached to the tip, the styloglossus muscle to the anterior aspect (lower part), the stylohyoid muscle to the posterior aspect (upper part), and the stylopharyngeus to the medial aspect.

tendon is then inserted into the hyoid bone at the junction of body and greater cornu (Fig. 5.8).

Nerve Supply and Action

The stylohyoid muscle is supplied by the facial nerve. It elevates the hyoid bone and retracts it.

Geniohyoid Muscle

The geniohyoid is a narrow muscle situated above the mylohyoid (Figs. 1.8, 5.9) and below the genioglossus. It arises from the posterior aspect of the symphysis menti below the genioglossus (Fig. 5.6) and runs backwards to be inserted into the anterior aspect of the hyoid bone (Fig. 5.8).

Nerve Supply and Action

The muscle is supplied by the first cervical nerve, but the fibres travel through the hypoglossal nerve (Fig. 9.87).

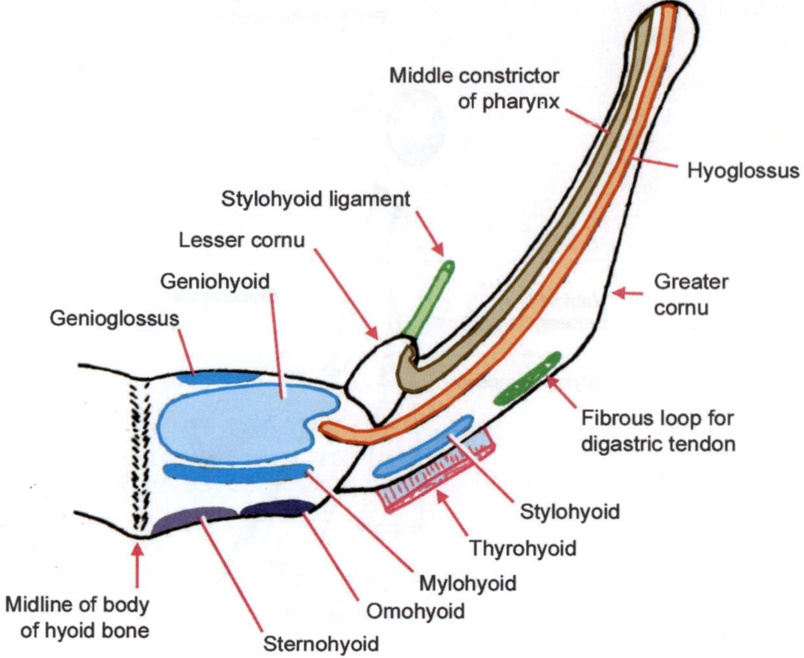

Fig. 5.8 Attachments on hyoid bone: anterosuperior aspect.

The muscle draws the hyoid bone upwards and forwards. When the hyoid bone is fixed (by other muscles) the geniohyoid can help to depress the mandible.

Mylohyoid Muscle

Oral Diaphragm

The mylohyoid muscles of the two sides bridge the gap between the two halves of the mandible. In the median plane the two muscles become continuous with each other at a median raphe. In this way the right and left muscles form the floor of the mouth. This floor is called the oral diaphragm (or diaphragma oris) (Figs. 5.4, 5.9). This diaphragm is strengthened. above by the geniohyoid muscle; and below by the anterior belly of the digastric muscle.

Attachments

On each side the mylohyoid muscle arises from the mylohyoid line on the medial surface of the body of the mandible (Fig. 5.5). From this origin the fibres pass medially. The most posterior fibres are attached to the anterior aspect of the body of the hyoid bone ((Fig. 5.8). The remaining fibres are inserted into a median fibrous raphe extending from the hyoid bone to the mandible.

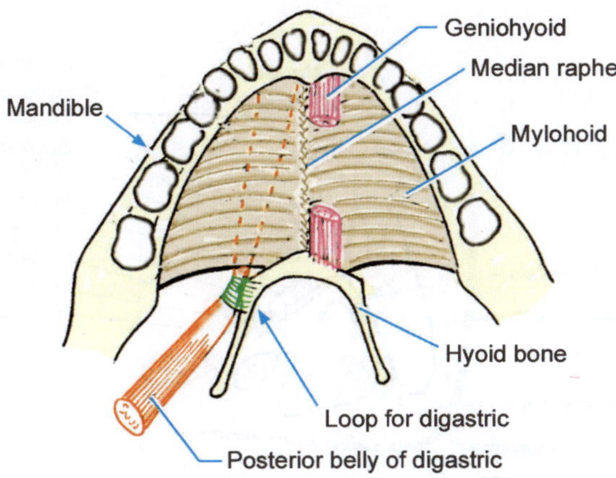

Fig. 5.9 Schematic diagram of floor of mouth seen from above. Note the layout of the mylohyoid and geniohyoid muscles.

Nerve Supply and Action

The mylohyoid muscle is supplied by the mylohyoid branch of the inferior alveolar nerve. The muscle helps in deglutition by raising the floor of the mouth.

Relations of Mylohyoid Muscle

The mylohyoid muscle has numerous relations. These are summarized in Fig. 5.10 which is a coronal section through the submandibular region. The figure is schematic and all structures shown may not actually be seen in one section. Compare with Fig. 5.15. Also see Figs. 1.6 to 1.8.

THE TONGUE

The tongue lies in the oral cavity. The anterior part of the tongue (or ***apex***) can be protruded out of the mouth. It has free upper and lower surfaces. The greater part of the tongue is attached below to the floor of the mouth. The attached part is called the ***root*** of the tongue. This part of the tongue has a free upper surface or ***dorsum***. On either side, the tongue has ***lateral edges*** that are also free. The free surfaces of the tongue are lined by mucous membrane.

The substance of tongue is made up mainly of muscle. Some of the muscles of the tongue are ***intrinsic*** i.e., they are confined to the tongue; while others which are ***extrinsic*** enter the tongue from outside. It is through the root that the various extrinsic muscles enter the substance of the tongue. Through these muscles the tongue is anchored to the hyoid bone behind (through the hyoglossus muscle) and to the mandible in front (through the genioglossus muscle).

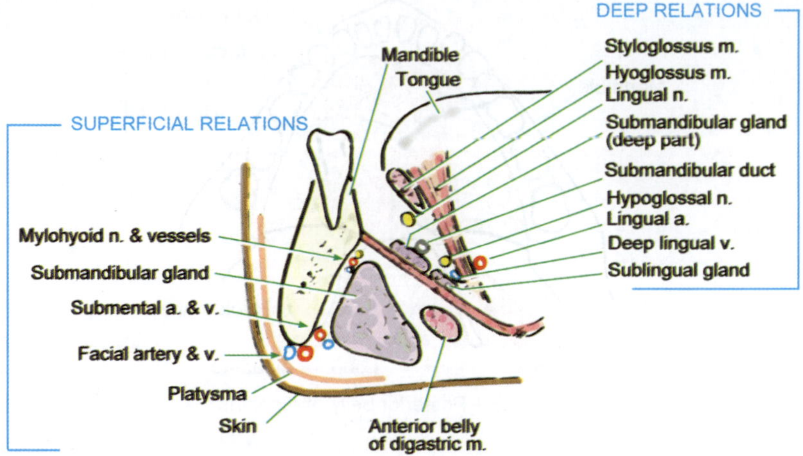

Fig. 5.10 Schematic coronal section of the submandibular region to show the relations of the mylohyoid muscle.

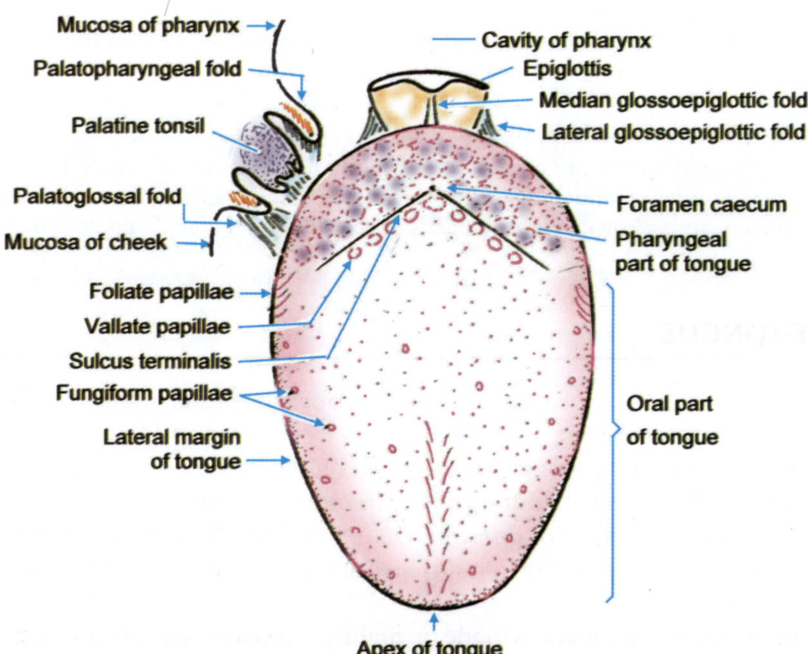

Fig. 5.11 Tongue and some related structures seen from above.

Features on the Dorsum of the Tongue

The features seen when the tongue is viewed from above are shown in Fig. 5.11. The upper surface (or dorsum) is seen. Identify the anterior end or apex, and the lateral edges.

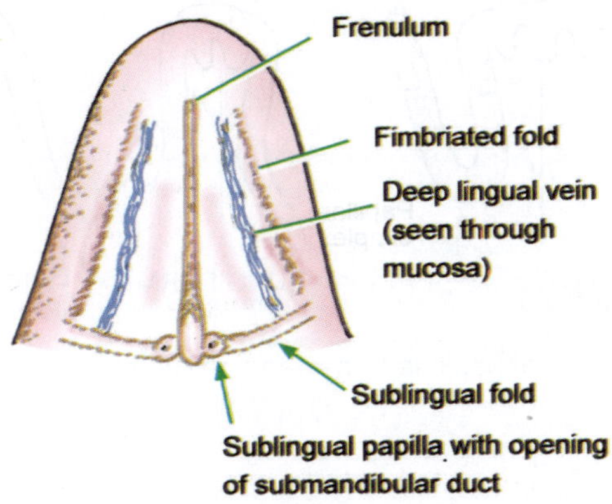

Fig. 5.12 Some structures seen on the undersurface of the anterior part of the tongue.

Near its posterior end the dorsum of the tongue is marked by a V-shaped groove called the ***sulcus terminalis***. The apex of the 'V' points backwards and is marked by a depression called the ***foramen caecum***. The limbs of the sulcus terminalis runs forwards and laterally to the lateral margin of the tongue. The sulcus terminalis divides the dorsum into an anterior larger part (two thirds) and a posterior smaller part (one third). The anterior part lies in the oral cavity and is, therefore, called the ***oral part.*** It faces upwards and comes into contact with the palate. The posterior one third faces backwards and is called the ***pharyngeal part***.

The mucous membrane covering the oral part of the dorsum of the tongue is rough because of the presence of numerous finger like projections or ***papillae***. The largest of these papillae are seen in a row just in front of the sulcus limitans. These are the ***vallate*** papillae. [They are so called because each of them is surrounded by a deep groove. Compare 'vallate' and 'valley']. Other papillae present on the tongue are described as ***fungiform***. They are present at the apex and along the sides of the tongue. The most numerous papillae are small and conical in shape. They are called ***filiform*** papillae (Fig. 5.13). On the posterior part of the lateral margin of the tongue, there are vertical folds that are called the ***foliate*** papillae (because they look like papillae on section: they are not true papillae). Another type of papillae sometimes mentioned in relation to the tongue are the papillae ***simplex***. Unlike the other papillae which can be seen with the naked eye these are microscopic and are quite different from the other papillae. They are not surface projections but are present at the junction of the lining epithelium with underlying tissues (see Fig. 5.13). They are the equivalent of dermal papillae seen in the skin. For further details about the mucosa of the tongue see the author's HUMAN HISTOLOGY.

The ***pharyngeal part of the tongue*** faces backwards and forms part of the anterior wall of the oropharynx. Its surface is not covered by papillae. However,

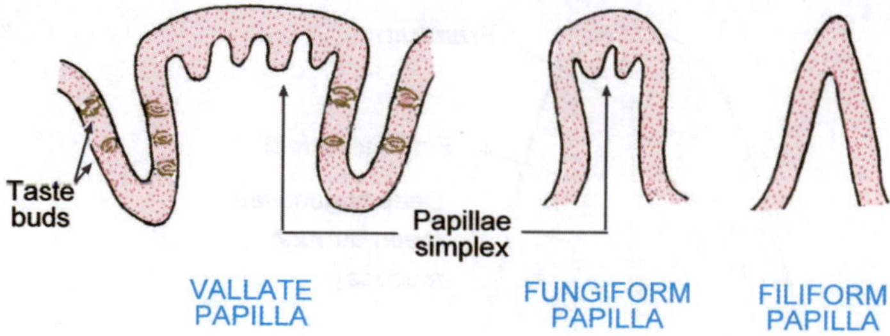

Fig. 5.13 Various kinds of papillae to be seen on the surface of the tongue.

it shows a number of rounded elevations which are produced by collections of lymphoid tissue lying deep to the mucosa. This lymphoid tissue is referred to, collectively, as the ***lingual tonsil***.

The posterior part of the tongue is connected to the palate (on either side) by a fold of mucous membrane called the ***palatoglossal fold***. Immediately posteriorly to this fold we see the palatine tonsil (Fig. 5.11). The mucous membrane lining the pharyngeal part of the tongue is continuous laterally with the mucosa of the palatoglossal folds and the mucosa covering the palatine tonsils.

Posteriorly, the tongue is closely related to the epiglottis (a part of the larynx). The mucosa of the tongue is connected to the anterior aspect of the epiglottis by a ***median glossoepiglottic fold***; and to its lateral edges by two ***lateral glossoepiglottic folds***. The space between the tongue and epiglottis on either side of the median glossoepiglottic fold is called the ***vallecula***.

Some features to be seen on the lower surface of the anterior part of the tongue are shown in Fig. 5.12. We have seen that this part of the tongue is not attached to the floor of the mouth, and that is why it can be protruded out of the mouth. In Fig. 5.12 note the ***frenulum linguae*** lying in the middle line. It is a delicate fold of mucosa passing from the tongue to the floor of the mouth. On either side of the posterior end of the frenulum notice a rounded projection. This is the ***sublingual papilla***. The submandibular duct opens on the summit of the papilla. Running laterally from the papilla we see the ***sublingual fold***. This fold is produced by the underlying sublingual salivary gland.

A little lateral to the frenulum a darkish line can be seen running towards the tip of the tongue. This line is produced by the deep lingual vein seen through the mucosa. Further laterally we see an irregular fold of mucosa called the ***fimbriated fold***.

MUSCLES OF THE TONGUE

The ***extrinsic muscles*** of the tongue enter it from the outside. They are the styloglossus, the palatoglossus, the genioglossus, and the hyoglossus. The ***intrinsic muscles*** lie within the substance of the tongue.

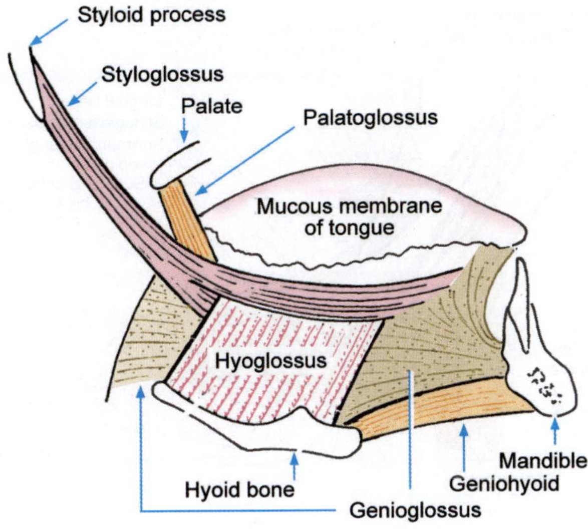

Fig. 5.14 Drawing to show the extrinsic muscles of the tongue. Also see Figs. 1.7, 1.8.

Styloglossus

The styloglossus arises from the anterior and lateral aspects of the styloid process, and from the upper part of the stylomandibular ligament (Fig. 5.14). It runs downwards and forwards to merge with the side of the tongue. Here it divides into two slips one lying superficial to the hyoglossus and the other deep to it.

Palatoglossus

The palatoglossus muscle arises from the anterior (oral) side of the palatine aponeurosis (a sheet of fibrous tissue in the soft palate). The muscle passes downwards and forwards to be inserted into the side of the tongue. Along with the mucous membrane covering it, it forms the ***palatoglossal arch,*** which lies anterior to the tonsil.

Genioglossus

The genioglossus lies next to the median plane. It arises from the upper genial tubercles on the posterior surface of the symphysis menti (Fig. 5.6). The fibres spread out to be inserted into the whole length of the ventral aspect of the tongue (Fig. 5.14, 5.15B). The lowest fibres of the muscle are attached to the body of the hyoid bone (5.8).

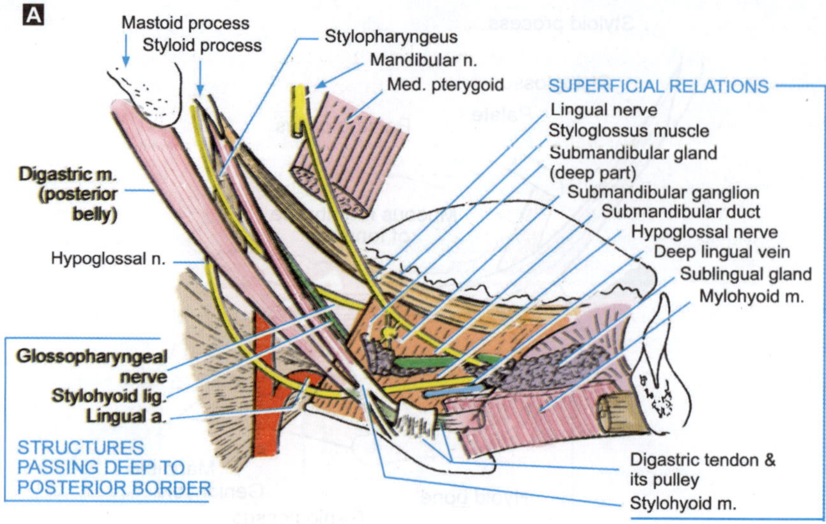

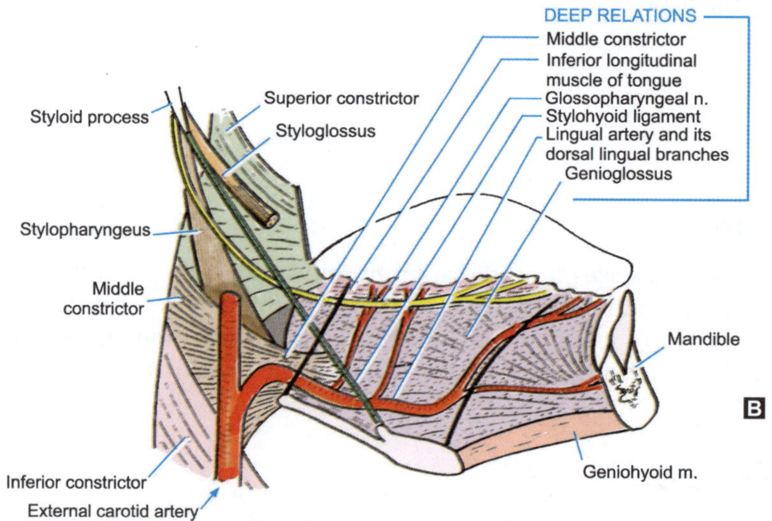

Fig. 5.15 Relations of the hyoglossus muscle. Also see Figs. 1.7, 1.8.

Hyoglossus

The hyoglossus arises from the hyoid bone (Fig. 5.8). The area of origin includes (i) the greater cornu, and (ii) the lateral part of the body. The fibres pass upwards to enter the side of the tongue. Here the styloglossus lies lateral to it and the inferior longitudinal muscle (see below) lies medial to it. The relations of the hyoglossus are summarized in Fig. 5.15.

Some deep fibres of the hyoglossus arising from the lesser cornu of the hyoid bone are sometimes described as a separate muscle, the ***chondroglossus.***

Intrinsic Muscles:

Apart from the muscles entering the tongue from the outside the tongue contains intrinsic fibres that are arranged in several groups viz., ***superior longitudinal***, ***inferior longitudinal***, ***transverse*** and ***vertical***.

Nerve Supply of Muscles of the Tongue:

All muscles of the tongue are supplied by the hypoglossal nerve except the palatoglossus which is supplied by the cranial part of the accessory nerve.

Actions:

The muscles of the tongue move the tongue and alter its shape for movements concerned with speech, mastication and swallowing. The hyoglossus depresses the tongue; the styloglossus pulls it upwards and backwards; and the genioglossus protrudes the tongue out of the mouth by pulling the posterior part forwards. The palatoglossal muscles of the two sides acting together bring the palatoglossal arches together, thus shutting the oral cavity from the oropharynx. The intrinsic muscles alter the shape of the tongue.

BLOOD VESSELS, LYMPHATICS, AND NERVES OF THE TONGUE

The main artery to the tongue is the ***lingual artery***. The venous drainage of the tongue is shown in Fig. 5.16. ***Dorsal lingual veins*** from the dorsum and sides of the tongue end in the ***lingual vein*** which accompanies the lingual artery and ends in the internal jugular vein. Other veins including the ***deep lingual vein*** (see above) drain through veins that accompany the hypoglossal nerve. These veins may join the lingual vein, or the facial vein, or may enter the internal jugular veins directly.

The ***lymphatic drainage*** of the tongue is very important because of the frequent occurrence of cancer in this organ. It is described in detail in Chapter 13.

The ***nerves supplying the tongue*** are of the three functional types.

(a) Nerves of Ordinary Sensation:

Sensations like touch, pain and temperature are carried from the anterior two thirds of the tongue by the ***lingual nerve***, and from the posterior one third by the ***glossopharyngeal nerve***.

(b) Nerves of Taste:

Sensations of taste from the anterior two thirds of the tongue are carried by fibres of the lingual nerve. These fibres pass into the chorda tympani branch of the facial nerve. For further course of these fibres see Fig. 9.67.

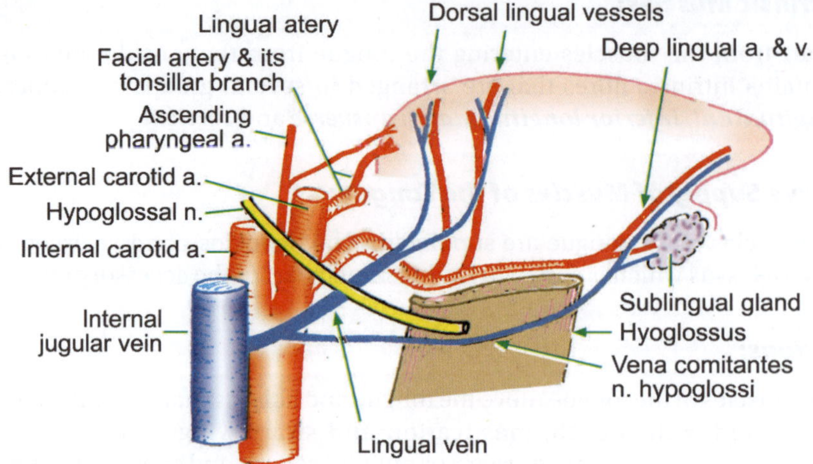

Fig. 5.16 Scheme to show the arteries and veiins that supply the tongue. Also see Figs. 1.8 and 8.16.

Sensations of taste from the posterior one third of the tongue are carried by the glossopharyngeal nerve (Fig. 9.80). Taste fibres from the posterior-most part of the tongue (just in front of the epiglottis) are carried by the ***superior laryngeal branch of the vagus nerve.***

(c) Nerves Supplying Muscles

The musculature of the tongue is supplied by the ***hypoglossal nerve.***

Clinical correlations of the tongue are discussed in Chapter 65. For development of the tongue, and its correlation with nerve supply see the author's HUMAN EMBRYOLOGY.

CHAPTER

6

Cranial Cavity and Vertebral Canal Joints of the Head and Neck

The cranial cavity and vertebral canal form one functional unit that houses the central nervous system: it is, therefore, useful to study them together. As a preliminary to this study it is essential that the student be familiar with the anatomy of the skull, and specially with the features to be seen within the cranial cavity. It is important to be able to identify the various foramina of the skull; and the bones taking part in forming the cranial fossae.

It is equally important to know the structure of the vertebral column including that of its joints. Joints of the skull and of upper cervical vertebrae will be considered in Chapter 7.

Contents of the Cranial Cavity and Vertebral Canal

The most important content of the cranial cavity is the brain; and that of the vertebral canal is the spinal cord.

The brain and spinal cord are surrounded by three membranes called the ***meninges***. The meninges are the ***dura mater***, the ***arachnoid mater*** and the ***pia mater***. Between the arachnoid mater and the pia mater there is the ***subarachnoid space*** which contains ***cerebrospinal fluid***. In relation to the dura mater there are a series of venous sinuses which drain intracranial structures including the brain.

The cranial cavity is lined on the inside by a periosteum-like membrane called the ***endocranium***. The segment of the vertebral canal lying within each vertebra is lined by periosteum. Some intervertebral ligaments take part in forming the walls of the vertebral canal.

In addition to the brain and meninges the cranial cavity contains the proximal parts of ***cranial nerves*** as they travel from their attachment to the surface of the brain to foramina in the skull through which they leave the cranial cavity. The cranial cavity also contains ***blood vessels*** that supply the brain, the meninges and other intracranial structures.

Lying in close relationship to the brain there are two endocrine glands of great importance. These are the ***hypophysis cerebri*** and the ***pineal gland***.

Apart from the spinal cord, meninges and cerebrospinal fluid, the vertebral canal contains the roots of spinal nerves. It also contains blood vessels. The veins form an elaborate ***vertebral venous plexus***. Some ligaments of intervertebral joints are also present over the walls of the vertebral canal.

We will consider the contents of the cranial cavity and vertebral canal listed above one by one. The hypophysis cerebri and the pineal gland are considered in Chapter 12.

The Endocranium

This a fibrous membrane (similar to periosteum) lining the inside of the cranial cavity. At the foramen magnum, and at smaller apertures in the skull, it becomes continuous with periosteum lining the exterior of the skull. At the superior orbital fissure it becomes continuous with the periosteum lining the orbit.

The endocranium is adherent to skull bones, the degree of adherence being variable. The union is better over the cranial fossae rather than over the vault of the skull.

At places where cranial nerves leave the cranial cavity the endocranium extends over them for some distance in the form of a tubular sheath. (However, the optic nerve is covered by sheaths derived from the meninges).

At sites of sutures the endocranium blends with sutural ligaments. It is, therefore, firmly anchored here. (The sutural ligaments connect the endocranium with the pericranium).

In the past the endocranium has been referred to as the ***outer layer of dura mater***. Certain terms that continue to be in use are meaningful only this fact is kept in mind. Most intracranial venous sinuses are bounded both by endocranium and dura mater. They are, however, called ***dural*** venous sinuses. An ***extradural haemorrhage*** is a bleeding into the potential space between the endocranium and skull bones, not between the dura mater and the endocranium.

THE MENINGES

We have seen above that term meninges is applied to three membranes that surround the brain and spinal cord, namely the dura mater, the arachnoid mater and pia mater.

The Cerebral Dura Mater

The dura mater is a thick fibrous membrane. It can be divided into a ***cerebral part*** lying in the cranial cavity and a ***spinal part*** lying in the vertebral canal. In this section we will consider the cerebral dura mater. The spinal dura mater is considered later in this Chapter.

Over the greater part of its extent the cerebral dura mater is closely adherent to the endocranium (and through the latter to the skull). At places the dura mater separates from endocranium forming double layered folds that play an essential role in supporting brain tissue (see below). At places where such folds are formed triangular spaces are left between the endocranium and the dura mater. These spaces are lined by endothelium forming venous sinuses. (See superior sagittal sinus and transverse sinus in Fig. 1.7). [As we shall see below all venous sinuses are not triangular in section, and some of them are bounded only by dura mater, the endocranium not taking part.]

The two largest folds of dura mater are seen in Fig. 1.17. These are the ***falx cerebri*** and the ***tentorium cerebelli***. Two smaller folds the ***falx cerebelli*** and the ***diaphragma sellae*** are also present. These folds are described below.

The Falx Cerebri

The falx cerebri lies in the sagittal plane. It is sickle shaped. It has a convex upper edge that is attached to the vault of the skull, in the middle line (i.e., along the sagittal suture). Its lower edge, which is free, is markedly concave downwards. The anterior end of the falx cerebri is narrow and pointed. It is attached to the crista galli. At its posterior end the falx cerebri has a straight lower edge which is attached to the upper surface of the tentorium cerebelli (Fig. 1.17A). Note the backward and downward slope of this edge.

A coronal section through the falx cerebri near its middle is shown in Fig. 6.1. Note that near its upper end the two layers of dura mater that form it diverge to enclose a triangular space. The third side of the triangle is formed by endocranium. This space is the ***superior sagittal sinus***. It is an example of a sinus walled partly by dura mater and partly by endocranium. Next, note that at the lower end of the falx cerebri the dura mater folds on itself to form the free lower edge. An oval space is left in the fold along the lower edge. This space is the ***inferior sagittal sinus***. The wall of this sinus is formed all round by dura mater (there being no participation of endocranium).

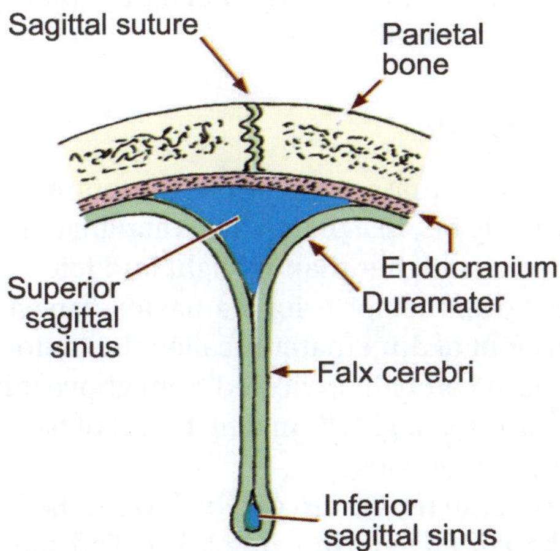

Fig. 6.1 Coronal section through falx cerebri midway between its anterior and posterior ends. For some details see Fig. 6.6.

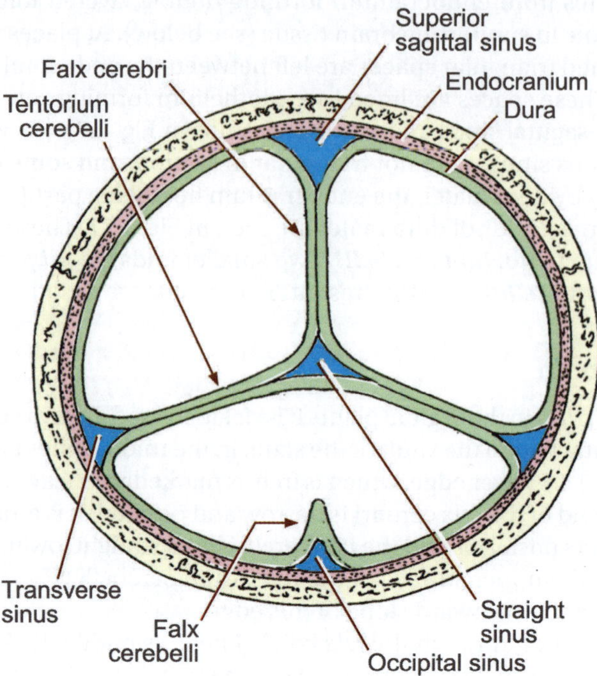

Fig. 6.2 Coronal section through posterior part of falx cerebri, and tentorium cerebelli. The falx cerebelli is also shown.

In Fig. 6.2 we see a coronal section through the posterior part of the falx cerebri. Observe that here the lower edge of the falx is attached to the upper surface of the tentorium cerebelli. At this junction we have a triangular space which is occupied by the ***straight sinus***.

The falx cerebri occupies the longitudinal fissure that (partially) separates the right and left cerebral hemispheres.

The Tentorium Cerebelli

In Fig. 1.17 and 6.2 observe that, on the whole, the tentorium cerebelli is placed more or less transversely i.e., in a plane that is at right angles to that of the falx cerebri. Its central part is higher than its right and left margins. It, therefore, forms a tent-like roof over the posterior cranial fossa in which the cerebellum lies. That is why this fold of dura mater is called the tentorium cerebelli.

When the tentorium cerebelli is viewed from above it has the appearance shown in Fig. 6.3. (Also see Fig. 1.16 in which part of the tentorium has been removed). Observe the following.

a. The anterior part of the tentorium cerebelli is marked by a deep ***tentorial notch***. The U-shaped edge of this notch is called the ***free margin*** of the tentorium cerebelli. Traced anteriorly, the free margin extends into the middle cranial fossa and gains attachment to the ***anterior*** clinoid process.

b. Anteriorly and laterally, each half of the tentorium cerebelli is attached to the superior border of the petrous temporal bone. Medially this edge is prolonged to reach the ***posterior*** clinoid process.

c. Posterolaterally, the tentorium cerebelli has a curved edge. Along this edge the two layers of dura mater forming the tentorium separate and gain attachment to the lips of a broad groove (transverse sulcus) present over the internal surface of the occipital bone. The anterior part of this groove extends on to the internal aspect of the posteroinferior angle of the parietal bone. From Fig. 6.2 it will be seen that along this attachment the two layers of dura mater forming the tentorium cerebelli separate to leave a triangular interval which forms the transverse sinus. As in the case of the superior sagittal sinus, the third side of the triangle (lateral) is formed by endocranium.

d. We have seen that the posterior part of the falx cerebri has a lower edge that is attached to the upper surface of the tentorium cerebelli. Note the manner of this attachment in Fig. 6.2. Observe that the falx cerebri has right and left layers, while the tentorium cerebelli has upper and lower layers. The right and left layers of the falx cerebri becomes continuous with the corresponding half of the upper layer of the tentorium cerebelli. The lower layer of the tentorium cerebelli passes transversely across the midline without interruption. We have already seen that the triangular interval at the junction of the falx cerebri and the tentorium cerebelli is occupied by the straight sinus.

A few additional facts about the tentorium cerebelli may now be noted.

1. The tentorium cerebelli divides the cranial cavity into an ***infratentorial compartment*** which is equivalent to the posterior cranial fossa. This compartment is occupied by the cerebellum and brainstem. The rest of the cranial cavity is the ***supratentorial compartment***. It is occupied mainly by the cerebral hemispheres.
2. The tentorial notch is the only communication between the two compartments. It is occupied by the midbrain and surrounding meninges. The narrow gap between the midbrain and the edge of the tentorial notch is a site at which flow of CSF through the subarachnoid space can be obstructed following inflammation..
3. In Fig. 6.2 observe that anteriorly the free margin of the tentorium cerebelli crosses above the attached margin. Just in front of the crossing, we see a triangular depression of dura mater.
4. The relationship of the tentorium cerebelli to the straight sinus and the right and left transverse sinuses has been explained. The ***superior petrosal sinus*** is situated along the anterolateral attachment of the tentorium cerebelli.

Near the medial part of this attachment, the dura mater forming the lower layer of the tentorium cerebelli is prolonged forwards onto the anterior surface of the petrous temporal bone to form a pouch-like extension (Fig. 9.39). This pouch is called the ***trigeminal cave***, because the trigeminal ganglion lies in it.

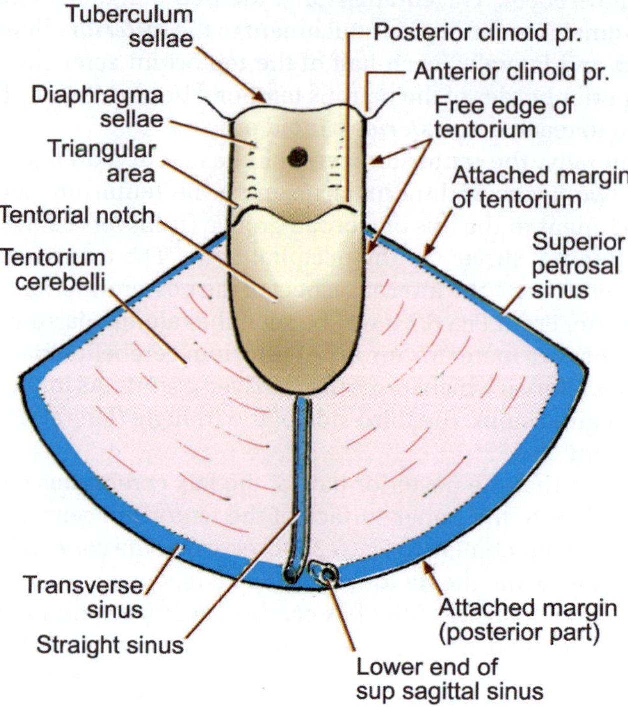

Fig. 6.3 Scheme to show the tentorium cerebelli and its attachments.

Falx Cerebelli

In Fig. 6.2 note that in the median plane, over the floor of the posterior cranial fossa, there is a short fold of dura mater called the falx cerebelli. The fold is crescentic in shape and is placed in the sagittal plane. It has an anterior edge that is free and a posterior edge that is attached to the occipital bone in the middle line. At its upper end (or base) it is attached to the undersurface of the tentorium cerebelli. Its lower end (or apex) reaches the posterior edge of the foramen magnum. Here is may divide into two parts that pass forwards on either side of the foramen. The occipital sinus lies along the posterior attachment of the ***falx cerebelli***.

The falx cerebelli occupies the median groove (vallecula cerebelli) that separates the lower part of the right and left cerebellar hemispheres.

Diaphragma Sellae

The median region of the middle cranial fossa is formed by the body of the sphenoid bone. The hypophyseal fossa is a depression over this bone.

The diaphragma sellae is a horizontal fold of dura mater that roofs over the hypophyseal fossa. At its centre there is an aperture. Anteriorly the diaphragma is attached to the tuberculum sellae, and posteriorly to the dorsum sellae.

The manner of formation of this fold is shown in Fig. 6.4 that is a coronal section across the median part of the middle cranial fossa. Observe that on either side of the body of the sphenoid bone the dura mater is widely separated from the endocranium to form a space that is occupied by the ***cavernous sinus***. The dura mater forming the lateral wall of the sinus turns medially to form the roof of the sinus, and then continues medially over the hypophyseal fossa to form the upper layer of the diaphragma sellae. Reaching the central aperture in the diaphragma sellae the dura mater curves on itself to form the lower layer of the diaphragma. The dura then descends forming the upper part of the medial wall of the cavernous sinus, and passes medially lining the hypophyseal fossa. In this way the dura forms a sac within which the hypophysis cerebri lies. We have already seen that the stalk of the organ passes through the aperture in the diaphragma sellae.

Blood Supply and Nerve Supply of Cerebral Dura Mater

A large number of meningeal arteries take part in supplying the cerebral dura mater. They also supply the endocranium and the skull bones (specially the marrow within them). Although they are called meningeal artery ***they do not supply*** the arachnoid mater and pia mater.

The largest meningeal artery is the middle meningeal branch of the maxillary artery. It is responsible for supplying the dura lining the vault of the skull.

The dura mater lining the anterior cranial fossa receives meningeal branches from the anterior ethmoidal, posterior ethmoidal and ophthalmic arteries.

The dura mater lining the middle cranial fossa is supplied by branches from the middle meningeal, accessory meningeal, and ascending pharyngeal arteries. Some branches arise directly from the internal carotid artery.

The dura mater lining the posterior cranial fossa is supplied by branches from the vertebral, occipital and ascending pharyngeal arteries.

The nerves to the dura mater are derived from various branches of the trigeminal nerve, and by some branches from the glossopharyngeal, vagus and upper three spinal nerves.

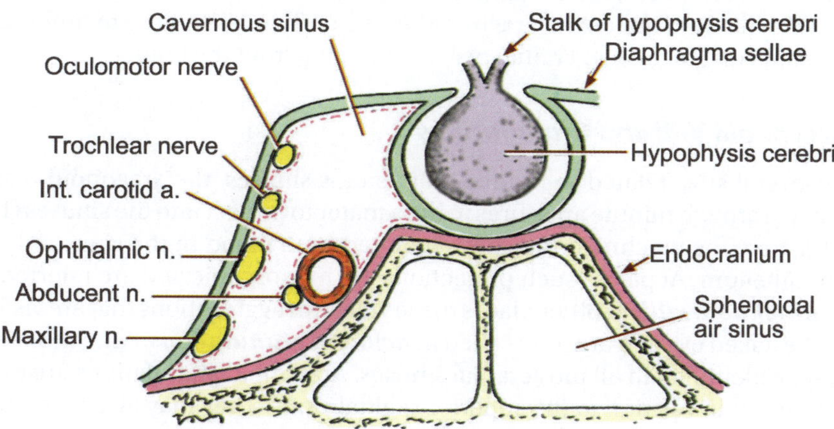

Fig. 6.4 Coronal section through hypophyseal fossa, cavernous sinus and diaphragma sellae

Arachnoid Mater and Pia Mater

The ***arachnoid mater*** is a thin membrane. There are no blood vessels in it. The arachnoid mater is separated from the dura mater by the ***subdural space***. On both sides (dural and arachnoid) the surface lining this capillary interval is smooth. This facilitates slight movement between the dura and arachnoid.

The ***pia mater*** is thicker than the arachnoid mater. In contrast to the arachnoid mater it is highly vascular, and the blood vessels in it are important for supply of the underlying brain.

The pia and arachnoid are separated by the ***subarachnoid space***. This space is filled in by ***cerebrospinal fluid***. Traversing the subarachnoid space there are numerous trabeculae that connect the pia and arachnoid, so that at many places the space resembles a sponge.

We have seen that the falx cerebri extends into the longitudinal fissure separating the right and left cerebral hemispheres; and that the tentorium cerebelli extends into the space betweem the posterior parts of the cerebral hemispheres and the cerebellum. It will be obvious that the arachnoid mater also extends into these intervals along with the folds of dura.

The surface of the brain is marked by several grooves or ***sulci*** that are of varying depth. At such sites the piamater extends into the sulci lining them, but the arachnoid does not do so. In other words the piamater is closely adherent to the brain surface at all places, but the arachnoid jumps across the sulci. This means that the subarachnoid space extends into the sulci. At places where pial blood vessels penetrate the brain substance the tube like extensions of pia are carried along them for some distance. Between these pial extensions and the blood vessels these are narrow ***perivascular spaces*** into which cerebrospinal fluid extends. The perivascular spaces are extensions of the subarachnoid space.

At some sites where there are deep depressions on the brain surface, the arachnoid is separated from the floor of these depressions by relatively large spaces. Such spaces, filled with cerebrospinal fluid, are called ***cisterns***.

Like the dura mater, the arachnoid mater and the piamater are prolonged for some distance on to cranial nerves emerging from the brain.

Arachnoid Villi and Granulations

At several sites related to intracranial venous sinuses, the arachnoid mater passes through minute apertures in dura mater to project into the sinuses (Fig. 6.6). Here the arachnoid mater is separated from blood in the sinus only by endothelium. At places such projections are microscopic and are referred to as ***arachnoid villi***. At other places these villi form aggregations that are visible to the naked eye and are then called ***arachnoid granulations***. Arachnoid villi can be identified in all intracranial sinuses. Arachnoid granulations are most numerous in relation to the superior sagittal sinus. They may also be seen in lateral extensions (lateral lacunae) present in relation to this sinus.

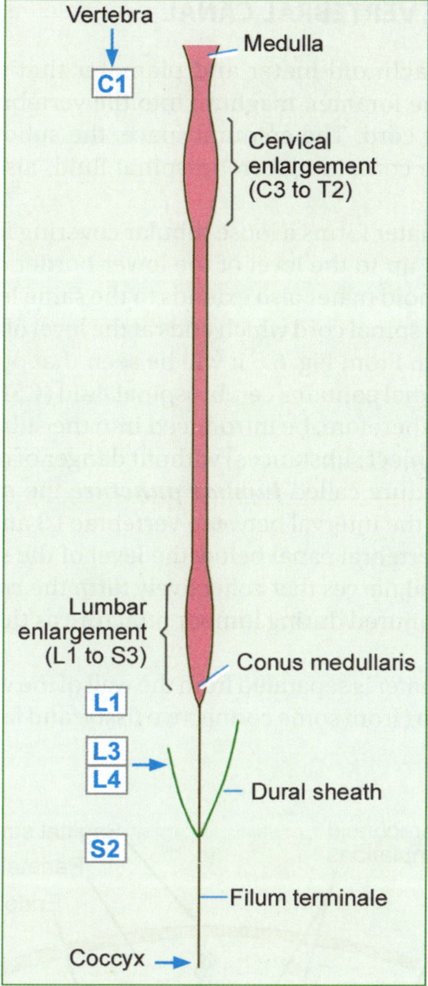

Fig. 6.5 Important vertebral levels in relation to the spinal cord

In children only arachnoid villi are present. Arachnoid granulations appear later in life and are most prominent in old persons in which they may produce depressions on the skull bones.

The importance of arachnoid villi is that these are sites at which cerebrospinal fluid is absorbed into the blood stream.

Choroid Plexuses

At certain sites in relation to the ventricles of the brain folds of piamater (or ***tela choroidea***) project into the ventricles. Enclosed within the fold there are tufts of capillaries. This highly vascular piamater is covered by ***ependyma*** which lines the inside of each ventricle. The masses of vascular piamater covered by ependyma are referred to as ***choroid plexuses***. They are sites at which cerbrospinal fluid is secreted into the ventricles of the brain.

MENINGES IN THE VERTEBRAL CANAL

The dura mater, arachnoid mater and piamater that surround the brain continue through the foramen magnum into the vertebral canal where they surround the spinal cord. The epidural space, the subdural space, and the subarachnoid space containing cerebrospinal fluid, also continue into the vertebral canal.

The spinal duramater forms a loose tubular covering for the spinal cord. It extends downwards up to the level of the lower border of the second sacral vertebra. The arachnoid mater also extends to the same level. The piamater is coextensive with the spinal cord which ends at the level of the lower part of the first lumbar vertebra. From Fig. 6.5 it will be seen that opposite vertebrae L2 to S2 the vertebral canal contains cerebrospinal fluid (CSF), but not the spinal cord. A needle can, therefore, be introduced into the subarachnoid space (to withdraw CSF or to inject substances) without danger of damage to the spinal cord. For this procedure called ***lumbar puncture*** the needle is most often introduced through the interval between vertebrae L3 and L4.

The part of the vertebral canal below the level of the spinal cord contains several roots of spinal nerves that collectively form the ***cauda equina***. These nerve roots are not injured during lumbar puncture as they are easily pushed aside by the needle.

The spinal dura mater is separated from the wall of the vertebral canal by the ***epidural space***. Apart from some connective tissue and fat this space contains

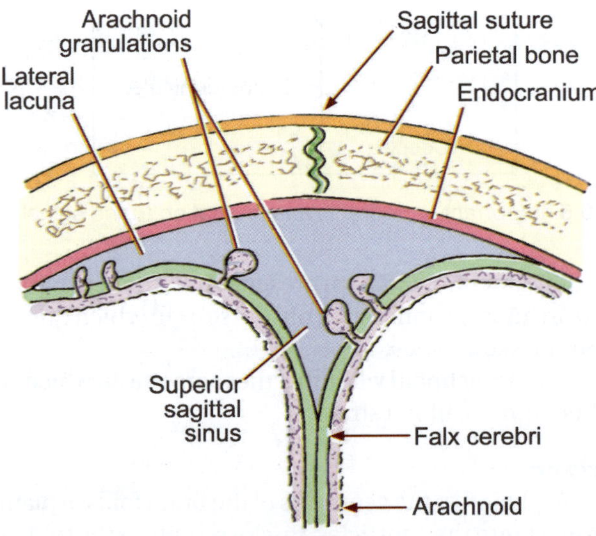

Fig. 6.6 Coronal section to show arachnoid granulations present in relation to the superior sagittal sinus

the ***internal vertebral venous plexus***. Spinal arteries entering the vertebral canal also traverse this space.

Filum Terminale

Below the level of the spinal cord pia mater becomes continuous with a fibrous cord called the filum terminale. (The upper part of the filum terminale may contain some nerve fibres, and a small extension of the cavity within the spinal cord). The filum terminale consists of an upper part, the ***filum terminale internum*** that lies within the dural sheath (i.e., up to the level of the second sacral vertebra); and a part that lies in the sacral canal below this level (***filum terminale externum***).

Ligamentum Denticulatum

Running longitudinally along each lateral margin of the spinal cord there is a thickening of piamater that projects laterally. This thickening is the ligamentum denticulatum. It lies midway between the lines along which ventral and dorsal nerve roots of spinal nerve emerge from the spinal cord. A number of pointed projections extend laterally from this ligament: that is why it is called the ligamentum denticulatum. In the vertical plane each projection lies in the interval between two spinal nerves. Its pointed end passes through arachnoid mater to fuse with the dura mater. In all the ligementum denticulatum bears 21 projections. The highest of these lies at the level of the foramen magnum (i.e., above the emergence of the first cervical nerve). The lowest projection lies between spinal nerves T12 and S1. The ligamentum denticulatum helps to keep the spinal cord at the centre of the vertebral canal.

Linea splendens

This term is applied to a narrow thickening of piamater present over the anterior median line of the spinal cord. Deep to the linea splendens the pia extends into the anterior longitudinal fissure of the spinal cord.

This completes our consideration of the cranial and vertebral meninges. The ***cerebrospinal fluid*** is described in Chapter 24.

INTRACRANIAL VENOUS SINUSES

While considering the folds of duramater mention has been made of a number of venous sinuses that lie within these folds. These are called ***intracranial or dural venous sinuses***. The superior and inferior sagittal sinuses have been seen in relation to the falx cerebri, and the transverse, straight, and superior petrosal sinuses have been mentioned in relation to the tentorium cerebelli. The cavernous sinus has been referred to while describing the diaphragma sellae.

Detailed descriptions of these sinuses, and of some others not mentioned here, are given in Chapter 8. All venous blood from within the cranial cavity (including that from the brain) drains into these sinuses and from them into the internal jugular vein.

NERVES AND ARTERIES IN THE CRANIAL CAVITY

Cranial Nerves

We have noted that the brain gives attachment to twelve pairs of ***cranial nerves***. Parts of these nerves traverse the cranial cavity. They are shown in Fig. 1.6.

In this figure observe the following. In the left half of this drawing the dura mater is intact and some structures are shown shining through the dura. In the right half of the drawing most of the dura lining the anterior and middle cranial fossae has been cut away. The greater part of the tentorium cerebelli has been removed on the right side to reveal structures lying over the floor of the posterior cranial fossa.

1. In the anterior cranial fossa note the median crista galli (a bony projection). To its right side we see the cribriform plate of the ethmoid bone bearing numerous foramina. Bundles of olfactory nerve fibres enter the cranial cavity through these foramina and end in the ***olfactory bulb*** (shown in the left half of Fig. 1.16). Posteriorly, the olfactory bulb continues into the ***olfactory tract*** which is attached to the cerebral hemisphere.
2. Medial to the anterior clinoid process observe the ***optic nerve***. It reaches the cranial cavity from the orbit by passing through the optic canal. The terminal part of the internal carotid artery lies posterolateral to the optic nerve.
3. Just behind the dorsum sellae observe the cut surface of the midbrain. Observe that the ***oculomotor nerve*** emerges from the anterior aspect of the midbrain (see left side) and passes forwards through the subarachnoid space. It penetrates the dura in the triangular interval between the free and attached margins of the tentorium cerebelli, and enters the lateral wall of the cavernous sinus (right side of drawing. Also see Fig. 6.4). It runs forwards and enters the orbit through the superior orbital fissure (Figs. 1.19, 1.20).
4. In the left half of Fig. 1.16 observe the ***trochlear nerve*** lying a short distance posterior to the oculomotor nerve. This nerve emerges from the ***posterior aspect*** of the midbrain, and winds around its lateral side to reach the front of the midbrain. The nerve runs forwards and penetrates the duramater just below the free margin of the tentorium cerebelli, a little behind the posterior clinoid process. The nerve then enters the lateral wall of the cavernous sinus (right half of drawing) and runs in it up to the superior orbital fissure through which it enters the orbit.
5. The ***trigeminal ganglion*** lies in a depression over the anterior apect of the petrous temporal bone, near its apex. We have already seen that the ganglion lies within a recess of dura called the ***trigeminal cave***. Posteriorly, the ganglion is continuous with the sensory root of the ***trigeminal nerve***. Anteriorly, it is continuous with the ophthalmic, maxillary and mandibular divisions of the same nerve. These divisions pierce the dura of the cave to emerge from it. The trigeminal ganglion (and cave) are closely related to the posterior end of the cavernous sinus.

   The ***ophthalmic nerve*** runs forwards in the lateral wall of the cavernous sinus, below the trochlear nerve (Fig. 6.4). It divides into three branches (lacrimal, frontal, nasociliary) that enter the orbit by passing through the superior orbital fissure.

The ***maxillary nerve*** pierces the distal edge of the trigeminal cave and comes to lie in the lowest part of the lateral wall of the cavernous sinus (Fig. 6.4). It runs forwards and enters the foramen rotundum through which it leaves the cranial cavity.

The mandibular nerve is formed by the union of two roots. The sensory root arises from the lateral part of the trigeminal ganglion and leaves the cranial cavity through the foramen ovale. The motor root passes forwards deep to the trigeminal ganglion, passes through the foramen ovale and then joins the sensory root outside the skull.

6. The ***abducent nerve*** runs upwards and laterally over the anterior wall of the floor of the posterior cranial fossa. It pierces the dura a little lateral to the dorsum sellae of the sphenoid bone. It then runs upwards to reach the upper border of the petrous temporal bone and bends round it to enter the middle cranial fossa. The nerve now comes to lie within the cavernous sinus where it is closely related to the internal carotid artery (Fig. 6.4). At the anterior end of the cavernous sinus the nerve passes through the superior orbital fissure to enter the orbit.
7. In Fig. 1.16 identify the ***facial nerve*** and the ***vestibulocochlear nerves***. They are seen entering the internal acoustic meatus located on the posterior aspect of the petrous temporal bone.
8. A short distance below and medial to the internal acoustic meatus we see the jugular foramen. Passing into it we see the ***glossopharyngeal nerve*** (medially), the ***vagus nerve*** (in the middle) and the ***spinal part of the accessory nerve*** (laterally). The spinal part of the accessory nerve is formed by union of a number of rootlets that emerge from the lateral aspect of the upper part of the spinal cord. The nerve ascends through the upper part of the vertebral canal, lateral to the spinal cord (between the dorsal nerve roots and the ligamentum denticulatum). It enters the cranial cavity through the foramen magnum and leaves it through the jugular foramen.
9. A little above the lateral margin of the foramen magnum observe the ***hypoglossal nerve*** passing through the hypoglossal (anterior condylar canal).

Other Nerves to be seen in the Cranial Fossae

Running downwards and medially over the anterior surface of the petrous temporal bone we see the ***greater and lesser petrosal nerves***. The ***deep petrosal nerve*** lies in the foramen lacerum.

In addition to these we have already seen that a number of small meningeal branches are given off by some cranial nerves.

Arteries to be seen in the Cranial Cavity

1. ***Intracranial Part of Internal Carotid Artery***

The internal carotid artery enters the skull through the carotid canal (opening on the base of the skull and passing through the petrous temporal bone).

After passing through the carotid canal the artery enters the foramen lacerum through which it enters the cranial cavity. As the foramen lacerum is closely related to the posterior end of the cavernous sinus the artery enters this sinus directly and runs forwards within it (Fig. 1.16, right half). Near the anterior end of the cavernous sinus the artery turns upwards, pierces the dura mater forming the roof the cavernous sinus and comes into relationship with the cerebrum (Fig. 1.16, left half). Note that the artery now lies medial to the anterior clinoid process, lateral to the optic nerve and optic chiasma. The artery ends here by dividing into the anterior and middle cerebral arteries that supply the brain. It also gives off the ophthalmic artery that runs forwards into the orbit through the optic canal.

2. ***Vertebral Artery***

In Fig. 1.16 the vertebral artery is seen ascending into the cranial cavity through the foramen magnum. This artery arises from the subclavian artery in the lower part of the neck, ascends through the foramina transversaria of the upper six cervical vertebrae, passes through the the suboccipital region and then enters the upper part of the vertebral canal.

After entering the cranial cavity the vertebral arteries of both sides anastomose in the middle line to form the basilar artery. The vertebral and basilar give branches that supply the brain and spinal cord.

3. ***The Meningeal Arteries***

These are the middle meningeal artery, and several other small arteries.

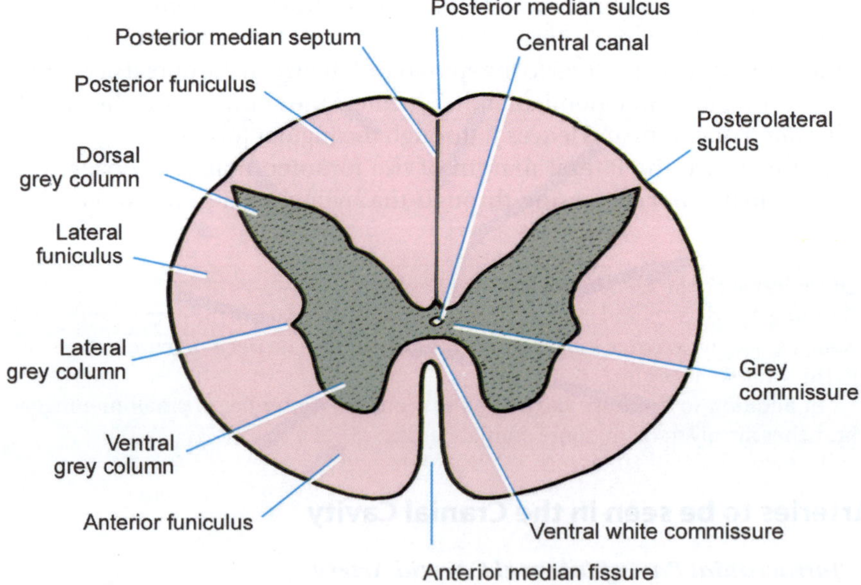

Fig. 6.7 Main features to be seen in a transverse section through the spinal cord.

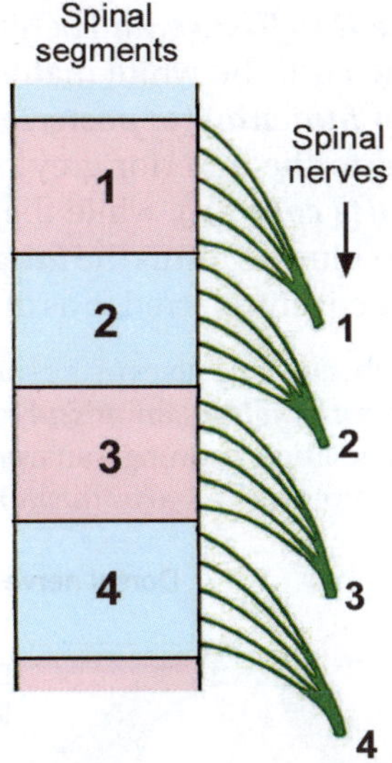

Fig. 6.8 Scheme to illustrate the concept of spinal segments.

THE SPINAL CORD

The spinal cord (or spinal medulla) is the most important content of the vertebral canal. Many facts of importance about the spinal cord will be considered in the section on the brain. Here we will consider its gross anatomy in relation to other structures within the vertebral canal.

The upper end of the spinal cord becomes continuous with the medulla oblongata at the level of the upper border of the first cervical vertebra. [A corollary of this fact is that it is the medulla oblongata that passes through the foramen magnum, not the spinal cord]. The lower end of the spinal cord lies at the level of the lower border of the first lumbar vertebra. The level is, however, variable and the cord may terminate one vertebra higher or lower than this level. The level also varies with flexion or extension of the spine.

The lowest part of the spinal cord is conical and is called the ***conus medullaris***. The conus is continuous with the filum terminale (described above).

When seen in transverse section the grey matter of the spinal cord forms an H-shaped mass (Fig. 6.7). In each half of the cord the grey matter is divisible into a larger ventral mass, the ***anterior (or ventral) grey column***, and a narrow elongated ***posterior (or dorsal) grey column***. The anterior and posterior grey columns are frequently miscalled the anterior and posterior ***horns***). In some parts of the spinal cord a small lateral projection of grey matter is seen between the ventral and dorsal grey columns. This the lateral grey column. The grey matter of the right and left halves of the spinal cord is connected across the middle line by the ***grey commissure*** which is traversed by the ***central canal***. The lower end of the central canal expands to form the ***terminal ventricle*** which lies in the conus medullaris. The cavity within the spinal cord continues for a short distance into the filum terminale.

The white matter of the spinal cord is divided into right and left halves, in front by a deep ***anterior median fissure***, and behind by the ***posterior median septum***. In each half of the cord the white matter medial to the dorsal grey column forms the ***posterior funiculus*** (or ***posterior white column***). The white matter medial and ventral to the anterior grey column forms the ***anterior funiculus*** (or ***anterior white column***), while the white matter lateral to the anterior and posterior grey columns forms the ***lateral funiculus***. [The anterior and lateral funiculi are collectively referred to as the ***anterolateral funiculus***].

The white matter of the right and left halves of the spinal cord is continuous across the middle line through the ***ventral white commissure*** which lies anterior to the grey commissure. Some myelinated fibres running transversely in the grey commissure, posterior to the central canal are referred to as the ***dorsal white commissure***.

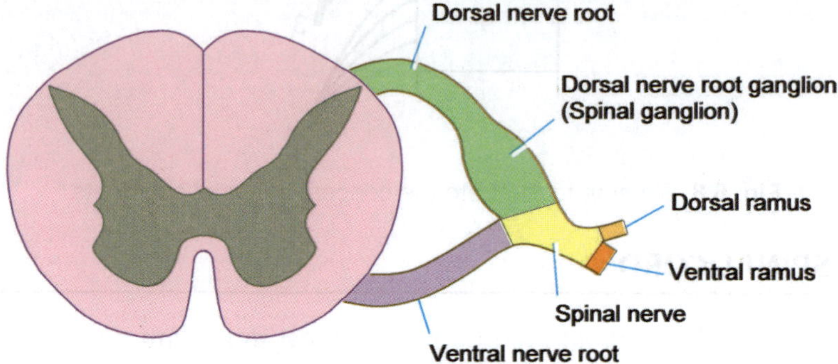

Fig. 6.9 Relationship of a spinal nerve to the spinal cord.

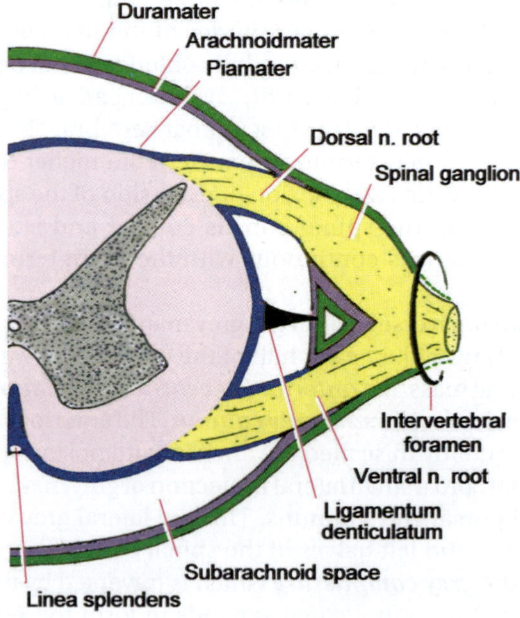

Fig. 6.10 Transverse section through spinal cord to show formation of meningeal sheaths over the roots of a spinal nerve.

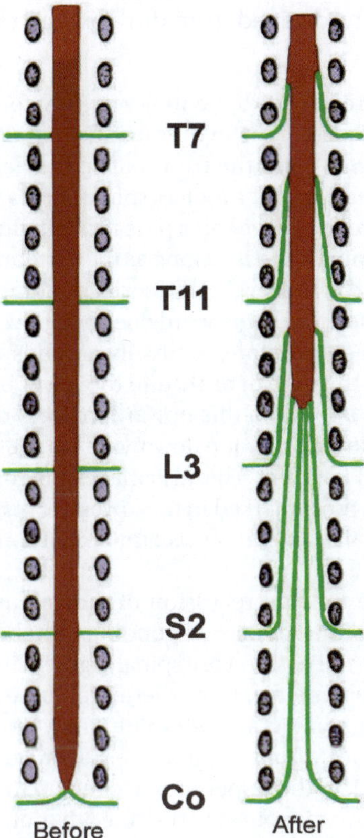

Fig. 6.11 Scheme to show the effect of recession of the spinal cord on course and length of the roots of spinal nerves.

SPINAL NERVES AND SPINAL SEGMENTS

The spinal cord gives attachment, on either side, to a series of spinal nerves. Each spinal nerve arises by two roots, anterior (or ventral) and posterior (or dorsal) (Fig. 6.7). Each root is formed by aggregation of a number of rootlets that arise from the cord over a certain length (Fig. 6.8). The length of the spinal cord giving origin to the rootlets of one spinal nerve constitutes one ***spinal segment***. The spinal cord is made up of thirty one segments: 8 cervical, 12 thoracic, 5 lumbar, 5 sacral and one coccygeal. (Note that in the cervical and coccygeal regions the number of spinal segments, and of spinal nerves, does not correspond to the number of vertebrae).

The rootlets that make up the dorsal nerve roots are attached to the surface of the spinal cord along a vertical groove (called the posterolateral sulcus) opposite the tip of the posterior grey column (Fig. 6.7). The rootlets of the ventral nerve roots are attached to the anterolateral aspect of the cord opposite the anterior grey column. The ventral and dorsal nerve roots join each other to form a spinal nerve. Just proximal to their junction the dorsal root is marked by a swelling called the ***dorsal nerve root ganglion***, or ***spinal ganglion*** (Fig. 6.9).

The dorsal and ventral roots of spinal nerves pass through the spinal dura mater separately. Sheaths derived from dura extend over the nerve roots (Fig. 6.10).

These dural sheaths reach up to the intervertebral foramina and are attached to the margins of these foramina. The dorsal and ventral nerve roots unite ***in the intervertebral foramina*** to form the trunks of spinal nerves. The pia mater and arachhoid mater also extend on to the roots of spinal nerves as sheaths. These sheaths reach up to the site where the nerve roots pass through dura mater.

In early fetal life the spinal cord is as long as the vertebral canal, and each spinal nerve arises from the cord at the level of the corresponding intervertebral foramen. In subsequent development the spinal cord does not grow as much as the vertebral column and its lower end, therefore, gradually ascends to reach the level of the third lumbar vertebra at the time of birth, and the lower border of the first lumbar vertebra in the adult. As a result of this upward migration of the cord the roots of spinal nerves have to follow an oblique downward course to reach the appropriate intervertebral foramen (Fig. 6. 11). This also makes the roots longer. The obliquity and length of the roots is most marked in the lower nerves and many of these roots occupy the vertebral canal below the level of the spinal cord. These roots constitute the ***cauda equina***.

Another result of the upward recession of the spinal cord is that the spinal segments do not lie opposite the corresponding vertebra. This fact is clinically important. For estimating the position of a spinal segment in relation to the surface of the body it is important to remember that a vertebral spine is ***always lower*** than the corresponding spinal segment. As a rough guide it may be stated that in the cervical region there is a difference of one segment (e.g., the 5th cervical spine overlies the 6th cervical segment); in the upper thoracic region there is a difference of two segments (e.g., the 4th thoracic spine overlies the 6th thoracic segment); and in the lower thoracic region there is a difference of three segments (e.g., the 9th thoracic spine lies opposite the 12th thoracic segment).

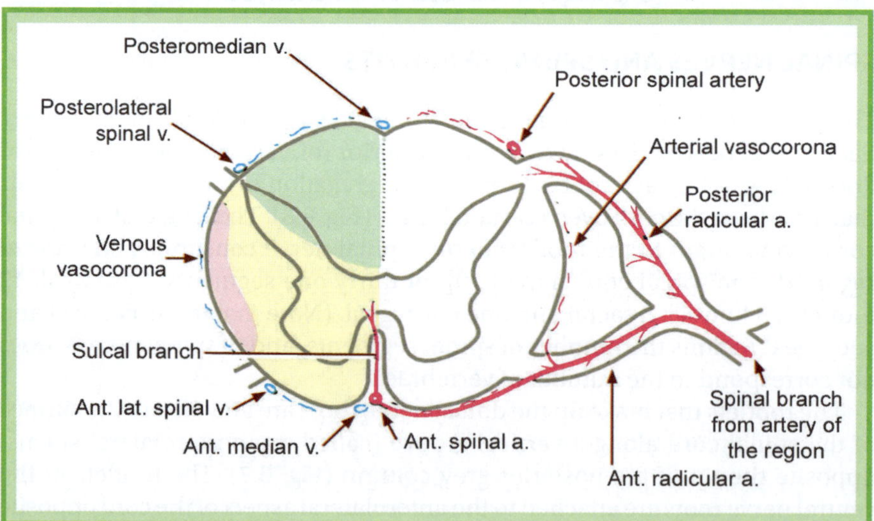

Fig. 6.12 Blood vessels supplying the spinal cord. In the left half of the figure, the area shaded green is supplied by the posterior spinal artery; the areas shaded pink is supplied by the arterial vasocorona; and the area shaded yellow is supplied by the anterior spinal artery.

The spinal cord is not of uniform thickness. The spinal segments that contribute to the nerves of the upper limbs are enlarged to form the ***cervical enlargement*** of the cord. Similarly, the segments innervating the lower limbs forms the ***lumbar enlargement*** (Fig. 6.5).

In addition to spinal nerves the upper five or six cervical segments of the spinal cord give origin to a series of rootlets that emerge on the lateral aspect (midway between the anterior and posterior nerve roots of spinal nerves). These rootlets join to form the spinal root of the accessory nerve.

The meninges surrounding the spinal cord have been described above.

Blood Supply of the Spinal Cord

The spinal cord receives its blood supply from three longitudinal arterial channels that extend along the length of the spinal cord (Fig. 6.12). The ***anterior spinal artery*** is present in relation to the anterior median fissure. Two ***posterior spinal arteries*** (one on each side) run along the posterolateral sulcus (i.e., along the line of attachment of the dorsal nerve roots). In addition to these channels the pia mater covering the spinal cord has an arterial plexus (called the ***arterial vasocorona***) which also sends branches into the substance of the cord.

The main source of blood to the spinal arteries is from the vertebral arteries (from which the anterior and posterior spinal arteries take origin). However, the blood from the vertebral arteries reaches only up to the cervical segments of the cord. Lower down the spinal arteries receive blood through ***radicular arteries*** that reach the cord along the roots of spinal nerves. These radicular arteries arise from spinal branches of the vertebral, ascending cervical, deep cervical, intercostal, lumbar and sacral arteries (Fig. 6.13).

Many of these radicular arteries are small and end by supplying the nerve roots. A few of them, which are larger, join the spinal arteries and contribute blood to them. Frequently, one of the anterior radicular branches is very large and is called the ***arteria radicularis magna***. Its position is variable. This artery may be responsible for supplying blood to as much as the lower two-thirds of the spinal cord.

The greater part of the cross sectional area of the spinal cord is supplied by branches of the anterior spinal artery (Fig. 6.12, left half). These branches enter the anterior median fissure (or sulcus) and are, therefore, called ***sulcal branches.*** Alternate sulcal branches pass to the right and left sides. They supply the anterior and lateral grey columns and the central grey matter. They also supply the anterior and lateral funiculi. The rest of the spinal cord is supplied by the posterior spinal arteries. As already mentioned branches from the arterial vasocorona also supply the cord.

The veins draining the spinal cord are arranged in the form of six longitudinal channels. These are ***anteromedian*** and ***posteromedian*** channels that lie in the midline; and ***anterolateral*** and ***posterolateral*** channels that are paired (Fig. 6.12). These channels are interconnected by a plexus of veins that form a ***venous vasocorona.*** The blood from these veins is drained into radicular veins that open into a venous plexus lying between the dura mater and the bony vertebral canal (***epidural*** or ***internal vertebral venous plexus***) and through it into various segmental veins.

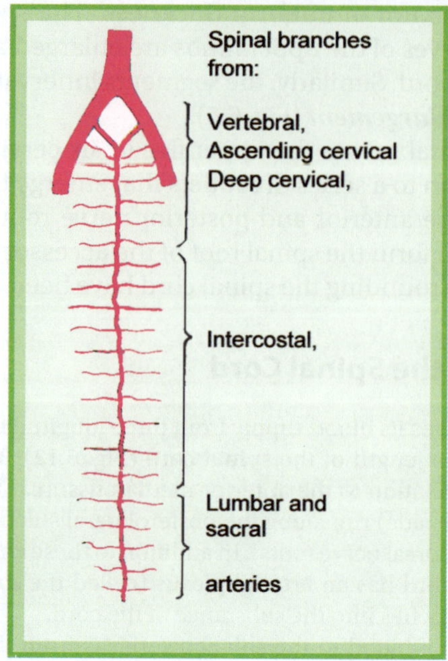

Fig. 6.13 Radicular arteries that contribute blood to spinal arteries

VERTEBRAL VENOUS PLEXUS

The vertebrae are surrounded by a dense plexus of veins. The plexus is divisible into an ***external part*** on the outer surface; and an ***internal part*** lining the vertebral canal. Each of these parts is divided into anterior and posterior divisions. A basivertebral vein from each vertebral body drains into the anterior internal plexus. It also communicates with the anterior external plexus. Apart from veins draining blood from the vertebrae, the plexus receives veins from the meninges and from the spinal cord. Opposite each intervertebral foramen

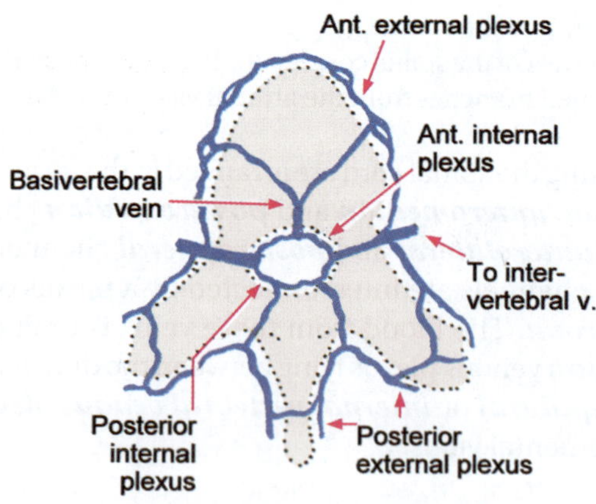

Fig. 6.14 The vertebral venous plexus.

the plexus drains into an intervertebral vein. The intervertebral veins end in the vertebral, intercostal and lumbar veins. In the pelvis the plexuses communicate with veins from some pelvic viscera.

The veins of the vertebral plexus do not have valves, and direction of blood flow in them is controlled by differences in venous pressure in different regions. Tumours of some viscera (e.g., of the prostate) may spread to vertebral bodies, and even into the skull through the communications.

JOINTS OF HEAD AND NECK

The joints to be seen in the head and neck are as follows.

1. **Joints between bones of the skull**
   Adjacent edges of bones of the skull are united to each other by fibrous joints called ***sutures***.
   The bodies of the occipital and sphenoid bones are united by a ***synchondrosis***. A synchondrosis is also present between the body of the sphenoid and the apex of the petrous temporal bone. At such a joint the two articulating surfaces are united by a plate of hyaline cartilage. As age increases the cartilage is gradually invaded by bone and the union becomes bony.
2. **The temporomandibular joint**
   At this joint the head of the mandible articulates with the articular fossa present on the temporal bone. This joint has been described on page 81.
3. **The atlanto-occipital joints**
   These are the joints between the occipital bone and the atlas. They are described below.
4. **Joints between cervical vertebrae.**
   Of these the joints between the atlas and axis vertebrae are atypical, and are described below. The remaining intervertebral joints are similar to typical intervertebral joints.
5. **Other joints**
   Highly specialized joints are present between ossicles of the middle ear, and between the cartilages of the larynx. These will be considered along with the respective organs.

THE ATLANTOAXIAL JOINTS

The atlas and axis vertebrae articulate with each other at three joints, one median, and two lateral.

The ***median atlantoaxial joint*** is a synovial joint of the pivot variety. The dens of the axis (the pivot) lies in the ring formed by the anterior arch of the atlas and its transverse ligament. In this situation there are really two synovial joints with independent capsules: one between the anterior surface of the dens and the posterior aspect of the anterior arch, and the other between the posterior surface of the dens and the transverse ligament.

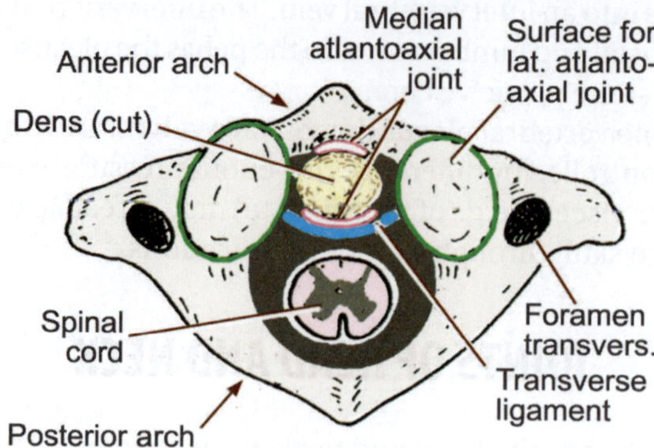

Fig. 6.15 Schematic view of the inferior aspect of the atlas to show the atlantoaxial joints.

The transverse ligament is attached at each end to the medial surface of the lateral mass of the atlas.

The ***lateral atlantoaxial joints*** are synovial joints of the plane variety.

The ligaments connecting the atlas and axis, and the movements at the atlanto-axial joints are considered below along with those of the atlanto-occipital joints.

THE ATLANTO-OCCIPITAL JOINTS

We have seen that on either side of the foramen magnum there is a large convex occipital condyle. The long axis of the condyle is directed forwards and medially. The condyle is convex both anteroposteriorly and from side to side. Each condyle articulates with a facet on the upper surface of the lateral mass of the atlas. This facet is concave and corresponds in size and direction to the occipital condyle.

These articular surfaces are enclosed in capsules to form synovial joints. From a functional point of view the right and left atlanto-occipital joints together form an ellipsoid joint.

Ligaments Uniting the Atlas, The Axis and The Occipital Bone

Apart from their capsules the atlas and axis are united to each other and to the occipital bone by a number of ligaments that are considered below. Before reading the descriptions of these ligaments it will be useful to recall the ligaments present in typical intervertebral joints.

1. The ***anterior longitudinal ligament*** (continued upwards from lower vertebrae) is attached to the front of the body of the axis; to the anterior arch of the atlas; and to the basilar part of the occipital bone (Fig. 6.16A).
2. Between the atlas and the occipital bone, the anterior longitudinal ligament is incorporated in the ***anterior atlanto-occipital membrane*** (Fig. 6.16A).

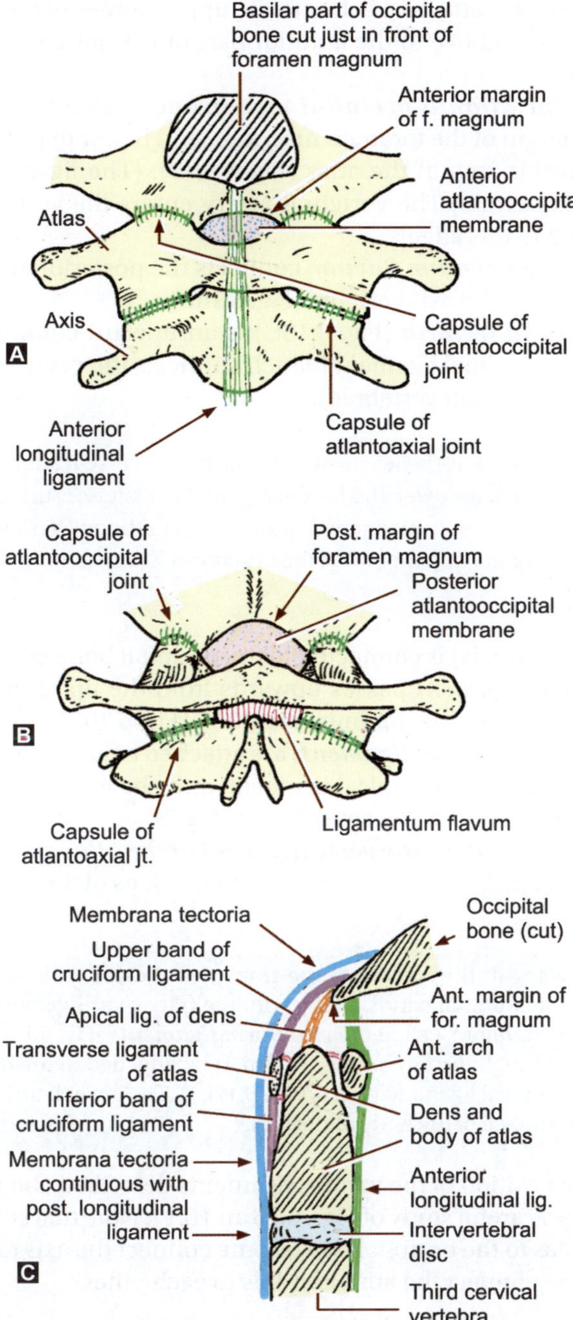

Fig. 6.16. Region of atlanto-occipital and atlantoaxial joints. A. Seen from the front. B. Seen from behind. C. Median section.

This membrane is attached below to the upper border of the anterior arch of the atlas, and above to the anterior part of the margin of the foramen magnum.

3. The ***posterior atlanto-occipital membrane*** is attached above to the posterior margin of the foramen magnum, and below to the upper border of the posterior arch of the atlas (Fig. 6.16B). [The ligament has a free inferolateral margin. The vertebral artery enters the vertebral canal by passing deep to this edge].
4. The highest ***ligamentum flavum*** connects the posterior arch of the atlas to the laminae of the axis vertebra (Fig. 6.16B).
5. The ***membrana tectoria*** (Fig. 6.16C) is an upward continuation of the posterior longitudinal ligament (which connects the posterior surfaces of the bodies of adjacent vertebrae).

The membrana tectoria lies posterior to the transverse ligament of the atlas (Figs. 6.16C, 6.17D). Its lower end is attached to the posterior surface of the body of the axis. Its upper end is attached to the occipital bone (basiocciput) above the attachment of the upper band of the cruciform ligament (See below and Fig. 6.16C).

6. The dens (of the axis) is connected to the occipital bone by the following:
   a. The ***apical ligament*** passes upwards from the tip of the dens to the anterior margin of the foramen magnum (Fig. 6.16C).
   b. The right and left ***alar ligaments*** are attached below to the upper part of the dens lateral to the apical ligament, and above to the occipital bone on the medial side of the condyle (Fig. 6.17B).
7. We have seen that the ***transverse ligament of the atlas*** stretches between the two lateral masses of the bone, behind the dens of the axis (Figs. 6.16C, 6.17C).

Continuous with the middle of the transverse ligament there are superior and inferior longitudinal bands. Along with the transverse ligament they form a cross and are, therefore, called the ***cruciform ligaments*** (Fig. 6.17C). The upper band passes through the foramen magnum to be attached to the occipital bone anterior to the apical ligament (Fig. 6.16C, 6.17C)). The lower band is attached to the posterior surface of the body of the axis.

The relative position of the various ligaments described above can be best appreciated by a careful study of Figs. 6.16 and 6.17. Note that some ligaments connect the atlas to the occipital bone, some connect the axis to the occipital bone, and some connect the atlas and axis to each other.

Movements at The Atlanto-occipital and Atlantoaxial Joints

Being a pivot joint the median atlantoaxial joint allows the atlas (and with it the skull) to rotate around the axis provided by the dens. This is accompanied by gliding movements at the lateral atlantoaxial joints. The extent of rotation is

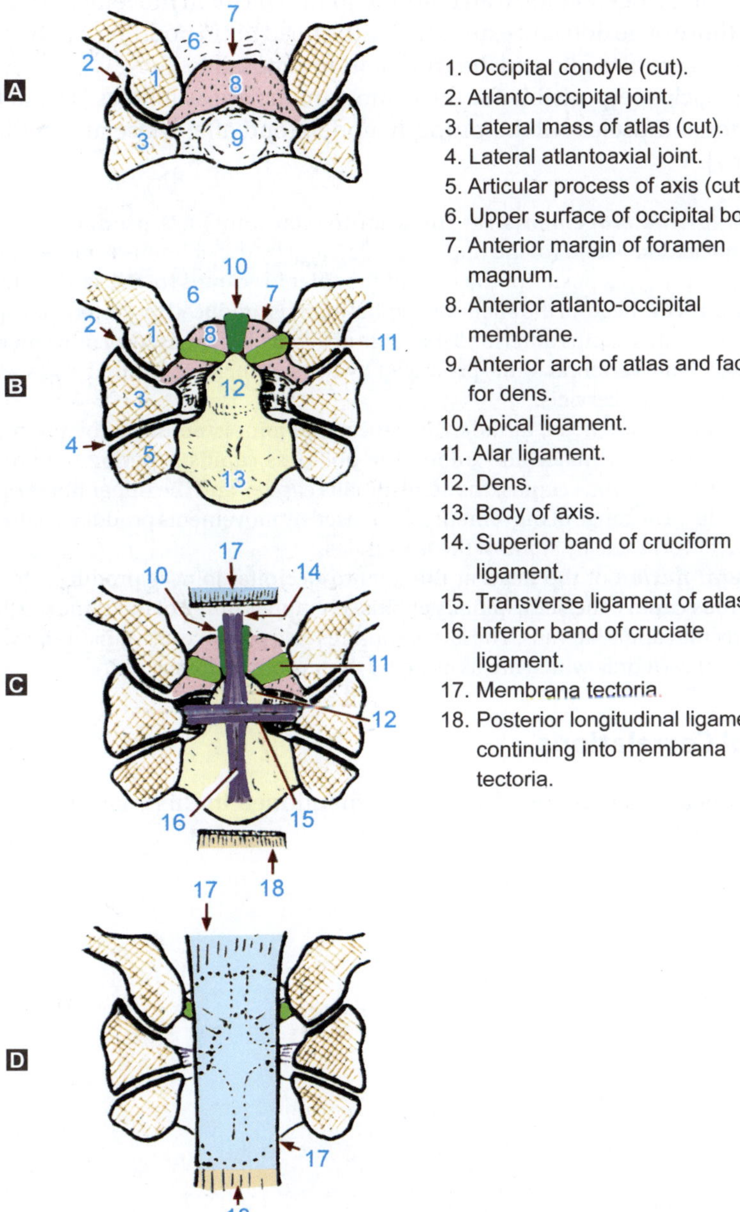

1. Occipital condyle (cut).
2. Atlanto-occipital joint.
3. Lateral mass of atlas (cut).
4. Lateral atlantoaxial joint.
5. Articular process of axis (cut).
6. Upper surface of occipital bone.
7. Anterior margin of foramen magnum.
8. Anterior atlanto-occipital membrane.
9. Anterior arch of atlas and facet for dens.
10. Apical ligament.
11. Alar ligament.
12. Dens.
13. Body of axis.
14. Superior band of cruciform ligament.
15. Transverse ligament of atlas.
16. Inferior band of cruciate ligament.
17. Membrana tectoria.
18. Posterior longitudinal ligament continuing into membrana tectoria.

Fig. 6.17 Schematic figures to show some ligaments connecting the axis, the atlas and the occipital bone. The anterior parts of the axis and atlas, and the anterior margin of the foramen magnum are seen from behind after making a coronal section through the lateral atlantoaxial and atlanto-occipital joints. The most anterior structures are shown in 'A', and the most posterior in 'D'.

limited by the alar ligaments. From a functional point of view the two atlanto-occipital joints together form an ellipsoid joint. The main movements allowed by it are those of flexion and extension (of the head) as in nodding. Slight lateral movements are also allowed, but no rotation is possible.

The muscles responsible for these movements are as follows [The actions of individual muscles will be properly understood after these are studied in Chapter 7].

1. ***Side to side movements*** (at the atlantoaxial joint) are produced by the sternocleidomastoid (of the opposite side); and by the obliquus capitis inferior, the rectus capitis posterior major, and the splenius capitis (of the same side).
2. ***Flexion*** of the head, at the atlanto-occipital joints is produced by the longus capitis and the rectus capitis anterior. The range of flexion is increased by movement at cervical intervertebral joints produced by the sternocleidomastoid, the scaleni and the longus cervicis.
3. ***Extension*** of the head, at the atlanto-occipital joint is produced by the rectus capitis posterior major and minor, the obliquus capitis superior, the erector spinae, the splenius capitis, the semispinalis capitis, and the upper fibres of the trapezius. The range of movement is increased by movements produced between cervical vertebrae by some of these muscles.
4. ***Lateral flexion*** of the head at the atlanto-occipital joint is produced by the splenius capitis, the semispinalis capitis, the upper fibres of the trapezius, and the rectus capitis lateralis. The larger muscles also produce movements between cervical vertebrae which are assisted by the sternocleidomastoid.

Clinical Correlations

Some clinical correlations of structures mentioned in this chapter are given in detail in Chapter 15.

CHAPTER

7

Muscles of the Neck, Triangles of the Neck, Deep Cervical Fascia

MUSCLES OF THE NECK

The Platysma

This is the most superficial muscle in the neck. Like the muscles of the face it lies in the superficial fascia (Fig. 1.21). It is a remnant of an extensive sheet of subcutaneous muscle (called the ***pannulus carnosus***) to be seen in somc animals.

Origin: The muscle arises from the deep fascia covering the upper part of the pectoralis major (f in Fig. 7.1) and the anterior part of the deltoid (g). The fibres form a broad thin sheet that passes upwards and forwards across the clavicle, and then across the sternocleidomastoid.

Insertion: The most anterior fibres end by interlacing with those of the opposite side below the chin (h). The remaining fibres cross the lower border of the mandible, some of them being attached to it (m). The fibres end by merging with muscles at the angle of the mouth (specially risorius and depressor anguli oris) (Fig. 1.2).

Nerve Supply: The muscles is supplied by the cervical branch of the facial nerve.

Action: The platysma produces wrinkles over the skin of the neck. [The much better developed subcutaneous sheet of muscle present in some animals e.g., the horse, enables them to move their skin over underlying structures.]

From Fig. 1.21 it will be seen that deeper tissues in the neck are overlapped by two large muscles, the sternocleidomastoid and the trapezius. These two muscles lie between the two layers of the investing fascia of the neck. The trapezius is a muscle of the upper limb. The sternocleidomastoid is described below.

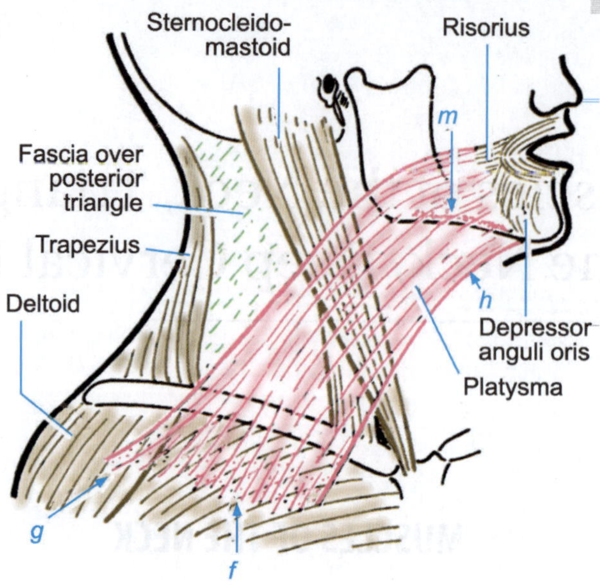

Fig. 7.1 The platysma muscle.

STERNOCLEIDOMASTOID

Origin:

The muscle arises by two heads (Fig. 7.2).

1. The ***sternal head*** arises from the anterior surface of the manubrium sterni (a).
2. The ***clavicular head*** arises from the upper surface of the medial part of the clavicle (b).

The two heads are separated at their origin by a triangular interval (c). Higher up the clavicular head blends with the deep aspect of the sternal head.

Insertion:

The muscle is inserted into the:

1. Lateral half of the superior nuchal line (d); and
2. The lateral surface of the mastoid process from its apex to the upper border (e) (Also see Fig. 7.14).

Nerve Supply:

The sternocleidomastoid is supplied by the accessory nerve (spinal part) and by branches from the ventral rami of spinal nerves C2, C3.

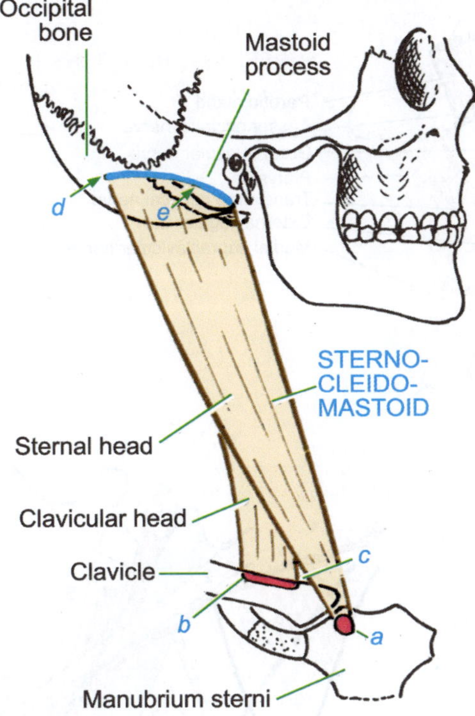

Fig. 7.2 Scheme to show the attachments of the sternocleidomastoid muscle.

Actions:

When the muscle of one side contracts the head is tilted to the same side, and the face is rotated to the opposite side. When the muscles of both sides act together the head and neck are flexed.

Relations:

The sternocleidomastoid forms an important landmark in the neck, and divides it into anterior and posterior triangles (Fig. 2.5). The muscle has numerous relations that are shown in Fig. 7.3. Also see Figs. 1.9, 1.10 and 1.21. Observe that the infrahyoid muscles separate the anterior part of the muscle from the thyroid gland.

INFRAHYOID MUSCLES

These are the sternohyoid, the sternothyroid, the thyrohyoid and the omohyoid muscles (Figs. 1.9, 1.10, 1.12 and 7.4). The sternohyoid passes from the sternum to the hyoid bone. The sternothyroid passes from the sternum to the thyroid cartilage (of the larynx). The thyrohyoid passes from the thyroid cartilage to the hyoid bone. The omohyoid is made up of upper and lower bellies united

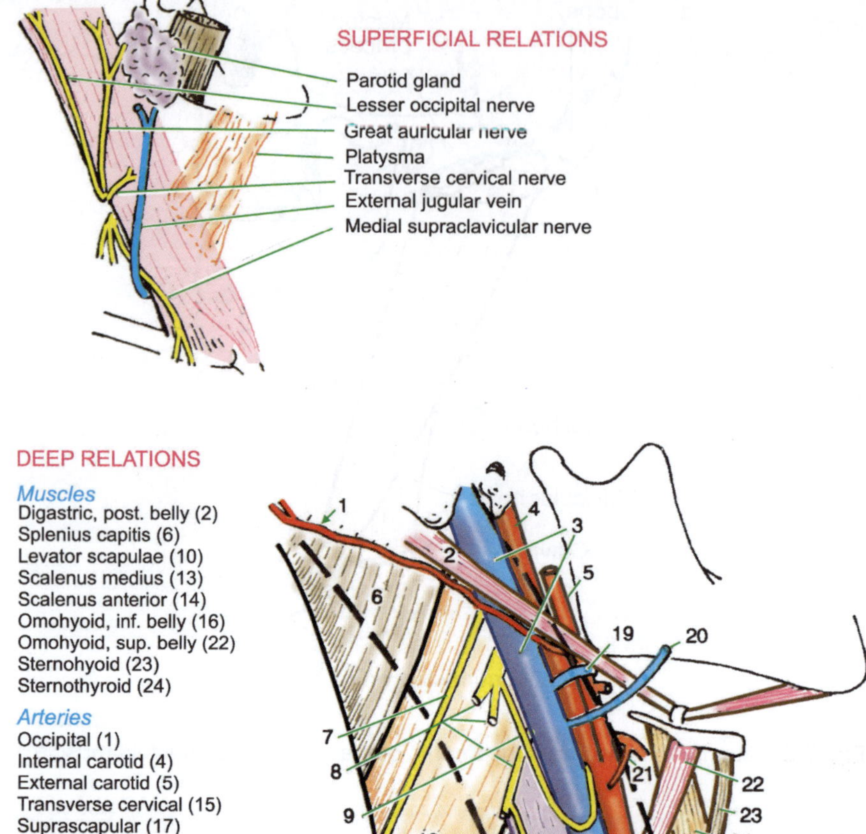

Fig. 7.3 Scheme to show the relations of the sternocleidomastoid muscle. (The outline of the muscle is shown in interrupted line). The superficial lamina of the investing layer of deep fascia, and skin, are additional superficial relations.

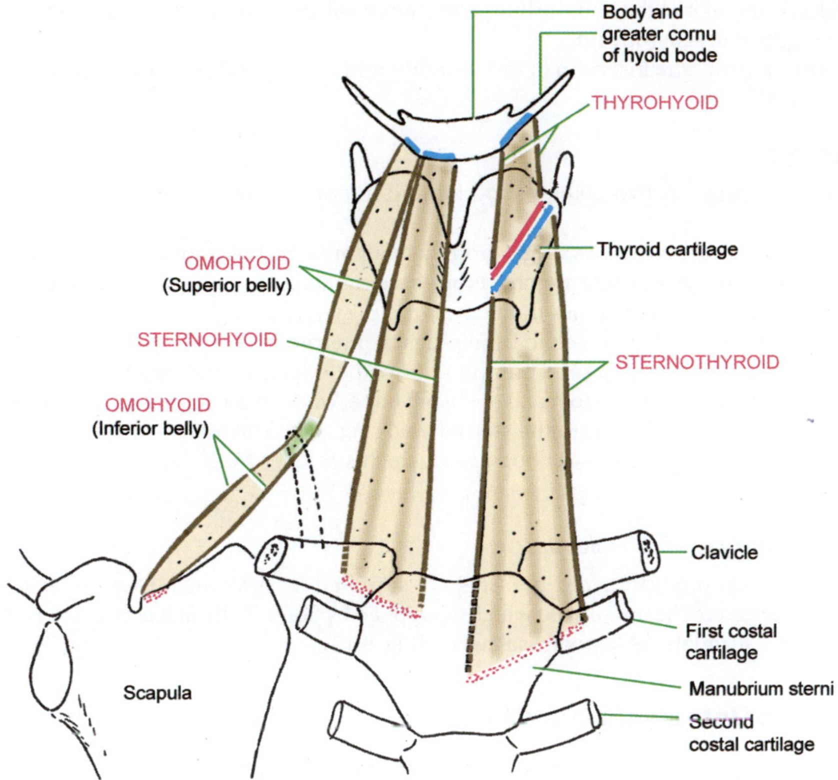

Fig. 7.4 Scheme to show the attachments of the infrahyoid muscles.

by an intermediate tendon. The lower belly is attached to the scapula, and the upper belly to the hyoid bone.

Sternohyoid

The sternohyoid takes origin from:

a. The posterior aspect of the manubrium sterni (upper part);
b. The medial end of the clavicle (posterior aspect); and
c. The capsule of the sternoclavicular joint.

The fibres of the muscle pass upwards and somewhat medially to be inserted into the body of the hyoid bone (lower border) (Fig. 5.8).

Thyrohyoid

The thyrohyoid muscle takes origin from the oblique line on the lamina of the thyroid cartilage. It is inserted into the lower border of the greater cornu of the hyoid bone.

Sternothyroid

The sternothyroid takes origin from the posterior surface of the manubrium sterni below the sternohyoid, and from the medial end of the first costal cartilage.

It is inserted into the oblique line on the lamina of the thyroid cartilage just below the origin of the thyrohyoid.

Observe that the insertion of the sternothyroid corresponds to the origin of the thyrohyoid.

Omohyoid

The omohyoid has two bellies, superior and inferior, joined by an intermediate tendon.

The ***inferior belly*** takes origin from a small area on the upper border of the scapula (near the scapular notch). From here the inferior belly passes forwards, upwards and medially across the floor of the posterior triangle (Fig. 2.5). It ends deep to the sternocleidomastoid by joining the intermediate tendon.

The ***superior belly*** arises from the intermediate tendon and passes upwards (and somewhat medially) to reach the hyoid bone, where it is inserted on the lower border of the body, lateral to the sternohyoid (Fig. 5.8). The intermediate tendon is kept in place by a band of deep fascia which stretches from the tendon to the clavicle (Fig. 7.4).

Nerve Supply of Infrahyoid Muscles

All the foregoing infrahyoid muscles are supplied by branches from the ansa cervicalis except the thyrohyoid which is supplied by fibres of the first cervical nerve that travel through the hypoglossal nerve (Fig. 9.13).

Actions of Infrahyoid Muscles

The sternohyoid, the omohyoid and the thyrohyoid depress the hyoid bone. The sternothyroid pulls the larynx downwards, whereas the thyrohyoid can raise it when the hyoid bone is fixed.

THE LATERAL VERTEBRAL MUSCLES

These are the ***scalenus anterior***, the ***scalenus medius***, the ***scalenus posterior*** and the ***scalenus minimus***. Each muscle is attached at one end to the transverse processes of one or more cervical vertebrae, and at the other end to the first or second rib.

Scalenus Anterior

The scalenus anterior arises from the anterior tubercles of the transverse processes of vertebrae C3 to C6 (Fig. 7.5). It passes downwards and laterally to be inserted into the inner border of the first rib (scalene tubercle) and to a ridge on its upper surface.

Nerve Supply and Action

It is supplied by the ventral rami of spinal nerves C4, C5, and C6. It bends the neck forwards and laterally and rotates it so that the face turns to the opposite side.

Scalenus Medius

The scalenus medius takes origin from the transverse process of the axis, and from the transverse processes (posterior tubercles) of vertebrae C3 to C7 (Fig. 7.8). The muscle passes downwards and laterally to be inserted into the upper surface of the first rib between its tubercle and the groove for the subclavian artery.

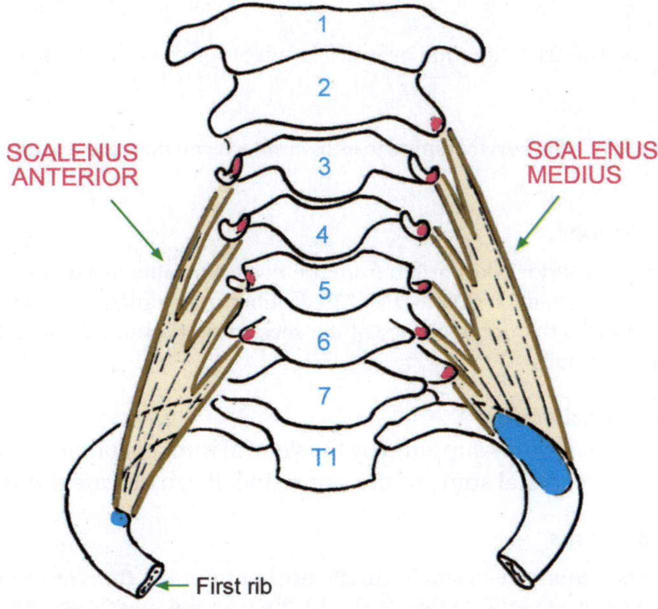

Fig. 7.5 Attachments of the scalenus anterior and scalenus medius muscles.

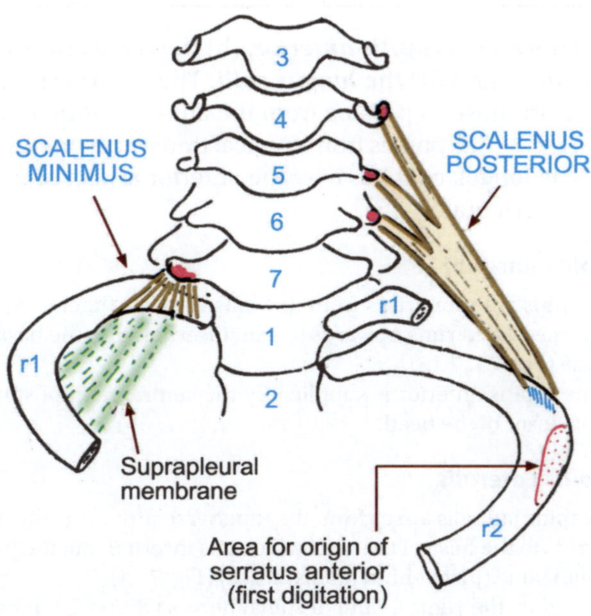

Fig. 7.6 Attachments of the scalenus posterior and scalenus minimus muscles.

Nerve supply

The scalenus medius is supplied by ventral rami of spinal nerves C3 to C8.

Action

The muscle bends the cervical spine to its own side. It can raise the rib during forced inspiration.

Scalenus Posterior

The scalenus posterior takes origin from the posterior tubercles of the transverse processes of vertebrae C4, C5, C6 (Fig. 7.6). Its fibres pass downwards and laterally to be inserted into the outer surface of the second rib (behind the attachment of the serratus anterior).

Nerve supply and action

The scalenus posterior is supplied by the ventral rami of spinal nerves C6, C7, C8. It bends the cervical spine to the same side. It can elevate the second rib.

Scalenus Minimus

The scalenus minimus is a small muscle arising from the transverse process of the seventh cervical vertebra (Fig. 7.6). The fibres of the muscle spread out to be inserted into the inner border of the first rib in its posterior part. Some of its fibres are continuous with the suprapleural membrane, which is sometimes considered to be an expansion of the muscle.

ANTERIOR VERTEBRAL MUSCLES (PREVERTEBRAL MUSCLES)

These are (a) the ***rectus capitis anterior***, (b) the ***rectus capitis lateralis***, (c) the ***longus capitis***, and (d) the ***longus colli***. The rectus capitis anterior and lateralis are short muscles passing from the atlas vertebra to the base of the skull. The longus capitis passes from cervical transverse processes to the base of the skull. The longus colli lies over the anterior aspect of the cervical and upper thoracic vertebrae.

Rectus Capitis Anterior

The rectus capitis anterior arises from the atlas vertebra (lateral mass and root of transverse process) and runs upwards to gain insertion into the basilar part of the occipital bone (Fig. 7.7, 7.15).

The rectus capitis anterior is supplied by the ventral rami of spinal nerves C1 and C2. It is a flexor of the head.

Rectus Capitis Lateralis

The rectus capitis lateralis arises from the transverse process of the atlas (Fig. 7.7). It runs upwards to the base of the skull where it is inserted into the jugular process of the occipital bone (just behind jugular fossa) (Fig. 7.14).

It is supplied by the ventral rami of spinal nerves C1 and C2. It bends the head to its own side.

Longus Colli

The longus colli is placed in front of the vertebral column (Figs. 1.14, 7.7). It extends vertically from the atlas above, to the third thoracic vertebra below. It consists of an upper oblique part, a middle vertical part, and a lower oblique part.

The ***upper oblique part*** runs upwards and medially from the transverse processes (anterior tubercles) of vertebrae C3, C4, and C5 to the anterior arch of the atlas.

The ***vertical part*** arises from the bodies of vertebrae C5, C6, C7 and T1, T2, T3. It runs upwards to be inserted into the bodies of vertebrae C2, C3, C4.

The ***inferior oblique part*** arises from the bodies of upper thoracic vertebrae and passes upwards and laterally to the transverse processes (anterior tubercles) of vertebrae C5 and C6.

Nerve Supply and Action

The longus colli is supplied by the ventral rami of cervical nerves C2 to C6. It is a flexor of the neck. It can help in lateral flexion and in rotation of the neck.

Longus Capitis

The longus capitis arises from the transverse processes (anterior tubercles) of cervical vertebrae (C3 to C6) and runs upwards and medially to be inserted into the base of the skull, on the basilar part of the occipital bone (Figs. 7.7, 7.14).

Nerve supply and action

The longus capitis is supplied by the ventral rami of spinal nerves C1, C2 and C3. It is a flexor of the head.

Note: The exact areas of attachment of the two recti and the longus capitis to the base of the skull are depicted in Fig. 7.14.

DEEP MUSCLES OF THE BACK

Deep Muscles of the Back and their Layout

The deep muscles of the back come into view after the superficial muscles that cover them (namely the trapezius, the latissimus dorsi, the levator scapulae, rhomboids, and the serratus posterior superior and inferior) are removed. They are arranged in layers (from superficial to deep) as follows (Figs. 1.21, 7.8, 7.9):

a. The ***splenius*** group is confined to the upper thoracic and cervical region. It consists of the ***splenius capitis*** and the ***splenius cervicis***.

b. Deep to the splenius group we have the ***erector spinae***, a large muscle mass extending vertically from the back of the sacrum and ilium up to the skull; and transversely from the spines of the vertebrae to the angles of the ribs.
   It is subdivided longitudinally into three parts as follows (Fig. 7.10):
   1. The ***spinalis*** is most medial;
   2. the ***longissimus*** is intermediate in position; and
   3. the ***iliocostocervicalis*** is most lateral.

c. Deep to the erector spinae we have a group of muscles that are collectively called the ***transversospinalis***. They occupy the interval between the spines and transverse processes of the vertebrae.

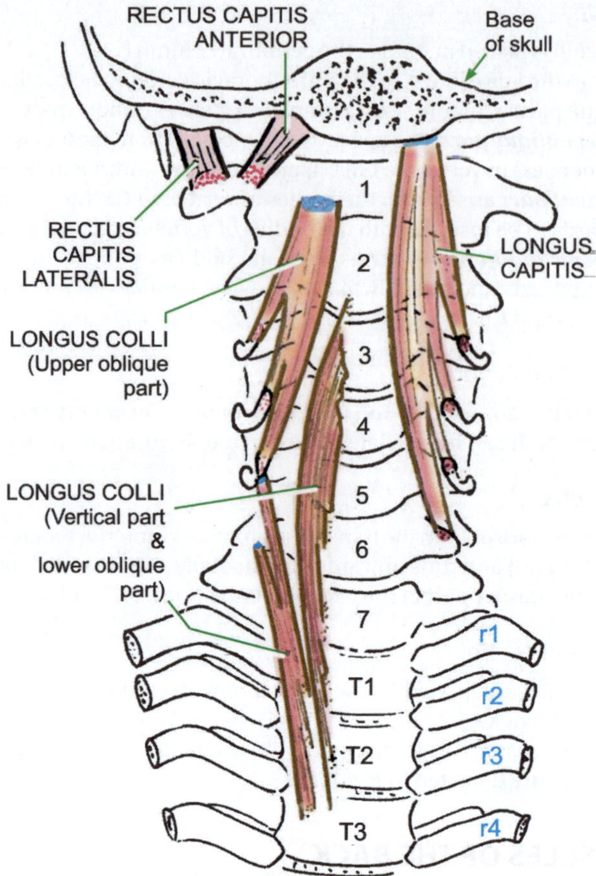

Fig. 7.7 The prevertebral muscles.

The transversospinalis is made up of three sub-groups placed one over the other. These (from superficial to deep) are as follows (Figs. 7.8, 7.9):

1. The ***semispinalis*** group (consisting of semispinalis thoracis, cervicis and capitis) is most superficial.
2. The ***multifidus*** is intermediate in position.
3. The ***rotatores*** are deepest.

A good idea of the relative depth at which the various muscle groups mentioned above lie can be had by examining a transverse section (Figs. 7.8, 1.21). The vertical extend of the various muscles is shown in Fig. 7.9 in which the deepest level is shown in 'A' and progressively more superficial layers are shown in 'B' to 'F'.

Some of these muscles are seen on the back of the neck in Figs. 1.15 A to D (superficial to deep).

In the descriptions that follow we will consider only three muscles in detail. These are the splenius capitis, the erector spinae and the semispinalis capitis. The remaining muscles will be mentioned briefly.

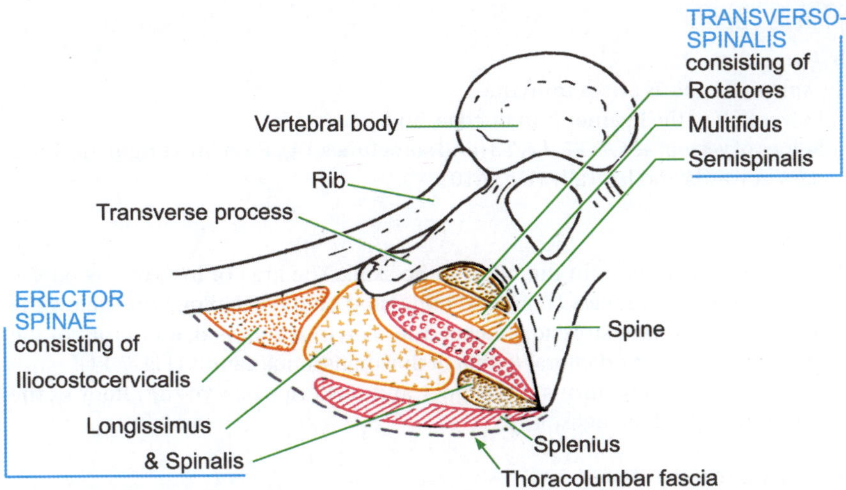

Fig. 7.8 Schematic transverse section to show the arrangement of deep muscles of the back.

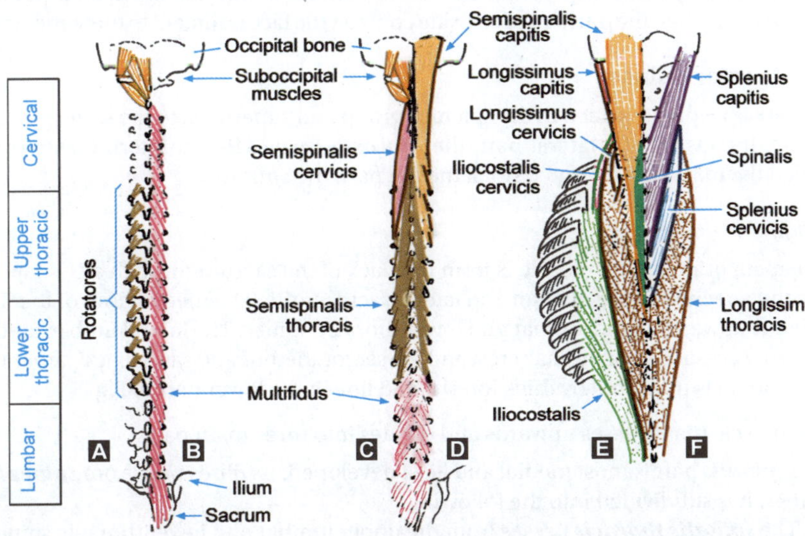

Fig. 7.9 A to F Deep muscles of the back. The deepest layer is shown in 'A' and the most superficial in 'F'.

Splenius Group

This group consists of the splenius capitis and the splenius cervicis. The fibres of the muscles of this group arise from vertebral spines and pass upwards and laterally.

Splenius Capitis

Origin:

The splenius capitus arises from the

a. Lower half of the ligamentum nuchae, and
b. Spines of vertebrae C7, T1, T2, T3 (and sometimes T4). From this origin the fibres pass upwards and laterally (Fig. 7.10).

Insertion

The muscle is inserted into the back of the skull. The area of insertion is on the back of the mastoid process (temporal bone) and on the occipital bone below the lateral one third of the superior nuchal line. The insertion is deep to that of the sternocleidomastoid and lateral to that of the longissimus capitis (Fig. 7.14).

The splenius capitis forms the (upper and posterior part of the) floor of the posterior triangle of the neck.

Splenius Cervicis

The splenius cervicis arises from spines T3 to T6 and is inserted into the transverse processes of upper cervical vertebrae (C1, C2 and sometimes C3).

Nerve Supply and Actions of Splenius Muscles

The splenius capitis and cervicis are supplied by dorsal rami of cervical nerves.

When the splenius capitis and cervicis of both sides contract the head is pulled backwards. When the muscles of one side contract the face is rotated to the same side.

The Erector Spinae

The erector spinae is deep to the splenius group and superficial to the semispinalis group. It consists of a lateral part, the ***iliocosto-cervicalis;*** an intermediate part called the ***longissimus;*** and a small medial part, the ***spinalis.***

Origin

The main origin of the muscle is from the back of the sacrum through a U-shaped tendon attached to the median and lateral sacral crests. The medial limb of the 'U' extends upwards to the lumbar and lower thoracic spines. The lateral limb extends on to the dorsal part of the iliac crest and the sacrotuberous and sacroiliac ligaments. (The origin is indicated by thick interrupted line in the lower part of Fig. 7.11).

The muscle mass passes upwards and divides into three main parts.

The ***spinalis*** part is most medial and least developed. Its fibres pass from ***spines to spines.*** It is subdivided into the following:

a. The ***spinalis thoracis*** passes from the upper lumbar and lower thoracic spines to the upper thoracic spines.
b. The ***spinalis cervicis*** passes from the ligamentum nuchae and upper thoracic spines to the spine of the axis vertebra.
c. The ***spinalis capitis*** passes from the lower cervical spines to the occipital bone (along with the semispinalis capitus).

The ***longissimus*** is the largest division of the erector spinae. It is subdivided into the following:

a. The fibres of the ***longissimus thoracis*** arise mainly from the sacrum. They are inserted into the transverse processes of lumbar and thoracic vertebrae, and into the ribs.

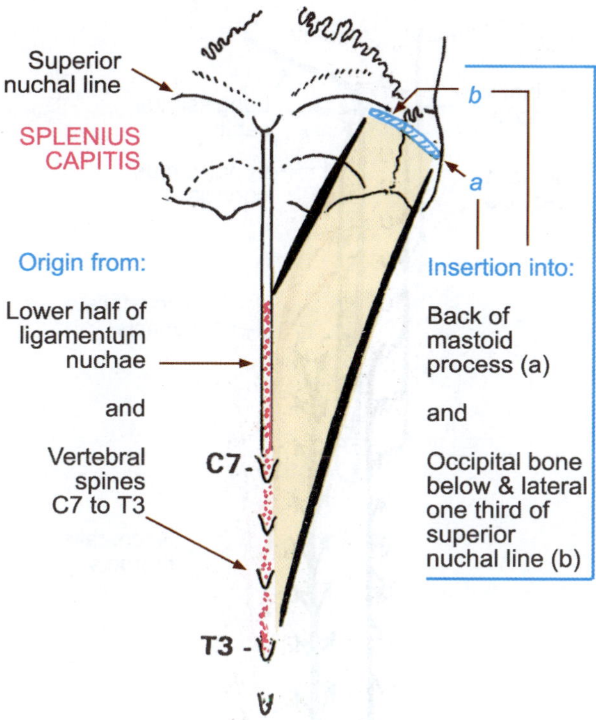

Fig. 7.10 Attachments of the splenius capitis muscle.

b. The ***longissimus cervicis*** arises from the upper thoracic transverse processes (and upper ribs) and is inserted into the transverse processes of the cervical vertebrae.
c. The ***longissimus capitis*** arises from the transverse processes of the upper thoracic vertebrae, and from the articular processes of the lower cervical vertebrae. It is inserted into the mastoid process deep to the splenius capitis (Fig. 7.14).

The ***iliocostocervicalis*** lies lateral to the longissimus and consists of:

a. The ***iliocostalis lumborum*** which arises mainly from the ilium and is inserted into the lower ribs;
b. The ***iliocostalis thoracis*** which passes from the lower ribs to the upper ribs; and
c. The ***iliocostalis cervicis*** which passes from the upper ribs to the lower cervical transverse processes.

Note that out of the large muscle mass of the erector spinae only three slender slips (namely the ***iliocostalis cervicis, longissimus cervicis*** and ***longissimus capitis***) reach the neck.

Nerve Supply and Actions of Erector Spinae

The erector spinae is supplied by ***dorsal*** primary rami of spinal nerves.

As a whole the erector spinae is an extensor and lateral flexor of the vertebral column. The longissimus capitis turns the face to its own side.

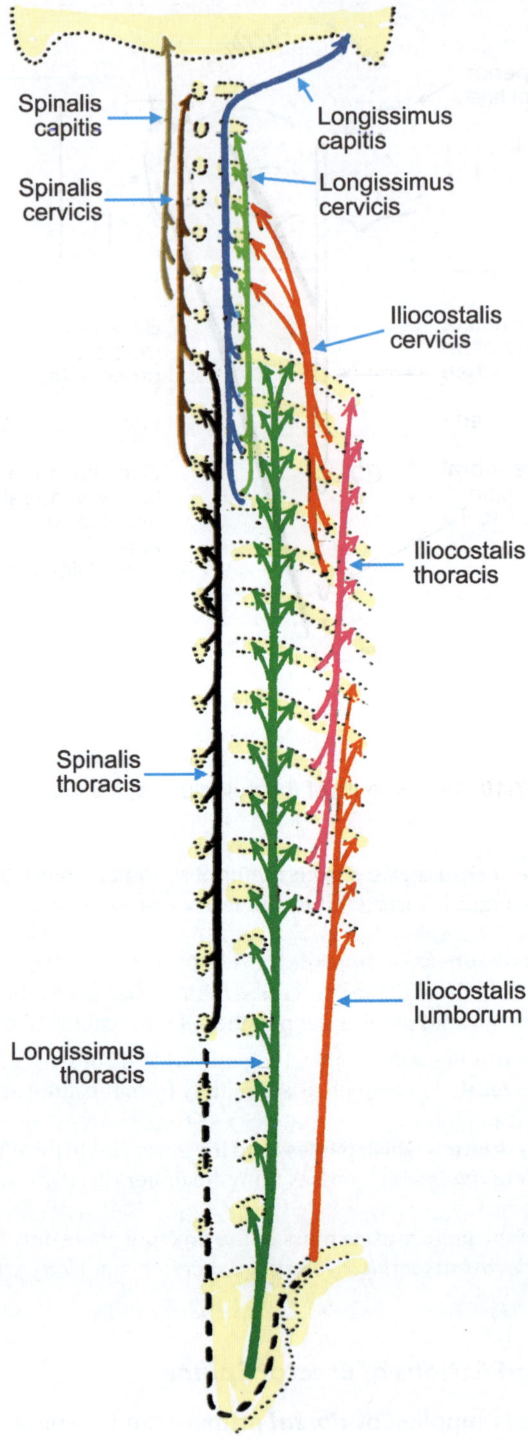

Fig. 7.11 Scheme to show the components of the erector spinae muscle.

The erector spinae is a very important postural muscle. In persons who lead a sedentary life, and with old age, the muscle becomes weak. The vertebral column then tends to bend forwards. This puts excessive strain on ligaments of the vertebral column and also predisposes to prolapse of intervertebral discs. These are common causes of back ache. Tone in the erector spinae can be maintained by exercises and also by brisk walking.

Semispinalis Group

This group consists of the semispinalis capitis, semispinalis cervicis, and semispinalis thoracis.

The ***semispinalis thoracis*** arises from the transverse processes of lower thoracic vertebrae and is inserted into the spines of upper thoracic and lower cervical vertebrae.

The ***semispinalis cervicis*** arises from the transverse processes of upper thoracic vertebrae and is inserted into the cervical (2nd and 5th) spines.

Semispinalis Capitis

Origin:

The semispinalis capitis arises from:

a. The transverse processes of the upper thoracic and seventh cervical vertebrae; and
b. The articular processes of the fourth, fifth and sixth cervical vertebrae.

Insertion:

The muscle is inserted into the occipital bone on the medial part of the area between the superior and inferior nuchal lines. (Also see Figs. 7.13, 7.14).

From these attachments it will be noted that the lateral margin of the muscle is fixed, while the medial margin can be lifted up. The muscle forms the roof of the suboccipital triangle (Fig. 1.15D).

Nerve Supply and Actions:

The semispinalis group is supplied by dorsal rami of cervical and thoracic spinal nerves.

The main action of the semispinalis capitis is to extend the head. It also has a slight rotatory action turning the face to the opposite side.

Multifidus and Rotatores

The ***multifidus*** extends from the sacrum to the axis vertebra. It consists of numerous short oblique slips each arising from a transverse process and passing to the spines of higher vertebrae.

The ***rotatores*** are well formed only in the thoracic region. Each muscle consists of a slip that arises from the transverse process of one thoracic vertebra and is inserted into the lamina of the vertebra next above it. There are thus eleven muscles on either side, but the number is variable.

The rotatores, multifidus and semispinalis are rotators of the vertebral column. The multifidus and semispinalis are, in addition, extensors and lateral flexors. However, their main function is postural.

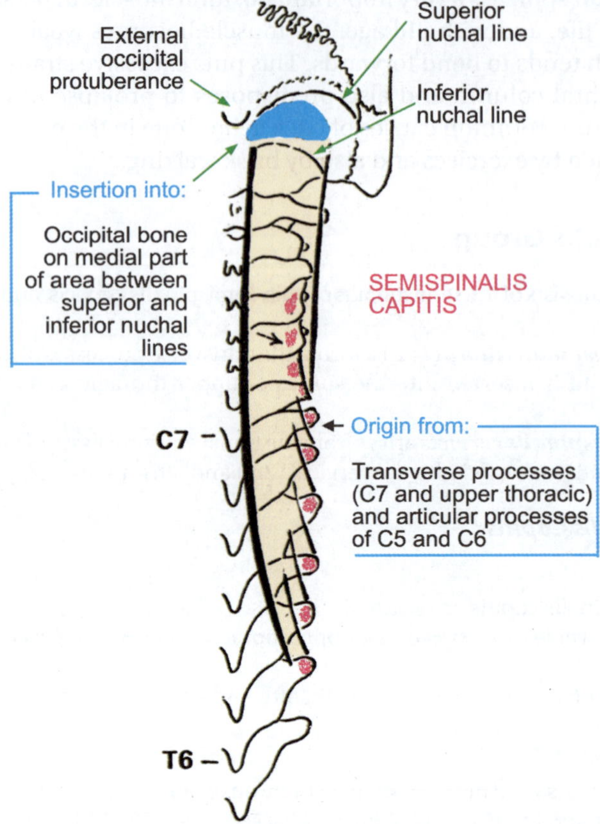

Fig. 7.12 Scheme to show the attachments of the semispinalis capitis muscle.

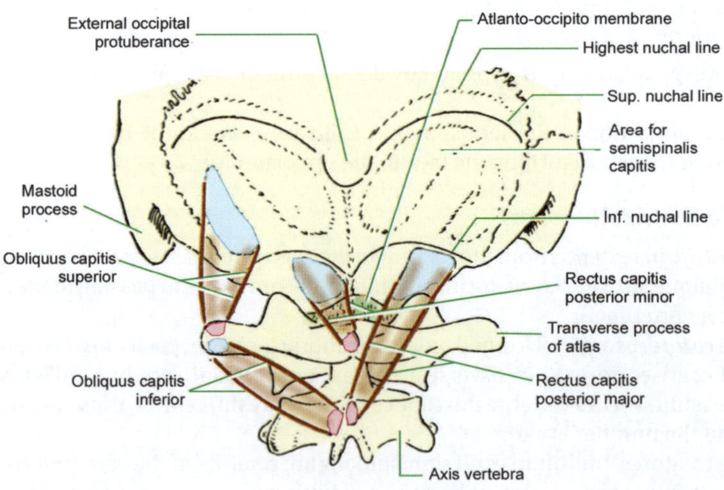

Fig. 57.13 Schematic diagram to show the attachments of the suboccipital muscles.

Other Muscles in the Back

Apart from the deep muscles of the back described above there are small muscles that bridge the intervals between adjacent spines (***interspinales***) and between adjacent transverse processes (***intertransversarii***).

The ***suboccipital muscles*** are considered below.

It may be noted that all the deep muscles of the back (rotatores, multifidus, semispinalis, erector spinae and splenius) are supplied by dorsal primary rami of the spinal nerves of the levels concerned. The muscles can be cut transversely, without denervating parts above or below the incision.

Suboccipital Muscles

This is a group of small muscles placed in the uppermost part of the back of the neck, deep to the semispinalis capitis. They form the boundaries of the suboccipital triangle (Fig. 7.13, 1.15D).

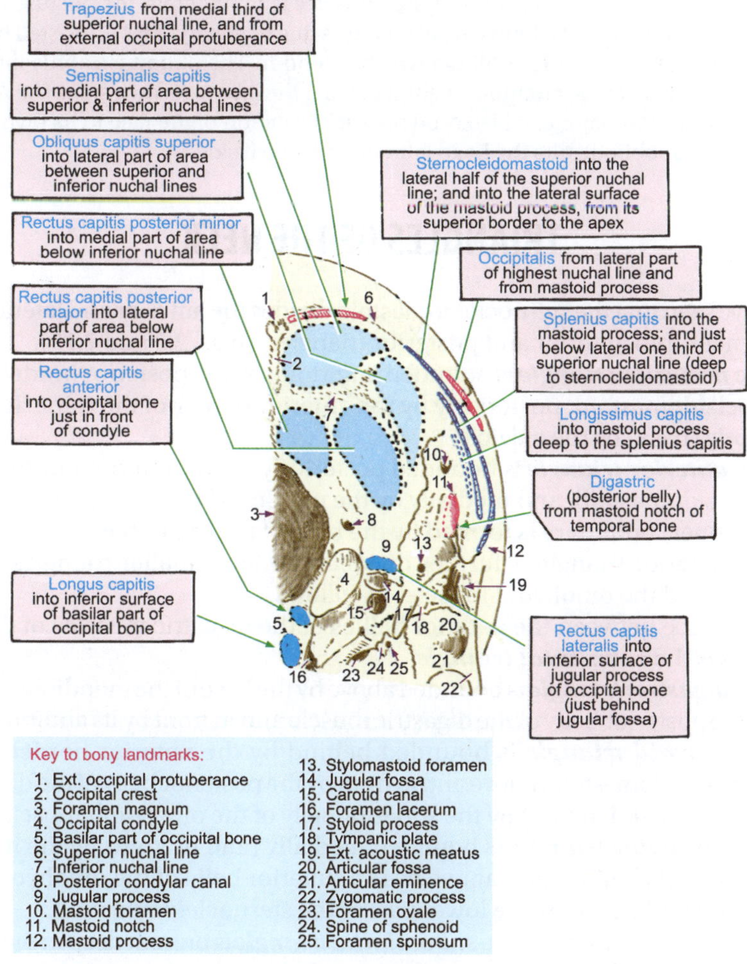

Fig. 7.14 Attachments of muscles of the neck to the base of the skull.

The ***rectus capitis posterior minor*** arises from the posterior arch of the atlas. Its fibres pass upwards to be inserted into the occipital bone in the medial part of the area below the inferior nuchal line (i.e., between the line and the foramen magnum) (Fig. 7.14).

The ***rectus capitis posterior major*** arises from the spine of the axis vertebra. Its fibres pass upwards and laterally to be inserted into the lateral part of the area below the inferior nuchal line.

The ***obliquus capitis inferior*** arises from the spine of the axis vertebra. Its fibres pass laterally and somewhat upwards to be inserted into the transverse process of the atlas vertebra.

The ***obliquus capitis superior*** arises from the transverse process of the atlas. Its fibres pass upwards (and somewhat medially) to be inserted into the lateral part of the area between the superior and inferior nuchal lines.

Nerve Supply and Actions:

The suboccipital muscles are supplied by the dorsal ramus of the first cervical nerve.

The main action of the suboccipital muscles is to maintain the posture of the head. Note that the head tends to fall forwards due to gravity. This is resisted by the two recti and the superior oblique which extend it. The obliquus capitis inferior rotates the head at the atlantoaxial joint turning the face to its own side. The rectus capitis posterior major can also produce slight rotation of the face to its own side. The superior oblique tilts the head laterally to its own side.

TRIANGLES OF THE NECK

We have seen that the sternocleidomastoid divides the anterior and lateral sides of the neck into anterior and posterior triangles (Figs. 2.5 and 7.15).

The ***posterior triangle*** is bounded anteriorly by the posterior border of the sternocleidomastoid, posteriorly by the anterior border of the trapezius, and inferiorly (base) by the clavicle.

The ***anterior triangle*** is bounded posteriorly by the anterior border of the sternocleidomastoid, and medially by the midline of the front of the neck. Its third (upper) boundary is formed by the base of the mandible.

The anterior triangle is further divided into four smaller triangles by the digastric and the omohyoid muscles as follows.

1. The space between the anterior bellies of the digastric muscles of the two sides is the ***submental triangle***.
2. The ***digastric triangle*** is bounded above by the base of the mandible, behind by the posterior belly of the digastric muscle and in front by its anterior belly.
3. The ***carotid triangle*** is bounded behind by the anterior border of the sternocleidomastoid, above and in front by the posterior belly of the digastric, and below and in front by the superior belly of the omohyoid muscle.
4. The ***muscular triangle*** is bounded medially (and in front) by the midline of the neck, behind and above by the superior belly of the omohyoid, and behind and below by the lower part of the sternocleidomastoid.
5. In addition to the above the ***suboccipital triangle*** is present deep in the upper part of the back of the neck, and is bounded by the suboccipital muscles.

We will consider some important aspects of these triangles in the paragraphs that follow.

THE POSTERIOR TRIANGLE

Boundaries

As stated above the posterior triangle is bounded anteriorly by the posterior border of the sternocleidomastoid, posteriorly by the anterior border of the trapezius, and inferiorly (base) by the clavicle.

Floor

The floor of this triangle is formed mainly by the splenius capitis, the levator scapulae, and the scalenus medius. Other muscles that may occasionally be seen in the floor are the semispinalis capitis, the scalenus posterior, and the scalenus anterior.

The lower part of the posterior triangle is crossed by the inferior belly of the omohyoid muscle which divides the triangle into an upper part (also called the ***occipital triangle***), and a lower part (also called the ***supraclavicular triangle***).

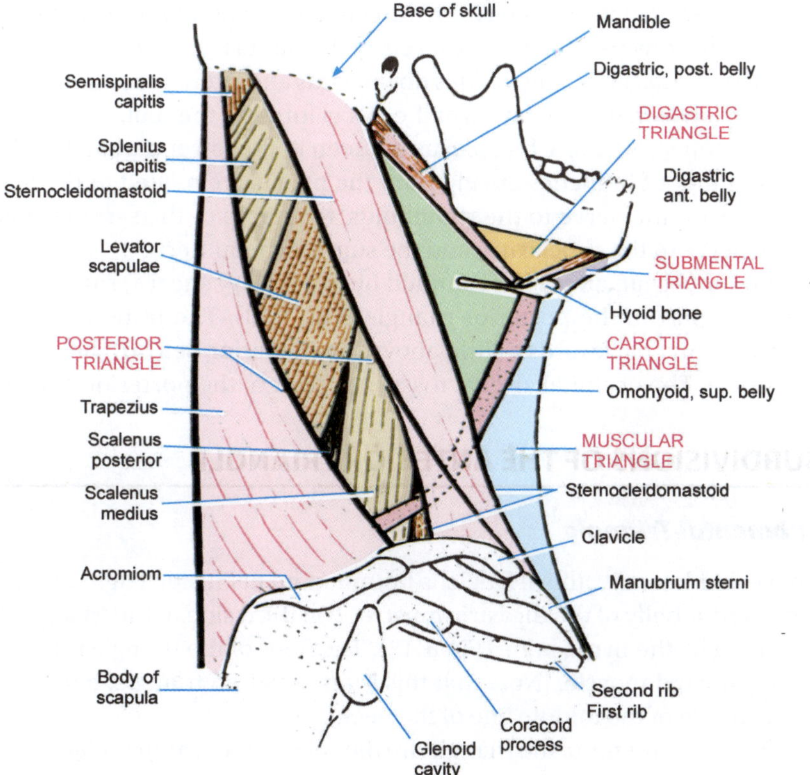

Fig. 7.15 Triangles of the neck. Also see Fig. 2.5.

The muscles forming the floor are covered by the prevertebral layer of deep cervical fascia.

Roof

The roof of the posterior triangle is formed by the investing layer of deep cervical fascia. This is best appreciated by examining a transverse section through the neck (Fig. 1.21). Superficial to the deep cervical fascia the posterior triangle is covered by superficial fascia and skin.

Several nerves and vessels are present in relation to the roof of the posterior triangle (Fig. 1.9). These include the supraclavicular, lesser occipital, great auricular, and transverse cutaneous nerves; the external jugular vein and some of its tributaries; several unnamed arteries; and lymph vessels.

Contents

1. Cutaneous branches of the cervical plexus (supraclavicular, lesser occipital, great auricular and transverse cutaneous) enter the posterior triangle by piercing the fascia over its floor, and run for some distance between the floor and roof, before piercing the latter to become subcutaneous.
2. Muscular branches arising from the cervical plexus for the levator scapulae and trapezius run deep to the fascia of the floor (Fig. 1.10).
3. The spinal accessory nerve runs downwards and laterally across the triangle lying between the two layers of the fascia forming the roof.
4. The trunks of the brachial plexus are seen in the lower part of the triangle. A number of branches arising from the plexus are related to the triangle. These are the nerve to the rhomboids, the nerve to the serratus anterior, the nerve to the subclavius, and the suprascapular nerve. .
5. The subclavian artery (surrounded by the axillary sheath) runs across the lowest part of the posterior triangle (Fig. 1.10). The transverse cervical artery runs backwards a little above the posterior belly of the omohyoid muscle. The occipital artery crosses the apex of the posterior triangle.

SUBDIVISIONS OF THE ANTERIOR TRIANGLE

Submental Triangle

Above and laterally, this triangle is bounded on each side (right and left) by the anterior belly of the digastric muscle. The third side of the triangle (base) is formed by the hyoid bone (Fig. 1.12). The floor of the triangle is formed by the mylohyoid muscle. [Note that this is an unpaired triangle, half of it lying on each side of the middle line of the neck].

The only contents of the triangle are the submental lymph nodes, and some small blood vessels.

Digastric Triangle

This triangle is bounded above by the base of the mandible, and below by the anterior and posterior bellies of the digastric muscle. Its floor is formed by the mylohyoid and hyoglossus muscles, and by the anterior part of the middle constrictor of the pharynx (Fig. 1.7). The roof of the triangle is formed by skin, superficial fascia (containing the platysma, the cervical branch of the facial nerve and some cutaneous nerves) and the investing layer of deep fascia. The main content of this triangle is the submandibular gland.

The contents of this triangle have been studied in detail in the submandibular region (Chapter 5).

Carotid Triangle

This triangle is bounded posteriorly by the anterior margin of the sternocleidomastoid muscle, superiorly by the posterior belly of the digastric muscle, and anteroinferiorly by the superior belly of the omohyoid muscle (Figs. 2.5, 8.12). Its roof is formed by skin, superficial and deep fascia. The floor of the triangle is formed by the thyrohyoid and hyoglossus muscles, and the middle and inferior constrictors of the pharynx (Fig. 1.10).

The carotid triangle contains several important blood vessels and nerves. These are as follows.

1. Common carotid artery, along with carotid sinus and carotid body.
2. Internal carotid artery.
3. External carotid artery and the following branches arising from it.
   a. Superior thyroid artery.
   b. Lingual artery.
   c. Facial artery.
   d. Ascending pharyngeal artery.
   e. Occipital artery.
4. Internal jugular vein, and some tributaries draining into it.
5. Vagus nerve and its superior laryngeal branch dividing into external and internal laryngeal nerves.
6. Spinal accessory nerve.
7. Hypoglossal nerve and upper root of ansa cervicalis.
8. Sympathetic trunk.

The common carotid and internal carotid arteries, the internal jugular vein and the vagus nerve are surrounded by the carotid sheath.

Muscular Triangle

This triangle is bounded posteroinferiorly by the sternocleidomastoid muscle, posterosuperiorly by the superior belly of the omohyoid muscle, and anteriorly (or medially) by the anterior middle line of the neck.

The triangle contains the infrahyoid muscles. Deep to these muscles it contains the thyroid gland, the larynx and the trachea. On either side of the trachea we see the carotid sheath and its contents. Part of the brachiocephalic artery may occasionally be present in front of the trachea just above the manubrium sterni.

SUBOCCIPITAL TRIANGLE

Boundaries

The suboccipital muscles have been described earlier in this Chapter. They form the boundaries of the suboccipital triangle as follows (Fig. 1.15).

1. Medially and above, there are the rectus capitis posterior major and minor muscles.
2. Laterally and above, there is the obliquus capitis superior.
3. Inferiorly, there is the obliquus capitis inferior.

Roof

The roof of the suboccipital triangle is formed by the semispinalis capitis muscle. Deep to the semispinalis capitis the triangle is covered by dense fascia. From Figs. 1.5 A to D it will be seen that to reach the suboccipital triangle we have to remove the trapezius, the splenius capitis, and the semispinalis capitis muscles. The longissimus capitis lies over the lateral part of the triangle.

Floor

The floor of the suboccipital triangle is formed by the posterior arch of the atlas, and the posterior atlantooccipital membrane (Figs. 6.16, 8.35).

Contents

1. The third part of the vertebral artery enters the suboccipital region after emerging from the foramen transversarium of the atlas. It then runs medially over the posterior arch of the atlas and disappears under the lateral free edge of the posterior atlantooccipital membrane.
2. The dorsal ramus of the first cervical nerve runs backwards above the posterior arch of the atlas, lying below the vertebral artery (Fig. 9.3). It gives branches to the suboccipital muscles and to the semispinalis capitis.
3. The greater occipital nerve winds round the lower border of the obliquus capitis inferior. It then runs upwards (and slightly medially) across the suboccipital triangle. It leaves the triangle by piercing the semispinalis capitis.

Other Nerves and Vessels on the Back of the Neck

These are the third occipital nerve, the occipital artery and the deep cervical artery. They will be described in Chapters 8 and 9.

DEEP CERVICAL FASCIA

As in other parts of the body, all muscles, blood vessels and nerves of the neck are surrounded by some connective tissue. However, we find that in several planes in the neck the connective tissue is condensed to form recognisable sheets that are collectively referred to as deep cervical fascia.

A good idea of the layers of the deep cervical fascia can be obtained by examining a transverse section through the neck (Fig. 1.21). The layers are as follows.

1. Investing Layer

Deep to the skin, superficial fascia and platysma we see the investing layer of deep fascia. This layer is made up of two laminae (shown in pink in Fig. 1.21) that go right round the neck enclosing all structures deep to them. Anteriorly, near the middle line of the neck the two laminae are fused to each other. Traced laterally, the laminae separate to enclose the sternocleidomastoid muscle. At the posterior edge of this muscle the layers meet again and form the roof of the posterior triangle. Passing posteriorly they again separate to enclose the trapezius, and end by gaining attachment to the ligamentum nuchae.

The vertical extent of the investing layer is as follows. When traced upwards over the front of the neck, the fascia gets attached to the hyoid bone, and then passes over the submental triangle to reach the lower border of the body of the mandible. When traced upwards over the sternocleidomastoid muscle the fascia reaches the mastoid process; and when traced upwards over the trapezius it reaches the superior nuchal line and the external occipital protuberance. (In other words the investing layer extends as far up as the muscles it covers).

Traced downwards on the front of the neck the investing layer of fascia reaches the manubrium sterni. More laterally it reaches the clavicle. Traced downwards over the trapezius the fascia reaches the lateral part of the clavicle, the acromion, and the spine of the scapula (again being coextensive with the muscles).

Note the following additional points about the investing layer of deep cervical fascia.

1. When traced upwards over the submandibular region the two laminae separate to enclose the submandibular gland.
2. In the interval between the mandible and the mastoid process the two laminae enclose the parotid gland. Here the superficial lamina is thick and forms the parotid fascia. The deep lamina forms the ***stylomandibular ligament*** which intervenes between the parotid gland and the submandibular gland (Fig. 5.2).
3. Just above the manubrium sterni the two laminae enclose the ***suprasternal space.***

   This space contains the sternal heads of the right and left sternocleidomastoid muscles, the interclavicular ligament, the jugular arch joining the right and left anterior jugular veins, and a lymph node.

4. Above the clavicle (near the base of the posterior triangle) the two laminae of the investing layer enclose the ***supraclavicular space.***

This space contains a part of the external jugular vein and the supraclavicular nerves.

5. The accessory nerve runs across the posterior triangle lying between the two laminae.

2. Pretracheal Fascia

In Fig. 1.21 note that the thyroid gland is enclosed in a layer of fascia (shown in green). When traced downwards this fascia lies in front of the trachea and is, therefore, called the pretracheal fascia.

It passes along the trachea into the superior mediastinum of the thorax to reach the arch of the aorta. When traced upwards the pretracheal fascia is attached to the hyoid bone, and more laterally to the oblique line of the thyroid cartilage. [Note that this line is also the upper limit of the lobe of the thyroid gland]. Laterally, the pretracheal fascia fuses with the carotid sheath.

3. Prevertebral Fascia

This layer of deep cervical fascia lies behind the oesophagus and pharynx. It covers the prevertebral muscles. Traced laterally, it passes onto the scalene muscles and levator scapulae, and then over the deep muscles of the back to reach the ligamentum nuchae. The prevertebral fascia covers the floor of the posterior triangle.

When traced upwards the prevertebral fascia reaches the base of the skull. Inferiorly, it passes into the thorax in front of the upper thoracic vertebrae. Some additional features of interest about the prevertebral fascia are as follows.

1. From Fig. 1.21 it will be obvious that the cervical nerves emerging from intervertebral foramina must lie deep to the prevertebral fascia. The cervical and brachial plexuses formed by union of the ventral rami of these nerves are also deep to this fascia. Branches from these plexuses to muscles remain deep to the fascia, but cutaneous nerves have to pierce it to become superficial.
2. The axillary sheath is an extension of this fascia around the subclavian artery and brachial plexus. The sheath extends into the axilla.

4. Carotid Sheath

The tubular sheath of fascia surrounding the common and internal carotid arteries, and the internal jugular vein, is also described as part of the deep cervical fascia. It extends from the lower end of the neck to the base of the skull. The vagus nerve lies within the sheath behind the interval between the common (or internal) carotid artery and the internal jugular vein. The sympathetic trunk descends just outside the sheath posterior to the arteries. The ansa cervicalis is closely related to the front of the carotid sheath.

CLINICAL CORRELATIONS

Various clinical correlations of the neck, relevant to topics discussed in this chapter are described in Chapter 15.

CHAPTER

8

Blood Vessels of Head and Neck

ARTERIES

THE COMMON CAROTID ARTERIES

On the right side the common carotid artery is a branch of the brachiocephalic trunk, while on the left side it is a direct branch of the arch of the aorta. It follows that the left common carotid artery runs parts of its course in the thorax.

The courses and relations of the cervical parts of the right and left common carotid arteries are similar (See Figs. 1.8, 1.10 to 1.13). Starting behind the corresponding sternoclavicular joint each artery runs upwards and somewhat laterally up to the level of the upper border of the thyroid cartilage (Fig. 8.1). Here it terminates by dividing into the internal and external carotid arteries. It (normally) gives no other branches. In its upward course each common carotid artery lies in a triangular area bounded behind by the transverse processes of the cervical vertebrae (fourth to sixth); medially in the lower part, by the oesophagus and trachea, and higher up by the pharynx and larynx; and anterolaterally by the sternocleidomastoid muscle (Fig. 8.3). The artery is enclosed in a fibrous ***carotid sheath*** which also encloses the internal jugular vein (lateral to the artery) and the vagus nerve (lying posterior to the interval between the artery and the vein).

Additional relations of the artery are as follows. Running vertically behind the carotid sheath there are the sympathetic trunk (Fig. 8.3), the ascending cervical artery (Fig. 8.1), the vertebral artery, a part of the subclavian artery, and the thoracic duct (on the left side only).

The inferior thyroid artery runs transversely behind the lower part of the artery (Fig. 8.1). On the right side only, the artery is crossed posteriorly by the recurrent laryngeal nerve; and on the left side only, by the thoracic duct. Apart from the sternocleidomastoid muscle the structures covering the artery anterolaterally are the sternohyoid and sternothyroid muscles (in its lower part, deep to the sternocleidomastoid), the deep cervical fascia, platysma

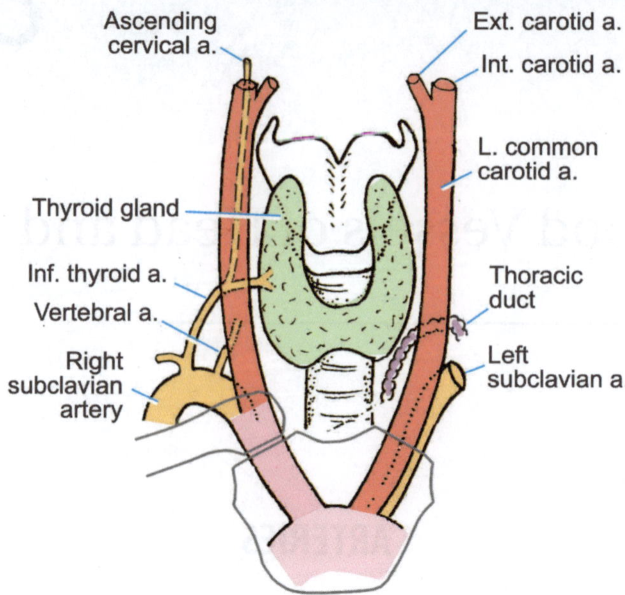

Fig. 8.1 Relationship of common carotid artery to the larynx, trachea and thyroid. Some structures deep to the artery are also shown.

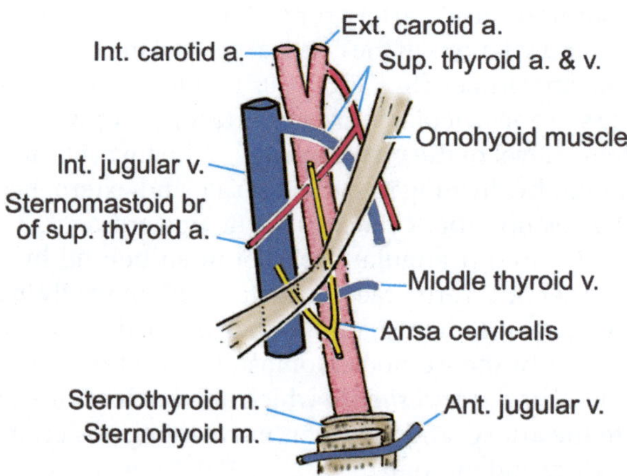

Fig. 8.2 Right lateral view showing structures crossing superficial to the common carotid artery.

and skin. Deep to the sternocleidomastoid the artery is crossed superficially by (Fig. 8.2): (i) the superior belly of the omohyoid muscle (at the level of the cricoid cartilage); (ii) the sternomastoid branch of the superior thyroid artery (above the omohyoid); (iii) the ansa cervicalis (a nerve loop); (iv) the superior thyroid vein (near the upper end of the artery), and the middle thyroid vein (below the omohyoid); and (v) the anterior jugular vein (just above the clavicle).

Other structures on the medial side of the artery are the recurrent laryngeal nerve (running vertically between the trachea and the oesophagus), the corresponding lobe of the thyroid gland, and a part of the inferior thyroid artery.

INTERNAL CAROTID ARTERY

Internal Carotid Artery in the Neck

The internal carotid arteries begin at the upper border of the thyroid cartilage and ascend to reach the base of the skull where they enter the carotid canal (Study Figs. 1.5, 1.6, 1.10 to 1.13). Each artery may be considered as the main upward continuation of the common carotid artery and occupies a similar position (Compare Figs. 8.3 and 8.4).

Like the latter it is surrounded by a carotid sheath along with the internal jugular vein and the vagus nerve. It lies on the transverse processes of the upper cervical vertebrae being separated from them by the longus capitis and the superior cervical sympathetic ganglion. On the medial side the artery is related to the pharynx.

Additional relations are as follows. At its upper end the internal jugular vein lies posterior to the artery; and the glossopharyngeal, vagus, accessory and hypoglossal nerves lie between them. The artery is crossed posteriorly by the superior laryngeal nerve (Fig. 8.5). Medially, it is related to the same nerve, the ascending pharyngeal artery and pharyngeal veins as they lie on the pharynx. Superficially the artery is crossed by a large number of structures that are shown in Fig. 8.5.

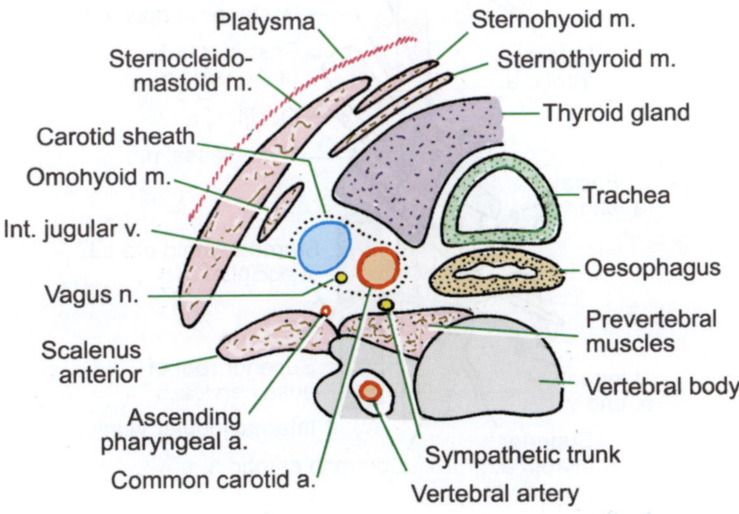

Fig. 8.3 T.S. neck to show some relations of the common carotid artery.

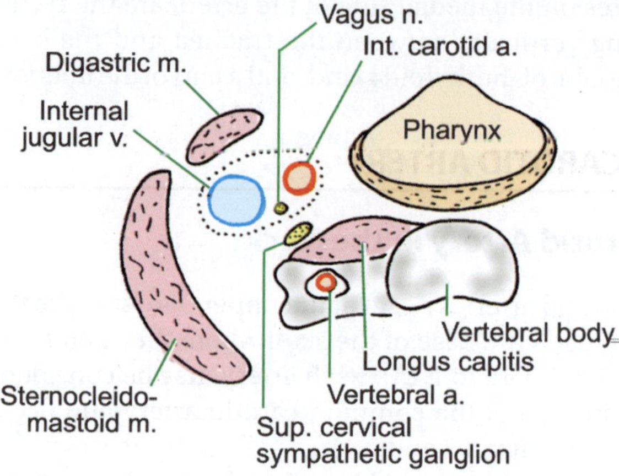

Fig. 8.4 T.S. neck to show some relations of the internal carotid artery.

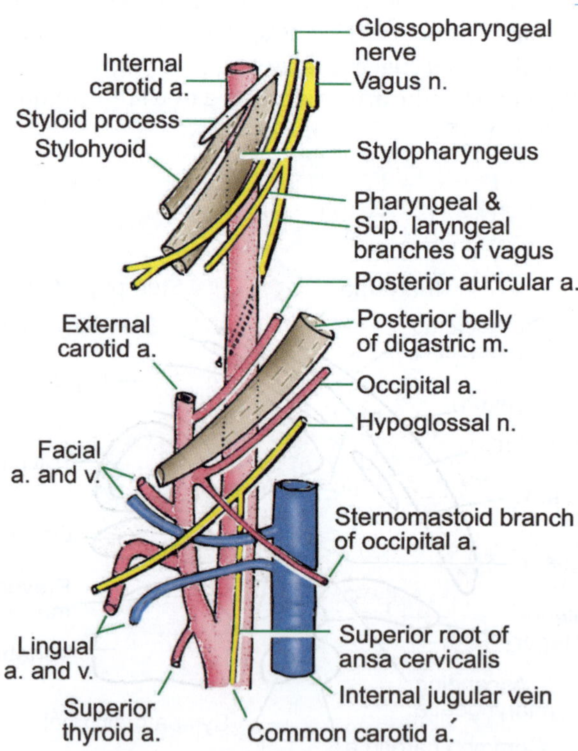

Fig. 8.5 Diagram showing some structures superficial to the internal carotid artery. The superior laryngeal nerve which crosses deep to the artery is also shown.

Cranial Part of the Internal Carotid Arteries

The cranial part of the internal carotid artery has a complicated course. Successive parts of the artery run vertically and horizontally (Fig. 8.6). On reaching the base of the skull the artery enters the petrous part of the temporal bone through the external opening of the carotid canal.

It then bends sharply (Fig. 8.6, first bend) to run horizontally forwards and medially through the carotid canal to reach the foramen lacerum. It now undergoes a second bend to run vertically through the upper part of this foramen to enter the cranial cavity. It then lies within the cavernous sinus.

Here it undergoes a third bend to run forwards on the side of the body of the sphenoid bone. Near the anterior end of the body it again bends upwards (fourth bend) on the medial side of the anterior clinoid process. Here it pierces through the duramater forming the roof of the cavernous sinus and comes into relationship with the cerebrum. The artery now turns backwards (fifth bend) to reach the anterior perforated substance of the brain. The artery terminates here by dividing into the anterior and middle cerebral arteries. From the above it is seen that the cranial part of the internal carotid artery can be divided into a ***petrous part***, a ***cavernous part*** and a ***cerebral part***.

Additional relations of importance are as follows:

a. Throughout its course the artery is surrounded by a plexus of sympathetic nerves derived from the superior cervical sympathetic ganglion, and by a plexus of veins that connect the intracranial veins to those outside the skull.
b. As it lies in the carotid canal the artery is closely related to the middle ear, the auditory tube and the cochlea (Fig. 8.7).
c. As the artery passes through the cavernous sinus it is related to several cranial nerves that are embedded in the lateral wall of the sinus (Fig. 8.8). From above downwards these are the oculomotor, trochlear, ophthalmic

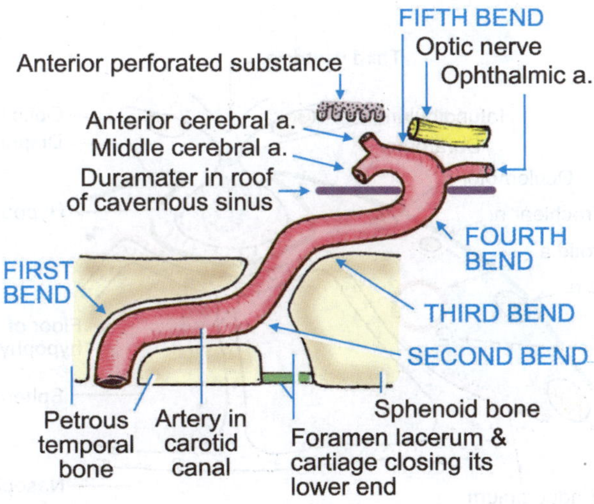

Fig. 8.6 Scheme to show the intracranial course of the internal carotid artery.

division of the trigeminal nerve, and the maxillary division of the same nerve. The artery has a more intimate relationship with the abducent nerve which runs in close contact with the inferolateral side of the artery.

d. After piercing the duramater the artery has the optic nerve above it and the oculomotor nerve below it.

The internal carotid artery gives off three large branches. These are the ***ophthalmic artery*** to the orbit, and the ***anterior and middle cerebral arteries*** to the brain. The ophthalmic artery is described in detail below. The cerebral arteries will be considered in the section on the brain (Chapter 25).

In addition to these, the internal carotid artery gives off several smaller branches that are shown in Fig. 8.9. The posterior communicating and the anterior choroidal artery are intimated related to the brain and will be described in Chapter 25. The other arteries are as follows.

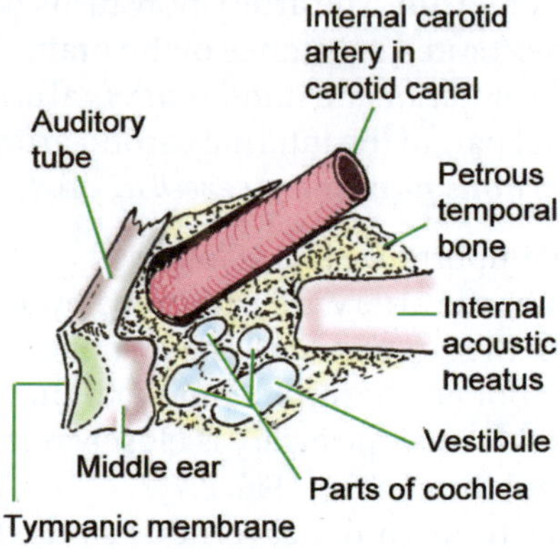

Fig. 8.7 Schematic diagram of the internal carotid artery as it lies in the carotid canal to show its relations to parts of the ear.

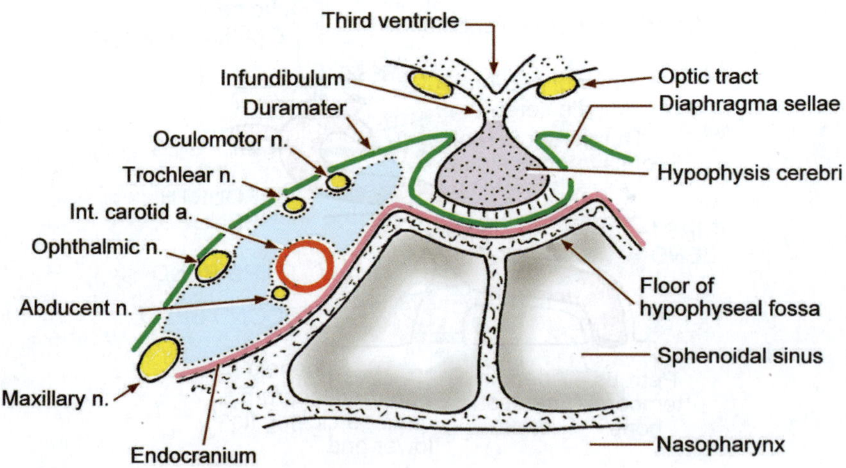

Fig. 8.8 Coronal section through the cavernous sinus showing the internal carotid artery and related structures.

THE OPHTHALMIC ARTERY

The ophthalmic artery passes forwards to enter the cavity of the orbit through the optic canal. In this canal it lies inferolateral to the optic nerve. Having entered the orbit the artery is at first lateral to the optic nerve (Figs. 1.20, 8.10). It then crosses above the nerve to reach the medial wall of the orbit and runs forwards along this wall.

Branches of the Ophthalmic artery

The branches of the ophthalmic artery are shown in Fig. 8.10.

1. The ***central artery of the retina*** is the first branch of the ophthalmic artery. It arises from the ophthalmic artery when the latter is still within the optic canal. It first lies below the optic nerve. It pierces the dural sheath of the nerve and runs forwards for a short distance between these two. It then enters the substance of the nerve and runs forwards in its centre to reach the optic disc. Here it divides into branches that supply the retina (Fig. 8.11).
2. The largest branch of the ophthalmic artery is the ***lacrimal artery*** which runs forwards along the lateral wall of the orbit. The further branches given off by the lacrimal artery are as follows.

   a. Just near its origin from the ophthalmic artery the lacrimal artery gives off a ***recurrent meningeal*** branch that runs backwards to enter the middle cranial fossa through the superior orbital fissure.
   b. The lacrimal artery gives off two ***zygomatic*** branches that enter canals in the zygomatic bone. One branch appears on the face through the zygomaticofacial foramen. The other appears on the temporal surface of the bone through the zygomaticotemporal foramen.
   c. Terminal ramifications of the lacrimal artery supply the lacrimal gland.
   d. The lateral palpebral branches supply the eyelids.

   The other branches of the ophthalmic artery arise from the main stem of the artery (Fig. 8.10).

3. The ***posterior ciliary arteries*** arise as the ophthalmic artery crosses the optic nerve. They run forwards around the optic nerve and supply the eyeball.
4. The ***supraorbital*** branch supplies the skin of the forehead.
5. The ***anterior*** and ***posterior ethmoidal*** branches enter foramina in the medial wall of the orbit to supply the ethmoidal air sinuses. They then enter the anterior cranial fossa. Their terminal branches (specially of the anterior artery) enter the nose and supply part of it.
6. The ***anterior ciliary arteries*** arise from the ophthalmic artery near the anterior part of the eyeball and supply it.
7. The ***medial palpebral*** branches supply the eyelids.
8. The ***supratrochlear artery*** is one of the terminal branches of the ophthalmic artery. It supplies the skin of the forehead (along with the supraorbital artery).
9. The ***dorsal nasal branch*** supplies the upper part of the nose.

   In addition to the branches shown in Fig. 8.10 the ophthalmic artery and its branches give off several ***muscular*** branches to muscles of the orbit.

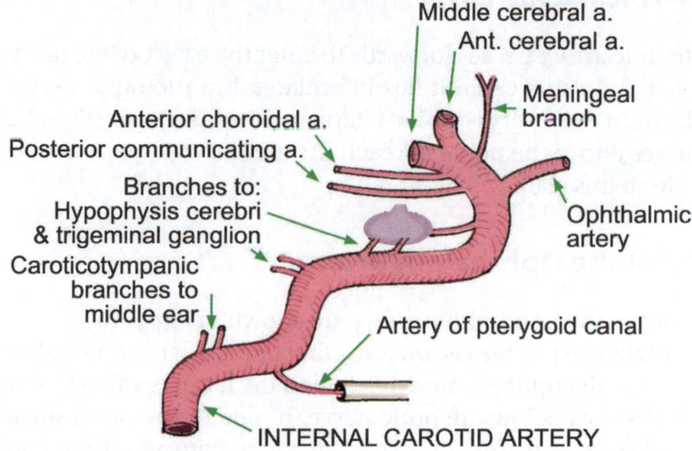

Fig. 8.9 Scheme to show the branches given off by the internal carotid artery.

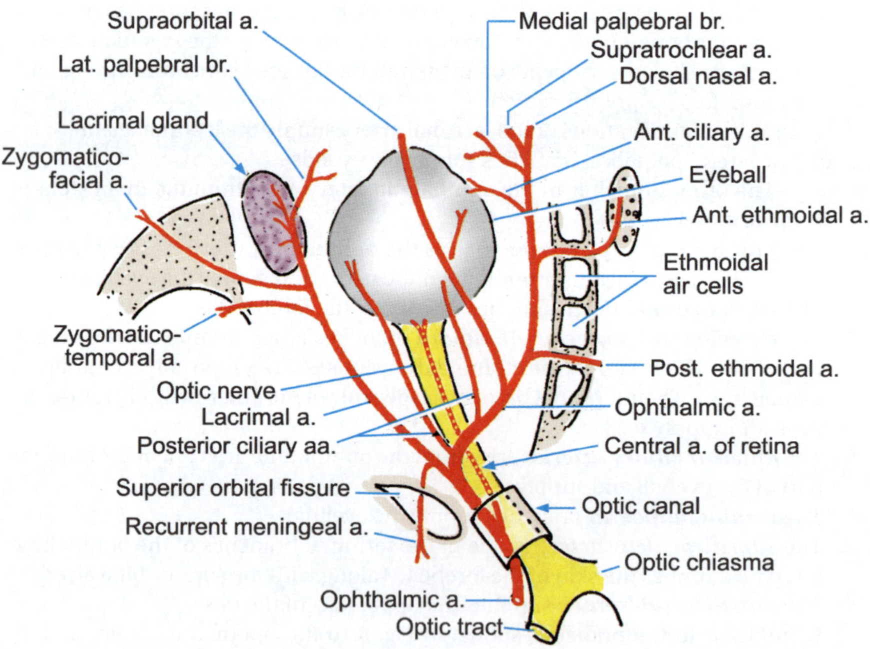

Fig. 8.10 Scheme to show the branches of the ophthalmic artery.

THE EXTERNAL CAROTID ARTERIES

Each external carotid artery arises from the common carotid at the level of the upper border of the thyroid cartilage (or the level of the disc between the third and fourth cervical vertebrae) (Figs. 1.5 to 1.13, 8.12). It gives off several branches through which it is widely distributed to structures of the head and neck outside the cranial cavity. From its origin the artery runs upwards and terminates behind the neck of the mandible. The lower part of the artery is anterior and medial to the internal carotid. Its upper part is lateral to the internal carotid. The lower part of the artery is located within the carotid triangle. (The boundaries of the triangle are shown in Fig. 8.12. Also see Fig. 2.11). Here it is relatively superficial being covered by skin, superficial and deep fascia and by the anterior margin of the sternocleidomastoid muscle. Above the triangle the artery lies deep to the posterior belly of the digastric muscle and the parotid gland. Deep to the artery there is the pharynx. The pharynx is separated from the upper part of the artery by the styloid process (and some muscles attached to it) and by the internal carotid artery. In addition to the relations mentioned above the external carotid artery is crossed by several structures that pass superficial or deep to it. These are shown in Fig. 8.13.

BRANCHES OF THE EXTERNAL CAROTID ARTERY

The branches of the external carotid artery and their levels of origin are as follows (in order of origin) (Figs. 1.6, 1.10, 8.12, 8.13).

1. The ***ascending pharyngeal*** artery arises from the deep aspect of the external carotid artery just above its lower end.
2. The ***superior thyroid*** artery arises from the front of the external carotid just below the level of the greater cornu of the hyoid bone.
3. The ***lingual*** artery arises from the front of the external carotid artery opposite the tip of the greater cornu of the hyoid bone.
4. The ***facial*** artery arises from the front of the external carotid a little above the origin of the lingual artery.
5. The ***occipital*** artery arises from the back of the external carotid opposite the origin of the facial artery.
6. The ***posterior auricular*** artery arises from the back of the external carotid just above the level at which the latter is crossed by the posterior belly of the digastric muscle.

7 and 8. The ***superficial temporal*** artery and the ***maxillary*** artery are terminal branches of the external carotid artery. They begin behind the neck of the mandible, in the substance of the parotid gland.

These branches will be considered one by one.

Ascending Pharyngeal Artery

The ascending pharyngeal artery runs upwards to the base of the skull, lying between the pharynx and the internal carotid artery. Its distribution is shown in Fig. 8.14

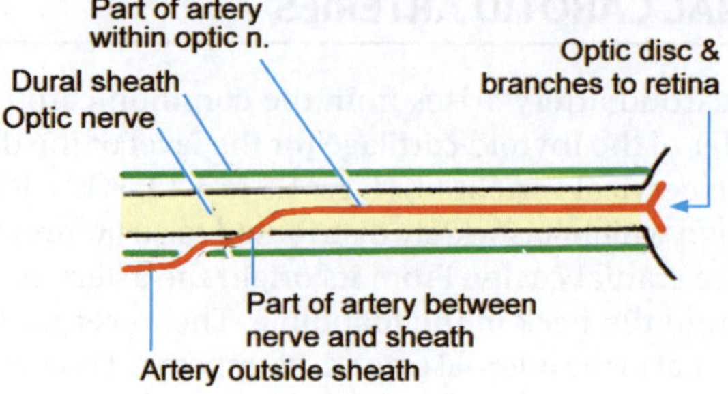

Fig. 8.11 Course of central artery of retina.

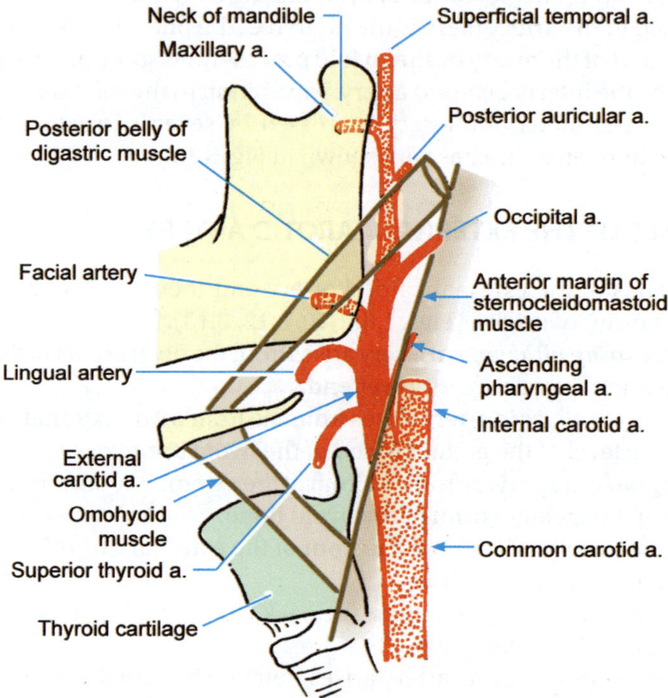

Fig. 8.12 Scheme to show the landmarks to which the external carotid artery, and its branches, are related. The boundaries of the carotid triangle are shown in interrupted line.

Superior Thyroid Artery

The superior thyroid artery runs downwards and medially to reach the upper pole of the thyroid gland. Here it divides into ***anterior*** and ***posterior thyroid branches*** (Figs. 1.11, 1.13, 8.15). These branches ramify over the corresponding surfaces of the gland. The terminal part of the anterior branch runs across the upper part of the isthmus of the gland to anastomose with the artery of the opposite side. The posterior branch runs downwards along the posterior border of the thyroid to anastomose with the inferior thyroid artery. Other branches of the superior thyroid artery are shown in Fig. 8.15.

Lingual Artery

The lingual artery arises from the external carotid artery opposite the tip of the greater cornu of the hyoid bone (Fig. 1.8). The ***first part*** of the artery lies in the carotid triangle, superficial to the middle constrictor of the pharynx (Fig. 8.16). It forms a characteristic upward loop which is crossed by the hypoglossal nerve. The ***second part*** of the artery lies deep to the hyoglossus muscle which separates it from the hypoglossal nerve. This part of the artery also lies on the middle constrictor. The ***third or deep part*** of the artery runs upwards along the anterior margin of the hyoglossus; and then forwards to the tip of the tongue. This part lies on the genioglossus muscle. The branches of the lingual artery are shown in Fig. 8.16.

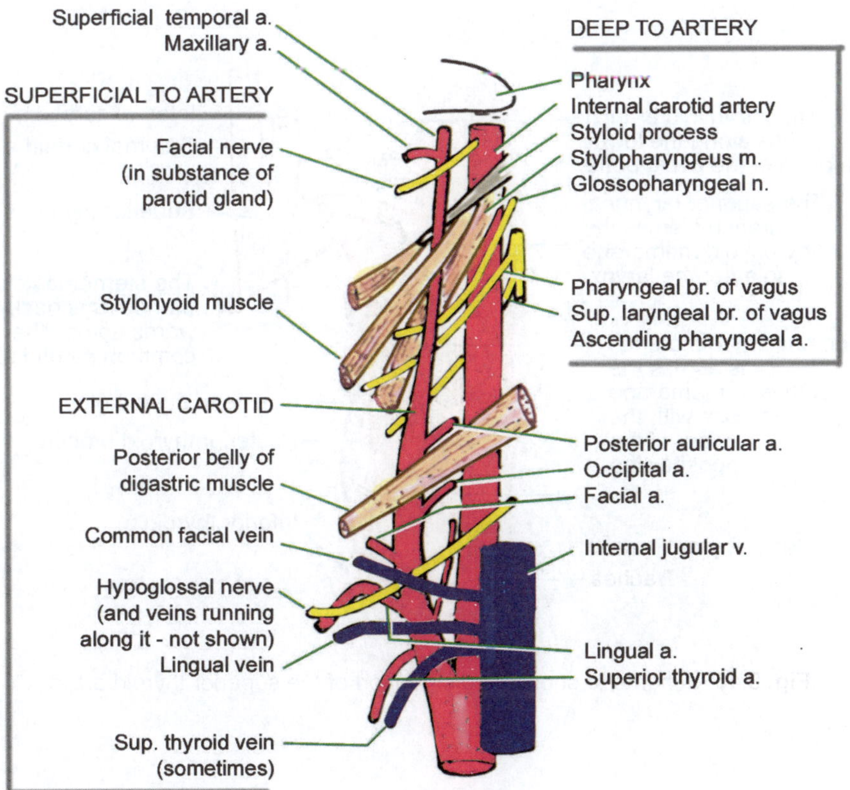

Fig. 8.13 Diagram to show structures crossing the external carotid artery.

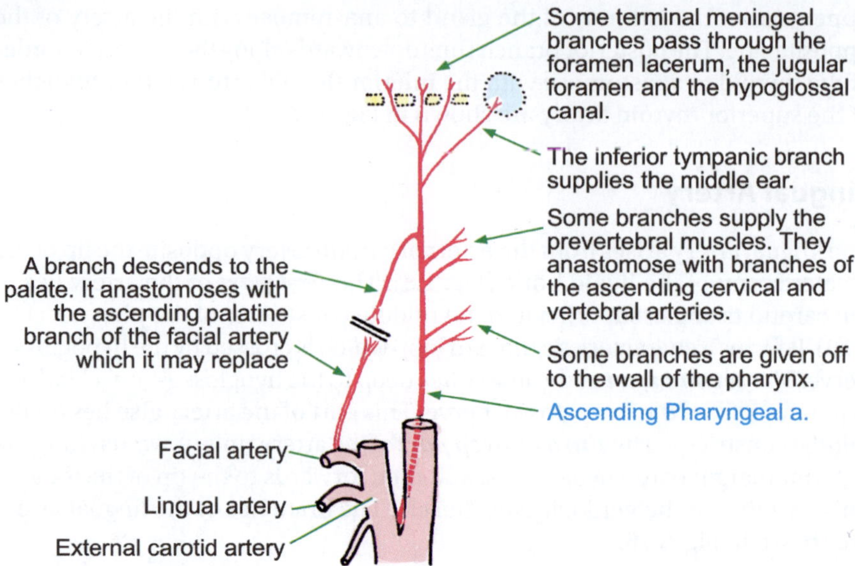

Fig. 8.14 Scheme to show the distribution of the ascending pharyngeal artery.

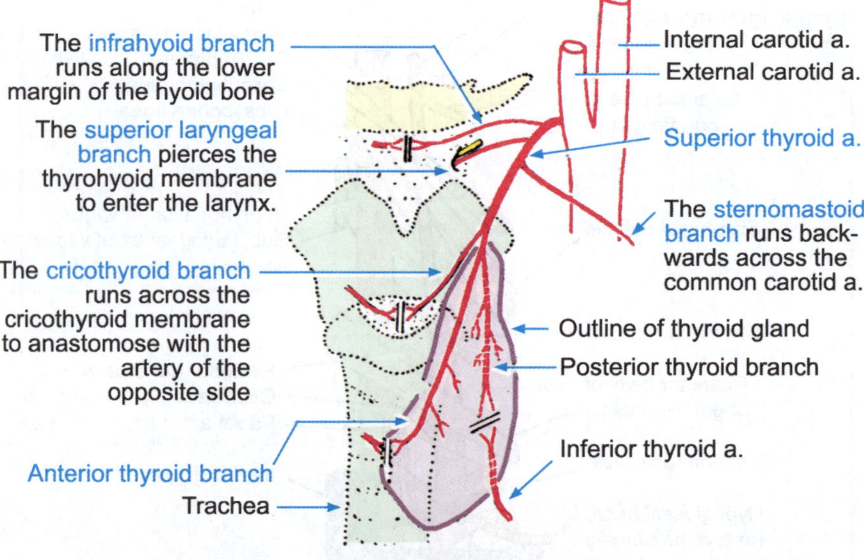

Fig. 8.15 Scheme to show the distribution of the superior thyroid artery.

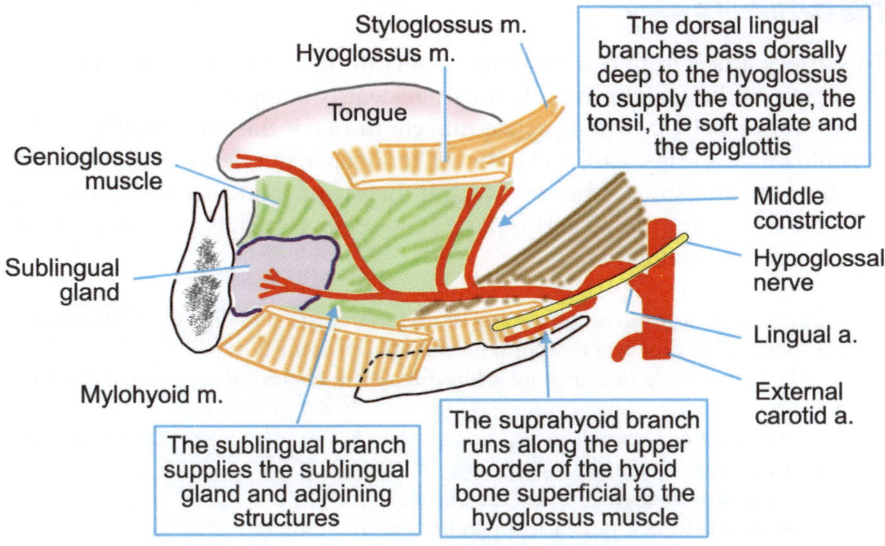

Fig. 8.16 Scheme to show the branches of the lingual artery.

The Facial Artery

The facial artery arises from the external carotid just above the greater cornu of the hyoid bone (Figs. 1.4, 1.5, 8.18). Its initial part lies deep to the ramus of the mandible, near the angle. This part is closely related to the submandibular gland. The artery first runs upwards along the posterior border of the gland and then downwards and forwards between the gland (deep to it) and the medial pterygoid muscle (superficial to it) (Fig. 8.17). It reaches the lower border of the mandible at the anterior edge of the masseter (Fig. 8.18). Curving round this border the artery runs upwards and forwards across the superficial aspect of the body of the mandible, and across the buccinator muscle to reach the angle of the mouth. It then runs upwards along the side of the nose to reach the medial angle of the palpebral fissure.

The branches of the facial artery are shown in Fig. 8.18. They are as follows:

1. The ***ascending palatine*** artery ascends on the side wall of the pharynx. It supplies the pharynx, the palate, the tonsil and the auditory tube.
2. The ***tonsillar*** branch reaches the tonsil by piercing the superior constrictor muscle.
3. Some branches are given off to the submandibular gland.
4. The ***submental*** artery runs forwards along the lower border of the mandible (over the mylohyoid muscle). It supplies muscles of the region including those of the chin and the lower lip.
5. The ***superior*** and ***inferior labial*** branches supply the lips.
6. The ***lateral nasal*** branch supplies the side of the nose.
7. The terminal part of the facial artery is called the ***angular*** artery.

The Occipital Artery

This artery arises from the posterior aspect of the external carotid opposite the origin of the facial artery. It runs backwards along the lower border of the posterior belly of the digastric muscle to reach the skull medial to the mastoid process (Figs. 1.10, 1.11). Here it lies deep to the sternocleidomastoid, the digastric and some other muscles. It then runs medially, and becoming superficial supplies the posterior part of the scalp. Here it is accompanied by the greater occipital nerve.

The occipital artery gives off several branches that are shown in Fig. 8.19. These are as follows. (Numbers correspond to those in the figure).

1, 2. Two branches ***to the sternocleidomastoid*** run backwards across the carotid sheath.
3. The ***stylomastoid branch*** enters the stylomastoid foramen to supply the middle ear and related structures.
4. The ***auricular branch*** supplies the pinna.
5. The ***mastoid branch*** passes through the mastoid foramen.
6. ***Meningeal branches*** enter the skull through the jugular foramen and the carotid canal.
7. The ***descending branch*** runs down through the deep muscles of the back of the neck. It divides into a superficial branch (7a) which anastomoses with the transverse cervical artery and a deep branch (7b) which anastomoses with branches of the vertebral and deep cervical arteries.
8. The ***occipital branches*** supply the posterior part of the scalp.
9. A ***meningeal branch*** may enter the cranium through the parietal foramen.

The Posterior Auricular Artery

This artery arises from the external carotid just above the posterior belly of the digastric muscle (and stylohyoid muscle). It passes backwards and upwards deep to the parotid gland to reach the mastoid process (Fig. 1.5). The branches of the artery are shown in Fig. 8.20.

The Maxillary Artery

This is one of the terminal branches of the external carotid artery. It begins behind the neck of the mandible, within the substance of the parotid gland. For convenience of description it is divided into three parts. The ***first part*** passes forwards deep to the neck of the mandible to reach the infratemporal fossa. Here it runs forwards along the lower border of the lateral pterygoid muscle (Figs. 1.6, 8.21). The ***second part*** of the artery runs forwards and upwards superficial to the lower head of the lateral pterygoid muscle. Frequently, the artery lies deep to the lower head and in that case it may form a loop that projects laterally between the two heads. The ***third part*** of the artery passes between the upper and lower heads of the lateral pterygoid muscle to pass through the pterygomaxillary fissure thus entering the pterygopalatine fossa.

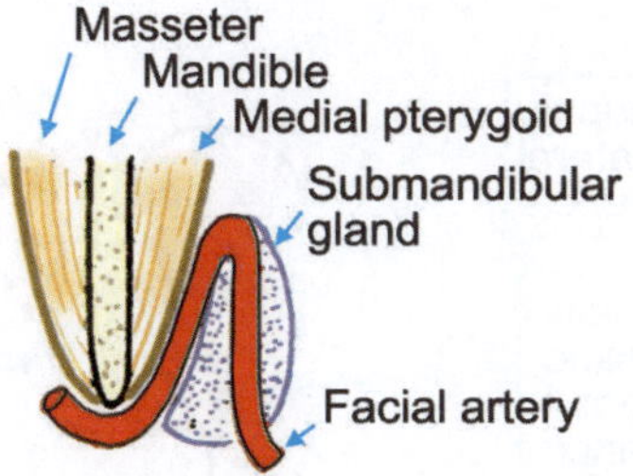

Fig. 8.17 Scheme to show the relationship of the facial artery to the submandibular gland.

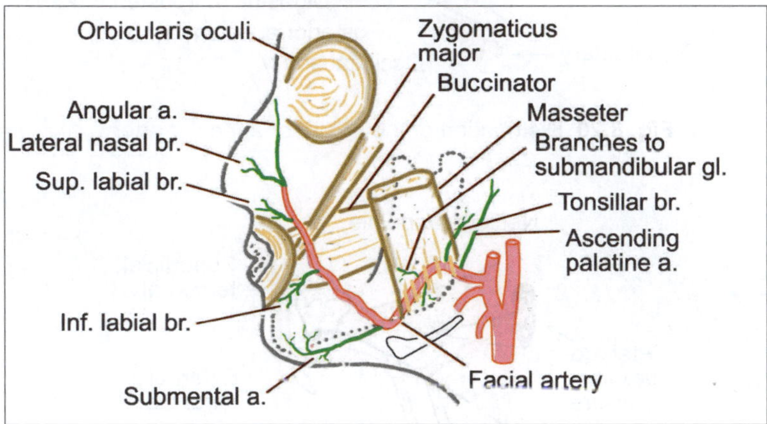

Fig. 8.18 Scheme to show branches of the facial artery.

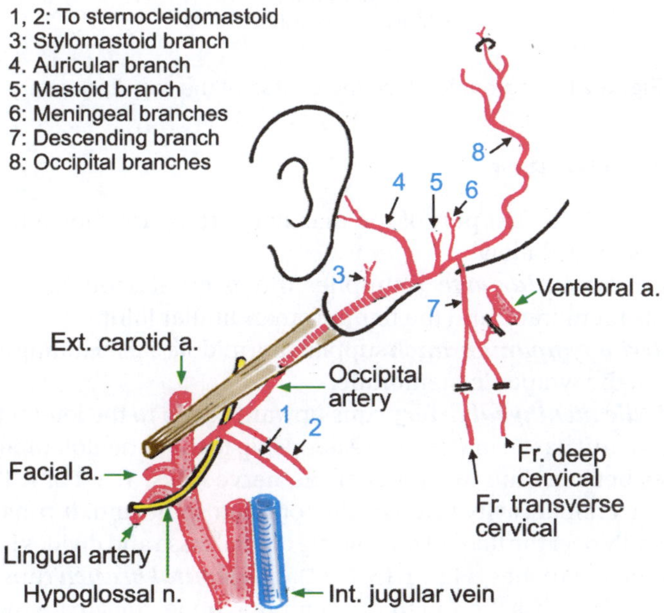

Fig. 8.19 Scheme to show the distribution of the occipital artery.

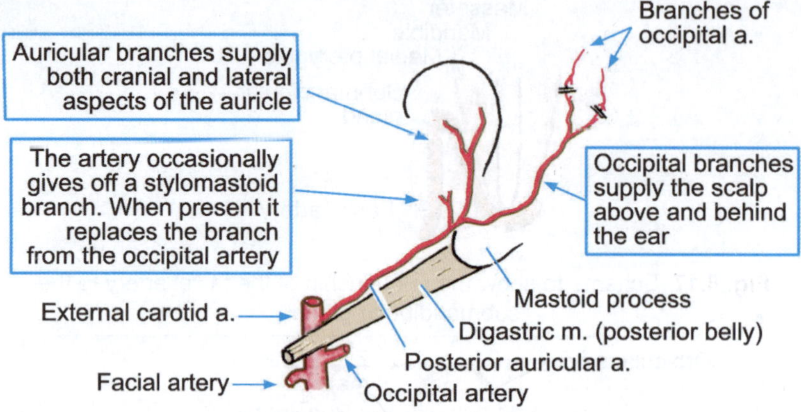

Fig. 8.20 Distribution of the posterior auricular artery.

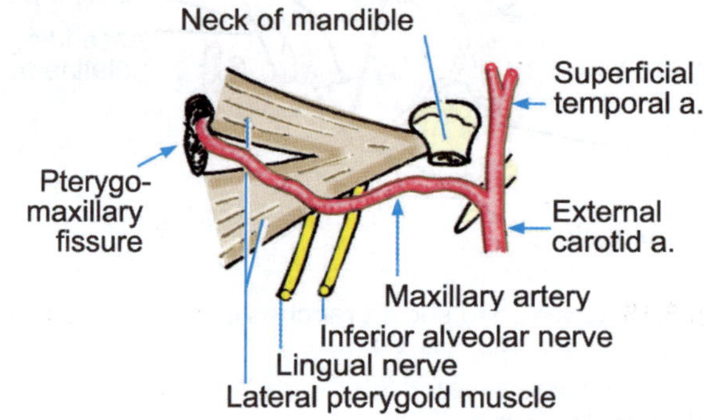

Fig. 8.21 Diagram to show the course of the maxillary artery.

Branches of First Part

The branches of the first part of the maxillary artery are shown in Fig. 8.22. They are described below.

1. The ***deep auricular artery*** supplies the external acoustic meatus, the tympanic membrane and the temporomandibular joint.
2. The ***anterior tympanic branch*** supplies the middle ear including the medial surface of the tympanic membrane.
3. The ***middle meningeal artery*** runs upwards deep to the lateral pterygoid muscle. Here it has an interesting relationship to the auriculotemporal nerve: it passes between the two roots of the nerve (Figs. 1.7, 8.22). The artery enters the cranial cavity through the foramen spinosum. It runs forwards and laterally over the floor of the middle cranial fossa and divides into frontal and parietal branches (Figs. 1.16, 8.23). The ***frontal branch*** runs forwards and upwards across the squamous temporal bone, the greater wing of the sphenoid and the anteroinferior angle of the parietal bone. It divides into branches that run predominantly upwards or backwards over the inner

surface of the parietal bone. The ***parietal branch*** first runs backwards on the squamous temporal bone and then over the parietal bone.

The following additional points about the middle meningeal artery are worth noting.

a. It is the largest artery supplying the meninges.
b. In Fig. 8.23 note that the frontal branch of the artery lies deep to the pterion (circular area at which the frontal, parietal, temporal and sphenoid bones meet); and it can be approached surgically by drilling a hole in the skull in this situation.
c. Apart from the meninges the artery supplies the skull bones over which it ramifies, the middle ear (and related structures: the facial nerve, the tensor tympani, the auditory tube) and the trigeminal ganglion.

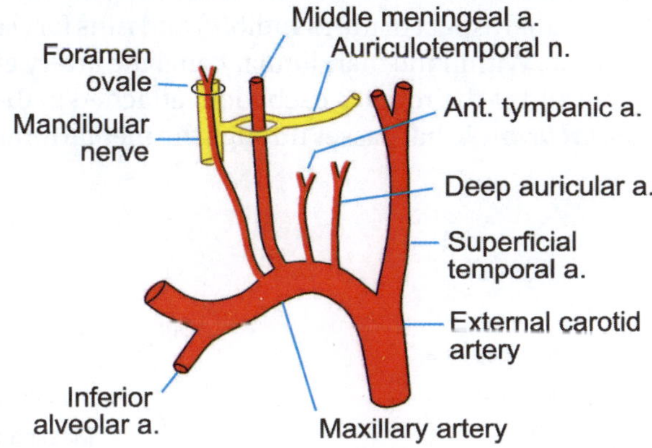

Fig. 8.22 Branches of the first part of the maxillary artery.

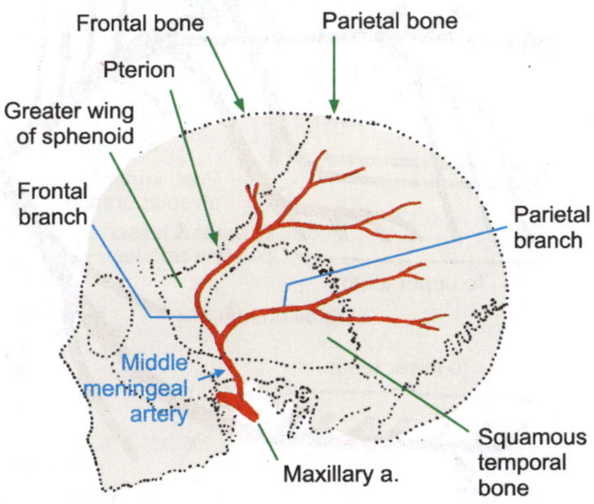

Fig. 8.23 Schematic diagram showing the course of the middle meningeal artery as projected on to the lateral aspect of the skull.

d. A branch of the artery passes through the inferior orbital fissure to anastomose with the recurrent meningeal branch of the lacrimal artery. Occasionally this anastomosis may be large and the lacrimal artery may then appear to be a branch of the middle meningeal.

4. The ***accessory meningeal branch*** enters the cranial cavity through the foramen ovale. Apart from the meninges it supplies structures in the infratemporal fossa (Fig. 8.22).

5. The ***inferior alveolar artery*** (Figs. 1.6, 8.24) runs downwards and forwards medial to the ramus of the mandible to reach the mandibular foramen. Passing through this foramen the artery enters the mandibular canal (within the body of the mandible) in which it runs downwards and then forwards. Before entering the mandibular canal the artery gives off a ***lingual branch*** to the tongue; and a ***mylohyoid branch*** that descends in the mylohyoid groove (on the medial aspect of the mandible) and runs forwards above the mylohyoid muscle. Within the mandibular canal the artery gives branches to the mandible and to the roots of each tooth attached to the bone. It also gives off a ***mental branch*** that passes through the mental foramen to supply the chin.

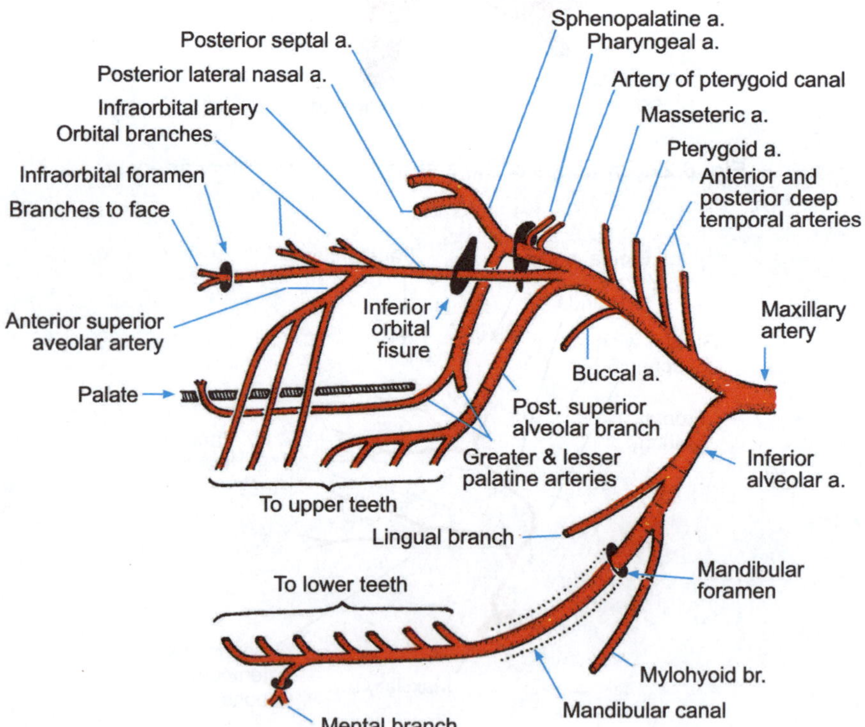

Fig. 8.24 Branches of the maxillary artery

Branches of Second Part

The branches of the second part of the maxillary artery (Fig. 8.24) are mainly muscular. The ***deep temporal*** branches (anterior and posterior) ascend on the lateral aspect of the skull deep to the temporalis muscle. Branches are also given off ***to the pterygoid muscles*** and ***to the masseter. A buccal branch*** supplies the buccinator muscle.

Branches of Third Part

The branches of the third part of the maxillary artery are shown in Fig. 8.24. They are as follows:

1. The ***posterior superior alveolar artery*** arises just before the maxillary artery enters the pterygomaxillary fissure. It descends on the posterior surface of the maxilla and gives branches that enter canals in the bone to supply the molar and premolar teeth, and the maxillary air sinus.
2. The ***infraorbital artery*** also arises just before the maxillary artery enters the pterygomaxillary fissure. It enters the orbit through the inferior orbital fissure. It runs forwards in relation to the floor of the orbit, first in the infraorbital groove and then in the infraorbital canal to emerge on the face through the infraorbital foramen. It gives off some orbital branches to structures in the orbit, and ***anterior superior alveolar*** branches that enter apertures in the maxilla to reach the incisor and canine teeth attached to the bone. After emerging on the face the infraorbital artery gives branches to the lacrimal sac, the nose and the upper lip.

   The remaining branches of the third part arise within the pterygopalatine fossa (the openings related to which should be reviewed to facilitate understanding.
3. The ***greater palatine artery*** runs downwards in the greater palatine canal to emerge on the posterolateral part of the hard palate through the greater palatine foramen.

   It then runs forwards near the lateral margin of the palate to reach the incisive canal (near the midline) through which some terminal branches enter the nasal cavity. Branches of the artery supply the palate and gums. While still within the greater palatine canal it gives off the ***lesser palatine arteries*** that emerge on the palate through lesser palatine foramina and run backwards into the soft palate and tonsil.
4. The ***pharyngeal branch*** runs backwards through a canal related to the inferior aspect of the body of the sphenoid bone (pharyngeal or palatinovaginal canal). It supplies part of the nasopharynx, the auditory tube and the sphenoidal air sinus.
5. The ***artery of the pterygoid canal*** runs backwards in the canal of the same name and helps to supply the pharynx, the auditory tube and the tympanic cavity.
6. The ***sphenopalatine artery*** passes medially through the sphenopalatine foramen to enter the cavity of the nose. It gives off ***posterolateral nasal*** branches to the lateral wall of the nose and the paranasal sinuses; and ***posterior septal branches*** to the nasal septum.

The Superficial Temporal Artery

This is the second terminal branch of the external carotid artery. It begins behind the neck of the mandible in the substance of the parotid gland. It runs upwards behind the temporomandibular joint and ramifies in the scalp over the temporal region. It is accompanied by the auriculotemporal nerve. The branches of the artery are shown in Fig. 8.25.

1. The ***frontal branch*** runs upwards and forwards in the part of the scalp overlying the temporal and frontal bones.
2. The ***parietal branch*** runs backwards in the scalp overlying the temporal and parietal bones.
3. The ***anterior auricular branch*** supplies part of the auricle and the external acoustic meatus.
4. The ***middle temporal artery*** supplies the temporalis.
5. The ***zygomatico-orbital branch*** runs forwards along the upper border of the zygomatic arch up to the lateral angle of the eye.
6. The ***transverse facial branch*** arises within the substance of the parotid gland. It runs forwards across the masseter above the parotid duct.

THE SUBCLAVIAN ARTERIES

We have seen that the right subclavian artery is a branch of the brachiocephalic trunk and begins behind the right sternoclavicular joint. The left subclavian artery is a direct branch of the aorta. It has a thoracic part which ends behind the left sternoclavicular joint. Thereafter, the course and relations of the right and left subclavian arteries are similar (with minor exceptions).

Each subclavian artery is the initial part of a long channel that supplies the upper limb. Entering the neck behind the corresponding sternoclavicular joint the artery loops upwards into the neck. It leaves the neck by passing into the axilla, where it becomes the axillary artery. The subclavian artery (whole of right, and cervical part of left) extends from the sternoclavicular joint to the outer border of the first rib. The artery has numerous relationships which are best understood by gradually building them up.

Because of the oblique placement of the inlet of the thorax the apex of the lung appears to extend for some distance into the neck. The pleura covering this part of the lung is called the cervical pleura. The cervical pleura is covered by the suprapleural membrane. The subclavian artery lies in front of these structures as it arches across the lower part of the neck (Fig. 8.26). In Fig. 8.27 it is seen that the artery is crossed anteriorly by the lower part of the scalenus anterior muscle (which gains insertion into the first rib just in front of the artery). It divides the artery in to the first part, medial to the muscle; the second part deep to it; and the third part lateral to it.

Some more structures covering the subclavian artery are shown in Fig. 1.13. The medial most part of the subclavian artery lies behind the common carotid artery. Immediately lateral to the latter the internal jugular vein runs vertically across the subclavian artery to join the subclavian vein (Fig. 1.12). The subclavian vein lies below and in front of the artery separated from it by the scalenus anterior muscle (Fig. 8.30). The artery is also crossed vertically by the vagus nerve which lies behind the internal jugular vein (Fig. 8.28). In other words the medial part of the subclavian artery is crossed by all structures

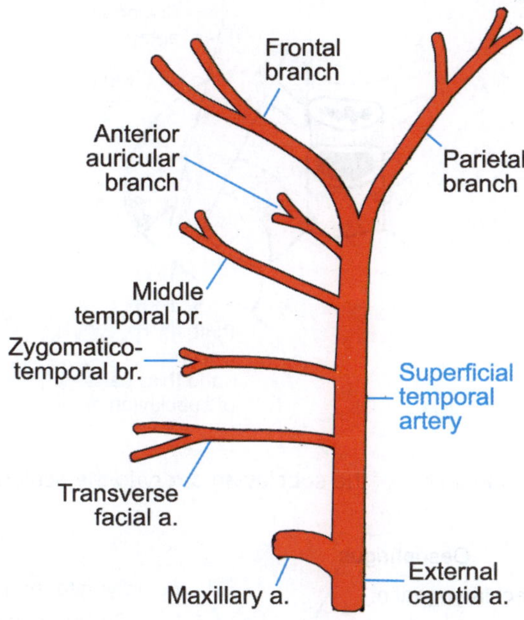

Fig. 8.25 Scheme to show the branches of the superficial temporal artery.

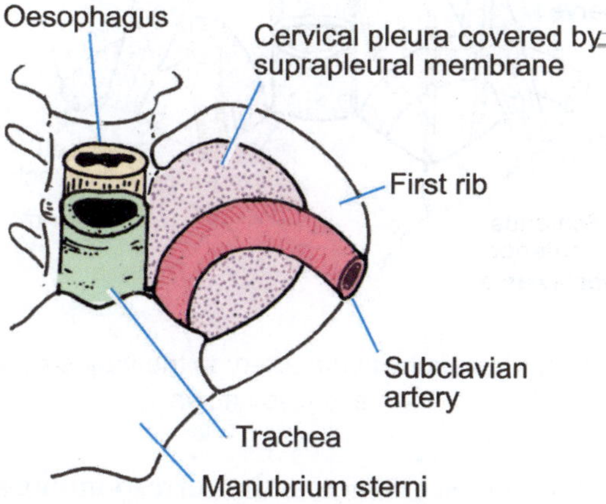

Fig. 8.26 Relationship of the subclavian artery to cervical pleura and to the first rib.

enclosed by the carotid sheath. The right vagus nerve gives off its recurrent laryngeal branch just as it reaches the lower margin of the subclavian artery. The recurrent laryngeal nerve curves around the inferior and posterior aspects of the artery and runs medially to reach the groove between the trachea and the oesophagus. Note that the left recurrent laryngeal nerve arises from the vagus below the arch of the aorta, winds round the ligamentum arteriosum and ascends in the groove between the trachea and the oesophagus. It is not closely related to the left subclavian artery in the neck.

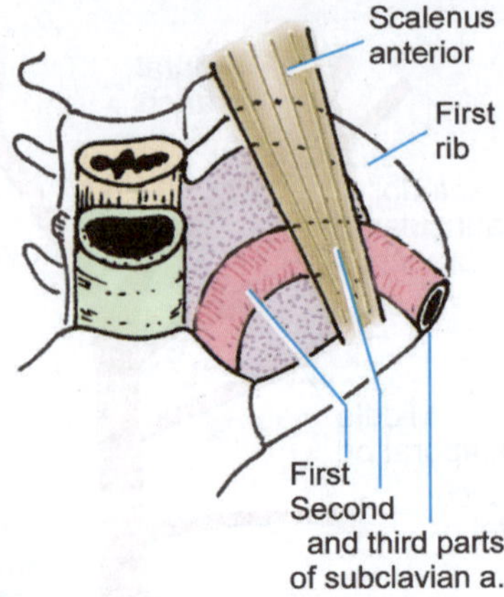

Fig. 8.27 Relationship of the subclavian artery to the scalenus anterior.

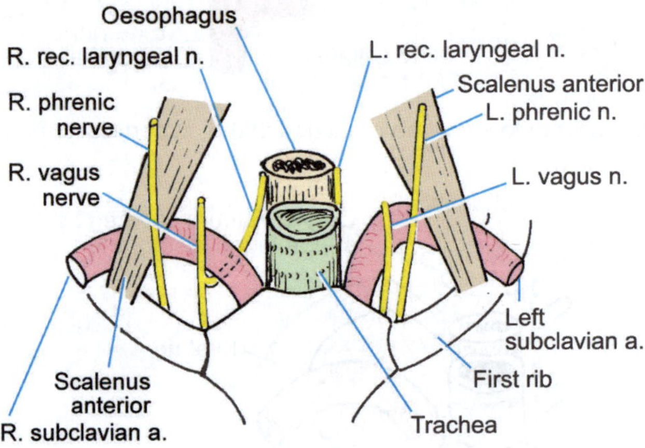

Fig. 8.28 Relationship of subclavian artery to the vagus nerve. The phrenic nerve is also shown.

Note that the nerves descend across the corresponding scalenus anterior muscle. On the left side the nerve passes across the medial border of the muscle on to the front of the first part of the subclavian artery. On the right side the nerve usually crosses the medial border of the muscle lower down so that the nerve does not come into direct contact with the first part of the subclavian artery, but is separated from the second part by the scalenus anterior. Occasionally, however, the relationship may be the same as on the left side.

The relationship of the subclavian artery to the brachial plexus is shown in the left half of Fig. 8.29. Observe that the plexus passes downwards and laterally across the lower part of the neck. The first part of the artery lies below the level of the plexus, but the second and third parts come into relationship with the trunks of the plexus. The lower trunk lies behind and below the second and third parts of the artery. The upper and middle trunks lie above the second part of the artery, and above and lateral to its third part.

The right half of Fig. 8.29 shows the relationship of the subclavian artery to the ansa subclavia. This is a nerve cord that descends from the middle cervical sympathetic ganglion to the front of the first part of the artery, and looping round it ascends behind it to reach the inferior cervical (cervicothoracic) sympathetic ganglion.

The terminal part of the thoracic duct comes into relationship with the first part of the left subclavian artery (Fig. 8.30). After ascending into the neck along the lateral side of the oesophagus the duct turns laterally forming a wide loop that is convex upwards. The terminal part of this loop descends in front of the artery (near the medial border of the scalenus anterior) to terminate by joining the junction of the left internal jugular and subclavian veins.

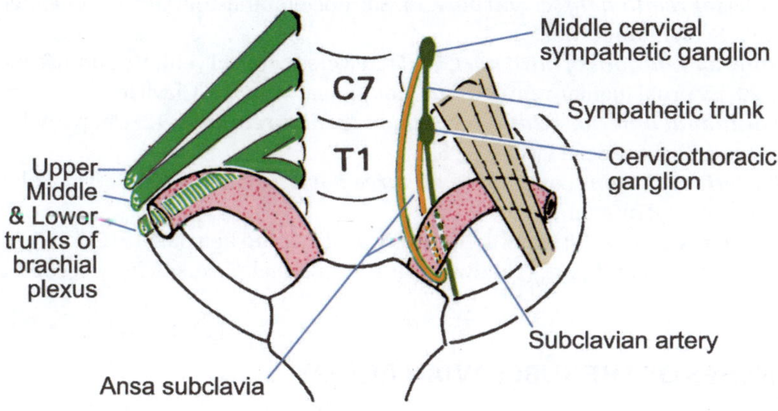

Fig. 8.29 Relationship of subclavian artery to the brachial plexus and to the ansa subclavia.

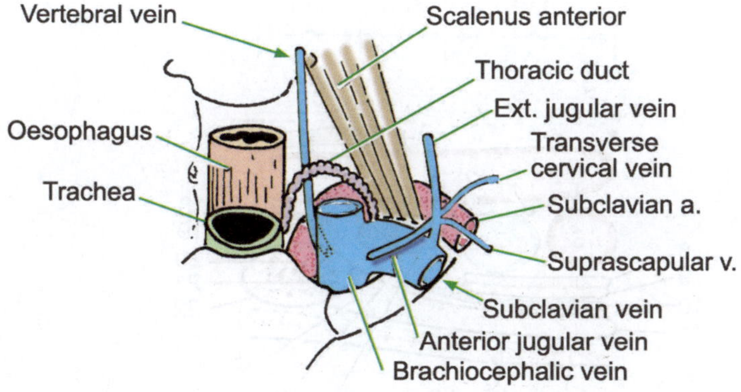

Fig. 8.30 Scheme to show the veins related to the subclavian artery. The thoracic duct is also shown.

The relationship of the subclavian artery to the internal jugular and subclavian veins has already been noted. Some other veins related to it are shown in Fig. 8.30. The vertebral vein descends across the first part of the artery to end in the brachiocephalic vein. The external jugular vein descends across the third part of the artery to end in the subclavian vein. In front of the artery it is joined by the transverse cervical, suprascapular and anterior jugular veins.

In the foregoing paragraphs we have considered numerous structures that cross in front of the subclavian artery. These and some additional relations are shown schematically in Fig. 8.31. They can be summarised as follows. Numbers correspond to those in the figure.

Anterior relations of first part: 1. Phrenic nerve. 2. Thoracic duct. 3. Vagus nerve. 4. Vertebral artery. 5. Ansa subclavia. 6. Common carotid artery. 7. Internal jugular vein. 8. Sternothyroid muscle. 9. Sternohyoid muscle. 10. Anterior jugular vein. 11. Sternocleidomastoid muscle.

Anterior relations of second part: 15. Sternocleidomastoid. 16. Anterior jugular vein. 17. Scalenus anterior.

Anterior relations of third part: 18. Transverse cervical vein. 19. Suprascapular vein. 20. External jugular vein. 21. Anterior jugular vein. 22. Clavicle.

Additional anterior relations common to all three parts: 12. Deep fascia. 13. Platysma and superficial fascia. 14. Skin.

Posterior relations common to all three parts: (a). Lung. (b) Cervical pleura. (c) Suprapleural membrane.

Other posterior relations: (d) Ansa subclavia behind first part. (e) Costocervical trunk behind second part. (f) Lower trunk of brachial plexus behind second and third parts.

BRANCHES OF THE SUBCLAVIAN ARTERY

The subclavian artery gives origin to several branches which are shown in Fig. 8.32. A brief introduction to these branches is given below. Each branch is considered in detail in subsequent pages.

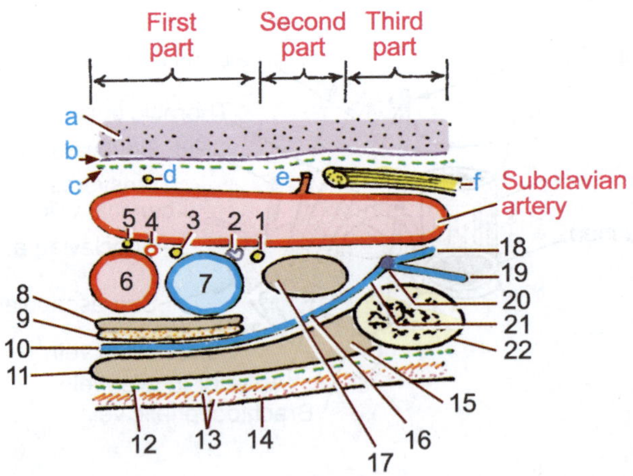

Fig. 8.31 Scheme to show the relations of the subclavian artery. For explanation of numbers see text.

1. The ***vertebral artery*** arises from the first part. It runs upwards to enter the foramen transversarium of the sixth cervical vertebra .
2. The ***internal thoracic*** artery arises from the first part and runs downwards into the thorax.
3. The ***thyrocervical trunk*** is a short vessel arising just medial to the scalenus anterior muscle i.e., from the first part. On the right side it usually arises behind the scalenus anterior (then being a branch of the second part). It divides into the inferior thyroid, suprascapular and transverse cervical arteries.
4. The ***costocervical trunk*** arises either from the first or second part. It runs backwards to reach the neck of the first rib. Here it divides into the deep cervical and superior intercostal arteries.
5. The ***dorsal scapular artery*** is an occasional branch of the third part. When present it replaces the deep branch of the transverse cervical artery.

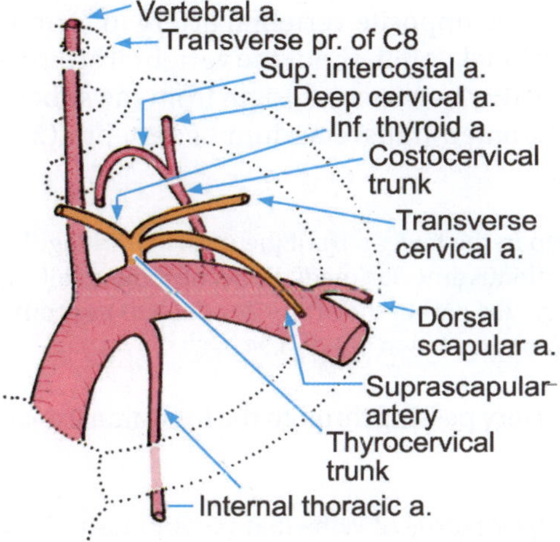

Fig. 8.32 Scheme to show the branches of the subclavian artery.

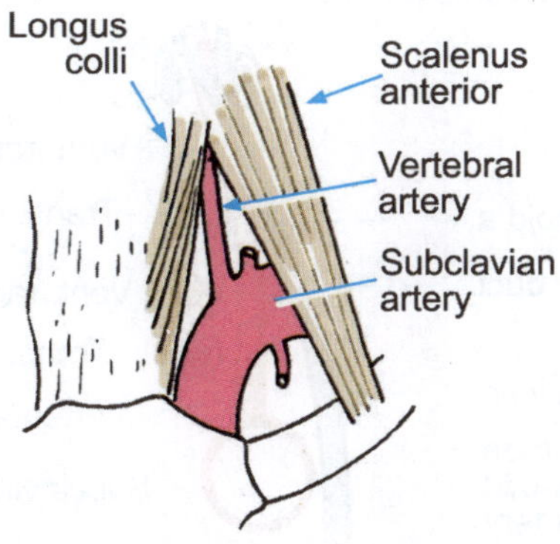

Fig. 8.33 Position of the first part of the vertebral artery.

The internal thoracic artery has been dealt with in the thorax. The other arteries are considered one by one below.

The Vertebral Artery

The Vertebral Artery arises from the first part of the subclavian artery (Figs. 1.11, 1.13, 1.14). It ascends to enter the foramen transversarium of the sixth cervical vertebra (not the seventh) and then continues upwards through the foramina of higher vertebrae. Emerging through the foramen transversarium of the atlas it winds round the lateral mass of this bone (Fig. 8.35). It then lies in the groove on the upper surface of the posterior arch of the atlas. Finally, it passes forwards into the vertebral canal and running upwards passes through the foramen magnum to enter the cranial cavity. Here it lies lateral to the lower end of the medulla oblongata. Continuing its ascent it gradually passes forwards and medially over the medulla and ends at the lower border of the pons by anastomosing with the opposite vertebral artery to form the ***basilar artery***. The following additional points about the vertebral artery may now be noted.

a. The part of the artery between its origin from the subclavian artery and its entry into the foramen transversarium of vertebra C6 constitutes its first part (Fig. 8.33).

This part lies deep in the lower part of the neck in a triangular interval bounded laterally by the scalenus anterior, medially by the longus colli, and inferiorly by the subclavian artery. This part of the artery lies deep to the common carotid. Other relations of this part are shown in Fig. 8.34.

b. The part of the artery passing through the foramina transversaria constitutes its second part.

It is surrounded by a plexus of veins that unite to form the vertebral vein; and by a plexus of sympathetic nerves derived from the cervicothoracic (or stellate) ganglion.

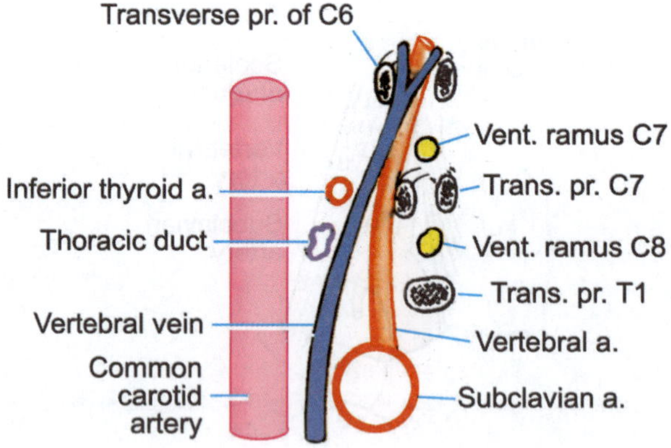

Fig. 8.34 Scheme to show anterior and posterior relations of the vertebral artery.

c. The part of the artery winding round the lateral mass of the atlas is its third part.

This part lies in the suboccipital triangle (Fig. 1.15). Its most important relation is the first cervical nerve. The dorsal ramus of the nerve runs backwards between the artery and the posterior arch of the atlas (Fig. 8.36). The ventral ramus runs forwards round the lateral mass of the atlas, where it lies medial to the artery. The vertebral artery enters the vertebral canal through an aperture bounded laterally by the lateral mass of the atlas and medially by the free lateral margin of the posterior atlanto-occipital membrane (Fig. 8.35).

The branches of the vertebral artery that supply structures in the neck are shown in Fig. 9.37. They are as follows.

1. Some ***muscular branches*** arise from the vertebral artery in the suboccipital triangle.
2. ***Spinal branches (s)*** pass through the intervertebral foramina to reach the vertebral canal. They help to supply the spinal cord and the vertebrae.
3. The ***anterior spinal arteries*** of the two sides join to form a single trunk which descends on the anterior aspect of the spinal cord, in the midline.
4. The ***posterior spinal artery*** descends along the posterolateral aspect of the spinal cord. It divides into two branches, one lying in front of the dorsal nerve roots (a) and one lying behind them (b).

The anterior and posterior spinal arteries are joined by spinal branches arising from the vertebral artery itself and from various other arteries.

In addition to the branches described above the vertebral artery gives off the ***posterior inferior cerebellar artery*** which takes part in supplying the brain. It will be considered in the section on the blood supply of the brain. The basilar artery and its branches will also be considered therein.

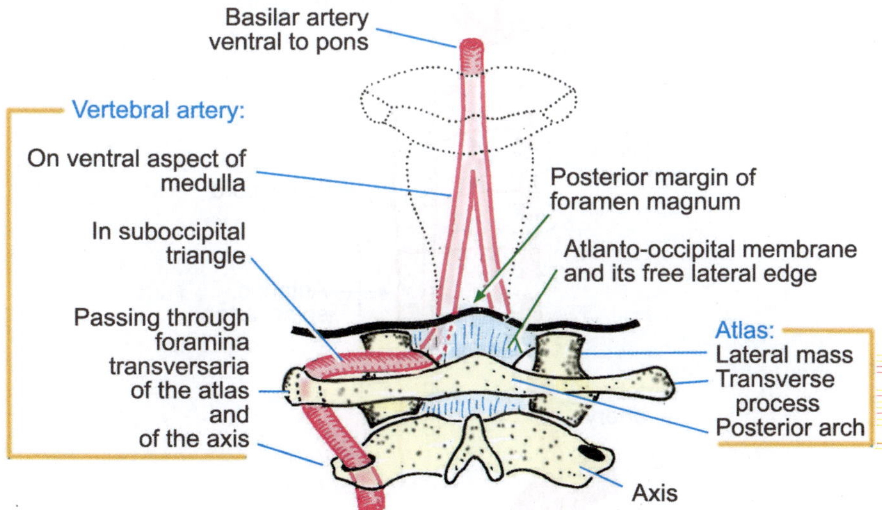

Fig. 8.35 Scheme to show the course of the upper part of the vertebral artery.

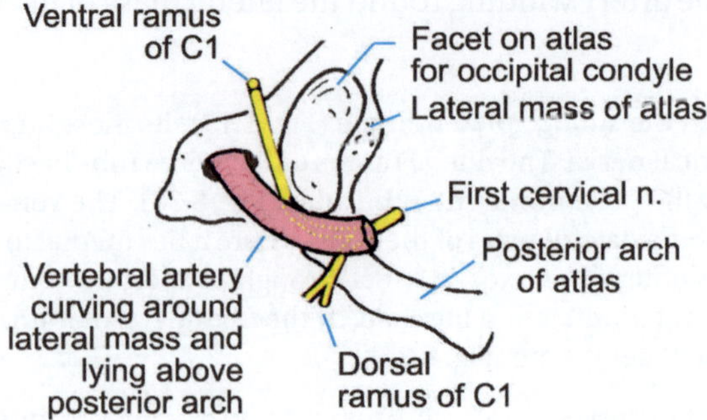

Fig. 8.36 Relationship of vertebral artery to atlas vertebra.

The Thyrocervical Trunk

The thyrocervical trunk is a short artery that arises near the junction of the first and second parts of the subclavian artery. On the left side it usually arises just medial to the scalenus anterior muscle i.e., from the first part of the subclavian artery. On the right side the trunk usually arises deep to the scalenus anterior, being a branch of the second part of the subclavian artery.

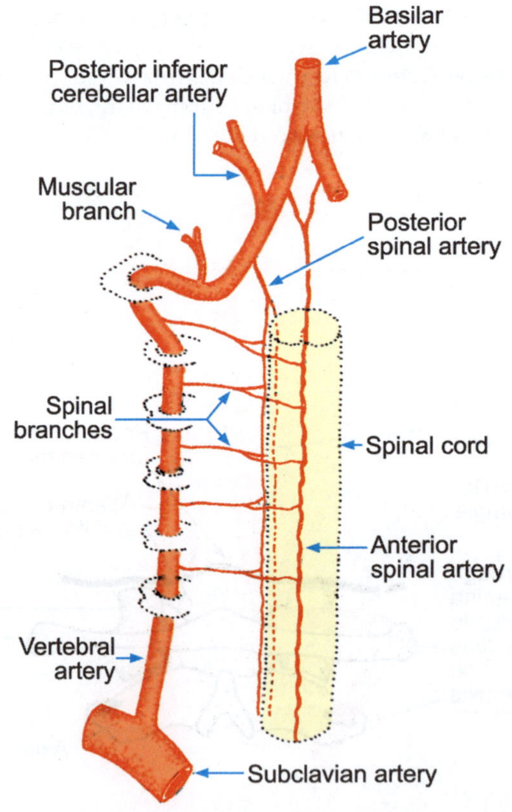

Fig. 8.37 Scheme to show the branches of the vertebral artery.

After a short course the trunk divides into three branches, namely the ***inferior thyroid*** artery, the ***suprascapular artery*** and the ***transverse cervical*** artery. The transverse cervical artery further divides into a ***superficial*** and a ***deep*** branch.

Quite frequently the deep branch arises directly from the third part of the subclavian artery. In that case the transverse cervical artery is represented only by its superficial branch and is called the ***superficial cervical*** artery. The deep branch, arising directly from the subclavian artery is called the ***dorsal scapular*** artery. The transverse cervical artery and the suprascapular artery are concerned mainly in supply of structures in the upper extremity. The inferior thyroid artery is described below.

The Inferior Thyroid Artery

This artery is a branch of the thyrocervical trunk. It runs upwards for some distance and then turns medially to reach the thyroid gland. The artery is distributed mainly to this gland through an ascending and a descending ***glandular branch.***

Other named branches arising from the inferior thyroid artery are the ***ascending cervical artery*** and the ***inferior laryngeal artery*** (Fig. 8.39). Several small branches are also given off to the pharynx, trachea, oesophagus and the infrahyoid muscles. The horizontal part of the artery is crossed by several important structures that are shown in Fig. 8.40. The relationship of the artery to the recurrent laryngeal nerve is particularly important. During the operation for removal of the thyroid (called thyroidectomy) the surgeon has to ligate the artery, and has to be careful that the nerve is not injured. In this connection it is important to remember that the nerve may (i) cross in front of the terminal branches of the artery; (ii) may pass behind them; or (iii) may have some branches in front of the nerve and some behind it (Fig. 8.41). Note that the artery comes into relationship with the nerve only near the thyroid gland and that it can be ligated safely some distance away from the gland. (In contrast the superior thyroid artery is closely related to the external laryngeal nerve some distance away from the gland and is safely ligated close to the gland.).

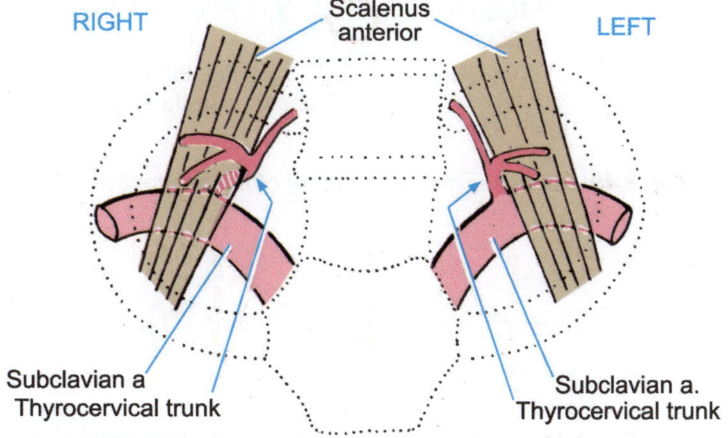

Fig. 8.38 Scheme showing the difference in the usual mode of origin of the thyrocervical trunk on the right and left sides.

The Costocervical Trunk

The costocervical trunk takes origin from the posterior aspect of the subclavian artery.

On the left side it arises from the first part, but on the right side the origin is from the second part. It runs backwards with an upward convexity following the curve of the cervical pleura to reach the neck of the first rib. Here it divides into the deep cervical and superior intercostal arteries.

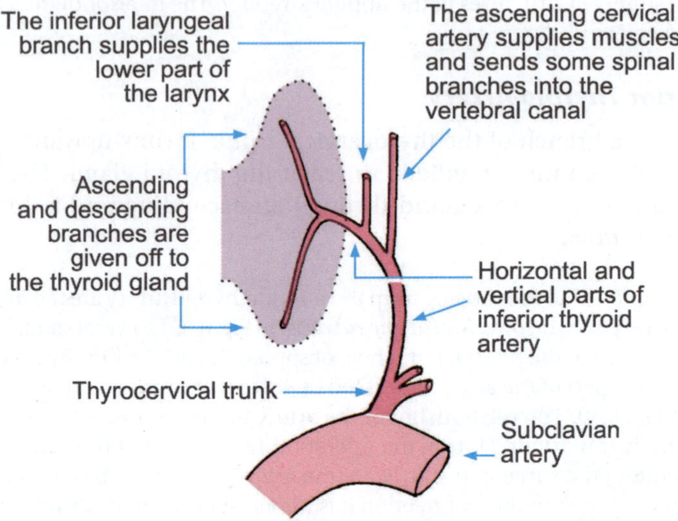

Fig. 8.39 Scheme to show the branches of the inferior thyroid artery.

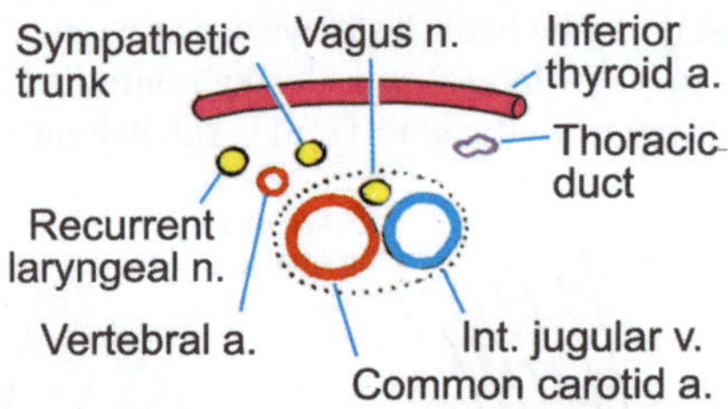

Fig. 8.40 Structures crossing in front of the inferior thyroid artery.

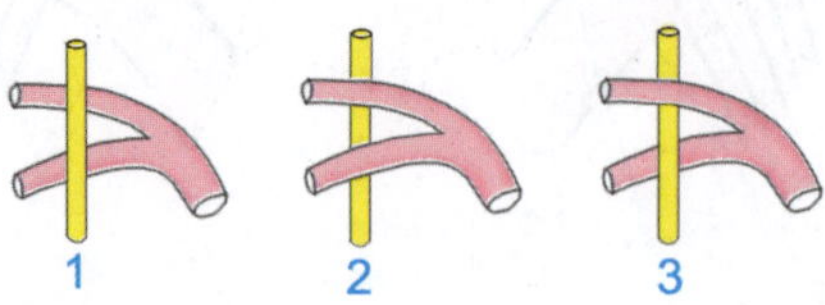

Fig. 8.41 Variations in relationship of the inferior thyroid artery to the recurrent laryngeal nerve.

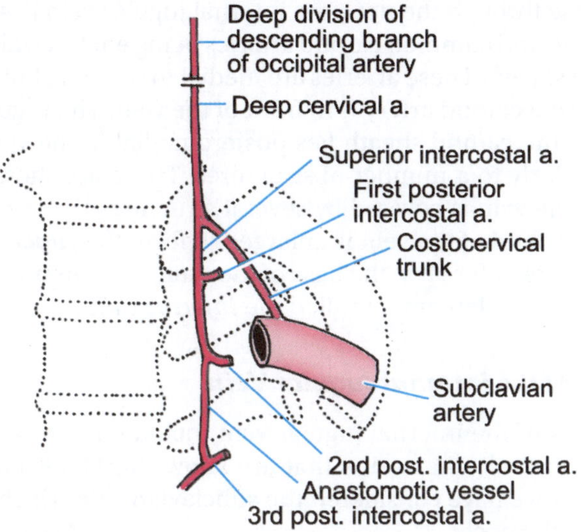

Fig. 8.42 Scheme to show the branches of the costocervical trunk.

The ***deep cervical artery*** passes backwards above the neck of the first rib to reach the back of the neck. Here it ascends through the deep muscles supplying them. It anastomoses with the deep division of the descending branch of the occipital artery.

The ***superior intercostal artery*** descends across the neck of the first rib to reach the first intercostal space.

The Dorsal Scapular Artery

The dorsal scapular artery is an occasional branch arising from the third part of the subclavian artery. When present it replaces the deep branch of the transverse cervical artery.

For ***clinical correlations*** of the arteries of the head and neck see Chapter 15.

THE VEINS

THE INTERNAL JUGULAR VEINS

The right and left internal jugular veins are the chief veins of the head and neck. On either side the upper end of the vein lies in the jugular foramen on the base of the skull. Here the internal jugular vein becomes continuous with the sigmoid sinus. The lower end of the vein lies behind the sternal end of the clavicle where the internal jugular joins the subclavian vein to form the corresponding brachiocephalic vein.

In its course through the neck the internal jugular vein lies alongside the internal carotid and common carotid arteries being enclosed along with them in the carotid sheath. These arteries are medial to the vein, but just below the skull the internal carotid artery is in front of the vein. The vagus nerve which is also within the carotid sheath lies posteromedial to the vein. The vein is related posteriorly to a number of structures. These are shown in Fig. 8.45. Superficially the vein is covered by several structures that are shown in Fig. 8.43. The upper end of the vein is enlarged to form the ***superior bulb*** which occupies the jugular fossa on the base of the skull. The inferior end of the vein may also show an enlargement called the ***inferior bulb***.

Tributaries of the Internal Jugular Vein

The tributaries of the internal jugular vein include the intracranial venous sinuses and several other veins that are shown in Fig. 8.44. They will be described after we have considered the subclavian vein which is the second largest vein of the neck.

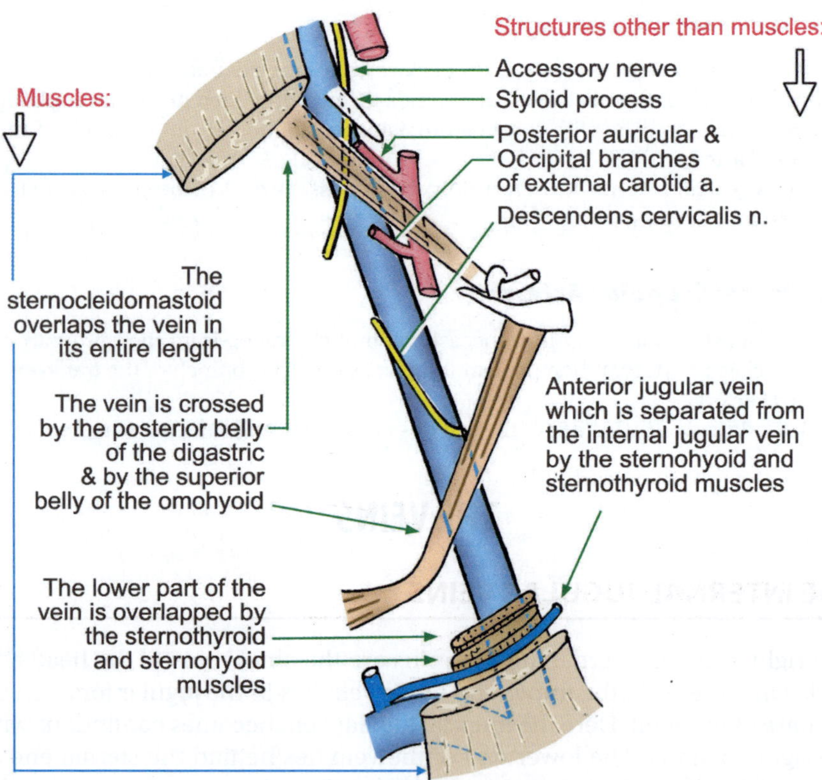

Fig. 8.43 Scheme to show the structures superficial to the internal jugular vein (lateral view). The parotid gland (not shown) is superficial to the vein above the posterior belly of the digastric muscle.

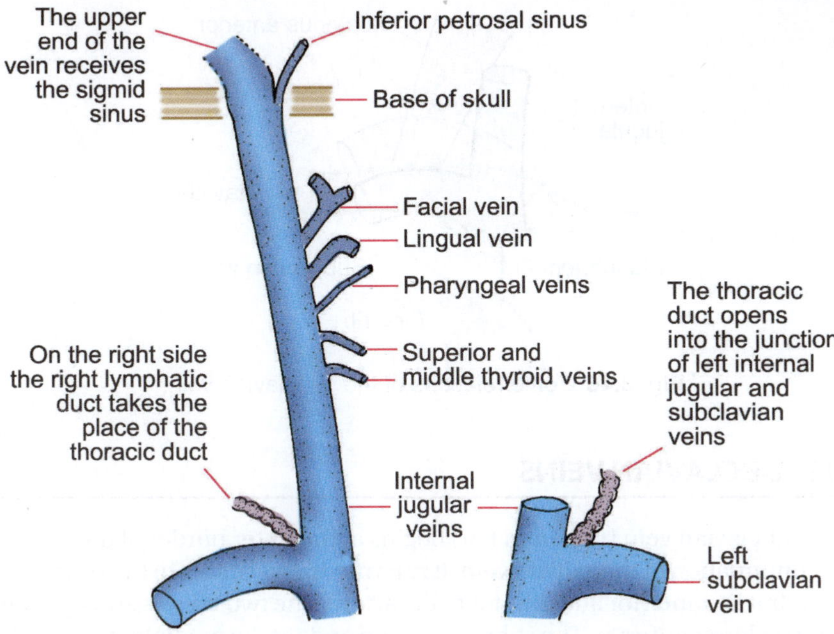

Fig. 8. 44 Scheme to show the tributaries of the internal jugular vein.

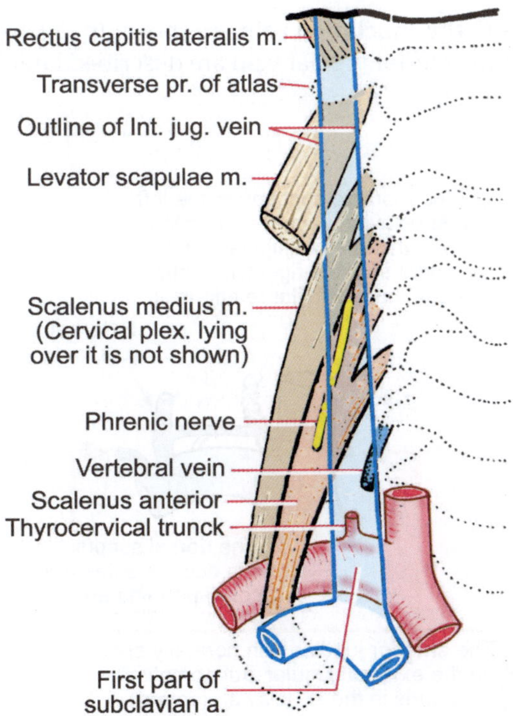

Fig. 8.45 Structures posterior to the internal jugular vein. The vein is drawn as if it was transparent. On the left side the thoracic duct is an additional relation.

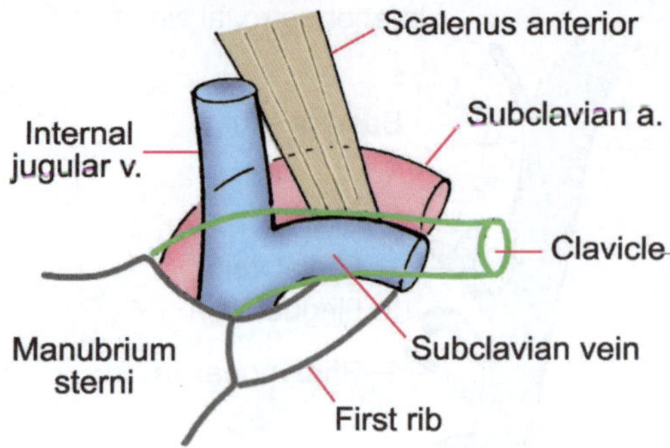

Fig. 8.46 Some relations of the subclavian vein.

THE SUBCLAVIAN VEINS

Each subclavian vein (right and left) begins at the outer border of the first rib, as a continuation of the axillary vein. It runs medially parallel to the subclavian artery, but lies anterior and inferior to the artery. The two vessels are separated by the scalenus anterior. The subclavian vein ends at the medial margin of this muscle by joining the internal jugular vein (Fig. 8.46). Anteriorly, the subclavian vein is related to the clavicle. Below, the vein rests on the first rib and on the cervical pleura.

The tributaries of the subclavian vein are shown in Fig. 8.47. The external jugular vein and the anterior jugular vein are described later in this Chapter.

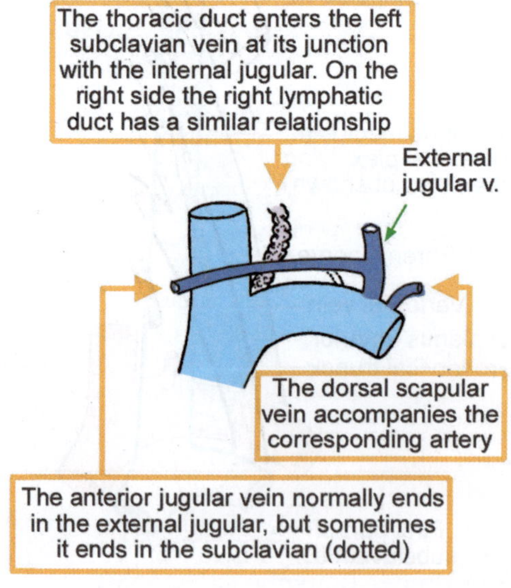

Fig. 8.47 Tributaries of the subclavian vein.

THE INTRACRANIAL VENOUS SINUSES

Within the cranial cavity there are venous channels of a special kind. Their walls are formed of duramater of which there are two layers. The outer layer of duramater (or endocranium) closely lines the inner wall of the cranial cavity. The inner layer is closely united to the outer layer over most of its extent. However, at some places the two layers are separated by spaces lined by endothelium. These spaces constitute the intracranial venous sinuses or dural venous sinuses. Various ways in which such a sinus may be formed are evident in Figs. 8.49 and 8.50. The main intracranial venous sinuses are shown schematically in Fig. 8.48 which is a left antero-lateral view. They are also seen in Figs. 8.49 and 59.50 which are coronal sections through the cranial cavity.

From the above it will be clear that the intracranial venous sinuses can be understood only after the skull and folds of duramater have been studied.

UNPAIRED SINUSES LYING IN THE MIDLINE

1. The ***superior sagittal sinus*** occupies the triangular space produced by the reflection of the inner layer of duramater to form the falx cerebri (Fig. 8.49). It begins anteriorly in front of crista galli. It then runs backwards deeply grooving the frontal bone (in the midline); the two parietal bones (where they join at the sagittal suture); and the occipital bone (again in the midline). The sinus ends at the internal occipital protuberance where it becomes continuous (usually) with the right transverse sinus (See below). Sometimes it is continuous with the left transverse sinus.
2. The ***inferior sagittal sinus*** lies within the lower free margin of the falx cerebri as shown in Fig. 8.49. It begins anteriorly and ends posteriorly by joining the straight sinus (Fig. 8.48).

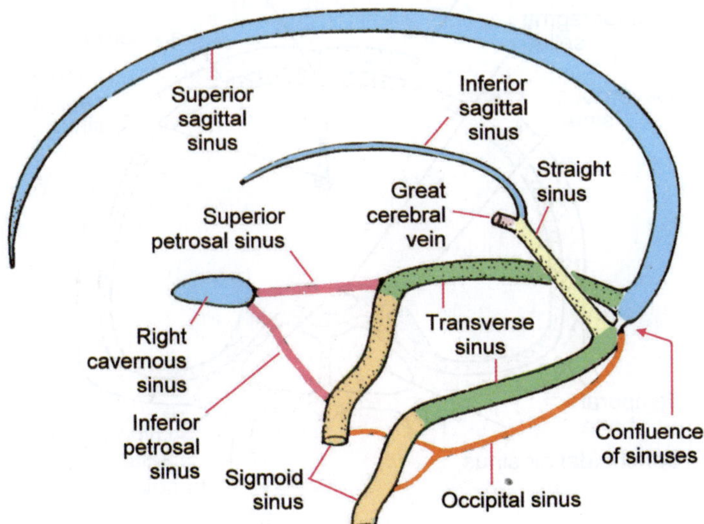

Fig. 8.48 Scheme to show the intracranial venous sinuses. The cavernous and petrosal sinuses are paired, but are shown only on one side for sake of clarity.

3. The ***straight sinus*** lies in the triangular interval where the lower edge of the posterior part of the falx cerebri joins the tentorium cerebelli. Anteriorly, it receives the inferior sagittal sinus, and a vein from the interior of the brain called the ***great cerebral vein*** (Chapter 25). Posteriorly the straight sinus ends by becoming continuous with the transverse sinus of the side opposite to that with which the superior sagittal sinus is continuous i.e., usually the left side.
   Note that several sinuses meet at the internal occipital protuberance. These are the superior sagittal sinus, the straight sinus and the right and left transverse sinuses (see below). This region is, therefore, called the ***confluence of sinuses.***
4. The ***occipital sinus*** lies in the midline in relation to the floor of the posterior cranial fossa. Here the dura is raised into a fold called the falx cerebelli; and the sinus lies within this fold. The anterior end of the occipital sinus bifurcates into two channels that pass round either side of the foramen magnum to join the corresponding sigmoid sinus. The occipital sinus ends posteriorly in the confluence of sinuses (Fig. 8.51).

LARGE PAIRED SINUSES

5. The right and left ***transverse sinuses*** lie horizontally as indicated by their names. Each sinus begins posteriorly at the internal occipital protuberance. The right sinus is usually a continuation of the superior sagittal sinus and the left sinus is usually a continuation of the straight sinus, but this arrangement is sometimes reversed. Each sinus runs in a curve at first laterally and then forwards, along the line of attachment of the tentorium cerebelli. It produces

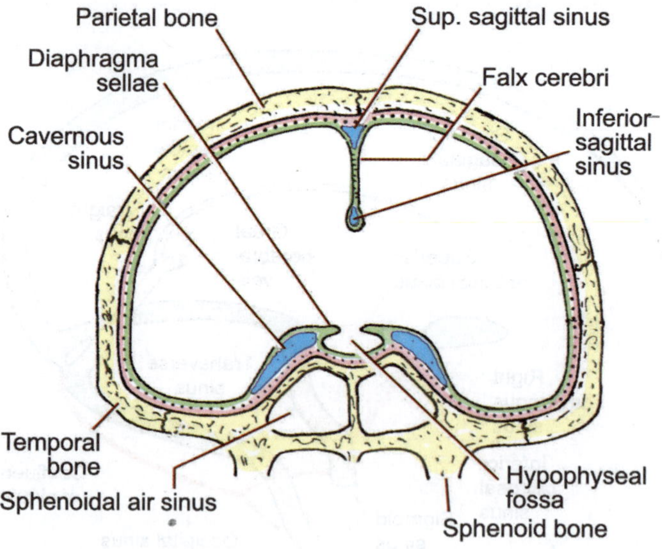

Fig. 8.49 Coronal section through middle cranial fossa to show the position of some intracranial venous sinuses.

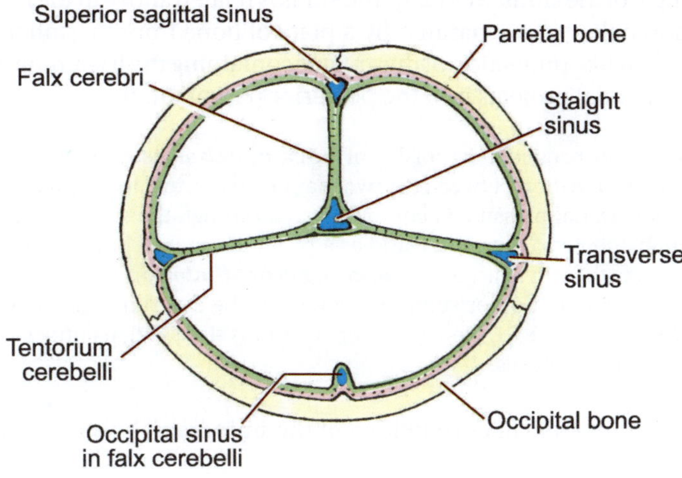

Fig. 8.50 Coronal section through the posterior cranial fossa (behind the foramen magnum) to show the position of some intracranial venous sinuses.

a transverse groove of the inner surface of the occipital bone, and on the posteroinferior angle of the parietal bone. Finally it reaches the petrous part of the temporal bone where it becomes continuous with the sigmoid sinus.

6. The right and left ***sigmoid sinuses*** are continuations of the corresponding transverse sinuses. As indicated by the name each sigmoid sinus is S-shaped. It first runs downwards and medially in a deep groove on the mastoid part of the temporal bone, and then across the jugular process of the occipital bone. Finally it runs forwards to reach the jugular foramen where it ends by becoming continuous with the upper end of the internal jugular vein.

> The upper part of the sinus is related anteriorly to the mastoid antrum from which it is separated only by a thin plate of bone. Infection can, therefore, travel from the mastoid antrum into the sigmoid sinus.

7. The right and left ***cavernous sinuses*** are so called because their cavities are traversed by delicate strands of tissue that appear to subdivide each sinus into a number of smaller spaces (or caverns). The sinuses lie in the middle cranial fossa. They are placed anteroposteriorly on either side of the body of the sphenoid bone. Anteriorly each sinus reaches the superior orbital fissure. Posteriorly it reaches the apex of the petrous part of the temporal bone (Fig. 8.51).

The cavernous sinus has important relations (Fig. 8.52). The internal carotid artery passes anteriorly within the cavity of the sinus. The artery is accompanied by the abducent nerve which lies below and lateral to it. Three cranial nerves are embedded in the lateral wall of the sinus. From above downwards these are the oculomotor nerve, the trochlear nerve, and the ophthalmic division of the trigeminal nerve. The maxillary division of the trigeminal nerve runs along the inferior angle of the sinus. Medially, the sinus is related above to the hypophysis cerebri, and below it is separated by a plate of bone from the sphenoidal air sinus. A pouch like projection of duramater containing the trigeminal ganglion (***trigeminal cave***) projects into the posterior part of the sinus.

Because of the peculiar relationship of the cavernous sinus to the internal carotid artery a communication between the two may occur as a result of injury. When this happens the arterial pressure is communicated through the sinus to veins of the orbit (which open into the sinus): and as a result the eyeball becomes prominent and pulsates with each heart beat (***pulsating exophthalmos***).

The tributaries and other communications of the cavernous sinus are shown in Fig. 8.53 and in Fig. 8.51. Note the intercavernous sinuses that connect the right and left cavernous sinuses.

For important clinical correlations of the intracranial venous sinuses see Chapter 15.

OTHER INTRACRANIAL SINUSES AND VEINS

We have now completed the consideration of the major intracranial venous sinuses. Brief mention will now be made of some smaller intracranial sinuses and veins.

Each ***sphenoparietal sinus*** (right or left) runs medially along the sharp posterior edge of the floor of the anterior cranial fossa (formed by the lesser wing of the sphenoid). The sinus ends by joining the anterior end of the cavernous sinus (Fig. 8.51).

Each ***superior petrosal sinus*** (right or left) begins at the posterior end of the cavernous sinus. It runs backwards and laterally along the sharp upper margin of the petrous temporal bone (i.e., along the attached margin of the tentorium cerebelli). It terminates by joining the junction of the sigmoid sinus and transverse sinus (Figs. 8.51, 8.53).

Each ***inferior petrosal*** sinus (right or left) begins at the posterior end of the cavernous sinus. It runs downwards and somewhat laterally in the groove between the petrous temporal bone and the basilar part of the occipital bone. It passes through the anterior part of the jugular foramen and terminates by joining the upper end of the internal jugular vein (Figs. 8.51, 8.53).

The inferior petrosal sinuses of the right and left sides are connected by a ***basilar plexus of veins*** lying on the basal parts of the sphenoid and occipital bones (Fig. 8.51).

The vein accompanying the middle meningeal artery is called the ***middle meningeal sinus.*** The sinus has frontal and parietal tributaries corresponding to those of the artery. The sinus often terminates in the cavernous sinus (a in Fig. 8.54), but occasionally it may end in the sphenoparietal sinus (b). Sometimes the parietal tributary may pass through the foramen spinosum (c) and the frontal tributary may pass through the foramen ovale (d) to end in the pterygoid plexus of veins.

VEINS DRAINING THE EYEBALL AND ORBIT

The ***superior ophthalmic vein*** accompanies the ophthalmic artery. Anteriorly it communicates with the facial vein. Posteriorly, it passes through the superior orbital fissure and ends in the cavernous sinus (Fig. 8.53). The vein acts as a

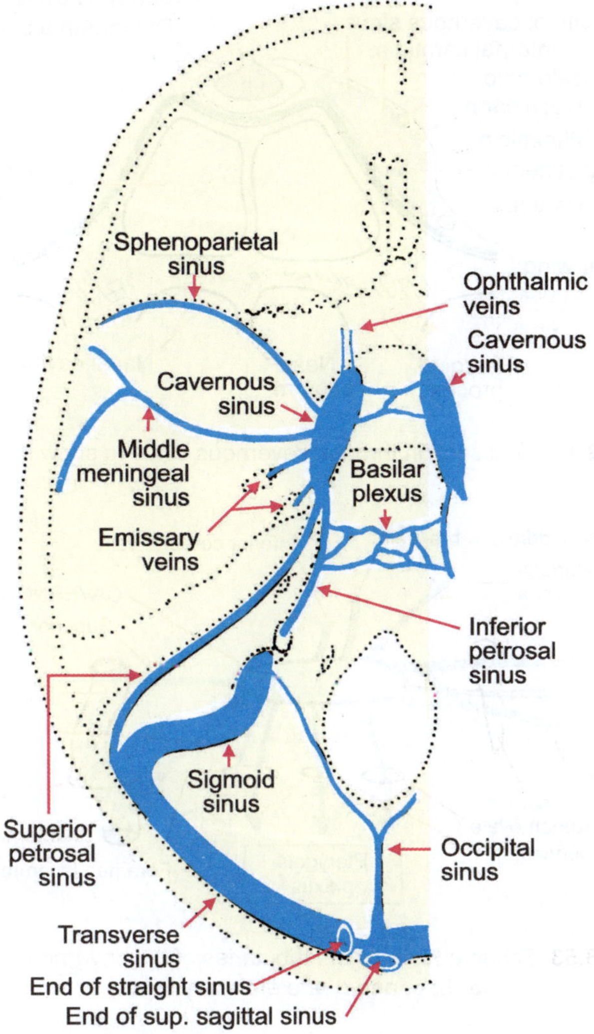

Fig. 8.51 Relationship of the cranial venous sinuses to the floor of the cranial cavity.

communication between the facial vein and the cavernous sinus. Infections on the face can spread to the cavernous sinus through this route.

The ***inferior ophthalmic vein*** lies below the eyeball. It terminates in the cavernous sinus either directly or by joining the superior ophthalmic vein (Fig. 8.53).

The ***central vein of the retina*** accompanies the artery of the same name. It ends in the cavernous sinus directly or through the superior ophthalmic vein (Fig. 8.53).

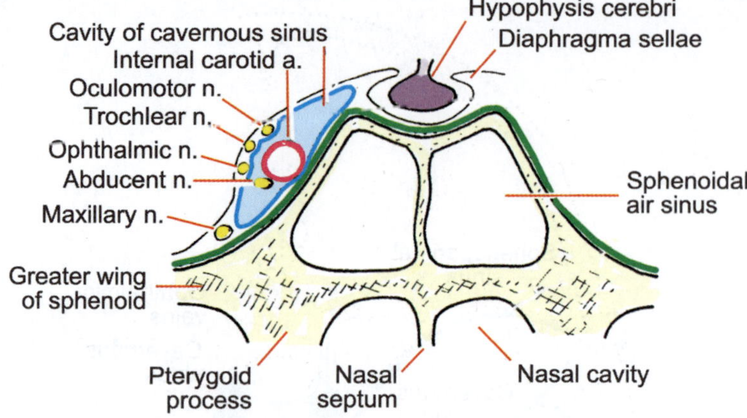

Fig. 8.52 Coronal section through cavernous sinus to show its relations.

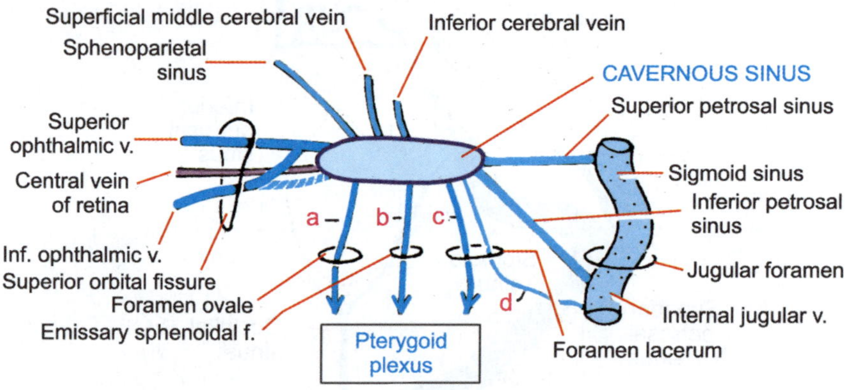

Fig. 8.53 Scheme to show the tributaries of the cavernous sinus. **a, b, c,** and **d** are emissary veins.

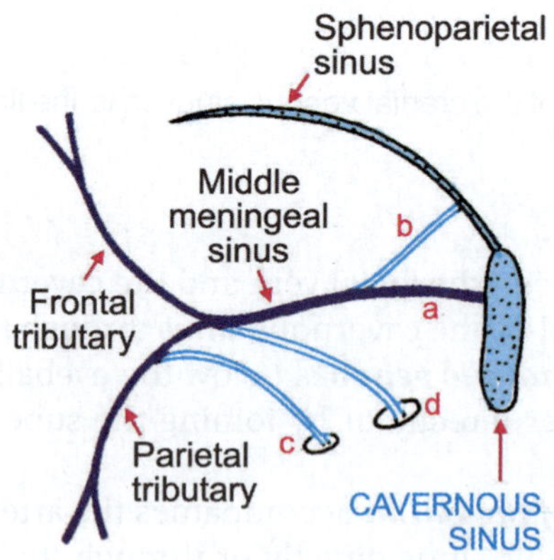

Fig. 8.54 Variations in mode of termination of the middle meningeal sinus.

Some venous channels are present within the thickness of the skull bones. They are called ***diploic veins.*** They drain mostly into the intracranial sinuses, but some end in the veins of the scalp.

Some ***meningeal veins*** lie in the duramater. The largest of these, the middle meningeal sinuses have already been considered above. Like the veins from the brain the meningeal veins also drain into the intracranial venous sinuses.

The ***emissary veins*** connect the intracranial venous sinuses to veins outside the skull. They are numerous and pass through various foramina of the skull.

TRIBUTARIES OF INTERNAL JUGULAR VEINS IN THE NECK

These are shown in Fig. 8.45. They will now be considered one by one

The Facial Vein

The facial vein begins near the medial angle of the eye by the union of two superficial veins of the forehead, namely, the ***supratrochlear*** and the ***supraorbital*** veins (Fig. 8.55). The vein runs downwards and backwards across the face and terminates by joining the anterior branch of the retromandibular vein to form the ***common facial vein*** which ends in the internal jugular vein.

Sometimes the common facial vein is described as part of the facial vein, which is then described as ending in the internal jugular vein

While running across the face the facial vein lies over the buccinator muscle, the body of the mandible and the lower part of the masseter. Below the mandible it crosses the submandibular gland (not shown), the posterior belly of the digastric and the stylohyoid muscles.

The terminal part of the vein (including the common facial part) crosses the internal and external carotid arteries, the hypoglossal nerve and the loop formed by the lingual artery (Fig. 8.56). The tributaries of the facial vein are shown in Fig. 8.55. The vein communicates with the superior ophthalmic veins and through them with the cavernous sinus.

The Lingual Vein

The lingual vein accompanies the lingual artery and joins the internal jugular vein near the greater cornu of the hyoid bone. Some veins of the tongue run along the hypoglossal nerve. They may join the lingual vein or the facial vein or may terminate directly in the internal jugular vein.

The Superior Thyroid Vein

The superior thyroid vein corresponds in its course and tributaries with the superior thyroid artery (Figs. 8.57, 8.15).

The Middle Thyroid Vein

The middle thyroid vein drains the lower part of the gland. It crosses the common carotid artery to enter the internal jugular vein (Fig. 8.57).

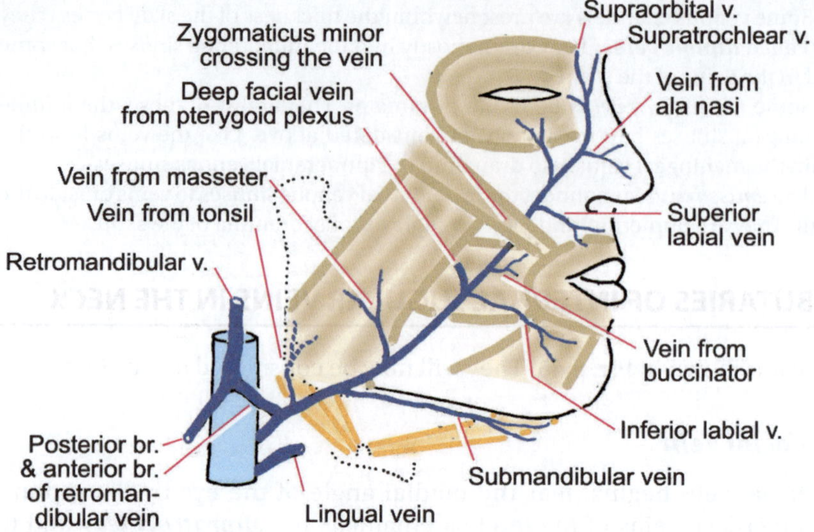

Fig. 8.55 Scheme to show the course and tributaries of the facial vein.

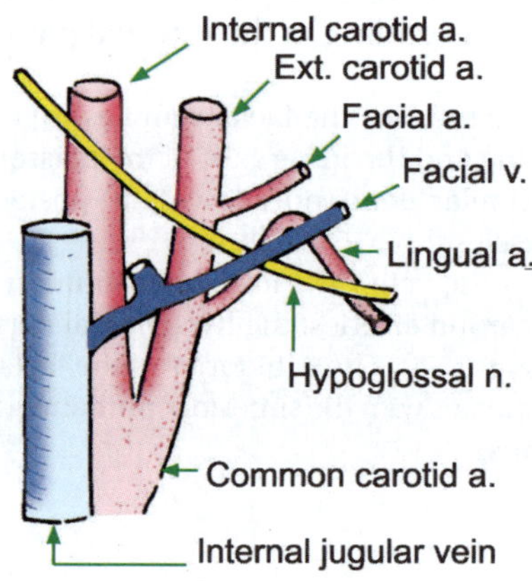

Fig. 8.56 Some relations of the terminal part of the facial vein.

The Inferior Thyroid Veins

The inferior thyroid veins are not tributaries of the internal jugular, but are described here for sake of convenience. They arise from the lower part of the thyroid gland and descend over the front of the trachea forming a plexus over it. The right and left veins end in the corresponding brachiocephalic veins (Fig. 8.57).

In addition to the tributaries described above the internal jugular vein also receives some veins from the pharynx.

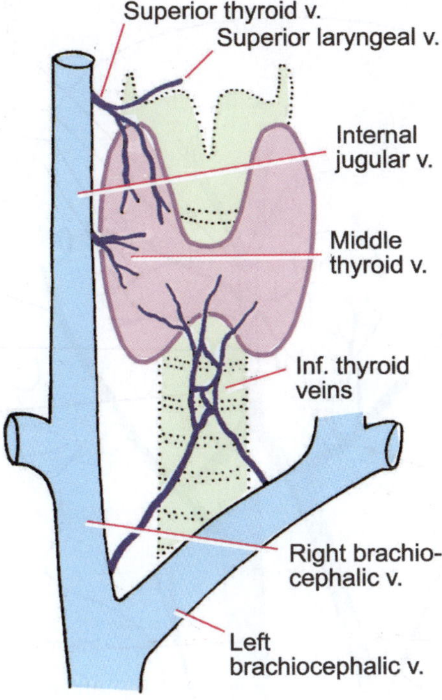

Fig. 8.57 Scheme to show the veins draining the thyroid gland.

OTHER VEINS OF THE HEAD AND NECK

Superficial Temporal Vein

The superficial temporal vein accompanies the corresponding artery. The vein is formed a little above the zygomatic arch by the union of numerous tributaries present in the scalp. A little below its formation it receives the ***middle temporal vein.*** After descending superficial to the zygomatic arch it is joined by the maxillary vein to form the retromandibular vein. The tributaries of the superficial temporal vein are shown in Fig. 8.58.

The Maxillary Vein

The maxillary vein runs alongside the first part of the maxillary artery. It has its origin in the ***pterygoid plexus*** of veins which is present in the infratemporal fossa. The veins corresponding to the branches of the maxillary artery drain into this plexus. The plexus is connected to the facial vein through the deep facial vein (Fig. 8.55). It is connected to the cavernous sinus by a number of emissary veins (Fig. 8.53). The plexus is drained by the maxillary vein which ends by joining the superficial temporal vein to form the retromandibular vein.

The Retromandibular Vein

The retromandibular vein lies behind the ramus of the mandible (as implied by its name). It is formed by union of the superficial temporal and maxillary veins.

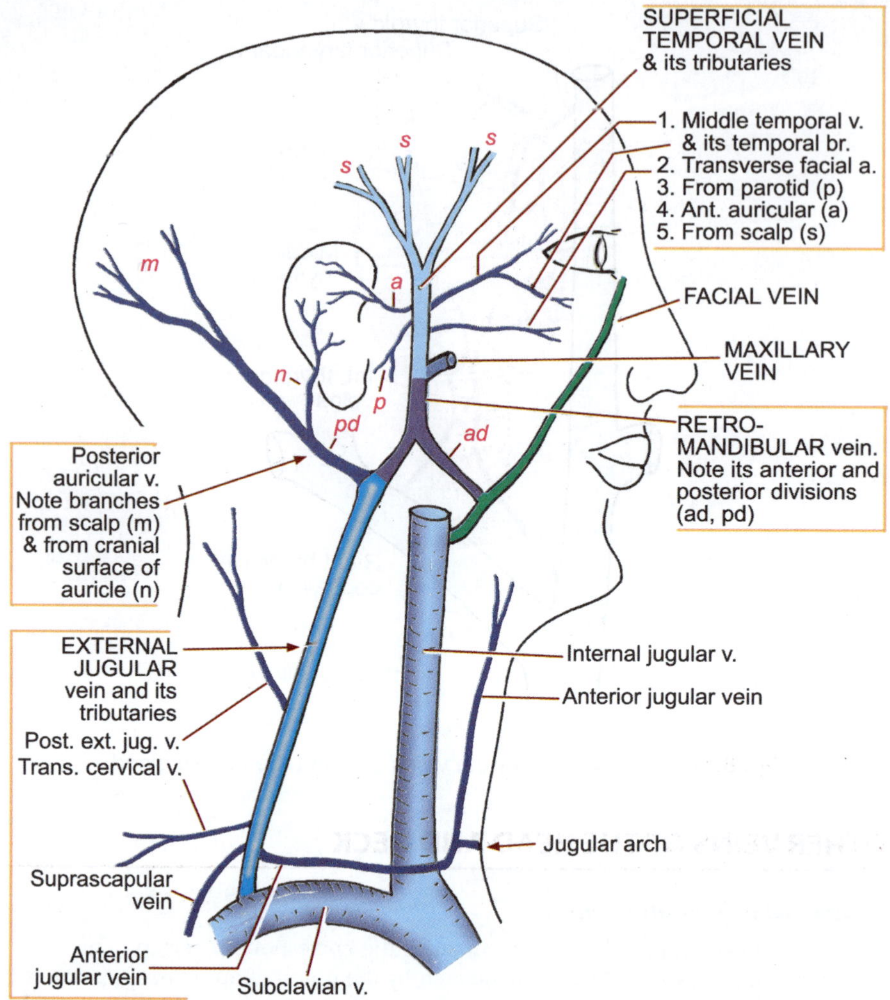

Fig. 8.58 Scheme to show some veins of the head and neck.

It is embedded in the parotid gland. Within the gland the vein is superficial to the external carotid artery and deep to the facial nerve (Fig. 1.4). Descending within the substance of the gland the vein divides into anterior and posterior branches. The anterior branch joins the facial vein. The posterior branch joins the posterior auricular vein (see below) to form the external jugular vein.

The Posterior Auricular Vein

The posterior auricular vein begins by union of tributaries present in the posterior part of the scalp. It passes downwards and forwards behind the auricle and receives veins from its cranial surface. Finally it ends by joining the posterior division of the retromandibular vein.

THE EXTERNAL JUGULAR VEIN

The external jugular vein is formed, as seen above, by union of the posterior division of the retromandibular vein with the posterior auricular vein (Fig. 8.58). The origin lies within the lower part of the parotid gland or just below it. The level corresponds to the angle of the mandible. From here the vein runs downwards and somewhat backwards and ends by joining the subclavian vein. The termination lies behind the middle of the clavicle, near the lateral margin of the scalenus anterior muscle.

The greater part of the vein is superficial being covered by skin, superficial fascia and platysma. As a result the vein can be clearly seen in the living. It pierces the deep fascia near its termination to reach the subclavian vein. The vein crosses the sternocleidomastoid obliquely running downwards and backwards across it (Fig. 1.9).

Apart from the veins that form it, the external jugular vein receives a number of tributaries. These are the ***posterior external jugular vein*** from the upper and posterior part of the neck, the ***transverse cervical*** and ***suprascapular veins*** that accompany the corresponding arteries, and the anterior jugular vein (Fig. 8.58).

The Anterior Jugular Vein

The anterior jugular vein runs down the front of the neck a short distance from the midline (Fig. 1.12, 8.58). It begins near the hyoid bone and extends downwards to a point a little above the sternoclavicular joint. Here the vein turns laterally deep to the sternocleidomastoid, but superficial to the sternohyoid and sternothyroid muscles (Fig. 8.44), and ends by joining the lower end of the external jugular vein. Sometimes it may end in the subclavian vein (Fig. 8.47). Just above the sternum the right and left anterior jugular veins are united by a transverse vein called the ***jugular arch*** (Fig. 1.12).

The Occipital Vein

The occipital vein begins by union of some veins draining the posterior part of the scalp (Fig. 8.59). It descends in the scalp a few centimetres behind the auricle. Reaching the attachment of the trapezius to the superior nuchal line it pierces it and becomes deep. It then reaches the suboccipital triangle where it ends in a plexus from which the deep cervical and vertebral veins begin.

The Deep Cervical Vein

The deep cervical vein begins in the venous plexus present in the suboccipital region. It accompanies the corresponding artery through the deep muscles of the back of the neck and ends by joining the lower part of the vertebral vein (Fig. 8.59).

The Vertebral Vein

The vertebral vein also begins in the suboccipital venous plexus (Fig. 8.59). It enters the foramen transversarium of the atlas and runs downwards in the form of a dense plexus around the vertebral artery. It is only at the foramen transversarium of the sixth cervical vertebra that the plexus takes the form of

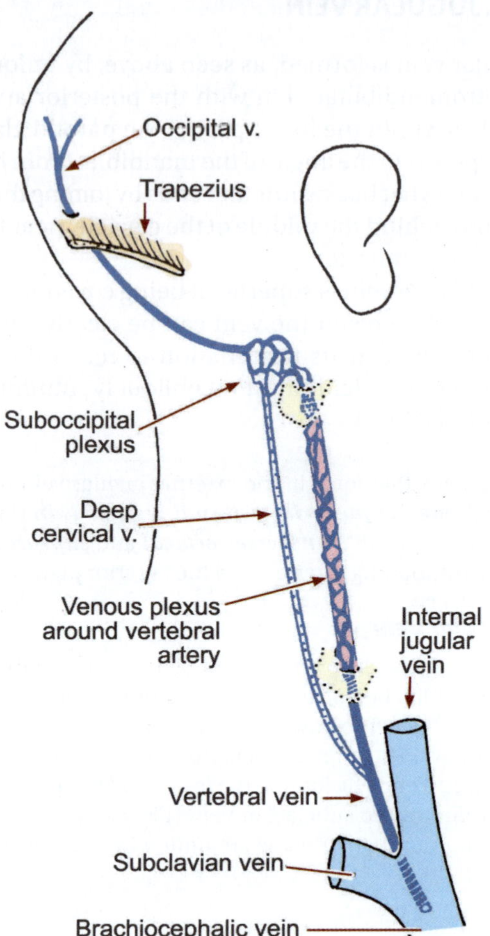

Fig. 8.59 Scheme to show the occipital, vertebral and deep cervical veins.

a single vessel. The vein runs downwards behind the internal jugular vein and ends in the upper part of the corresponding brachiocephalic vein.

CHAPTER

9

Nerves of the Head and Neck

CERVICAL NERVES

In the thoracic, lumbar and sacral regions the number of spinal nerves corresponds to that of vertebrae, each nerve lying ***below*** the numerically corresponding vertebra. However, in the neck we have seven cervical vertebrae, and eight cervical nerves. The reason for this will be clear from Fig. 9.1. Note that the ***upper seven cervical nerves lie above the numerically corresponding vertebrae***. The eighth cervical nerve lies below vertebra C7.

THE DORSAL RAMI OF CERVICAL NERVES

The dorsal ramus of a typical spinal nerve is smaller than the ventral ramus. It passes backwards and divides into medial and lateral branches which supply the deep muscles and skin of the back (Fig. 9.2). This is all that needs to be known about the dorsal rami of most spinal nerves. The dorsal rami of the upper three cervical nerves, however, have some atypical features and are briefly described below.

Dorsal Ramus of the First Cervical Nerve

The dorsal ramus of the first cervical nerve is larger than the ventral ramus. It is seen the suboccipital triangle which it reaches by passing above the posterior arch of the atlas (Fig. 9.3). Here the nerve lies between the arch and the vertebral artery. The dorsal ramus divides into branches that supply the rectus capitis posterior major and minor, the superior and inferior oblique muscles and the semispinalis capitis (Fig. 9.4). Some branches may reach the skin of the scalp.

Dorsal Ramus of the Second Cervical Nerve

The dorsal ramus of the second cervical nerve is large. It reaches the suboccipital region by passing below the posterior arch of the atlas, and below

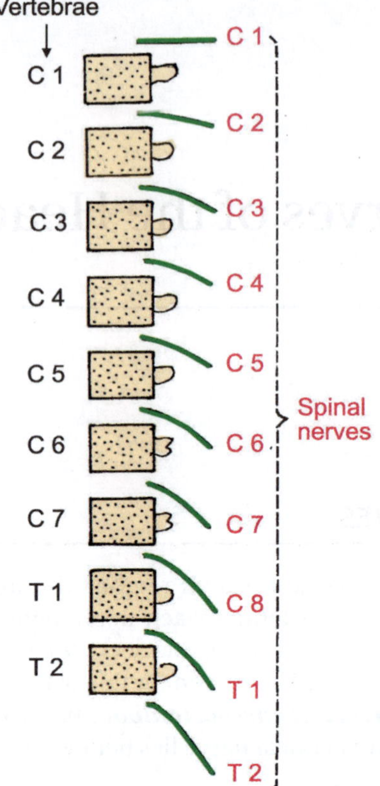

Fig. 9.1 Scheme to show the relationship of cervical and upper thoracic nerves to vertebrae.

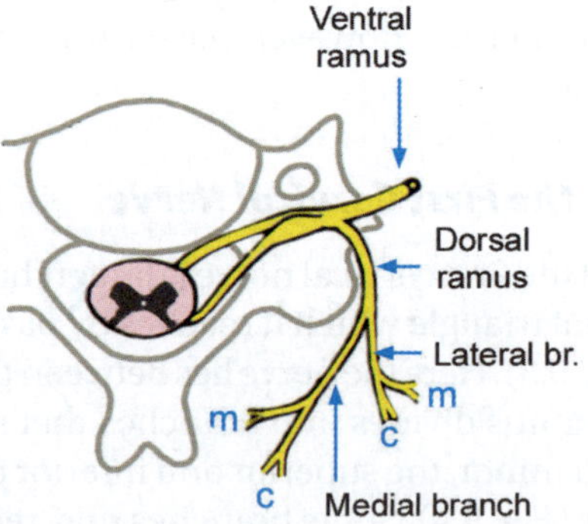

Fig. 9.2 Dorsal ramus of a typical spinal nerve.

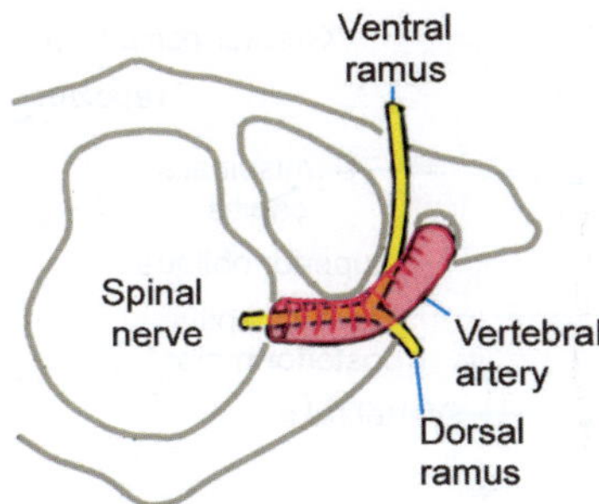

Fig. 9.3 Dorsal ramus of the first cervical nerve.

the inferior oblique muscle. of its medial and lateral branches, the medial branch is much more prominent and is called the ***greater occipital nerve*** (Fig. 9.5). Winding around the lower border of the inferior oblique muscle this nerve passes upwards and medially across the suboccipital triangle, lying deep to the semispinalis capitis. It becomes superficial by piercing first the semispinalis capitis and then the trapezius. Finally it divides into branches that ramify in the scalp supplying its posterior part. It also gives a branch to the semispinalis capitis muscle.

Dorsal Ramus of the Third Cervical Nerve

The dorsal ramus of the third cervical nerve behaves like a typical dorsal ramus. The only special feature about it is that it also gives a small branch to the skin of the occipital region. This branch is called the ***third occipital nerve.***

THE VENTRAL RAMI OF CERVICAL NERVES

The ventral rami of the first, second, third and fourth cervical nerves unite with each other to form the ***cervical plexus***. The ventral rami of the fifth, sixth, seventh and eighth cervical nerves, and the greater part of the ventral ramus of the first thoracic nerve, join one another to form the brachial plexus. The brachial plexus has been considered with the upper extremity. The cervical plexus is described below.

THE CERVICAL PLEXUS AND ITS BRANCHES

The cervical plexus is formed by the ventral rami of the first, second, third and fourth cervical nerves as follows (Fig. 9.6). With the exception of the ramus of the first cervical nerve each of them divides into ascending (***a***) and descending (***d***) branches. The ascending branch of the second nerve joins the first nerve; and its descending branch joins the ascending branch of the third nerve. Similarly the descending branch of the third nerve joins the ascending branch of the fourth nerve. The descending branch of the fourth nerve is small and joins the fifth cervical nerve.

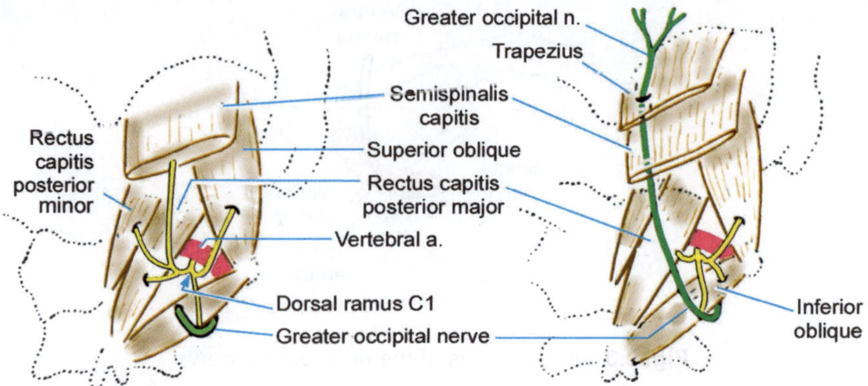

Fig. 9.4 Distribution of the dorsal ramus of the first cervical nerve.

Fig. 9.5 Course of the greater occipital nerve.

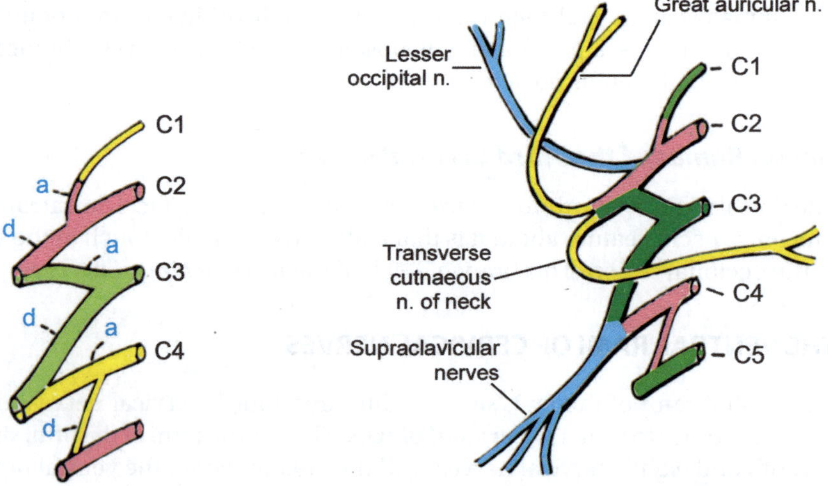

Fig. 9.6 Plan of cervical plexus.

Fig. 9.7 Cervical plexus and its cutaneous branches.

The cervical plexus gives off a large number of branches. The ***cutaneous branches*** are shown in Fig. 9.7 and are as follows. The ***lesser occipital*** nerve arises from the second cervical nerve. The ***greater auricular*** nerve and the ***transverse cutaneous nerve of the neck*** arise from the second and third nerves. The ***supraclavicular*** nerves arise from the third and fourth nerves. These nerves are considered in detail on pages that follow.

The ***muscular branches*** of the cervical plexus are numerous. For ease of visualisation they may be subdivided as follows (Fig. 9.8):

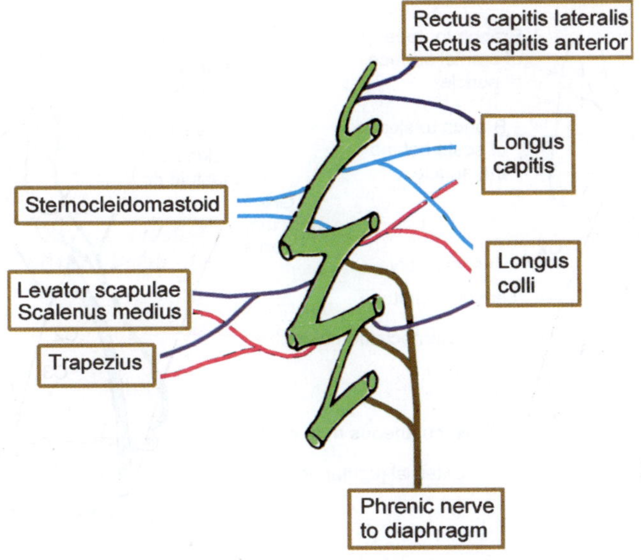

Fig. 9.8 Scheme to show the muscular branches of the cervical plexus.

1. ***Branches to prevertebral muscles:***
   The rectus capitis lateralis and the rectus capitis anterior receive branches from C1. The longus capitis receives branches C1, C2 and C3. The longus colli receives branches from C2, C3 and C4.
2. ***Branches to muscles forming boundaries of the posterior triangle:*** The sternocleidomastoid receives a branch from C2 (and sometimes from C3). The levator scapulae, the scalenus medius and the trapezius receive branches from C3 and C4.
3. The ***phrenic nerve*** (which supplies the diaphragm) arises by separate roots from C3, C4 and C5.
4. ***Branches to infrahyoid muscles*** reach them through the hypoglossal nerve and through the ansa cervicalis.
   We will now consider some of these branches one by one.

Lesser Occipital Nerve

The lesser occipital nerve arises from the descending branch of the ventral ramus of the second cervical nerve. The origin lies deep to the sternocleidomastoid muscle. The nerve forms a loop round the accessory nerve. It then runs upwards and backwards for some distance along the posterior border of the sternocleidomastoid. Higher up it lies superficial to the muscle between it and the deep fascia. It becomes subcutaneous behind the auricle and divides into branches which supply the skin of this region. It also gives off an ***auricular branch*** that supplies the upper part of the cranial surface of the auricle (Figs. 1.9, 9.7, 9.9, 9.11, 9.12).

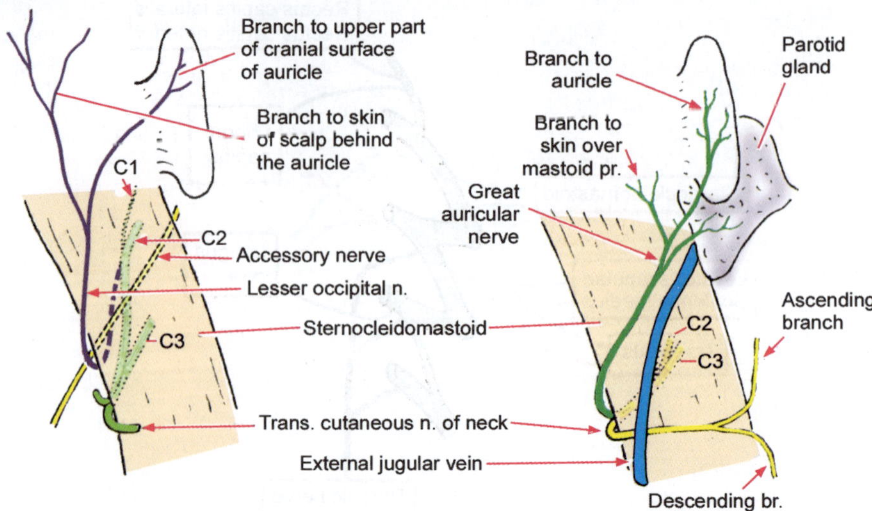

Fig. 9.9 Course and distribution of lesser occipital nerve

Fig. 9.10 Course and distribution of greater auricular and transverse cutaneous nerves

Greater Auricle Nerve

The greater auricular nerve arises from the ventral rami of the second and third cervical nerve. Its origin lies deep to the sternocleidomastoid. Winding around the posterior border of this muscle it reaches its superficial surface. It pierces the deep fascia and runs upwards and somewhat forwards over the surface of the sternocleidomastoid. Here it is accompanied by the external jugular vein. A little below the auricle it divides into anterior and posterior branches. The anterior branch supplies the skin over the parotid gland. The posterior branch supplies (i) most of the cranial surface of the auricle (except the part supplied by the lesser occipital); (ii) the posteroinferior part of the lateral surface of the auricle including the lobule and concha; and (iii) the skin over the mastoid process (Figs. 1.9, 9.7, 9.10 to 9.12).

Transverse Cutaneous Nerve of Neck

The transverse cutaneous nerve of the neck is also called the anterior cutaneous nerve. It arises from the ventral rami of the second and third cervical nerves. It first runs laterally deep to the sternocleidomastoid. Reaching the posterior border of this muscle it curves around it and then runs forwards across the muscle. The nerve becomes superficial and divides into ascending and descending branches which supply the skin on the front of the neck (Figs. 1.9, 9.7).

The Supraclavicular Nerves

The supraclavicular nerves arise (as a single ramus) from the third and fourth cervical nerves (Fig. 9.7). The origin lies deep to the sternocleidomastoid. The

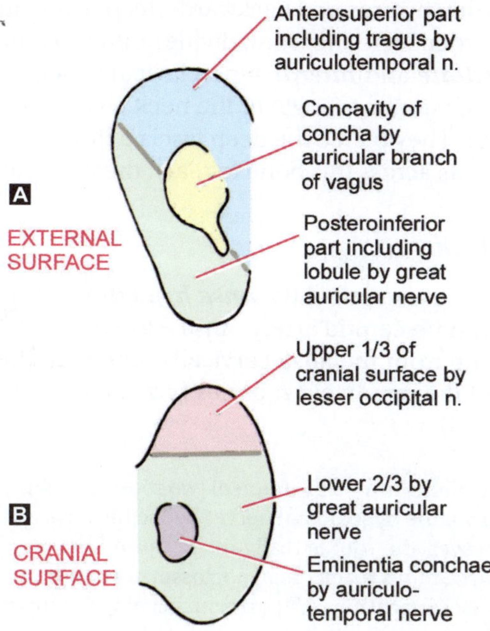

Fig. 9.11 Nerve supply of the external surface (A) and cranial surface (B) of the auricle.

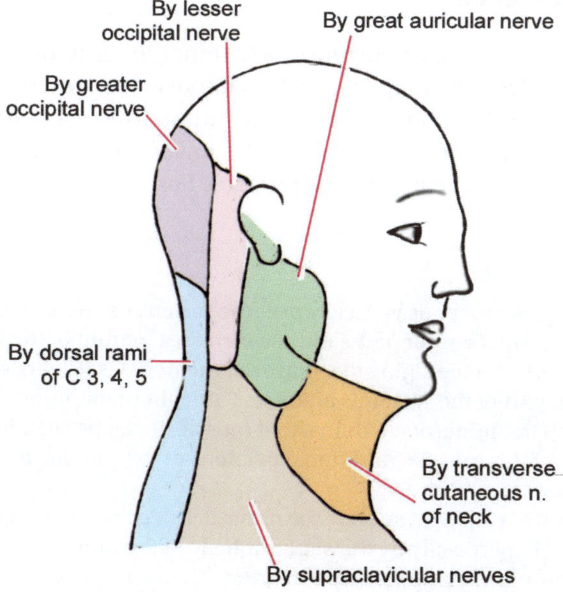

Fig. 9.12 Areas of skin of neck supplied by various cutaneous nerves.

nerve trunk runs downwards and backwards deep to the muscle and appears at its posterior border. Here the trunk divides into three branches called the ***medial, intermediate*** and ***lateral*** supraclavicular nerves. These branches descend over the posterior triangle of the neck giving some branches to the skin here (Fig. 1.9). They pierce the deep fascia a little above the clavicle and then run downwards across this bone to reach the pectoral region.

The Ansa Cervicalis

The ansa cervicalis is also called the ***ansa hypoglossi***. It is a nerve loop lying in front of the common carotid artery (ansa = loop).

Branches arising from the ansa cervicalis innervate the sternohyoid, the sternothyroid and the omohyoid muscles (viz., all infrahyoid muscles other than the thyrohyoid).

The ansa cervicalis is formed by union of two roots (Fig. 9.13). The superior root appears to arise from the hypoglossal nerve (hence the term ansa hypoglossi given to the loop). However, the root is really made up of fibres derived from the first cervical nerve. These fibres reach the hypoglossal nerve through a communicating branch from the first cervical nerve. Apart from forming the superior root of the ansa cervicalis these fibres from the first cervical nerve (travelling along the hypoglossal nerve) innervate the thyrohyoid and geniohyoid muscles (Also see Fig. 9.87). The inferior root of the ansa cervicalis arises from the second and third cervical nerves. It descends at first lateral to the internal jugular vein and then superficial to it to join the superior root superficial to the common carotid artery.

The Phrenic Nerve

The phrenic nerve is one of the most important nerves in the body as it is the only motor supply to the diaphragm. This nerve arises from the (ventral rami of) spinal nerves C3, C4 and C5 the contribution from C4 being the greatest. The nerve descends vertically through the lower part of the neck, and then through the thorax to reach the diaphragm. Some terminal branches enter the abdomen.

Relations in the neck:

The phrenic nerve descends vertically over the scalenus anterior muscle. Crossing the medial (or lower) border of the muscle it crosses in front of the first part of the subclavian artery. On the right side, however, the nerve is usually separated from the artery by a part of the scalenus anterior. Throughout its course in the neck the nerve lies deep to the sternocleidomastoid muscle. It can be seen by lifting up the lateral border of this muscle. Additional relations of the phrenic nerve in the neck are as follows.

1. While over the scalenus anterior the nerve lies deep to the prevertebral fascia. It is crossed superficially by the superior belly of the omohyoid, the transverse cervical artery and the suprascapular artery. On the left side it is also crossed by the thoracic duct (Fig. 9.14).
2. Lower down the nerve lies behind the lower end of the internal jugular vein. Still lower down the nerve passes behind the medial end of the subclavian vein.

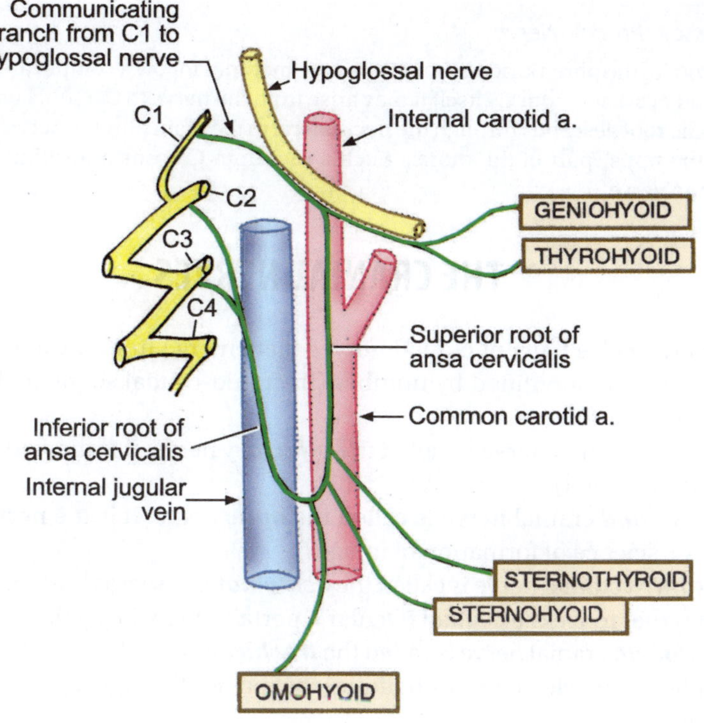

Fig. 9.13 Scheme to show the mode of innervation of the infrahyoid muscles from the cervical plexus.

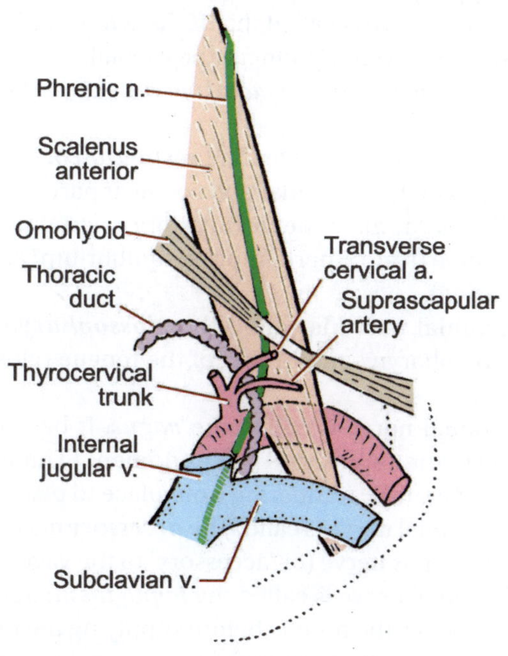

Fig. 9.14 Some relationships of the phrenic nerve.

Accessory Phrenic Nerve

The root of the phrenic nerve from C5 may sometimes follow a complicated course. Instead of arising from C5 itself it may arise from the nerve to the subclavius. From here the root descends through the neck lateral to the main phrenic nerve and joins it in the upper part of the thorax. Such a root from C5 constitutes the accessory phrenic nerve.

THE CRANIAL NERVES

There are twelve pairs of cranial nerves that emerge from the surface of the brain. They are identified by number (in cranio-caudal sequence) and also bear names as follows.

The ***first*** cranial nerve is called the ***olfactory*** nerve. It is the nerve of smell (Olfaction = smell).

The ***second*** cranial nerve is called the ***optic*** nerve. It is the nerve of sight (Optics = science of formation of images).

The ***third*** cranial nerve is called the ***oculomotor*** nerve as it supplies several muscles that move the eyeball (Ocular = pertaining to the eye).

The ***fourth*** cranial nerve is called the ***trochlear*** nerve. It is so called because it supplies a muscle (superior oblique) that passes through a pulley (trochlea = pulley).

The ***fifth*** cranial nerve is called the ***trigeminal*** nerve because it has three major divisions. These are ***ophthalmic*** division to the orbit, the ***maxillary*** division to the upper jaw, and the ***mandibular*** division to the lower jaw.

The ***sixth*** cranial nerve is called the ***abducent*** nerve because it supplies a muscle (lateral rectus) which 'abducts' the eyeball.

The ***seventh*** cranial nerve is the ***facial*** nerve because it supplies the muscles of the face.

The ***eighth*** cranial nerve is called the ***vestibulo-cochlear*** nerve because it supplies structures in the vestibular and cochlear parts of the internal ear. It is sometimes called the auditory nerve (auditory = pertaining to hearing) or the stato-acoustic nerve (stato = pertaining to equilibrium; acoustic = pertaining to sound or hearing).

The ***ninth*** cranial nerve is called the ***glossopharyngeal*** nerve as it is distributed to the pharynx and to part of the tongue (glossal = pertaining to the tongue).

The ***tenth*** cranial nerve is called the ***vagus***. It has an extensive course through the neck, the thorax and the abdomen. (The word vagus may be correlated with 'vagrant' = wandering from place to place).

The ***eleventh*** cranial nerve is called the ***accessory*** nerve because it appears to be a part of the vagus nerve (or 'accessory' to the vagus).

The ***twelfth*** cranial nerve is called the ***hypoglossal*** nerve (because it runs part of its course below the tongue before supplying the muscles in it (hypo = below; glossal = pertaining to tongue).

TYPES OF FIBRES IN PERIPHERAL NERVES

Both spinal and cranial nerves contain fibres than can be classified into several types on the basis of their function. It is necessary to consider this topic here as cranial nerves can contain some functional types of fibres not encountered in spinal nerves.

Fibres in a peripheral nerve are basically of two types.

a. Some fibres carry impulses from the spinal cord or brain to a peripheral organ like muscle. Impulses passing along such nerves cause the muscle to contract and thus result in movement. Such nerve fibres are called ***motor fibres.*** They are also called ***efferent fibres*** (efferent = go away from). Some efferent fibres end in glands and their stimulation produces secretion. They are therefore called ***secretomotor fibres.***
b. Other nerve fibres carry impulses in the opposite direction i.e., towards the spinal cord or brain. They are called ***afferent fibres*** (afferent = come towards). Fibres bringing the sensations of touch from the skin, of sight from the eye, or of hearing from the ear are examples of afferent fibres. It is through these nerve fibres that we become conscious of such sensations. They are, therefore, also called ***sensory fibres.*** Some afferent fibres carry impulses (e.g., from muscles or joints) of which we may not become conscious, but which are nevertheless very important for maintenance of posture and for proper control of movement. Such impulses are referred to as ***proprioceptive*** (as they have their origin within the body 'proper' and not from outside the body). Similar impulses arising from viscera also reach the brain. We are conscious of some of them (e.g., distension of the urinary bladder). Many of them do not reach our consciousness, but help to regulate the functions of the viscera.

Both afferent and efferent fibres can be further classified on the basis of the tissues supplied by them. The tissues and organs that make up the body can be broadly divided into two major parts, somatic and visceral. ***Somatic*** structures are those present in relation to the body wall (or soma); they include the tissues of the limbs (which represent a modified part of the body wall). Thus the skin, bones, joints and skeletal muscle of the limbs and body wall are classified as somatic. In contrast, the tissues that make up the internal organs like the heart, lungs or stomach are classified as ***visceral***. These include the lining epithelia of hollow viscera, and smooth muscle (including smooth muscle in the walls of blood vessels). A distinction between somatic and visceral structures may also be made on embryological considerations as follows.

a. Structures developing from specialised areas of ectoderm e.g., the retina or the membranous labyrinth, are classified as somatic; while the epithelium of the tongue (and the taste buds) which are of endodermal origin is classified as visceral.
b. Skeletal muscle may be derived embryologically from three distinct sources. These are (i) the somites developing in the paraxial mesoderm; (ii) the somatopleuric mesoderm of the body wall; and (iii) the mesoderm of the branchial arches. The musculature of the limbs and body wall develops partly from somites and partly in situ from the mesoderm of the body wall. The nerves

supplying this musculature are classified as somatic. The muscles that move the eyeball, and the muscles of the tongue are also derived from somites and the nerves supplying them are, therefore, also classified as somatic. However, skeletal muscle that develops in the mesoderm of the branchial arches is classified as visceral (or branchial).

Keeping in view the distinction between afferent and efferent fibres on one hand, and somatic and visceral structures on the other, we may divide fibres in peripheral nerves into four broad categories as follows:

a. Somatic efferent.
b. Visceral efferent.
c. Somatic afferent.
d. Visceral afferent.

With the exception of somatic efferent fibres each of the other categories is subdivided into a ***general*** and a ***special*** group. We thus have a total of seven functional components as follows:

1. ***Somatic efferent*** fibres supply skeletal muscle of the limbs and body wall. They also supply the extrinsic muscles of the eyeball and the muscles of the tongue.
2. ***General visceral efferent*** fibres supply smooth muscle and glands. The nerves to glands are called secretomotor nerves.
3. ***Special visceral efferent*** fibres supply skeletal muscle developing in branchial arch mesoderm. They are frequently called ***branchial efferent*** fibres. The muscles supplied include those of mastication, and of the face, pharynx and larynx.
4. ***General somatic afferent*** fibres are those that carry:
   a. sensations of touch, pain and temperature from the skin (exteroceptive sensations); and
   b. proprioceptive impulses arising in muscles, joints and tendons. These convey information regarding movement and position of joints.
5. ***Special somatic afferent*** fibres carry impulses of (a) vision, (b) hearing, and (c) equilibrium (from the vestibular apparatus).
6. ***General visceral afferent*** fibres carry sensations e.g., pain from viscera (visceroceptive sensations).
7. ***Special visceral afferent*** fibres carry the sensations of taste.

A typical spinal nerve contains fibres of the four general categories. The special categories are present in cranial nerves only.

We will now consider the general disposition of the neurons giving rise to each of the above varieties of fibres.

Each spinal nerve arises from the spinal cord by two roots, anterior (or ventral) and posterior (or dorsal). Each root is formed by aggregation of rootlets that arise from one segment of the spinal cord. The anterior and posterior nerve roots join each other to form a spinal nerve. Just proximal to the junction of the two roots the posterior root is marked by a swelling called the ***dorsal nerve root ganglion***.

Neurons Supplying Typical Skeletal Muscle

In the spinal cord the cell bodies of neurons supplying most skeletal muscle (derived from somites) lie in the ventral grey column. (They are, sometimes, called anterior horn cells). The axons of these neurons leave the spinal cord through the ventral nerve root. They then travel through the spinal nerve (and its branches) to reach a muscle and supply it. The axon may divide into several branches along its course, each of which ends by supplying one muscle fibre (Fig. 9.15).

In the case of cranial nerves the cell bodies of neurons supplying most skeletal muscle are situated in masses of grey matter present in the brainstem.

The neurons supplying most skeletal muscle are called ***somatic efferent*** neurons. In the case of cranial nerves the neurons are located in ***somatic efferent nuclei***.

Some skeletal muscle is derived from branchial arches. This includes the muscles of mastication and the musculature of the face, the pharynx and the larynx. Such muscle is innervated by neurons that are present in special visceral efferent nuclei of the brain stem, and are referred to as ***special visceral efferent neurons***, or ***branchial efferent neurons***.

Neurons Supplying Smooth Muscle and Glands

Nerve fibres innervating smooth muscle and glands are present in both spinal and cranial nerves. The pathway for supply of smooth muscle or gland always consists of two neurons that synapse in a ganglion (Fig. 9.16). The first neuron carries the impulse from the brain or spinal cord to the ganglion and is, therefore, called the ***preganglionic neuron.*** The second neuron carries the impulse from the ganglion to smooth muscle or gland and is called the ***postganglionic neuron.***

Neurons innervating smooth muscle or glands are ***general visceral efferent neurons***. They constitute the greater part of the autonomic nervous system.

Afferent Neurons

The cell bodies of neurons that give rise to afferent fibres are located outside the central nervous system. In the case of spinal nerves they lie in dorsal nerve root ganglia (Fig. 9.17). In the case of cranial nerves they lie in sensory ganglia (e.g., trigeminal ganglion) associated with these nerves. We may illustrate the arrangement with reference to a spinal nerve (Fig. 9.17). The cells of dorsal nerve root ganglia are of the unipolar type. The cell body gives off a single process that divides into a ***peripheral process*** (which is really a dendrite) and a ***central process*** (which is the axon). The peripheral process extends into the spinal nerve and courses through its branches to reach the tissue or organ supplied. It may branch repeatedly during its course. ***Such peripheral processes constitute the afferent fibres of peripheral nerves.*** The sensory impulses brought by these processes from various organs of the body are conveyed to the spinal cord by the central processes. The central processes pass through the dorsal roots of spinal nerves to enter the spinal cord. In the case of cranial nerves they pass into the brainstem through the sensory roots of these nerves.

We have seen that afferent nerve fibres can be divided into four categories viz., general somatic afferent, special somatic afferent, general visceral afferent, and special visceral afferent. The basic arrangement of neurons that give origin to all four categories of afferent fibres is similar and the description given above applies to all of them.

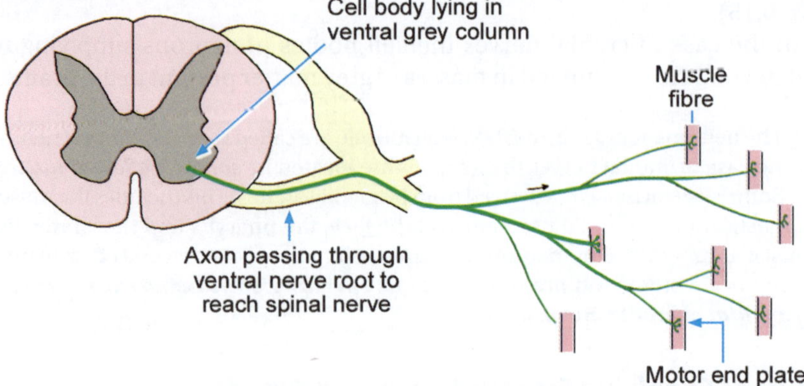

Fig. 9.15 Scheme to show the typical arrangement of a neuron supplying skeletal muscle (somatic efferent neuron).

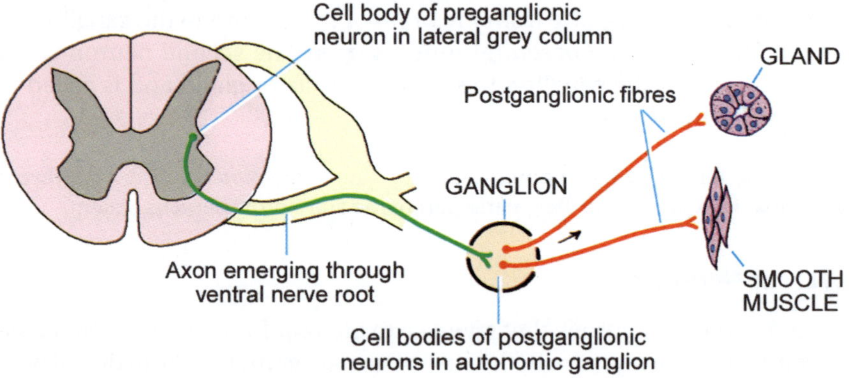

Fig. 9.16 Scheme to show the arrangement of neurons supplying smooth muscle or gland (general visceral efferent neurons).

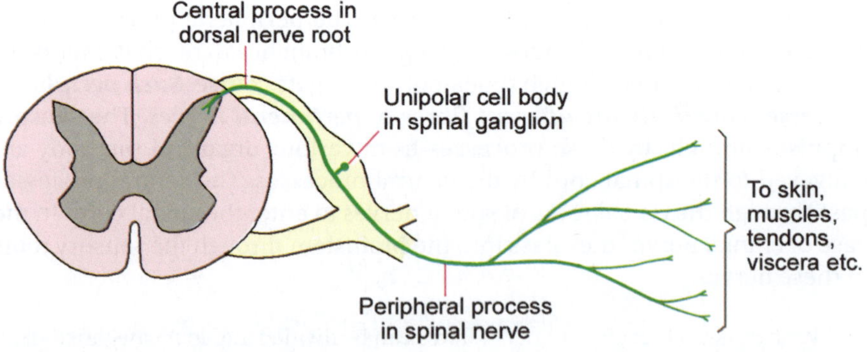

Fig. 9.17 Scheme to show the arrangement of an afferent neuron.

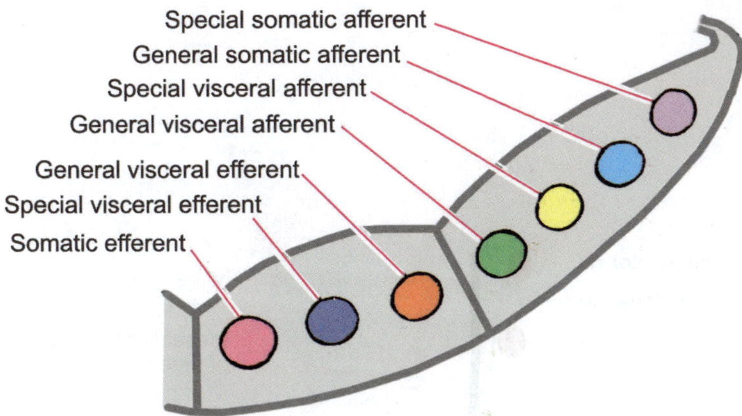

Fig. 9.18 Arrangement of the columns of cranial nerve nuclei as seen in the embryo.

CRANIAL NERVE NUCLEI

Cranial nerves begin or end in groups of neurons, or nuclei, present in the brain. The olfactory and optic nerves are present in relation to the cerebral hemispheres. The nuclei of remaining cranial nerves are located in the brainstem.

These cranial nerve nuclei are arranged in seven groups that correspond to the seven functional types of nerve fibres described above. As a preliminary to the study of cranial nerves it is necessary to briefly consider these nuclei.

In the early embryo the nuclei related to the various types of fibres present in cranial nerves are arranged in vertical rows (or columns). The sequence in which the nuclei for different functional components are arranged is shown in Fig. 9.18. As development proceeds parts of these columns disappear so that each column no longer extends through the whole length of the brainstem, but is represented by one or more discrete nuclei. These are shown schematically in Fig. 9.19. The nuclei are briefly considered below (For details see the author's HUMAN NEUROANATOMY). The position of the nuclei can be properly appreciated only after the brain has been studied. For the time being identify them in Figs. 1.19 and 1.20.

Somatic Efferent Nuclei

Somatic efferent nuclei supply skeletal muscle that is derived (embryologically) from somites. They are as follows.

1. The ***oculomotor nucleus*** is situated in the midbrain (upper part at the level of the superior colliculus). The nuclei of the two sides form a single complex that lies in the central grey matter, ventral to the aqueduct (Fig. 1.19, 9.20F).
2. The ***trochlear nucleus*** is situated in the midbrain (lower part, at the level of the inferior colliculus). The nucleus lies ventral to the aqueduct in the central grey matter (Fig. 9.19, 9.20E).
3. The ***abducent nucleus*** is situated in the lower part of the pons. It lies in the grey matter lining the floor of the fourth ventricle, near the midline (Figs. 9.19, 9.20C).
4. The ***hypoglossal nucleus*** lies in the medulla. It is an elongated column extending

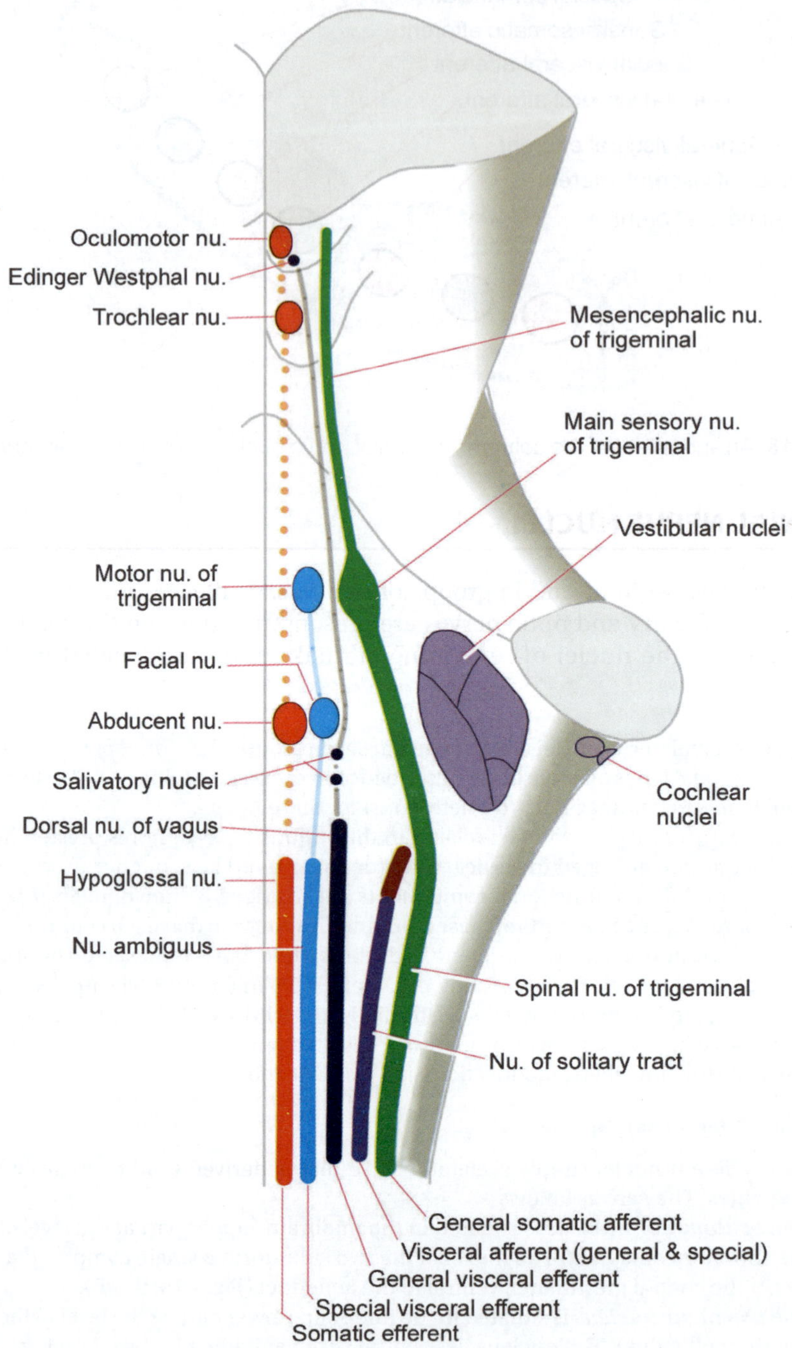

Fig. 9.19 Schematic view of cranial nerve nuclei projected on to the posterior aspect of the brainstem.

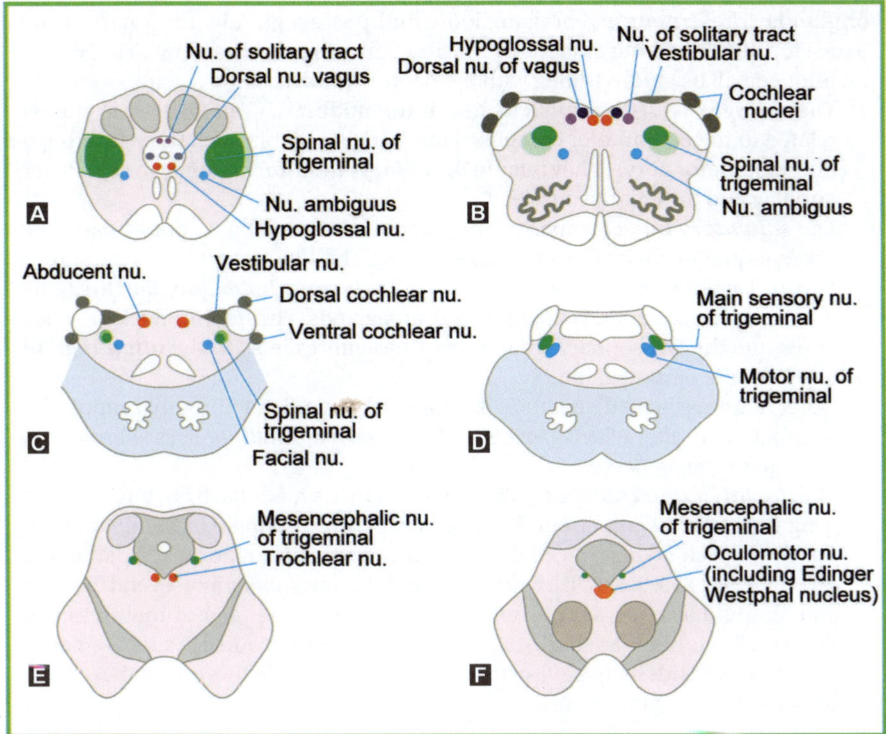

Fig. 9.20 Transverse sections through the brainstem to show the position of cranial nerve nuclei. A, B. Lower and upper parts of medulla. C, D. Lower and upper parts of pons. E, F. Lower and upper parts of midbrain.

into both the open and closed parts of the medulla. Its upper part lies deep to the hypoglossal triangle in the floor of the fourth ventricle. When traced downwards it lies next to the middle line in the central grey matter ventral to the central canal (Figs. 9.19, 9.20A, B).

Special Visceral Efferent Nuclei

These nuclei supply skeletal muscle derived from branchial arch mesoderm.

1. The ***motor nucleus of the trigeminal nerve*** lies in the upper part of the pons, in its dorsal part (Figs. 9.19, 9.20D).
2. The ***nucleus of the facial nerve*** lies in the lower part of the pons (Figs. 9.19, 9.20C).
3. The ***nucleus ambiguus*** lies in the medulla. It forms an elongated column that extends through both the open and closed parts of the medulla (Figs. 9.19, 9.20 A, B). It is a composite nucleus and contributes fibres to the glossopharyngeal, vagus and accessory nerves.

General Visceral Efferent Nuclei

The nuclei in this column give origin to preganglionic fibres that end in peripheral ganglia. Postganglionic fibres arising in these ganglia supply smooth muscle or glands. These neurons, preganglionic and postganglionic, form part of the parasympathetic nervous system. The nuclei of this group are as follows. The ganglia mentioned will be studied along with the nerves concerned.

1. The ***Edinger-Westphal nucleus*** lies in the midbrain (Fig. 9.19). It is closely related to the oculomotor complex. Fibres arising in this nucleus pass through the oculomotor nerve. They relay in the ***ciliary ganglion*** to supply the sphincter pupillae and the ciliaris muscle.
2. The ***salivatory nuclei*** (superior and inferior) lie in the pons (dorsal part) just above its junction with the medulla (Fig. 9.19). The superior nucleus sends fibres into the facial nerve. These fibres relay in the ***submandibular ganglion*** to supply the sub-mandibular and sublingual salivary glands. The inferior nucleus sends fibres into the glossopharyngeal nerve. These fibres relay in the ***otic ganglion*** to supply the parotid gland.
   Other neurons located near the salivatory nuclei send out fibres that supply the lacrimal gland, after relaying in the ***pterygopalatine ganglion***. These fibres travel through the facial nerve.
3. The ***dorsal (motor) nucleus of the vagus*** lies in the medulla. It is a long nucleus lying vertically. Its upper end lies deep to the vagal triangle in the floor of the fourth ventricle. When traced downwards it extends into the closed part of the medulla (Fig. 9.19, 9.20 A, B). Fibres arising in this nucleus supply several thoracic and abdominal viscera. They end in ganglia closely related to these viscera. Postganglionic fibres arising in these ganglia run a short course to supply smooth muscle and glands in these viscera. Some facts relevant to these fibres have been presented in Chapter 34 and 48.

General and Special Visceral Afferent Nuclei

Both these columns are represented by the ***nucleus of the solitary tract***, present in the medulla (Figs. 9.19, 9.20 A, B). Like other cranial nerve nuclei in the medulla, the cells of this nucleus form an elongated column extending into both the open and closed parts of the medulla. The nucleus of the solitary tract receives fibres carrying general visceral sensations through the vagus and glossopharyngeal nerves. Fibres of taste (special visceral afferent) carried by the facial, glossopharyngeal and vagus nerves end in the upper part of the nucleus. This part is sometimes called the ***gustatory nucleus.***

General Somatic Afferent Nuclei

The general somatic afferent column is represented by the sensory nuclei of the trigeminal nerve. These are as follows.

1. The ***main sensory nucleus*** lies in the upper part of the pons, lateral to the motor nucleus of the nerve (Figs. 9.19, 9.20D).
2. The ***spinal nucleus*** extends from the main nucleus down into the medulla (Figs. 9.19, 9.20 A, B) and into the upper two segments of the spinal cord. In addition to fibres of the trigeminal nerve it also receives general somatic sensations carried by the facial, glossopharyngeal and vagus nerves.
3. The ***mesencephalic nucleus*** of the trigeminal nerve extends from the upper end of the main sensory nucleus into the midbrain (Fig. 9.19, 9.20 E, F). Functionally this nucleus appears to be similar to sensory ganglia of cranial nerves, and to the dorsal nerve root ganglia, rather than to afferent nuclei. It is made up of unipolar cells. The peripheral processes of these cells are believed to carry proprioceptive impulses from muscles of mastication and possibly also from muscles of the

eyeball, face and tongue. The central processes of the neurons in the nucleus probably end in the main sensory nucleus of the trigeminal nerve.

Special Somatic Afferent Nuclei

These are the cochlear and vestibular nuclei. The ***cochlear nuclei*** are two in number, dorsal and ventral. They are placed dorsal and ventral to the inferior cerebellar peduncle (Figs. 9.20D, E) at the level of the junction of the pons and the medulla. These nuclei receive fibres from end organs in the cochlea that are concerned with hearing.

The ***vestibular nuclei*** lie in the grey matter underlying the lateral part of the floor of the fourth ventricle (Fig. 9.19, 9.20B, C). They lie partly in the medulla and partly in the pons. They receive fibres from end organs in the vestibular part of the internal ear. They are functionally related to the maintenance of equilibrium.

THE OLFACTORY NERVES

The olfactory (first cranial) nerves are purely sensory and are concerned with smell. The peripheral end organ for smell is the olfactory mucosa which lines the upper and posterior part of the nasal cavity (both on the lateral wall and on the septum). Nerve fibres arising in this mucosa collect to form about twenty bundles that together constitute an olfactory nerve.

The fibres of the olfactory nerves are processes of olfactory receptor cells located in the olfactory epithelium. Each cell gives off a short peripheral process directed towards the lumen of the nasal cavity; and a larger central process that passes into the mucosa forming one fibre of the olfactory nerve. These fibres collect to form about twenty bundles that together constitute an olfactory nerve. The bundles pass through foramina in the cribriform plate of the ethmoid bone to enter the cranial cavity (anterior cranial fossa) where they terminate in the ***olfactory bulb*** (Fig. 9.21). Olfactory impulses carried by these fibres pass to other neurons located in the olfactory bulb. From the bulb they pass into the olfactory tract and ultimately end in several small areas located on the inferior surface of the cerebral hemisphere.

The most important of these is the ***entorhinal area*** made up of the ***uncus*** and the anterior part of the ***parahippocampal gyrus*** (Fig. 9.22). Smell is perceived in this region of the brain.

As the olfactory mucosa is derived from ectoderm the olfactory nerves are classified as special somatic afferent (along with fibres for vision and hearing). However, smell is often regarded as a visceral sensation because of its close association to eating. Some authorities, therefore, classify the fibres of the olfactory nerves as special visceral afferent (like those of taste).

THE OPTIC NERVE

The optic nerve forms an important part of the visual pathway. It lies partly in the orbit and partly in the cranial cavity. Its anterior end is attached to the posterior pole of the eyeball. The attachment lies a little medial to the anteroposterior axis of the eyeball. From here the nerve passes backwards

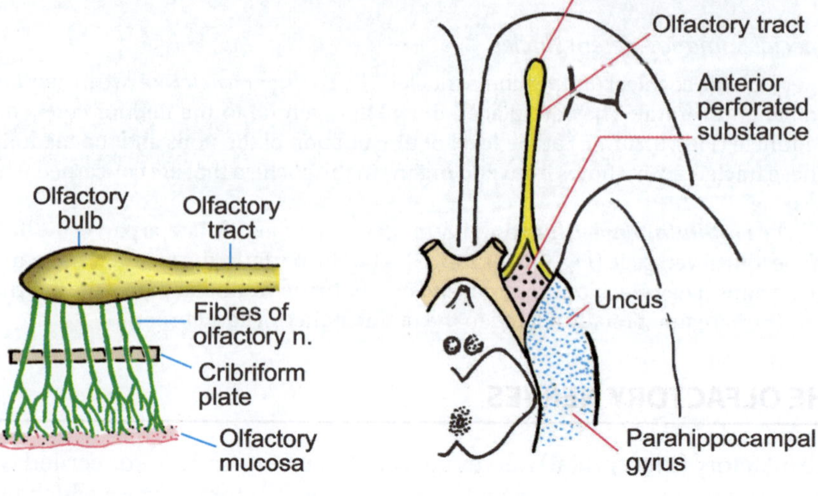

Fig. 9.21 Scheme to show the course of the olfactory nerve.

Fig. 9.22 Diagram showing the entorhinal area made up of the uncus and the anterior part of the hippocampal gyrus.

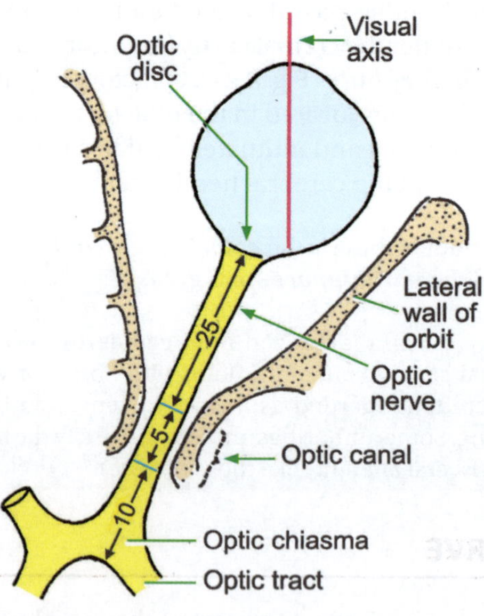

Fig. 9.23 Scheme to show course of the optic nerve.

and medially first through the orbit, next through the optic canal and finally through part of the cranial cavity. The nerve ends by joining the nerve of the opposite side to form the ***optic chiasma*** (Fig. 9.23). The total length of the nerve is about 40 mm. of this 25 mm is in the orbit, 5 mm in the optic canal and 10 mm in the cranial cavity.

The intraorbital part of the nerve is surrounded by the superior, inferior, medial and lateral recti (Fig. 9.24). The ciliary ganglion is placed between the optic nerve and the lateral rectus muscle. The relationship of the nerve to the ophthalmic artery is shown in Figs. 1.20B and 8.10. The artery is inferolateral to the nerve in the optic canal and in the posteriormost part of the orbit. The artery then crosses above the nerve from lateral to medial side. Apart from the ophthalmic artery the optic nerve is crossed from medial to lateral side by the nasociliary nerve which crosses above the nerve; and by the branch from the oculomotor nerve to the medial rectus muscle, which crosses below the nerve. The relationship of the nerve to the central artery of the retina is shown in Fig. 8.11. The artery first lies below the optic nerve. Piercing the dural sheath of the nerve it runs forwards for a short distance between these two. About 12 mm behind the eyeball the artery enters the substance of the nerve and runs forwards in its substance to reach the eyeball. The part of the optic nerve within the optic canal is related to the ophthalmic artery which lies below and lateral to it (Fig. 9.25). On the medial side the nerve is separated only by a thin plate of bone from the sphenoidal air sinus. The intracranial part of the optic nerve is related to the internal carotid artery which is on its lateral side; and to the anterior cerebral artery which crosses above it (Fig. 9.26).

The fibres of the optic nerve are classified as special somatic afferent (because the retina is derived from ectoderm).

The Visual Pathway

To understand the functional importance of the optic nerve it is necessary to briefly consider some facts about the visual pathway. The peripheral receptors for light are situated in the retina. Nerve fibres arising in the retina constitute the optic nerves. The two optic nerves join to form the optic chiasma in which many of their fibres cross to the opposite side. The uncrossed fibres of the optic nerve, along with the fibres that have crossed over from the opposite side form the ***optic tract.*** The optic tract terminates predominantly in the ***lateral geniculate body***. Fresh fibres arising in the lateral geniculate body form the ***geniculo-calcarine tract*** (or optic radiation) which ends in the ***visual areas*** of the cerebral cortex. Vision is actually perceived in the cerebral cortex.

Nerve fibres arising in the retina converge upon an area on the posteromedial part of the eyeball called the optic disc. Here the fibres pass through the thickness of the retina, the choroid and the sclera. In this situation the sclera has numerous perforations and is, therefore, called the ***lamina cribrosa*** (crib = sieve). The optic nerve is formed by the aggregation of fibres passing out through the lamina cribrosa.

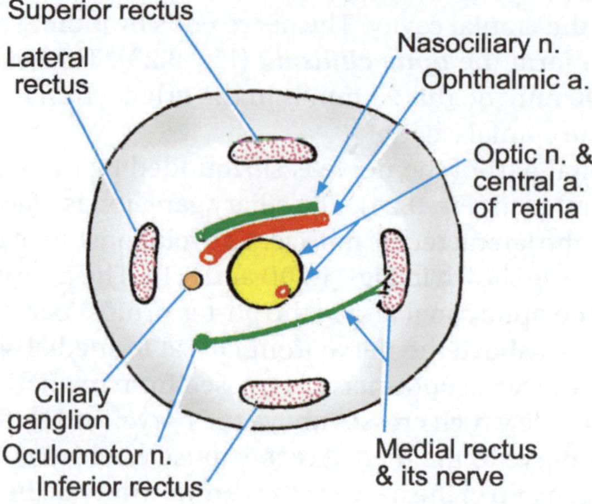

Fig. 9.24 Schematic coronal section to show some relations of the optic nerve.

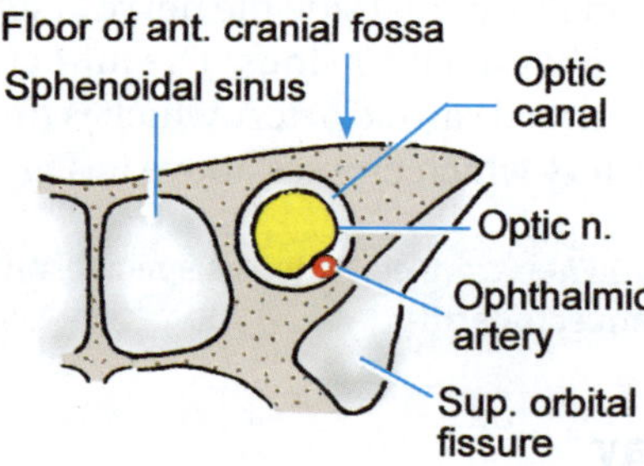

Fig. 9.25 Optic nerve in the optic canal.

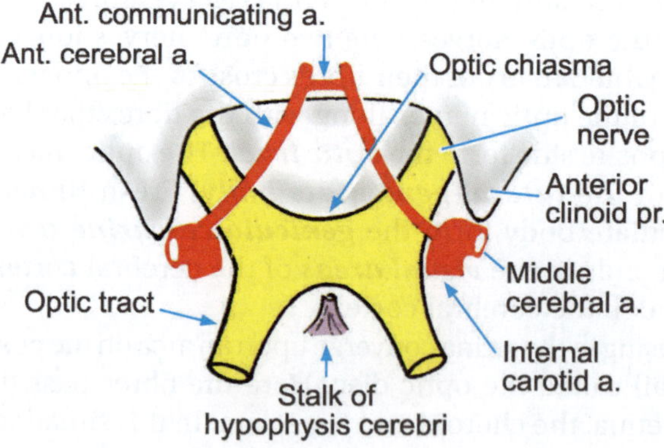

Fig. 9.26 Some relations of the optic nerve in its intracranial part.

The optic nerve contains about 1,200,000 fibres. Within the retina these fibres are unmyelinated, but come to be surrounded by myelin sheaths after they emerge through the lamina cribrosa.

The optic nerves are surrounded by sheaths formed by prolongation on to them of the duramater, the arachnoidmater and the piamater. This is one reason why the optic nerves are often regarded as parts of the brain rather than as peripheral nerves. Other reasons are the mode of development of the nerve (as a diverticulum from the brain) and the fact that the myelin sheaths for the fibres are formed not by Schwann cells (as in peripheral nerves) but by glial cells (as in the brain).

Fibres responsible for sharp vision arise from an area of the retina called the ***macula***. The fibres arising from the macula form the ***papillo-macular bundle.***

Close to the eyeball the macular fibres occupy the lateral part of the optic nerve, but by the time they reach the chiasma they lie in the central part of the nerve.

The fibres of the optic nerve arising in the medial (or nasal) half of each retina enter the optic tract of the opposite side after crossing in the optic chiasma. Fibres of the lateral (or temporal) half of each retina enter the optic tract of the same side. Thus the right optic tract comes to contain fibres from the right halves of both retinae; and the left tract from the left halves. The optic tract carries these fibres to the lateral geniculate body of the corresponding side. From here they are relayed to the corresponding cerebral hemisphere. (For details of the visual pathway see Chapter 23). For effects of damage see Chapter 15

THE OCULOMOTOR NERVE

The oculomotor is the third cranial nerve. Most of the fibres of this nerve arise from the oculomotor nuclear complex which is situated in the upper part of the midbrain (ventral to the aqueduct, Figs. 9.19, 9.20F). The right and left nuclei are fused to form a midline complex. Fibres arising in the complex supply all extrinsic muscles of the eyeball except the lateral rectus and the superior oblique. These fibres also supply the levator palpebrae superioris.

Some fibres of the oculomotor nerve arise from the Edinger-Westphal nucleus which forms part of the oculomotor complex. Fibres arising in this nucleus relay in the ciliary ganglion. Postganglionic fibres arising in this ganglion supply the sphincter pupillae and the ciliaris muscle.

Arising from these nuclei the fibres of the oculomotor nerve pass forwards through the substance of the midbrain and emerge on the anteromedial side of the cerebral peduncle (Figs. 9.28, 9.29). Just in front of the midbrain the nerve passes between the superior cerebellar artery (which lies below it) and the posterior cerebral artery (which lies above it). Here the nerve lies in the subarachnoid space. Passing forwards and laterally the nerve pierces the arachnoid. It then pierces the inner layer of dura mater in the triangular interval bounded by the free and attached margins of the tentorium cerebelli (Fig. 9.28). The nerve now comes to lie in the lateral wall of the cavernous sinus (Fig. 9.30). In the anterior part of this wall the nerve divides into superior and inferior rami (Fig. 9.35).

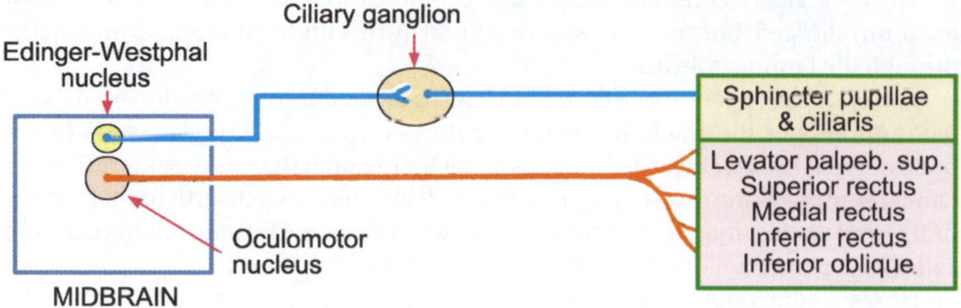

Fig. 9.27 Scheme to show the distribution of the oculomotor nerve.

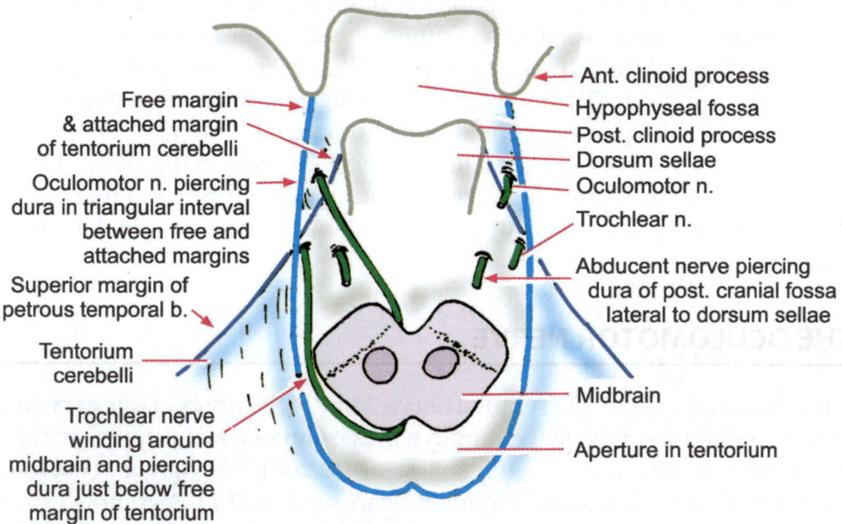

Fig. 9.28 Diagram to show the sites of penetration of duramater by the oculomotor, trochlear and abducent nerves.

The superior and inferior rami enter the orbit by passing through the superior orbital fissure (Fig. 9.32). They pass through the part of the fissure that lies within the tendinous ring that gives origin to the four recti of the eyeball. Within the orbit the superior ramus supplies the superior rectus and the levator palpebrae superioris. The inferior division supplies the medial rectus the inferior rectus and the inferior oblique (Figs. 1.19B, 9.31).

Preganglionic fibres arising from the Edinger Westphal nucleus travel through the trunk of the nerve, and then through its inferior division. They then pass into the nerve for the inferior oblique muscle. A short branch arising from this nerve conveys the fibres to the ciliary ganglion. This branch to the ciliary ganglion from the nerve to the inferior oblique constitutes the ***motor root*** of the ganglion. The cells of the ganglion give origin to postganglionic fibres which pass through the short ciliary nerves to reach the sphincter pupillae and the ciliaris muscles.

The ***ciliary ganglion*** lies lateral to the optic nerve (between it and the lateral rectus, Fig. 9.24). Posteriorly, it receives three roots: motor or parasympathetic, sympathetic, and sensory. The motor or parasympathetic root has been described above. The ***sympathetic root*** arises from the sympathetic plexus on the internal carotid artery. It carries postganglionic sympathetic fibres that begin in the superior cervical sympathetic ganglion. They pass through the ciliary ganglion, without relay, and enter the short ciliary nerves through which they reach the blood vessels of the eyeball. (The fibres for the dilator pupillae normally follow a separate route, as described below, but sometimes they may pass through the ciliary ganglion).

The sensory root of the ciliary ganglion is a branch of the nasociliary nerve. It carries sensory fibres that begin in the cornea, the iris and the choroid; pass through the short ciliary nerves and then through the ciliary ganglion; and finally enter the sensory root through which they reach the nasociliary nerve.

The effects of injury to the oculomotor nerve are considered in Chapter 15.

The fibres of the oculomotor nerve that supply skeletal muscle are classified as somatic efferent, while those that supply smooth muscle (sphincter pupillae, ciliaris) are general visceral efferent.

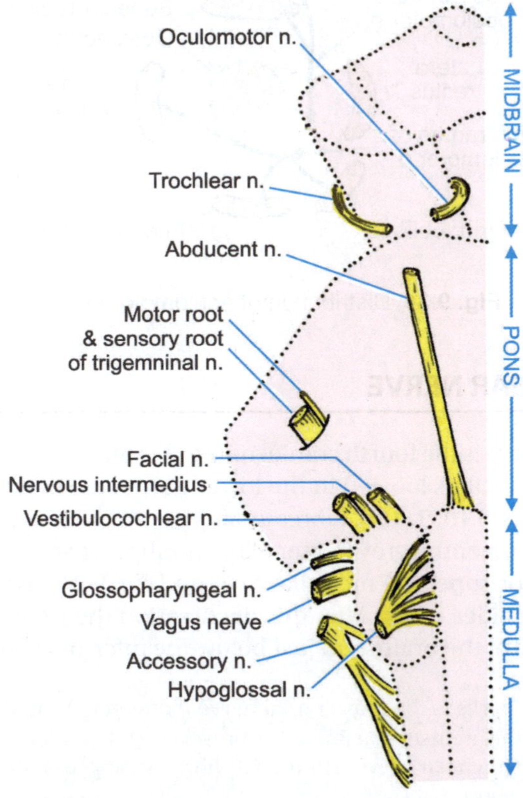

Fig. 9.29 Attachment of cranial nerves to the surface of the brainstem.

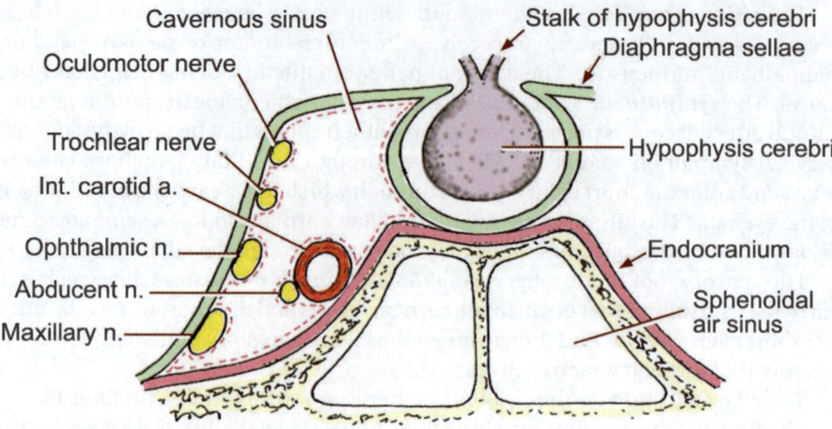

Fig. 9.30 Relationship of cranial nerves to the cavernous sinus.

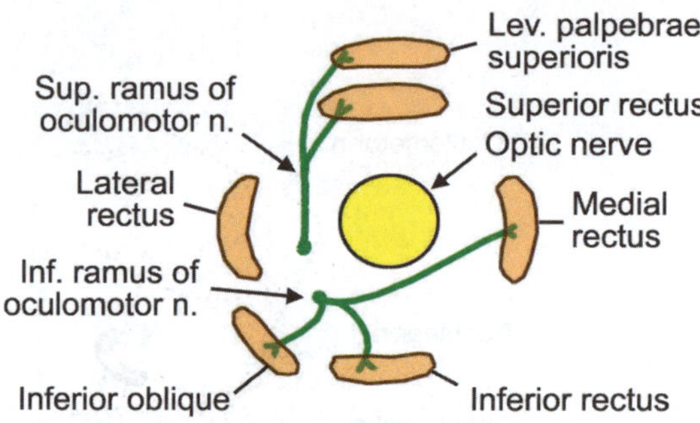

Fig. 9.31 Distribution of oculomotor nerve.

THE TROCHLEAR NERVE

The trochlear nerve is the fourth cranial nerve. It is made up of fibres that arise in the trochlear nucleus located in the lower part of the midbrain (ventral to the aqueduct, Figs. 9.19, 9.20E). Fibres arising in this nucleus pass ***backwards*** winding round the central grey matter of the midbrain to reach the upper part of the anterior (or superior) medullary velum (Fig. 9.34). Here the fibres of the right and left sides ***cross.*** After this decussation the fibres emerge on the posterior surface of the brainstem just below the inferior colliculus.

The trochlear nerve is the only cranial nerve that emerges on the posterior (or dorsal) aspect of the brainstem. It is also the only nerve that undergoes decussation. As a result the left trochlear nerve is formed by fibres arising from the right trochlear nucleus and vice versa.

Having emerged from the midbrain the nerve winds round the cerebral peduncle to reach the front of the brain stem (Fig. 9.29). While winding round the cerebral peduncle the nerve lies between the posterior cerebral artery (above it) and the superior cerebellar artery (below it). The nerve now runs forwards and pierces the dura mater just below the free margin of the tentorium cerebelli (Fig. 9.28). The point of penetration lies a little behind the posterior clinoid process. Having pierced the dura the nerve comes to lie in the lateral wall of the cavernous sinus, below the oculomotor nerve, but above the ophthalmic division of the trigeminal nerve (Fig. 9.30, 9.35).

Continuing forwards it crosses lateral to the oculomotor nerve to enter the upper part of the superior orbital fissure (Fig. 9.32). In the fissure it lies above the tendinous ring for origin of the recti of the eyeball (Fig. 9.32). Having entered the orbit the nerve runs forwards, above the orbital muscles, and ends in the superior oblique muscle (Fig. 1.19B).

> The fibres of the trochlear nerve are classified as somatic efferent
> The effects of injury to the trochlear nerve are considered in Chapter 15.

The next cranial nerve, in order of numerical sequence, is the fifth or trigeminal. However, the abducent nerve (sixth) is considered first as its course and distribution are similar to those of the oculomotor and trochlear nerves.

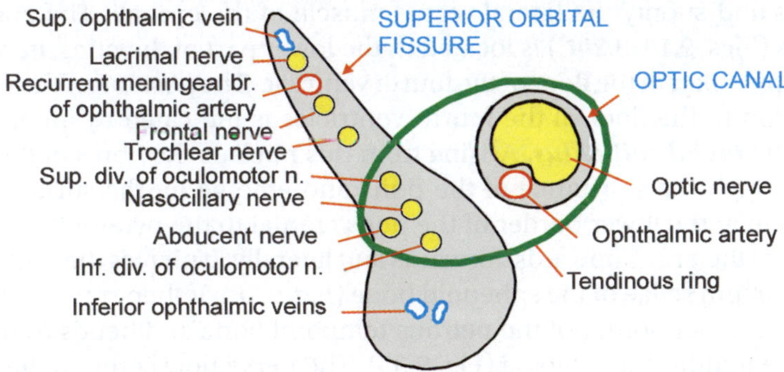

Fig. 9.32 Position of cranial nerves in the superior orbital fissure.

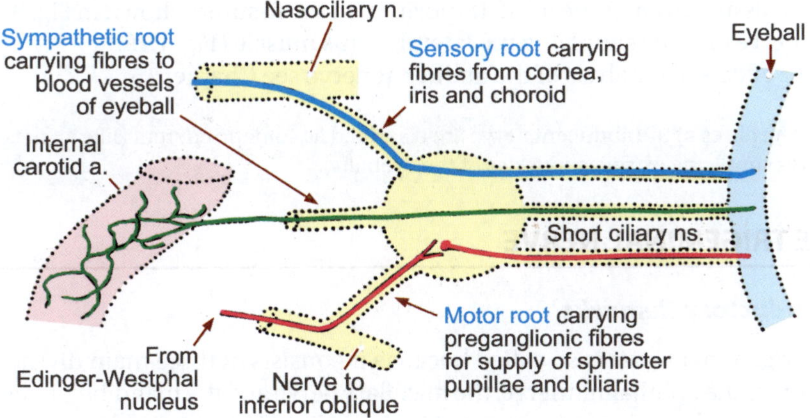

Fig. 9.33 Scheme to show the connections of the ciliary ganglion.

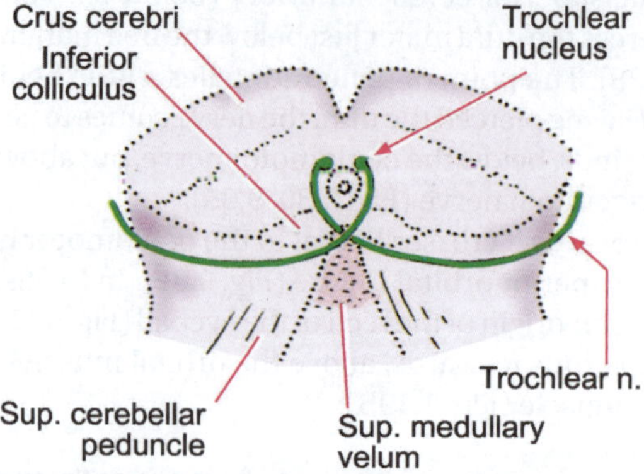

Fig. 9.34 Schematic posterior view of the course of the trochlear nerve.

THE ABDUCENT NERVE

This is the sixth cranial nerve. It is made up of fibres that arise in the abducent nucleus and supply the lateral rectus muscle of the eyeball. The abducent nucleus (Figs. 9.19, 9.20C) is located in the lower part of the pons, in relation to the upper part of the floor of the fourth ventricle. The position of the nucleus in relation to the floor of the fourth ventricles is indicated by an elevation called the ***facial colliculus.*** Arising from this nucleus the fibres of the nerve pass through the substance of the pons and emerge on the surface of the brainstem at the lower border of the pons cranial to the pyramid (Fig. 9.29). The nerve then runs upwards, forwards and laterally. It pierces the dura lateral to the dorsum sellae of the sphenoid bone (Fig. 9.28). It then runs upwards to reach the upper border of the petrous temporal bone and bends round it to enter the middle cranial fossa (Fig. 9.35). The nerve now comes to lie within the cavernous sinus, where it is closely related to the internal carotid artery. The nerve is first lateral to the artery and then inferolateral to it (Fig. 9.35). At the anterior end of the cavernous sinus the nerve passes through the superior orbital fissure to enter the orbit. Its position in the fissure is shown in Fig. 9.32. The nerve ends by supplying the lateral rectus muscle (Fig. 1.19B).

For effects of paralysis of the abducent nerve see Chapter 15.

The fibres of the abducent nerve are classified as somatic efferent (like all nerve fibres supplying extrinsic muscles of the eyeballs).

THE TRIGEMINAL NERVE

Introductory Remarks

The trigeminal nerve is so called because it consists of three main divisions. These are the ophthalmic nerve, the maxillary nerve and the mandibular nerve. These nerves arise from a large trigeminal ganglion. The ganglion is connected to the brain stem (pons) by a thick sensory root. The trigeminal nerve also has

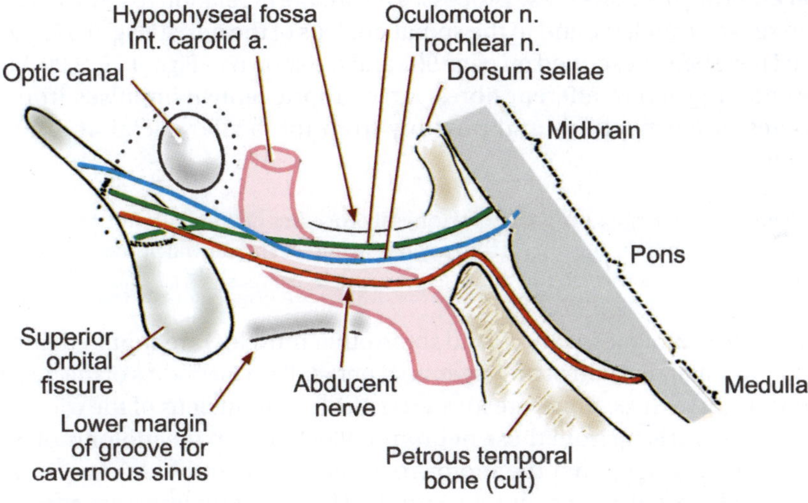

Fig. 9.35 Schematic lateral view of the region of the cavernous sinus to show the course of the oculomotor, trochlear and abducent nerves.

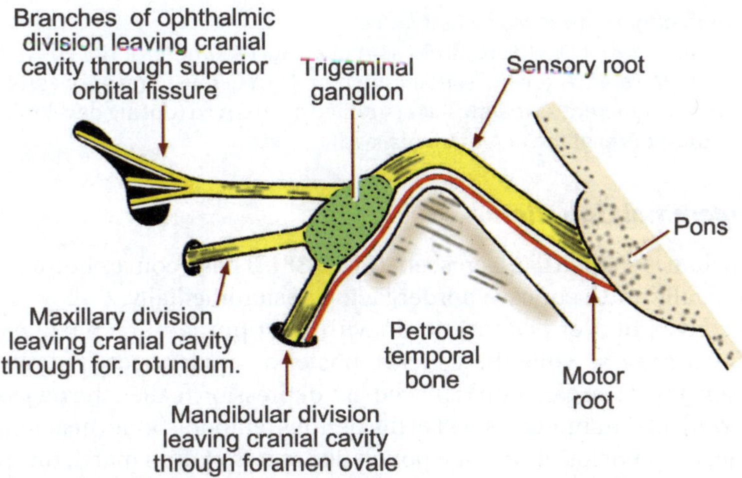

Fig. 9.36 Roots and divisions of the trigeminal nerve.

a motor root (Fig. 9.29) which emerges from the pons medial to the sensory root. (Note: M for motor and M for medial). The motor root passes deep to the trigeminal ganglion and joins the mandibular nerve (See Fig. 9.36).

The trigeminal nerve contains both afferent and efferent fibres.

Afferent fibres are peripheral processes of unipolar neurons located in the trigeminal ganglion. They are distributed through all three divisions of the nerve. They carry exteroceptive sensations from the skin of the face, the mucous membrane of the mouth, and the mucous membrane of the nose. The central processes of the neurons in the trigeminal ganglion form the sensory root.

After entering the pons these processes terminate in relation to neurons in the main sensory nucleus, and in the spinal nucleus of the nerve (Fig. 9.37). These nuclei have been described on page 903 and are shown in Figs. 9.19, 9.20 A to D.

Another group of afferent fibres carry proprioceptive impulses from the muscles of mastication (and possibly from the ocular, facial and lingual muscles).

These fibres are believed to be peripheral processes of unipolar neurons present in the mesencephalic nucleus of the trigeminal nerve. The central processes of these neurons end in relation to the main sensory nucleus.

The muscles of mastication (and some other muscles) are supplied through the mandibular division of the trigeminal nerve. The cell bodies of the neurons giving origin to these fibres are located in the motor nucleus of the trigeminal nerve. Axons arising from these neurons collect to form the motor root of the nerve. We have seen that the motor root joins the mandibular nerve and is distributed through it. The muscles supplied by the motor fibres are as follows:

A. ***Muscles of mastication***: Masseter, temporalis, medial and lateral pterygoids.
B. ***Other muscles***: Mylohyoid, anterior belly of digastric, tensor palati, tensor tympani.

Functional components of trigeminal nerve

The afferent fibres of the nerve (from skin and mucosa and proprioceptive from muscle) are classified as general somatic afferent. The efferent fibres are classified as special visceral efferent as the muscles supplied are derived (during development) from the mesoderm of the first branchial arch.

The Trigeminal Ganglion

This ganglion is shaped like a crescent (Fig. 9.38). It has a convex border facing anterolaterally and a concave border facing posteromedially.

The convex border is continuous with the ophthalmic, maxillary and mandibular nerves; while the concave posterior border is continuous with the sensory root. The ganglion is placed in a depression (called the ***trigeminal impression***) on the anterior aspect of the petrous temporal bone (near its apex). The ganglion is enclosed within a pouch like recess of dura mater. this recess is called the ***trigeminal cave*** (Fig. 9.39). It bulges into the posterolateral part of the cavernous sinus. The nerves arising from the ganglion pierce the dura forming the anterior end of the trigeminal cave.

Some relations of the trigeminal ganglion are shown in Fig. 9.40.

THE OPHTHALMIC NERVE

The fibres of the ophthalmic nerve are purely sensory. However, some sympathetic fibres for the eyeball travel for part of their course through the nerve and some of its branches.

The ophthalmic nerve arises from the anteromedial part of the trigeminal ganglion (Fig. 9.41). It pierces the dura of the trigeminal cave (and comes to

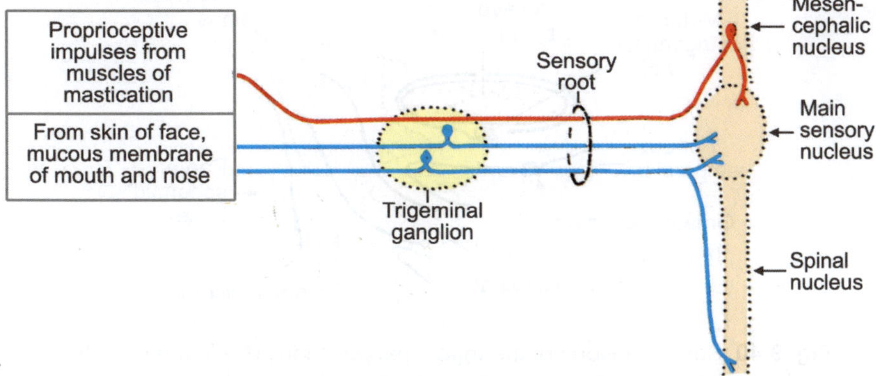

Fig. 9.37 Scheme to show the arrangement of afferent neurons of the trigeminal nerve. The fibres that descend along the spinal nucleus constitute the spinal tract of the nerve.

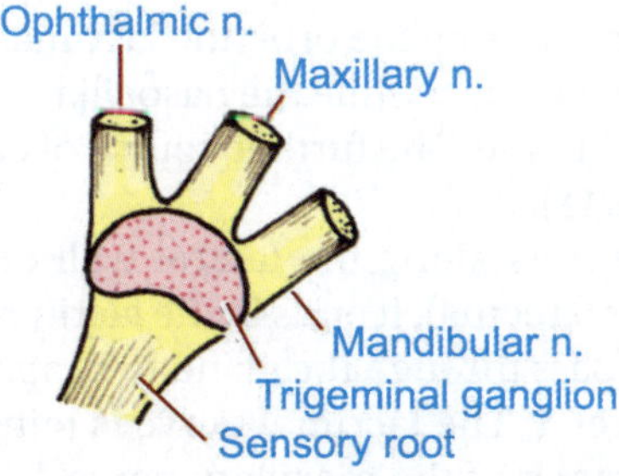

Fig. 9.38 Trigeminal ganglion seen from above.

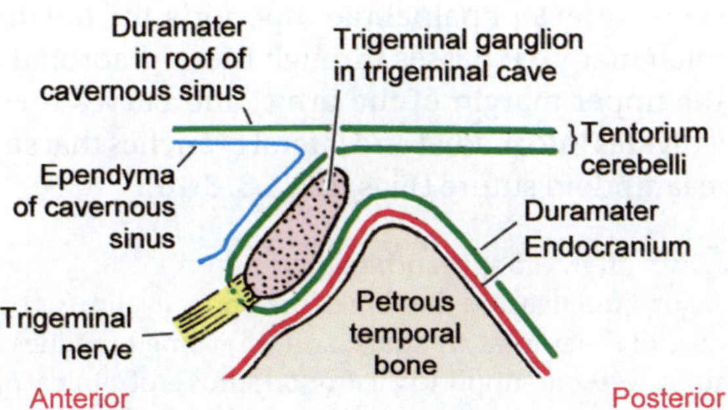

Fig. 9.39 Diagram showing formation of the trigeminal cave. The diagram represents a parasagittal section through the medial part of the petrous temporal bone.

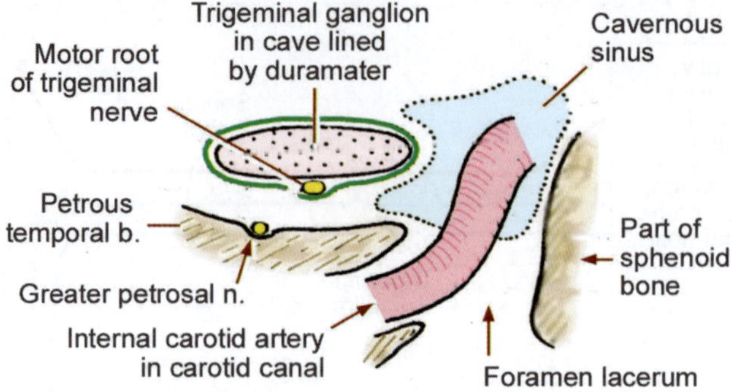

Fig. 9.40 Some relations of the trigeminal ganglion. The figure depicts a schematic coronal section through the foramen lacerum.

lie in the lateral wall of the cavernous sinus, below the trochlear nerve (Fig. 9.30). Passing forwards it divides into three branches. These are the ***lacrimal***, the ***frontal***, and the ***nasociliary*** nerves.

These branches enter the orbit by passing through the superior orbital fissure. Their positions in the fissure are shown in Fig. 9.32. From this figure it will be obvious that on entering the orbit the lacrimal and frontal branches will lie above the orbital muscles; while the nasociliary nerve will lie between them, lateral to the optic nerve. The further course of each of these branches is as follows (Fig. 1.20, 9.41).

The ***lacrimal nerve*** runs along the lateral wall of the orbit (along the upper border of the lateral rectus). It ends in the lacrimal gland (and hence its name). Some branches pass through the gland to supply the conjunctiva and the skin of the upper eyelid. The lacrimal nerve is joined by a twig from the zygomaticotemporal branch of the maxillary nerve. The ***frontal nerve*** runs forwards between the levator palpebrae superioris and the periosteum lining the roof of the orbit. It ends by dividing into supraorbital and supratrochlear branches.

The ***supraorbital nerve*** continues in the line of the frontal nerve (Fig. 9.41), lying between the levator palpebrae superioris and the roof of the orbit. Reaching the orbital margin it passes through the supraorbital notch (on the medial part of the upper margin of the orbit) and curves upwards into the forehead. Here it divides into medial and lateral branches that supply the scalp as far back as the lambdoid suture (Figs. 1.2, 1.3, 3.16).

Other branches given off by the supraorbital nerve are:
(i) branches to the conjunctiva and the skin of the upper eyelid; (ii) branches to the mucous membrane of the frontal air sinus; and (iii) some branches to the deeper tissues of the scalp. The nerve supply to the frontal sinus is of clinical importance. In frontal sinusitis pain is referred to the area of the scalp supplied by the supraorbital nerve (***frontal headache***).

The ***supratrochlear nerve*** runs forwards and medially above the orbital muscles, and medial to the supraorbital nerve. It passes above the trochlea

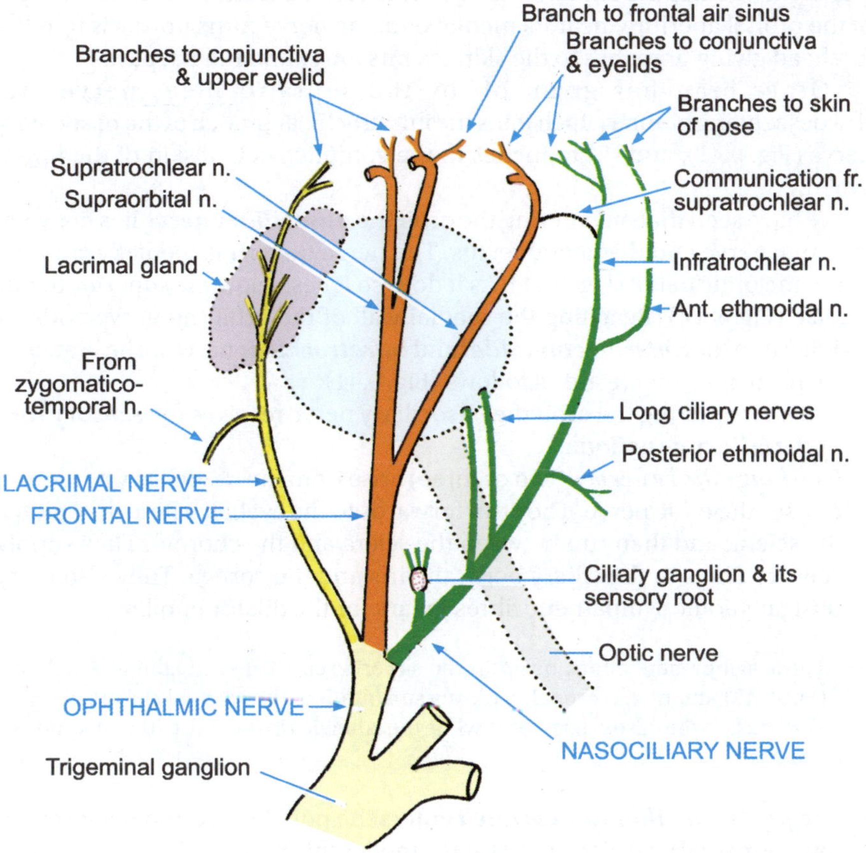

Branch to frontal air sinus
Branches to conjunctiva & upper eyelid
Branches to conjunctiva & eyelids
Branches to skin of nose
Supratrochlear n.
Supraorbital n.
Communication fr. supratrochlear n.
Lacrimal gland
Infratrochlear n.
Ant. ethmoidal n.
From zygomatico-temporal n.
Long ciliary nerves
Posterior ethmoidal n.
LACRIMAL NERVE
FRONTAL NERVE
Ciliary ganglion & its sensory root
Optic nerve
OPHTHALMIC NERVE
Trigeminal ganglion
NASOCILIARY NERVE

Fig. 9.41 Scheme to show the distribution of the ophthalmic nerve.

Supraorbital n.
Frontal sinus
Frontal n.
Roof of orbit
Eyelid
Eyeball
Optic nerve
Optic nerve
Lev. palpebrae superioris
Superior rectus

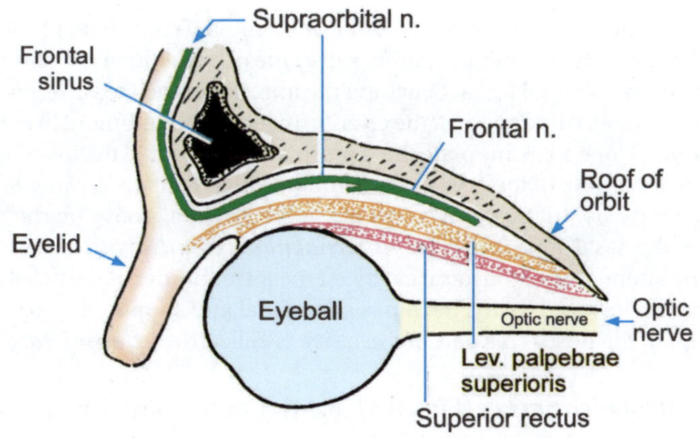

Fig. 9.42 Scheme to show the course of the frontal and supraorbital nerves.

(for the tendon of the superior oblique muscle). Reaching the upper margin of the orbital aperture, near its medial end, the nerve turns upwards into the forehead giving branches to the skin over its lower and medial part.

Other branches given off by the supratrochlear nerve are: (i) a descending branch which joins the infratrochlear branch of the nasociliary nerve (Fig. 9.41); and (ii) branches to the conjunctiva and skin of the upper eyelid.

We have seen that on entering the orbit the ***nasociliary nerve*** lies between the optic nerve and the lateral rectus. The nerve then runs medially crossing above the optic nerve (Fig. 9.41). As it does so it lies below the superior rectus muscle (Fig. 9.24). Reaching the medial wall of the orbit the nerve ends by dividing into the ***anterior ethmoidal*** and ***infratrochlear*** nerves. The branches of the nasociliary nerve are as follows (Fig. 9.41):

1. Just after entering the orbit the nasociliary nerve receives the ***sensory root of the ciliary ganglion.***.
2. The ***long ciliary nerves*** (two or three) arise from the nasociliary nerve as it crosses the optic nerve. They run forwards to the eyeball where they pierce the sclera; and then run between the sclera and the choroid. They supply sensory fibres to the ciliary body, the iris and the cornea. They also carry postganglionic sympathetic fibres meant for the dilator pupillae.

These sympathetic fibres begin in the superior cervical sympathetic ganglion (Fig. 9.43) and travel through a plexus surrounding the internal carotid artery. They pass to the nasociliary nerve while the latter lies in the wall of the cavernous sinus.

3. The ***posterior ethmoidal branch*** enters the posterior ethmoidal foramen (on the medial wall of the orbit) and supplies the ethmoidal and sphenoidal air sinuses (Fig. 9.44).
4. The ***anterior ethmoidal nerve*** has a complicated course through the orbit, the anterior cranial fossa, and the nasal cavity. Its terminal part is seen on the face as the external nasal nerve.

The first part of the nerve lies in the anterior ethmoidal canal (a in Fig. 9.44). One end of this canal opens on the medial wall of the orbit while the other end opens into the anterior cranial fossa. Reaching the anterior cranial fossa the nerve runs forwards for a short distance over the cribriform plate of the ethmoid (b in Fig. 9.44). Near the anterior end of this plate the nerve leaves the floor of the fossa by passing into a slit at the side of the crista galli through which it enters a canal (c) leading to the nasal cavity. In the nasal cavity the nerve lies in a groove on the posterior surface of the nasal bone (d). It gives ***internal nasal branches*** to the nasal septum and to the lateral wall of the nasal cavity. At the lower border of the nasal bone the nerve leaves the nasal cavity, becomes superficial and supplies the skin over the lower part of the nose. This part of the nerve is called the ***external nasal nerve***.

5. The ***infratrochlear nerve*** (Figs. 9.41; 9.44) runs forwards on the medial wall of the orbit and ends by supplying part of the skin of the upper and lower eyelids and over the upper part of the nose.

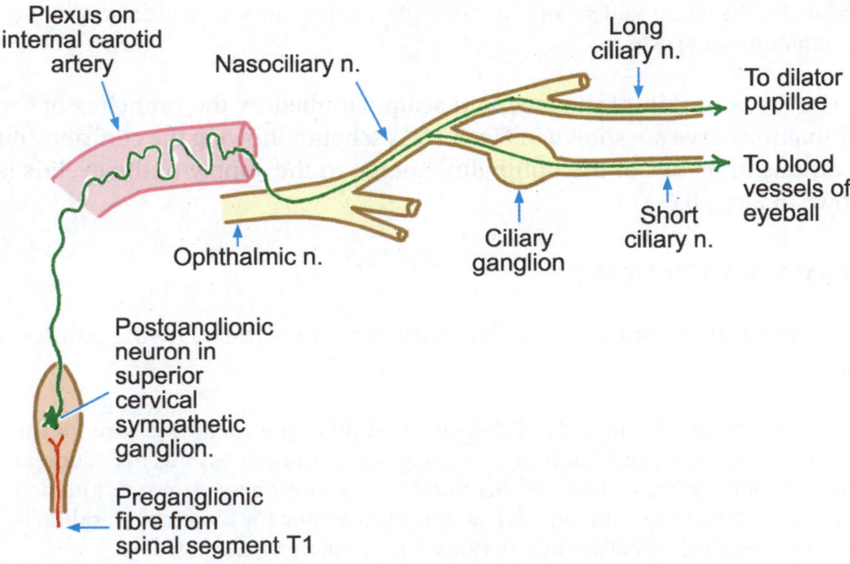

Fig. 9.43 Two pathways followed by sympathetic fibres for the eyeball. Occasionally, the fibres for the dilator pupillae may pass through the ciliary ganglion.

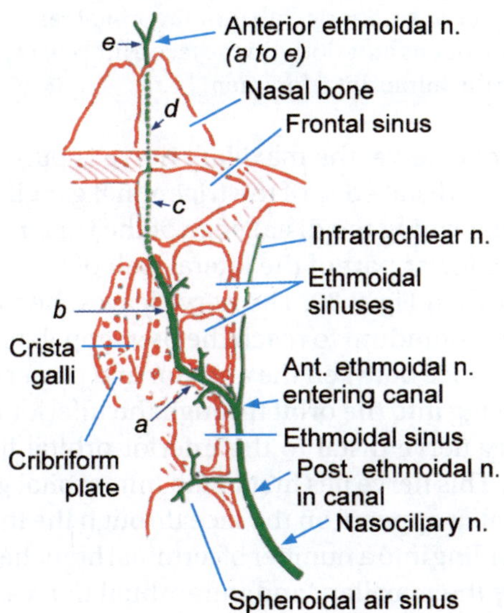

Fig. 9.44 Scheme to show the course of the anterior ethmoidal nerve. (a) in the anterior ethmoidal canal, (b) on the cribriform plate. (c) in the canal passing from the anterior cranial fossa to the nasal cavity. (d) on the deep surface of the nasal bone, (e) to skin over lower part of the nose. Superior view after removing bone covering the air sinuses shown.

The nerve also gives branches to the conjunctiva, the lacrimal sac and the lacrimal caruncle. The infratrochlear and supratrochlear nerves are joined to each other by a communicating twig.

The areas of skin of the face and scalp supplied by the branches of the ophthalmic nerve are shown in Fig. 3.16. A scheme showing the contribution of various branches of the ophthalmic nerve to the supply of the eyelids is shown in Fig. 3.6.

THE MAXILLARY NERVE

To understand the course of the maxillary nerve note the following points on a skull.

On either side of the body of the sphenoid there is a shallow groove for the cavernous sinus. Traced anteriorly the lower part of the groove ends in relation to the posterior opening of the foramen rotundum. If a wire is passed into this foramen and the skull is viewed from the lateral side it is seen that the foramen rotundum is really a canal. This canal opens anteriorly into the pterygopalatine fossa.

The pterygopalatine fossa is a narrow cleft having anterior, posterior and medial walls. The foramen rotundum opens on its posterior wall (Fig. 9.46). Anteriorly, the fossa communicates with the orbit through the inferior orbital fissure. The medial wall of the fossa has a large sphenopalatine foramen. The fossa is continued inferiorly into the greater and lesser palatine canals.

On the floor of the posterior part of the orbit there is a prominent infraorbital groove which is continuous anteriorly with the infraorbital canal. This canal traverses part of the maxilla and opens anteriorly on the face a little below the inferior margin of the orbit, through the infraorbital foramen.

Like the ophthalmic nerve, the maxillary nerve is purely sensory. It arises from the middle of the distal edge of the trigeminal ganglion (Fig. 9.36).

Piercing the dura forming the distal edge of the trigeminal cave (Fig. 9.39) it comes to lie in the lower part of the lateral wall of the cavernous sinus: its position here is shown in Fig. 9.30. The nerve leaves the middle cranial fossa through the foramen rotundum to reach the pterygopalatine fossa. The nerve crosses the short distance between the anterior and posterior wall of the fossa and leaves it by passing into the orbit through the inferior orbital fissure. The part of the maxillary nerve distal to the inferior orbital fissure is called the ***infraorbital nerve.*** This nerve lies first in the infraorbital groove, and then in the infraorbital canal. It appears on the face through the infraorbital foramen and ends here by dividing into a number of terminal branches. Several branches are also given off by the maxillary and infraorbital nerves along their course as follows.

A. Branch in middle cranial fossa:

Before entering the foramen rotundum the maxillary nerve gives off a ***meningeal branch*** to the dura mater of the middle cranial fossa (Fig. 9.47).

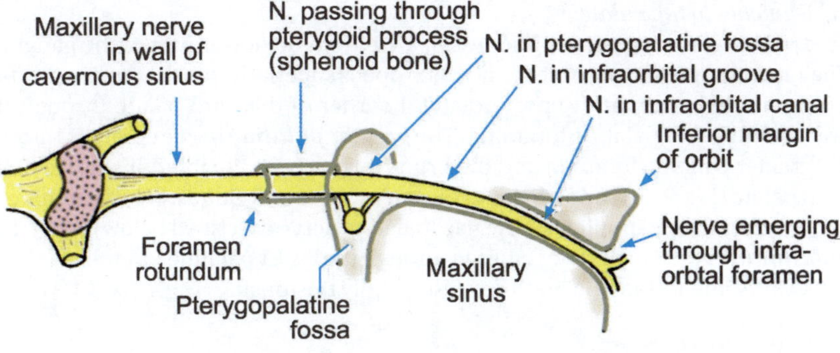

Fig. 9.45 Scheme to show the course of the maxillary nerve.

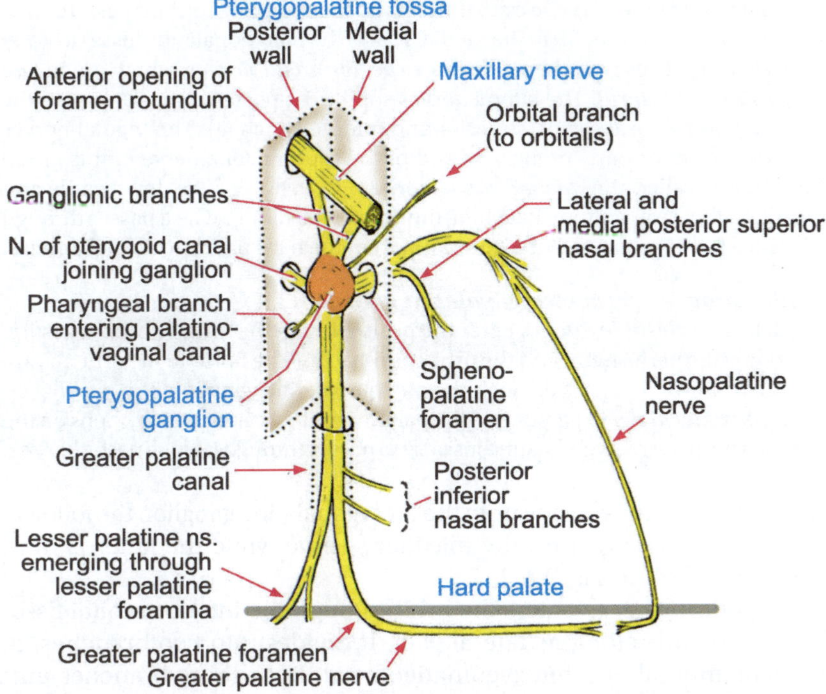

Fig. 9.46 Scheme to show branches of the pterygopalatine ganglion.

B. Branches arising in pterygopalatine fossa:

In the pterygopalatine fossa the maxillary nerve is connected to the pterygopalatine ganglion by two ***ganglionic branches*** (Figs. 9.26, 9.27). Many fibres of the maxillary nerve pass through these ganglionic branches to the ganglion. They, however, have no functional relationship to the ganglion and leave it through a number of branches which are as follows (Fig. 9.46).

(1) Branches to the palate:
Two palatine nerves, greater and lesser, arise from the lower part of the ganglion. They enter the greater palatine canal which opens superiorly into the pterygopalatine fossa; and inferiorly at the posterolateral corner of the hard palate through the greater and lesser palatine foramina. The ***greater palatine nerve*** emerges through the greater palatine foramen and then runs forwards on the inferior surface of the hard palate (Fig. 9.46) supplying mucous membrane and glands. (The anterior part of the hard palate is supplied by the nasopalatine nerve described below). The ***lesser palatine nerves*** (usually two) emerge through the lesser palatine foramina and run backwards into the soft palate. They also supply the tonsil.

(2) Branches to the nose:
Some ***posterior inferior nasal branches*** arise from the greater palatine nerve and pass through minute apertures in the medial wall of the canal to enter the nasal cavity. They supply the posterior and inferior part of the lateral wall of the nasal cavity (inferior concha, middle meatus, inferior meatus).

Several nasal branches arise from the pterygopalatine ganglion and pass through the sphenopalatine foramen (in the medial wall of the pterygopalatine fossa) to enter the nasal cavity. These are the ***posterior superior nasal nerves***, which are in two sets, ***medial*** and ***lateral***. The lateral nerves supply the posterosuperior part of the lateral wall of the nasal cavity (superior and middle conchae). The medial nerves supply the posterior parts of the roof and of the septum. One nerve of this group is large and is called the ***nasopalatine nerve*** (Fig. 9.46). It runs downwards and forwards on the nasal septum. Reaching the floor of the nasal cavity it passes through the incisive foramen to reach the anterior part of the hard palate which it supplies.

(3) Other branches from pterygopalatine ganglion:
A few delicate ***orbital branches*** enter the orbit through the inferior orbital fissure. They supply the periosteum and the orbitalis muscle. (The fibres to the orbitalis are sympathetic fibres that pass through the pterygopalatine ganglion.

The ***pharyngeal nerve*** passes into the palatinovaginal canal (which opens on the posterior wall of the pterygopalatine fossa) and passes through it to the nasopharynx.

Apart from branches arising from the pterygopalatine ganglion the following branches arise directly from the maxillary nerve while the latter is in the pterygopalatine fossa (Fig. 9.47).

The ***zygomatic nerve*** enters the orbit through the inferior orbital fissure and runs forwards along its lateral wall. It divides into two branches, the zygmaticotemporal and the zygomaticofacial. Both these branches enter foramina present on the orbital surface of the zygomatic bone. Travelling through the zygomatic bone the ***zygomaticotemporal nerve*** emerges from the temporal surface of the bone. The nerve ends by supplying the skin over the temple. The ***zygomaticofacial nerve*** also passes through the substance of the zygomatic bone. It emerges from the bone through the zygomaticofacial foramen present on the lateral surface of the bone and supplies the skin of the cheek.

The ***posterior superior alveolar nerve*** arises from the maxillary nerve in the pterygopalatine fossa. It runs down on the posterior surface of the maxilla (which forms the anterior wall of the pterygopalatine fossa) and then pierces it. The nerve

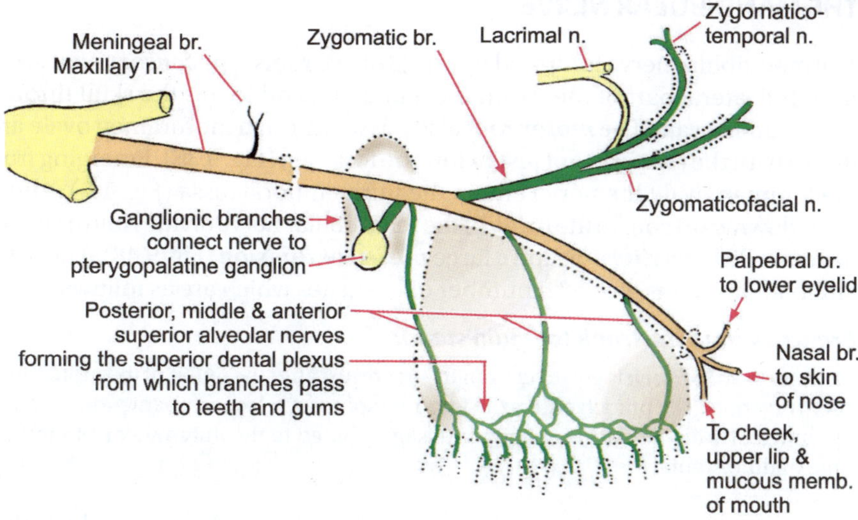

Fig. 9.47 Scheme to show direct branches arising from the maxillary nerve (including its infraorbital continuation). For indirect branches through the pterygopalatine ganglion see Fig. 9.46.

now comes to lie in the wall of the maxillary sinus which it supplies. It then divides into branches that form a plexus over the roots of the molar teeth. Branches from the plexus supply these teeth and the related gums.

C. Branches arising in the infraorbital groove and canal:

The ***middle superior alveolar nerve*** arises from the infraorbital nerve as the latter lies in the infraorbital groove. Entering a foramen in the floor of the groove it reaches the maxillary sinus and joins the posterior superior alveolar nerve in forming a plexus above the roots of the upper teeth. The fibres of this nerve supply the premolar teeth through the plexus.

The ***anterior superior alveolar nerve*** arises from the infraorbital nerve as the latter lies in the infraorbital canal. It then enters a bony canal that follows a complicated course through the maxillary bone (hence called the canalis sinuosis) to reach the incisor and canine teeth which it supplies. Branches from the posterior, middle and anterior superior alveolar nerves form a continuous plexus (***superior dental plexus***) in relation to the roots of the teeth borne on the maxilla. The anterior superior alveolar nerve also gives minute branches to the nasal cavity.

D. Branches of infraorbital nerve in the face:

The infraorbital nerve divides into the following branches after emerging from the infraorbital foramen.

The ***palpebral branches*** supply the lower eyelid. ***Nasal branches*** supply the skin on the lateral side of the nose. ***Superior labial*** branches supply the skin of the upper lip and part of the cheek. Some branches reach the mucous membrane of the mouth. The area of the skin of the face supplied by the maxillary nerve is shown in Fig. 3.16. The pterygopalatine ganglion is functionally related to the facial nerve and is considered later in this Chapter.

THE MANDIBULAR NERVE

The mandibular nerve is formed by union of two roots. The ***sensory root*** arises from the lateral part of the trigeminal ganglion, and leaves the skull through the foramen ovale. The ***motor root*** also passes through the foramen ovale and unites with the sensory root just below the foramen (Fig. 9.36). Emerging from the foramen ovale the nerve enters the infratemporal fossa (Fig. 1.7). After a short downward course the trunk of the mandibular nerve divides into a smaller ***anterior*** division ***division*** and a large ***posterior division*** (Fig. 9.48). The trunk and both divisions give off a number of branches which are as follows.

Branches from the trunk (or main stem):

A ***meningeal branch*** is given off from the nerve just after the union of the motor and sensory roots. The branch enters the foramen spinosum. It accompanies the middle meningeal artery and its branches and is distributed to the duramater (mainly) of the middle cranial fossa.

The ***nerve to the medial pterygoid*** supplies this muscle. It gives a branch to the otic ganglion. The fibres in this branch pass through the ganglion without relay and supply the tensor tympani and the tensor palati muscles (Fig. 9.49).

Branches from the anterior division:

The ***buccal nerve*** is sensory (Fig. 1.5). It runs downwards and forwards through the muscles of the infratemporal fossa to reach the surface of the buccinator muscle. Here it supplies the skin superficial to the muscle and the mucous membrane lining its deep surface. (Note: Take care not to confuse the buccal nerve with the buccal branch of the facial nerve).

The remaining branches of the anterior division of the mandibular nerve are motor. They supply the masseter, the lateral pterygoid and the temporalis as follows (Fig. 9.49).

The ***nerve to the masseter*** passes laterally in front of the neck of the mandible (i.e., in the posterior part of the mandibular notch) to reach the masseter (Fig. 1.6).

The ***nerve to the lateral pterygoid*** may be independent or may arise from the buccal nerve.

The temporalis is supplied through the ***anterior, middle and posterior deep temporal nerves*** (Fig. 1.6). These nerves pass upwards (above the lateral pterygoid) to reach the deep surface of the temporalis (Fig. 9.49). The anterior branch sometimes arises from the buccal nerve. The posterior branch may arise from the nerve to the masseter.

Branches from the posterior division:

The posterior division of the mandibular nerve gives rise to three important nerves. These are the auriculotemporal, the lingual and the inferior alveolar nerves.

The Auriculotemporal Nerve

The auriculotemporal nerve arises by two roots which form a ring through which the middle meningeal artery passes upwards (Figs. 9.48, 9.50). The nerve runs backwards deep in the infratemporal fossa; and crosses deep to the neck of the mandible. It then turns laterally behind the temporomandibular joint. In this part of its course it is closely related to the upper part of the parotid gland. The nerve finally turns upwards into the scalp and ends by dividing into branches that supply the skin over the temple (Figs. 1.6, 1.7). The other branches of the nerve are shown in Fig. 9.50.

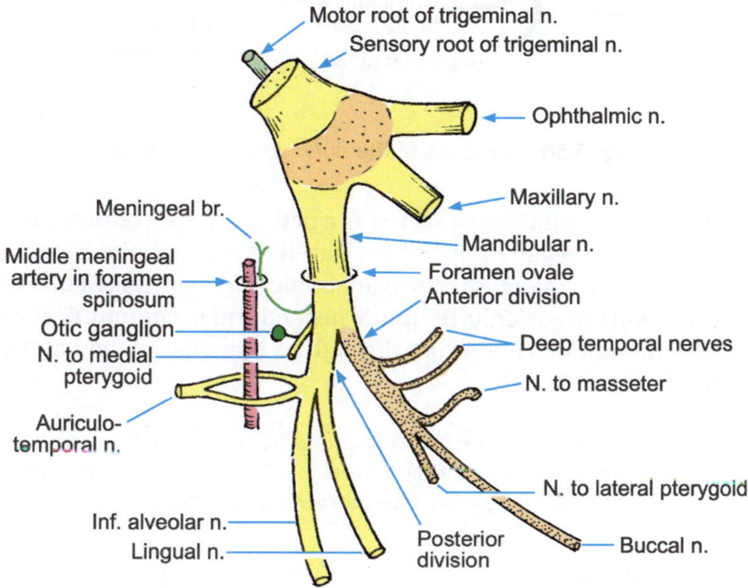

Fig. 9.48 Scheme to show the branches of the mandibular nerve.

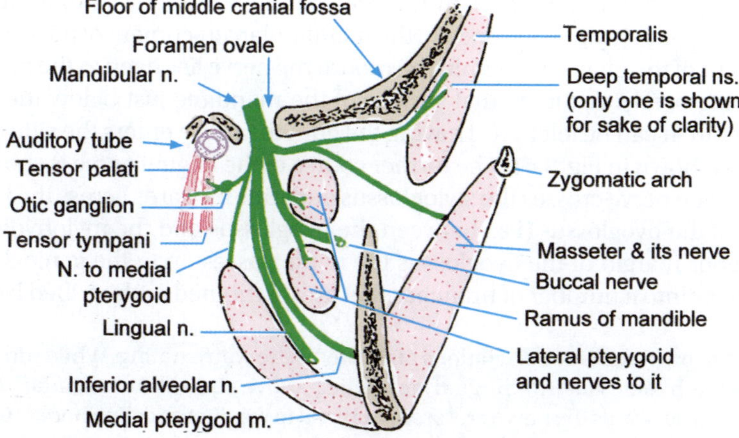

Fig. 9.49 Schematic coronal section through the infratemporal fossa to show the relationship of some branches of the mandibular nerve to the muscles of mastication

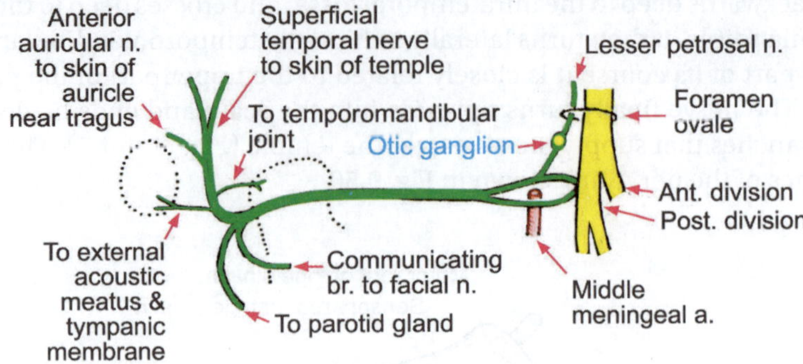

Fig. 9.50 Branches of the auriculotemporal nerve.

The auriculotemporal nerve serves as a pathway for secretomotor fibres to the parotid gland. Preganglionic fibres travelling through the lesser petrosal nerve relay in the otic ganglion. Postganglionic fibres starting in this ganglion reach the roots of the auriculo-temporal nerve through communicating twigs. They travel through this nerve and through its branches to the parotid gland (white dots in Fig. 9.50).

From Fig. 9.50 note that the auriculotemporal nerve supplies (i) ***skin*** (of the temple); (ii) a ***gland*** (parotid); (iii) a ***joint*** (temporo-mandibular); (iv) a ***tube*** (external acoustic meatus); and (v) a ***membrane*** (tympanic).

The Lingual Nerve

The lingual nerve arises from the posterior division of the mandibular nerve (Fig. 9.52). Its upper part runs downwards deep to the lateral pterygoid muscle (Fig. 9.49). It is joined here by the ***chorda tympani*** nerve (a branch of the facial nerve). Lower down the lingual nerve runs downwards and forwards between the medial pterygoid (deep to it) and the ramus of the mandible (superficial to it). It then enters the mouth (by passing deep to the mandibular attachment of the superior constrictor of the pharynx). Within the mouth the nerve lies deep to the mucous membrane overlying the medial surface of the mandible just below the third molar tooth. It can be felt here. Leaving the gum the nerve enters the side of the tongue as shown in Fig. 9.51. The further course of the lingual nerve is shown in Fig. 9.52. The nerve crosses the styloglossus and runs forwards across the lateral surface of the hyoglossus (i.e., between the hyoglossus and the mylohyoid). At the anterior margin of the hyoglossus the nerve passes on to the genioglossus and divides into a number of branches that are distributed as described below.

The following additional relations of the nerve are worth noting. While running across the hyoglossus the lingual nerve lies above the submandibular duct. Continuing forwards the nerve crosses superficial to the duct and then hooks round it to reach its medial side (Fig. 9.52). Lying on the hyoglossus, a little below the lingual nerve, there is the submandibular ganglion. The lingual nerve is connected to the ganglion by two or three branches. Still lower down the hypoglossal nerve runs across the hyoglossus. Also see Fig. 1.7.

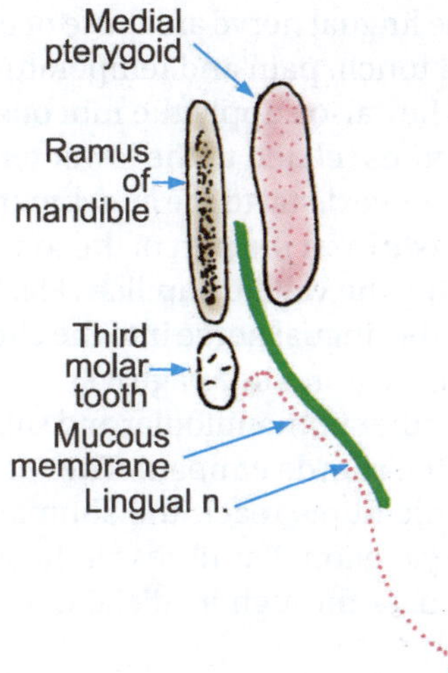

Fig. 9.51 Scheme to show how the lingual nerve passes from the infratemporal fossa to the mouth (schematic transverse section).

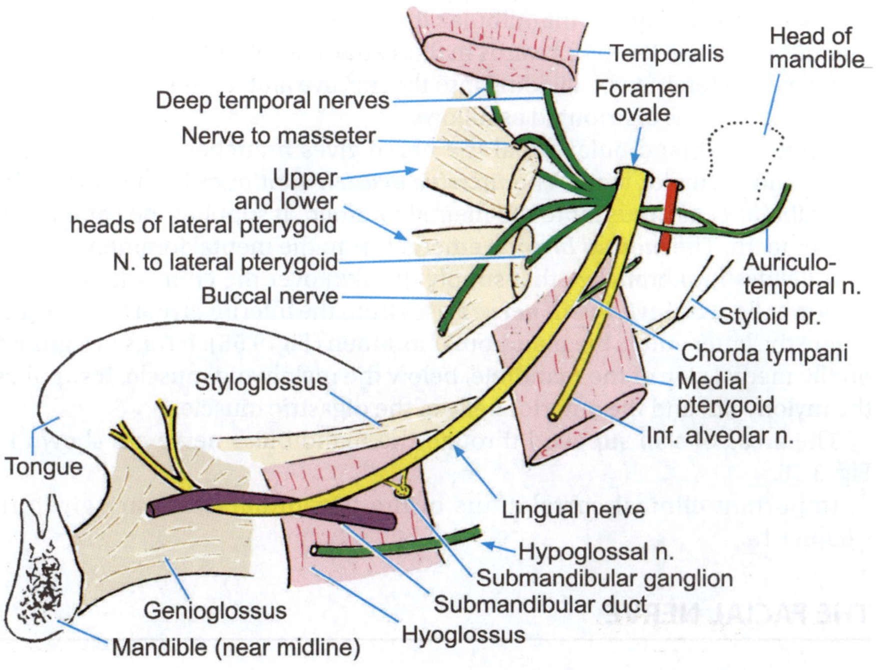

Fig. 9.52 Course and some relations of the lingual nerve and of some other branches of the mandibular nerve .

The lingual nerve carries three types of the fibres that are distributed as follows:

1. Most of the fibres of the lingual nerve are those of ordinary sensation. They carry the sensations of touch, pain and temperature from the anterior two thirds of the tongue. They also supply the mucous membrane of the floor of the mouth and the gums related to the lower teeth.
2. The part of the lingual nerve distal to the attachment of the chorda tympani carries the ***fibres for taste*** from the part of the tongue in front of the sulcus terminalis, but excluding the vallate papillae (Fig. 9.53).
   These fibres pass from the lingual nerve into the chorda tympani (Fig. 9.54). For further course of these fibres see page 853.
3. ***Secretomotor fibres*** for the submandibular and sublingual glands reach the lingual nerve through the chorda tympani. They end in the submandibular ganglion. Postganglionic fibres reach the submandibular gland through branches to it from the ganglion. The fibres for the sublingual gland re-enter the lingual nerve and pass through its distal part to reach the gland (Fig. 9.54).

The Inferior Alveolar Nerve

The ***inferior alveolar nerve*** is a branch of the posterior division of the mandibular nerve. At its upper end the nerve lies deep to the lateral pterygoid (Fig. 9.49). Emerging at the lower border of this muscle the nerve runs downwards and forwards deep to the ramus of the mandible (Fig. 9.52). Here it is separated from the medial pterygoid by the sphenomandibular ligament (Fig. 9.55). Reaching the mandibular foramen it passes through it into the mandibular canal. It runs forwards in this canal just below the teeth, and ends at the mental foramen by dividing into the incisive and mental branches (Fig. 9.57). The nerve is distributed as follows:

Within the mandibular canal the nerve gives branches that supply the molar and premolar teeth. The ***incisive branch*** continues in the part of the mandibular canal anterior to the mental foramen. It supplies the canine and incisor teeth. The ***mental branch*** emerges from the mental foramen.

It divides into branches that supply the skin over the chin, and that over the lower lip. The ***mylohyoid nerve*** arises from the inferior alveolar nerve just before the latter enters the mandibular foramen (Fig. 9.56). It runs in a groove on the medial side of the mandible, below the mylohyoid muscle. It supplies the mylohyoid, and the anterior belly of the digastric muscle.

The areas of skin supplied through the mandibular nerve are shown in Fig. 3.16.

Important clinical correlations of the trigeminal nerve are given in Chapter 15.

THE FACIAL NERVE

Preliminary Remarks:The facial nerve is the seventh cranial nerve. It is attached to the brainstem by two roots: a large ***motor root***, and a smaller ***sensory root.*** These roots are attached in the lateral part of the groove between

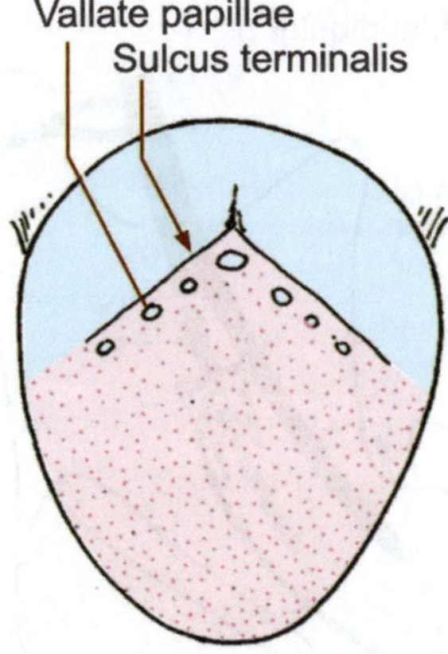

Fig. 9.53 Area of tongue supplied by the lingual nerve.

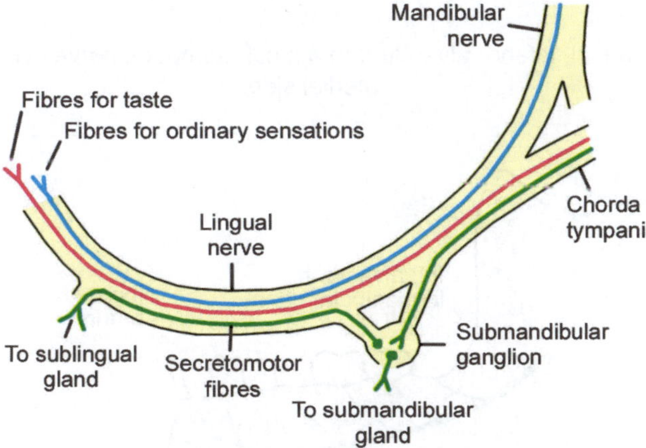

Fig. 9.54 Course of three types of fibres carried by the lingual nerve.

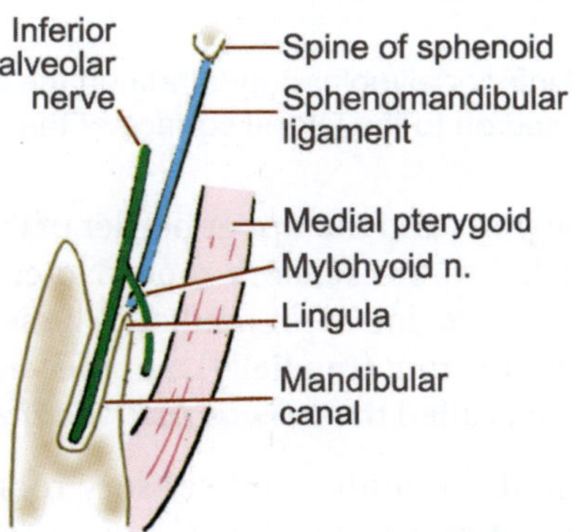

Fig. 9.55 Coronal section through ramus of mandible to show how the inferior alveolar nerve enters the mandibular canal.

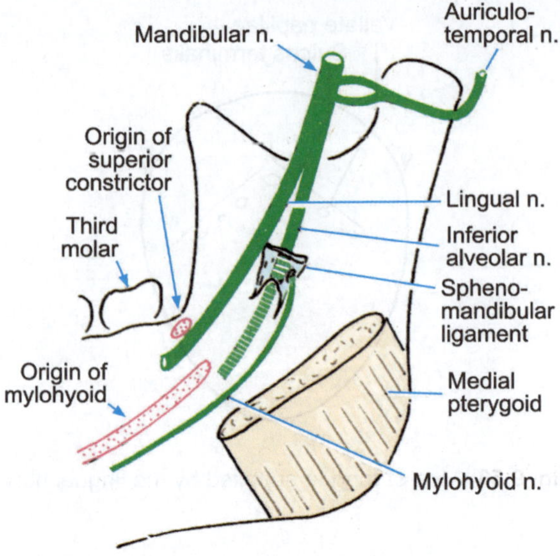

Fig. 9.56 Lingual, inferior alveolar and auriculo-temporal nerves viewed from the medial side.

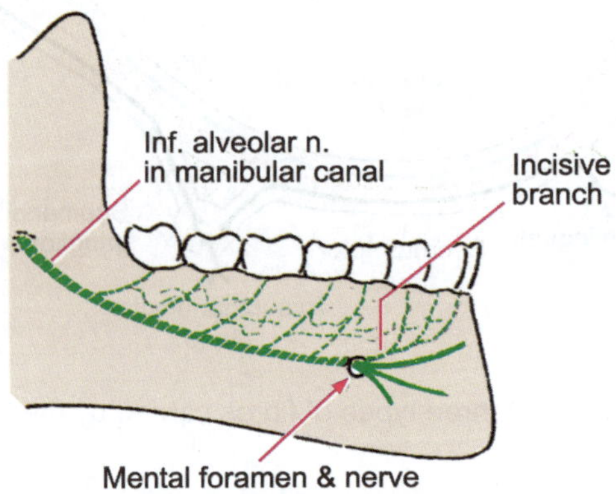

Fig. 9.57 Course of inferior alveolar nerve through the mandibular canal as projected on to the lateral surface of the bone.

the lower border of the pons and the upper border of the medulla (Fig. 9.29). The motor root is medial to the sensory root. (Note: As in the case of the trigeminal nerve, M for motor and M for medial). The sensory root is attached midway between the motor root (medially) and the vestibulocochlear nerve (laterally). It is, therefore, called the ***nervus intermedius.***

From this attachment the motor and sensory roots pass forwards and laterally and leave the posterior cranial fossa by entering the internal acoustic meatus (on the posterior aspect of the petrous temporal bone).

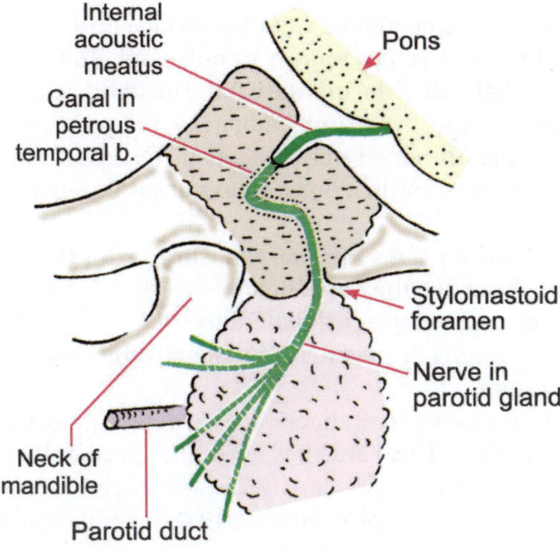

Fig. 9.58 Scheme to show the course of the facial nerve. Structures through which the nerve passes are shown as if transparent.

The nerve has a complicated course through the substance of the petrous temporal bone. This part of the nerve bears the ***genicular ganglion*** (so called because it is situated on a sharp bend of the nerve). The nerve emerges on the base of the skull through the stylomastoid foramen. It immediately enters the substance of the parotid gland and runs forwards within it and ends behind the neck of the mandible by dividing into several branches. Some details of the course of the nerve are considered below:

Intrapontine course:

(Note: The course of the facial nerve within the pons can be fully understood only after the internal structure of the pons has been studied. The main facts can be seen in Fig. 9.59).

The ***facial nucleus*** lies deep in the reticular formation of the pons, medial to the spinal nucleus of the trigeminal nerve (Figs. 9.19, 9.20C, and 9.59). The fibres arising in the nucleus follow an unusual course. They first run backwards and medially to reach the lower pole of the abducent nucleus. They then ascend on the medial side of that nucleus. Finally, the fibres turn forwards and laterally passing above the upper pole of the abducent nucleus. As they pass forwards the fibres lie between the facial nucleus, medially; and the spinal nucleus and tract of the trigeminal nerve laterally. The abducent nucleus and the facial nerve fibres looping round it together form a surface elevation, the facial colliculus, in the floor of the fourth ventricle.

Course through the petrous temporal bone:

Complete understanding of the course of the facial nerve through the petrous part of the temporal nerve requires a knowledge of the anatomy of the middle and internal ear. The salient facts can be seen in Fig. 9.60.

In this diagram some parts of the bony labyrinth and of the middle ear are shown. The region of the vestibule is drawn as if it was enclosed in a transparent cube. This cube has an anterolateral surface (facing the reader) which corresponds to the medial wall of the middle ear. The cube has an anteromedial surface through which the cochlea appears to project; and a superior surface through which the superior and posterior semicircular canals appear to bulge out. To the right of the square representing the medial wall of the middle ear the posterior wall of the middle ear is shown It has a large aperture, the ***aditus*** leading into the tympanic antrum. The facial nerve is shown passing from the internal acoustic meatus into the posteromedial aspect of the cube. We are now in a position to trace the course of the facial nerve.

On reaching the bottom of the internal acoustic meatus the facial nerve enters a bony canal. Within this canal the nerve first passes laterally above the vestibule (1) to reach the anterosuperior angle of the medial wall of the middle ear. At this point (2) the nerve bends sharply backwards. This bend is thickened by the presence of the ***genicular ganglion***.

The nerve then runs horizontally backwards in a canal projecting into the medial wall of the middle ear (3). This canal lies above the promontory and the fenestra vestibuli; and below the bulge produced by the lateral semicircular canal. Reaching the junction of the medial and posterior walls of the middle ear (4) the nerve turns downward. Here it lies medial to the aditus into the tympanic antrum.

Continuing downwards along the junction of the medial and posterior wall of the middle ear (5) the nerve reaches the stylomastoid foramen through which it leaves the skull.

Course through parotid gland:

As the facial nerve runs forwards through the parotid gland it crosses the styloid process, the retromandibular vein and the external carotid artery .

It divides into several branches while still within the gland. These branches emerge from the anteromedial surface of the gland and come into view along the anterior margin of the gland (Figs. 1.4, 9.61, 9.62).

Branches of the Facial Nerve:

The branches of the facial nerve are shown in Fig. 9.63. They are as follows:

1. The ***greater petrosal nerve*** arises from the genicular ganglion. It is described in detail below.
2. The ***nerve to the stapedius*** arises from the facial as the latter turns downwards along the junction of the medial and posterior walls of the middle ear. It runs forwards through a short canal in the petrous temporal bone to reach the stapedius (See Fig. 9.64).
3. The ***chorda tympani*** arises from the intrapetrous part of the facial nerve about 6 mm above the stylomastoid foramen. It is considered below:
4. The ***posterior auricular nerve*** is given off just after the facial nerve emerges from the stylomastoid foramen. It runs upwards into the scalp passing behind the external acoustic meatus. It divides into an ***auricular branch***, which supplies some muscles of the auricle; and an ***occipital branch*** which supplies the occipital belly of the occipitofrontalis.
5. The ***nerve to the posterior belly of the digastric muscle*** and the ***nerve to the stylohyoid*** arise near the stylomastoid foramen. They end by supplying the muscles concerned.

   The remaining branches of the facial nerve arise within the parotid gland.

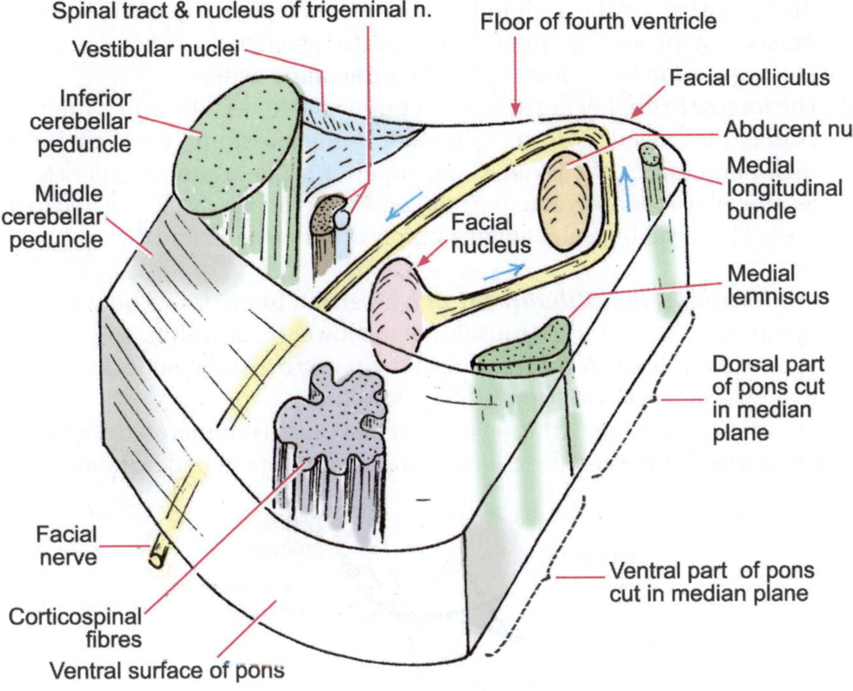

Fig. 9.59 Three dimensional diagram of the lower part of the pons to show the course of fibres of the facial nerve.

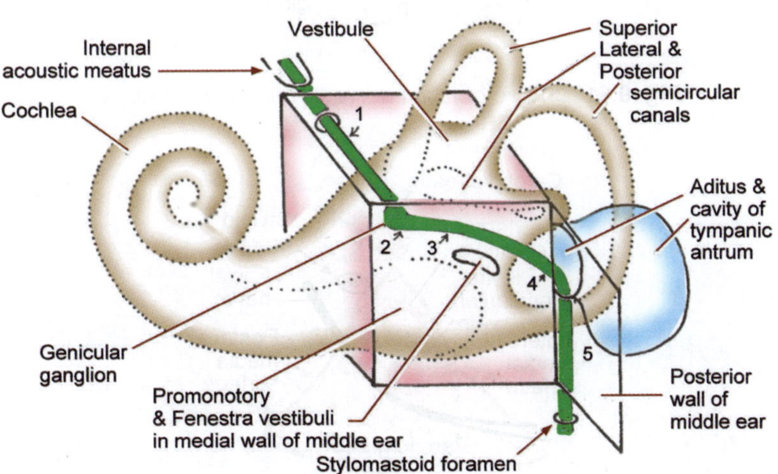

Fig. 9.60 Scheme to show the course of the facial nerve within the petrous temporal bone.

6. The ***temporal branches*** enter the scalp in the temporal region. They supply the frontal belly of the occipitofrontalis, the corrugator supercilii, and some muscles of the auricle. Some twigs are also given to the orbicularis oculi.
7. The ***zygomatic branches*** supply the orbicularis oculi.
8. The ***buccal branches*** are in two sets upper and lower. The upper branches (sometimes called the lower zygomatic branches) supply the zygomaticus major and minor, the levator labii superioris, the levator anguli oris, the levator labii superioris alaeque nasi, and some small muscles related to the nose. The lower buccal branches supply the buccinator and the orbicularis oris.
9. The ***marginal mandibular branch*** is related to the lower border of the mandible. It supplies the muscles of the lower lip and chin.
10. The ***cervical branch*** emerges from the parotid gland near its lower end. It enters the neck and supplies the platysma.

The various branches of the facial nerve have been enumerated above. The greater petrosal nerve and the chorda tympani are considered in detail below.

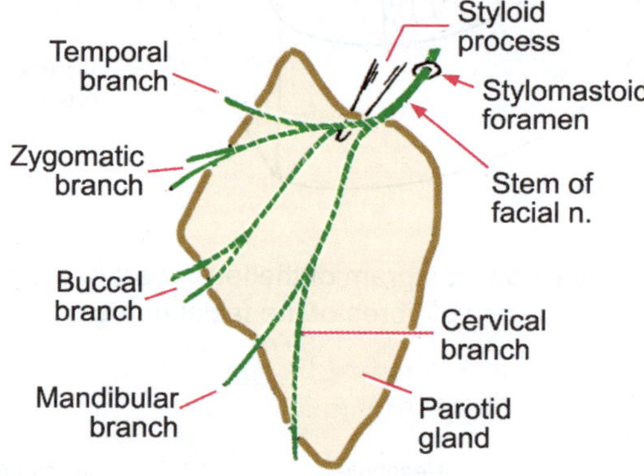

Fig. 9.61 Course of facial nerve through parotid gland.

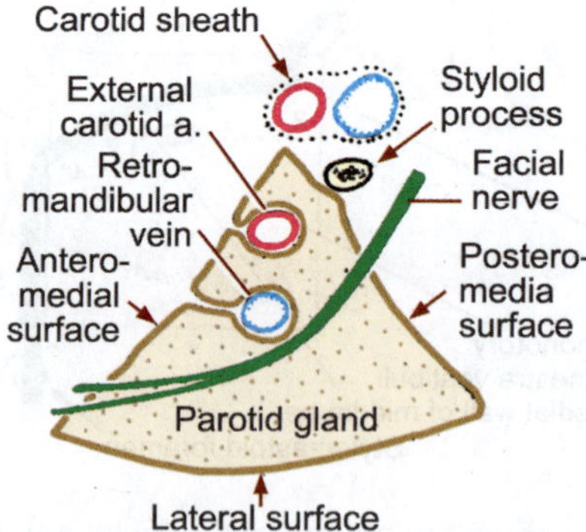

Fig. 9.62 Transverse section through the parotid gland to show relationship to the facial nerve.

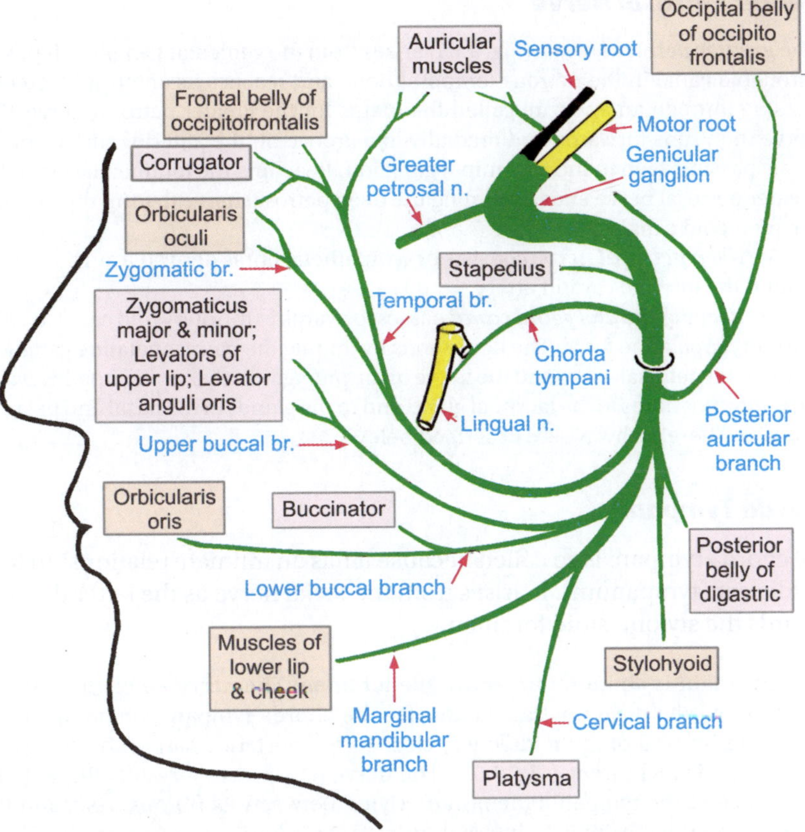

Fig. 9.63 Scheme to show the branches of the facial nerve.

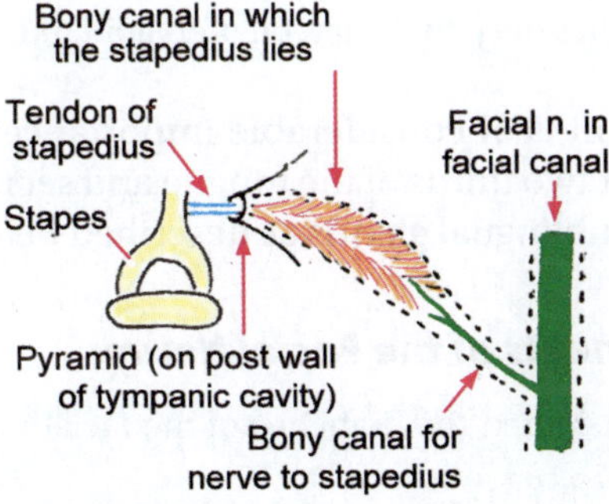

Fig. 9.64 Diagram of stapedius and its nerve seen from the medial side.

Greater Petrosal Nerve

The ***greater petrosal nerve*** (Fig. 9.65) arises from the genicular ganglion. It passes through a canal in the petrous temporal bone and reaches its anterior surface by passing through an aperture called the hiatus for the greater petrosal nerve. The nerve then runs forwards and medially in a groove on the anterior surface of the bone, passing deep to the trigeminal ganglion. Reaching the foramen lacerum the greater petrosal nerve ends by joining the deep petrosal nerve to form the nerve of the pterygoid canal.

The ***deep petrosal nerve*** consists of sympathetic fibres derived from the plexus around the internal carotid artery.

The ***nerve of the pterygoid canal*** passes forwards in the pterygoid canal to enter the pterygopalatine fossa. The nerve ends by joining the pterygopalatine ganglion. The greater petrosal nerve and the nerve of the pterygoid canal serve as pathways for secretomotor fibres to the lacrimal gland and to the glands of the nasal and palatine mucosa. These pathways are described below.

Chorda Tympani

The chorda tympani is so called because it has an intimate relationship to the middle ear (tympanum). It arises from the facial nerve as the latter descends towards the stylomastoid foramen.

The origin is about 6 mm above the foramen. The nerve enters the middle ear through the posterior canaliculus for the chorda tympani, which opens on the posterior wall of the middle ear, close to the posterior part of the margin of the tympanic membrane (Fig. 9.66). The nerve now passes forwards through the substance of the tympanic membrane (lying between its fibrous basis and the mucous membrane lining its internal surface). As it does so it crosses the handle of the malleus (which is embedded in the membrane). Reaching the anterior margin of the tympanic membrane the chorda tympani enters the anterior canaliculus (in the anterior wall of the middle ear). It passes through this canaliculus and emerges on the base of the skull through the medial end of the petrotympanic fissure. Passing medially, forwards and downwards the nerve crosses medial to the spine of the sphenoid. (Note: the auriculotemporal nerve passes lateral to the spine: See Fig. 9.66).

The chorda tympani ends by joining the lingual nerve from behind. To do so it has to pass deep to the inferior alveolar nerve. The junction of the chorda tympani with the lingual nerve lies deep to the lateral pterygoid muscle (Fig. 1.7).

The chorda tympani is of considerable importance as it carries fibres of taste from the anterior two thirds of the tongue and secretomotor fibres to the submandibular and sublingual glands as described below.

Functional Components of the Facial Nerve:

Now that we have considered the branches of the facial nerve we can review its functional components.

1. We have seen that most of the branches of the nerve are motor. Many of them supply the muscles of facial expression. Motor fibres also supply the occipitofrontalis, the muscles of the auricle, the stapedius, the platysma, the

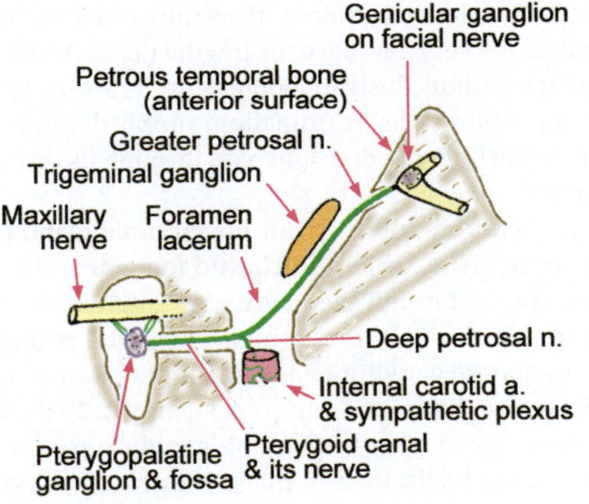

Fig. 9.65 Scheme to show the course of the greater petrosal nerve.

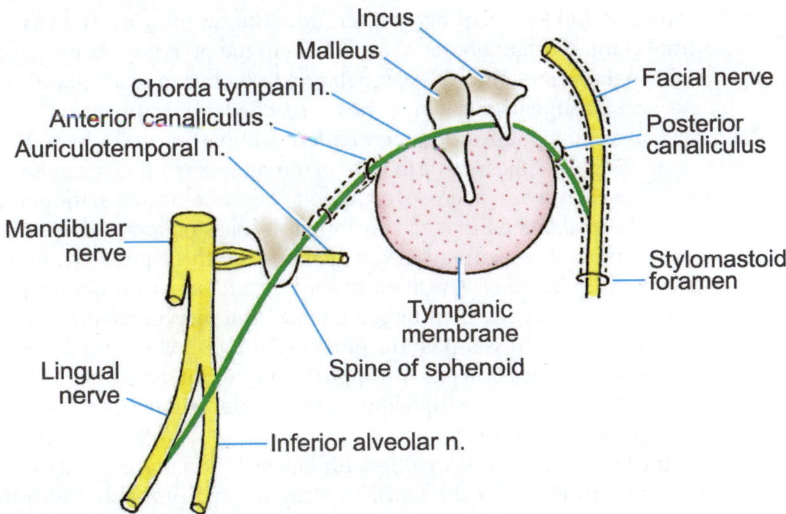

Fig. 9.66 Course of the chorda tympani as seen from the medial side.

stylohyoid and the posterior belly of the digastric. All these muscles are derived from the mesoderm of the second branchial arch. The nerve fibres concerned in their innervation arise in the facial nucleus which lies in the lower part of the pons, and belongs to the ***special visceral efferent*** column (Figs. 9.19, 9.20D). The axons of neurons located in this nucleus collect to form the motor root of the facial nerve.

2. The facial nerve also contains ***general visceral efferent*** fibres which are as follows:
   a. Preganglionic secretomotor fibres for the submandibular and sublingual glands (Fig. 9.67) arise from neurons located in the ***superior salivatory nucleus.*** (This nucleus lies in the lower part of the pons). The fibres leave the pons through the nervus intermedius and run for some distance in the

intrapetrous part of the facial nerve. They then enter the chorda tympani to reach the lingual nerve. They leave the lingual nerve through branches to the submandibular ganglion. Postganglionic neurons are located in this ganglion. Some of the nerve fibres arising from them supply the submandibular gland. Others re-enter the lingual nerve and pass through its distal part to reach the sublingual gland.

b. Preganglionic secretomotor fibres for the lacrimal gland (Fig. 9.68) arise in the lacrimatory nucleus, which is believed to lie near the salivatory nuclei. They leave the pons through the nervus intermedius, pass into the greater petrosal nerve and through it into the nerve of the pterygoid canal to end in the pterygopalatine ganglion. Postganglionic neurons are located in this ganglion. Fibres arising from them pass successively through a ganglionic branch connecting the pterygopalatine ganglion to the maxillary nerve; the maxillary nerve itself; its zygomatic branch; the zygomaticotemporal branch of the zygomatic nerve; the loop of communication between the zygomaticotemporal and lacrimal nerves; and finally through the lacrimal nerve to reach the lacrimal gland.

c. Preganglionic secretomotor fibres for glands in the nasal and palatine mucosa arise in neurons the location of which is uncertain. They probably lie near the salivatory nuclei. The preganglionic fibres follow the same path as for the lacrimal gland. Postganglionc fibres arising in the pterygopalatine ganglion pass through its greater and lesser palatine branches to reach glands in the palate; and through its nasal branches to reach glands in the nasal mucosa.

3. The facial nerve contains ***special visceral afferent*** fibres that carry the sensations of taste from the part of the tongue in front of the sulcus terminalis; and from the soft palate. These fibres are processes of unipolar neurons located in the genicular ganglion. Peripheral processes reach the tongue by passing successively through part of the intrapetrous segment of the facial nerve, the chorda tympani and the lingual nerve (Fig. 9.67). Those for the soft palate pass through the greater petrosal nerve, the nerve of the pterygoid canal, the pterygopalatine ganglion (without relay), and the lesser palatine nerves (Fig. 9.68). The central processes leaving the genicular ganglion pass through the nervus intermedius to reach the brainstem. Here they terminate in relation to the upper part of the nucleus of the solitary tract (Figs. 9.19, 9.20B).

4. Although the facial nerve gives no direct branches to skin there is evidence that some of its fibres reach part of the skin of the auricle. They probably pass through communications between the facial nerve and the auricular branch of the vagus.

   The evidence for this is as follows. There is a disease called herpes zoster in which a virus infects one or more sensory ganglia. When this happens vesicles appear on the skin over the region innervated by that ganglion. When such an infection occurs in the genicular ganglion vesicles appear over part of the auricle.

   These fibres are ***general somatic afferent*** and are peripheral processes of unipolar cells located in the genicular ganglion. Central processes arising in these neurons pass through the nervus intermedius and end in the nucleus of the spinal tract of the trigeminal nerve.

The Pterygopalatine Ganglion

Several features of this ganglion have already been noted. We have seen that it is located in the pterygopalatine fossa and is suspended from the maxillary nerve by two ganglionic branches (Fig. 9.46). The fibres passing through the ganglion are as follows:

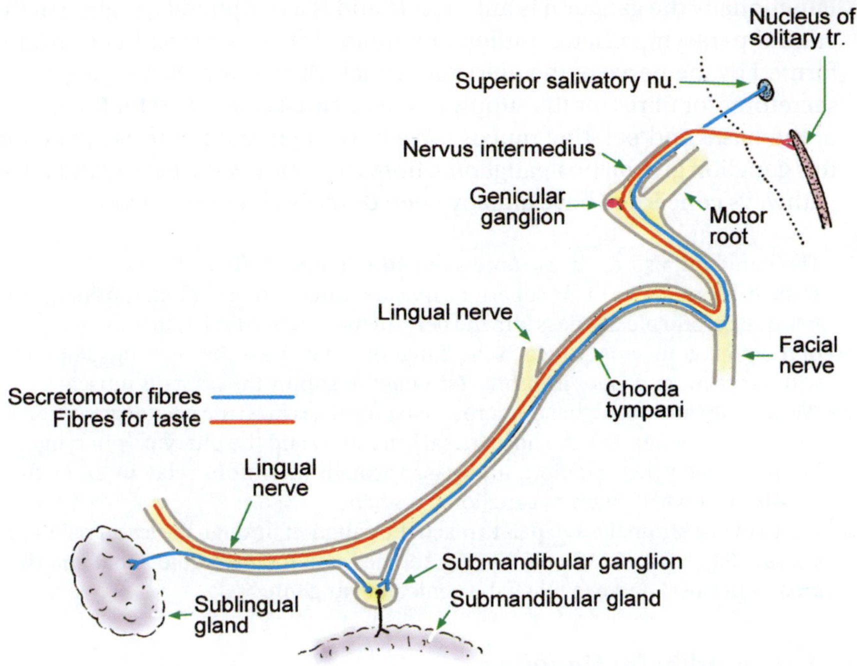

Fig. 9.67 Scheme to show the secretomotor pathway for the submandibular and sublingual glands. The pathway for taste from the anterior two thirds of the tongue is also shown.

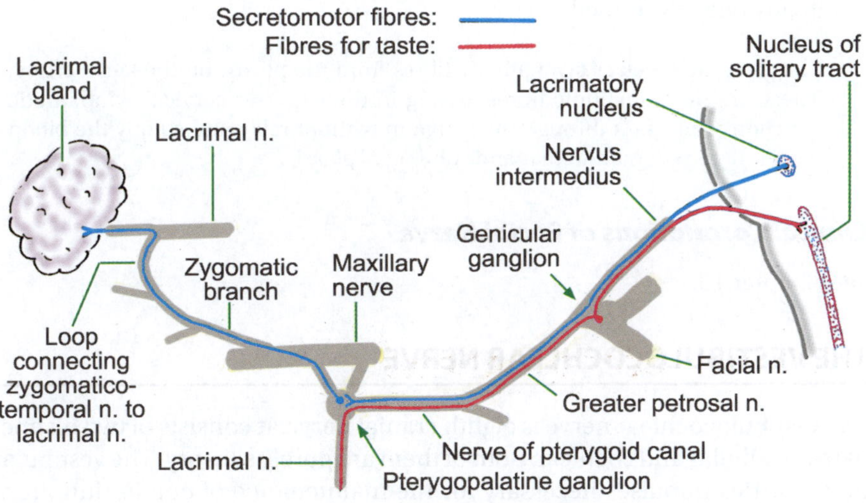

Fig. 9.68 Scheme to show (a) the secretomotor pathway for the lacrimal gland; and (b) the pathway for fibres of taste from the soft palate.

a. Functionally the ganglion is autonomic and is a peripheral ganglion of the cranial parasympathetic outflow. Its motor (or parasympathetic) root is formed by the nerve of the pterygoid canal which conveys pre-ganglionic secretomotor fibres for the supply of the lacrimal gland, and for the glands of the nasal and palatine mucosa. We have seen that neurons located in this ganglion give off postganglionic fibres that innervate these glands. The pathways concerned have already been described (figure above).

b. The ganglion also receives some sympathetic fibres. These fibres, which are postganglionic, arise in the superior cervical sympathetic ganglion, run along the internal carotid plexus, pass into the deep petrosal nerve and then into the nerve of the pterygoid canal to reach the ganglion. They pass through the ganglion, without relay, and enter its orbital branches to supply the orbitalis muscle.
c. We have already noted that numerous sensory fibres from the palate (greater and lesser palatine nerves), the nose (nasal branches) and the pharynx (pharyngeal branch) reach the ganglion, and pass through it without relay to enter the maxillary nerve through its ganglionic branches.
d. Fibres of taste from the soft palate reach the ganglion through the lesser palatine nerves (Fig. 9.68). They pass through the nerve of the pterygoid canal and the greater petrosal nerve to reach the genicular ganglion.

The Submandibular Ganglion

Several facts about this ganglion have already been noted. We have seen that it lies over the hyoglossus muscle, suspended from the lingual nerve by two or more roots (Fig. 9.52). It is an autonomic ganglion connected with the cranial parasympathetic outflow. The fibres passing through it are as follows:
a. Functionally the ganglion is concerned with the secretomotor innervation of the submandibular and sublingual salivary glands. These fibres are parasympathetic. The pathway concerned is shown in Fig. 9.67 and has already been described.

b. The ganglion receives sympathetic fibres from the plexus on the facial artery. These are postganglionic fibres arising in the superior cervical sympathetic ganglion. They pass through the ganglion without relay and supply the blood vessels of the submandibular and sublingual glands.

Clinical Correlations of Facial Nerve

See Chapter 15.

THE VESTIBULOCOCHLEAR NERVE

The vestibulocochlear nerve is eighth cranial nerve. It consists of two distinct parts, vestibular and cochlear. Both of them are purely sensory. The vestibular nerve carries impulses necessary for the maintenance of equilibrium from the vestibular part of the internal ear. The cochlear nerve carries impulses of hearing from the cochlear part of the internal ear.

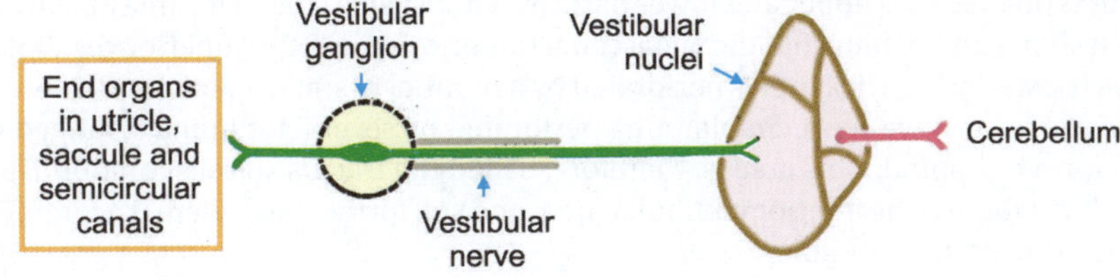

Fig. 9.69 Basic plan of the vestibular nerve.

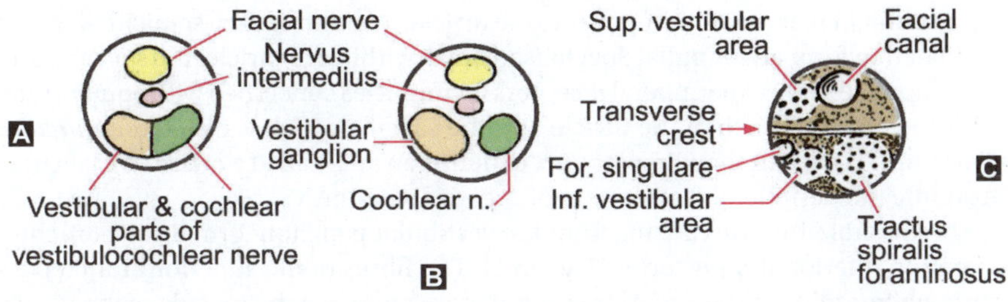

Fig. 9.70 (A). T. S through internal acoustic meatus near its opening into the posterior cranial fossa i.e., near its medial end. (B). T. S through the middle of the internal acoustic meatus. (C). Floor of the internal acoustic meatus. In each figure the right side of the figure is anterior.

The vestibulocochlear nerve is attached to the surface of the brainstem at the lower border of the pons, posterolateral to the attachment of the facial nerve (Fig. 9.29). From here the nerve passes forwards and enters the internal acoustic meatus along with the motor and sensory roots of the facial nerve. The relative position of the nerves near the opening of the meatus is shown in Fig. 9.70. Here the nerve divides into vestibular and cochlear parts.

The Vestibular Nerve

A plan of the vestibular nerve is shown in Fig. 9.69. The fibres of the nerve are processes of cells in the vestibular ganglion which is located within the internal acoustic meatus (Fig. 9.70B). The cells of this ganglion are bipolar (not unipolar as in typical sensory ganglia). Peripheral processes arising from neurons in the ganglion supply end organs in the vestibular part of the membranous labyrinth. These are shown in Fig. 9.71.

The central processes of neurons in the vestibular ganglion form the vestibular nerve. Entering the brainstem they end in relation to the vestibular nuclei (Figs. 9.19, 9.20 B, C). Fibres arising in the vestibular nuclei carry impulses for equilibrium to the cerebellum. Some fibres from the vestibular ganglion pass directly to the cerebellum.

We will now consider some details of the distribution of the peripheral processes of the vestibular nerve. For this purpose we must examine some features to be seen at the blind end (floor) of the internal acoustic meatus (Fig. 9.70C). We see that the floor is divided into upper and lower parts by a transverse crest. The area above the crest shows an opening into the facial canal (anteriorly); and the superior vestibular area (posteriorly). The latter is perforated by a number of small openings. Below the transverse crest we see a circular area perforated by several foramina arranged in the form of a spiral. This area is, therefore, called the tractus spiralis foraminosus. Behind it there is the inferior vestibular area, and still further back there is a foramen called the foramen singulare.

At this stage it is also necessary to note some features of the structure of the internal ear (Fig. 9.71). The internal ear consists of a bony space of complex shape called the bony labyrinth. Within it there is an equally complex membranous labyrinth which consists of a vestibular part and a cochlear part. The vestibular part consists of a sac called the utricle (UT); another sac called the saccule (SAC); and of three semicircular ducts that open into the utricle. One end of each semicircular duct is dilated to form an ampulla. Specialised areas within the utricle, the saccule, and the ampullae serve as peripheral receptors for impulses concerned with equilibrium. There is one area each in the utricle and the saccule which is called the ***macula***. The ampulla of each semicircular duct contains an area called a ***crista***. We can now examine the peripheral distribution of the vestibular nerve.

Peripheral processes arising from the vestibular ganglion form three branches, superior, inferior and posterior (Fig. 9.71). The fibres of the superior branch pass through foramina in the superior vestibular area to reach the macula of the utricle and the ampullae of the superior and lateral semicircular ducts. The inferior branch passes through foramina in the inferior vestibular area to reach the macula of the saccule. The posterior branch passes through the foramen singulare to reach the ampulla of the posterior semicircular duct.

The Cochlear Nerve

A plan of the cochlear nerve is shown in Fig. 9.72. The cochlear nerve is made up of the central processes of neurons located in the spiral ganglion (Also see Fig. 9.71). Peripheral processes of the neurons of the spiral ganglion reach the organ of Corti, which is the peripheral receptor for sound. Sound is ultimately perceived in the auditory area of the cerebral cortex. A simplified scheme of the pathway for hearing from the cochlear nuclei to the cerebral cortex is given in Fig. 9.73.

The spiral ganglion is so called because it has a spiral configuration parallel to the turns of the cochlea. The neurons in this ganglion are bipolar (like those of the vestibular ganglion). The fibres of the cochlear nerve pass through the foramina of the tractus spiralis foraminosus (Fig. 9.70C) to enter the internal acoustic meatus. On reaching the brain stem they terminate in the dorsal and ventral cochlear nuclei located respectively on the dorsal and ventral sides of the inferior cerebellar peduncle.

The fibres in both the vestibular and cochlear nerves are classified as special somatic afferent, as the epithelium of the membranous labyrinth is of ectodermal origin.

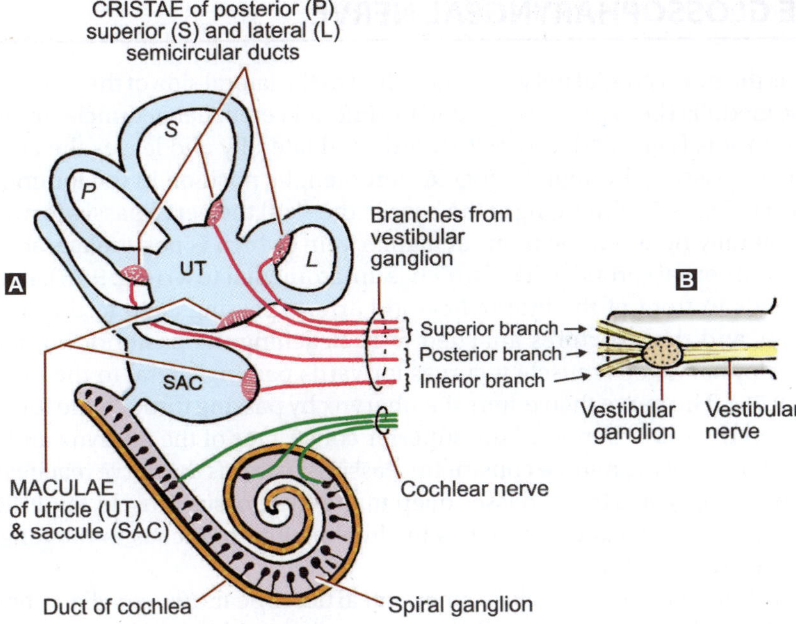

Fig. 9.71 (A). Scheme to show end organs in the membranous labyrinth. (B). Vestibular nerve and ganglion in the internal acoustic meatus.

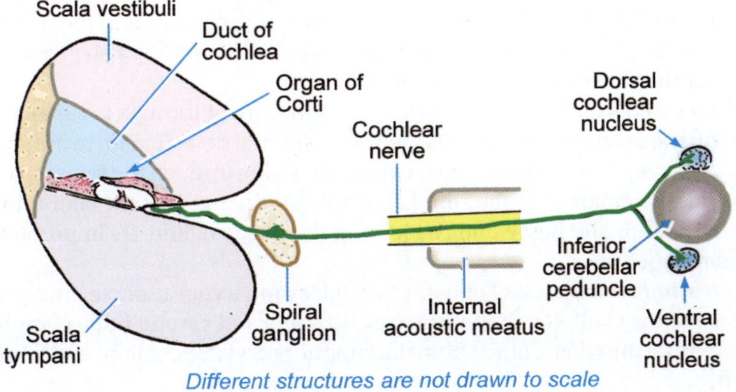

Fig. 9.72 Simplified scheme to show the course of the cochlear nerve.

THE GLOSSOPHARYNGEAL NERVE

This is the ninth cranial nerve. It is attached to the lateral side of the upper part of the medulla (between the olive and the inferior cerebellar peduncle) by three or four roots (Fig. 9.29). It runs forwards and laterally and leaves the cranial cavity by passing through the jugular foramen. Its position in the foramen is shown in Fig. 9.74. Emerging at the base of the skull the nerve passes forwards and laterally between the internal jugular vein (which is posterolateral to it) and the internal carotid artery (which is anteromedial to it) (Fig. 9.75). It then descends in front of the internal carotid artery, passing deep to the styloid process and the structures attached to it. Reaching the posterior border of the stylopharyngeus muscle it curves forwards passing lateral to the muscle (Fig. 9.76). The nerve then enters the pharynx by passing through the interval between the lower border of the superior constrictor of the pharynx and the upper border of the middle constrictor. Passing forwards the nerve reaches the side of the tongue. Here it passes deep to the hyoglossus muscle, superficial to the genioglossus and terminates by dividing into branches to the tongue. Also see Figs. 1.7 and 1.8.

The proximal part of the glossopharyngeal nerve bears two ganglia, superior and inferior. The ***superior ganglion*** is small and lies within the jugular foramen. The ***inferior ganglion*** is larger and lies just below the foramen (Fig. 9.77).

The branches of the glossopharyngeal nerve are shown in Fig. 9.77 and are considered below:

1. The ***tympanic branch*** arises from the inferior ganglion. It enters a canal (called the inferior tympanic canaliculus) within the petrous temporal bone. The lower opening of this canal is situated on the ridge of bone that separates the jugular fossa from the carotid canal. Passing through the canal the nerve reaches the tympanic cavity and forms a plexus (***tympanic plexus***) over the promontory. Branches arising from this plexus supply the mucous membrane of the tympanic cavity, the auditory tube, and the mastoid air cells. The plexus also gives rise to the lesser petrosal nerve described below.
2. The ***lesser petrosal nerve*** leaves the tympanic cavity through a canal which opens on the anterior surface of the petrous temporal bone (lateral to the greater petrosal nerve). It leaves the cranial cavity by passing through the foramen ovale (or through a small foramen, the canalis innominatus present lateral to the foramen ovale). The nerve ends by joining the otic ganglion. Its importance is considered below.
3. The ***carotid branch*** arises soon after the glossopharyngeal nerve emerges on the base of the skull. It supplies the carotid sinus and carotid body (forming a plexus with sympathetic fibres from the superior cervical ganglion, and from the vagus).
4. ***Pharyngeal branches*** are given off to the mucous membrane of the pharynx. Their fibres pass through the pharyngeal plexus (which is also joined by sympathetic fibres and by fibres from the vagus).

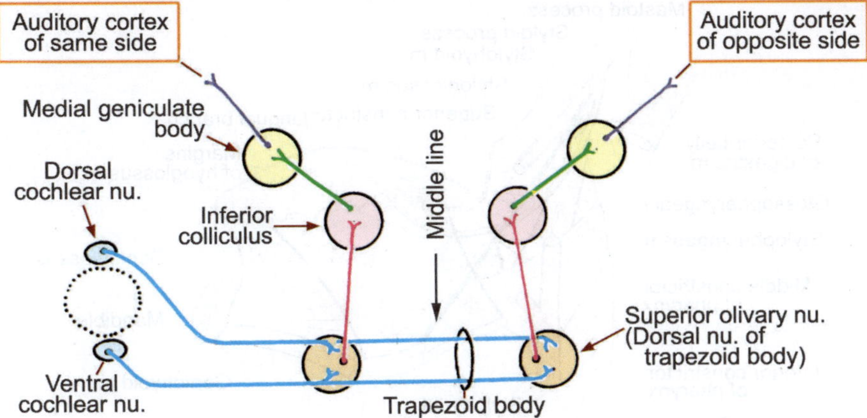

Fig. 9.73 Simplified scheme to show the pathway from cochlear nuclei to the auditory cortex.

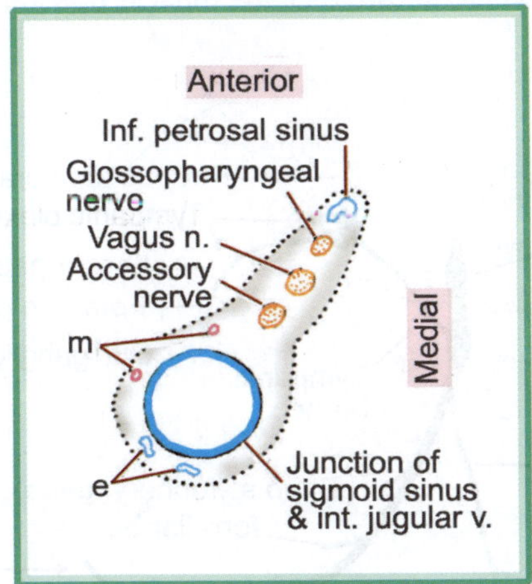

Fig. 9.74 Relative position of structures passing through the jugular foramen. m= meningeal arteries. e = emissary veins.

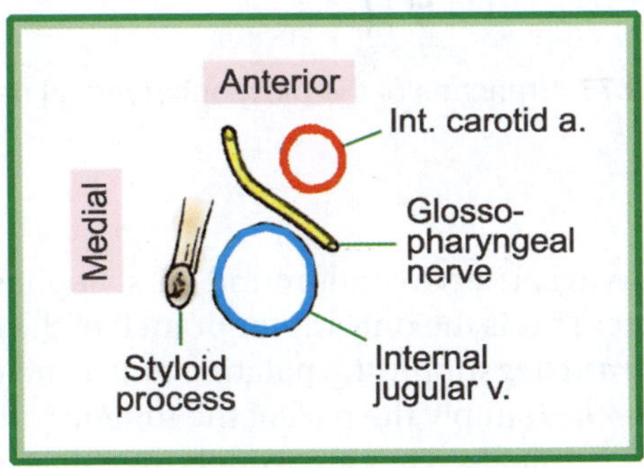

Fig. 9.75 Relationship of glossopharyngeal nerve to large vessels just below the base of the skull.

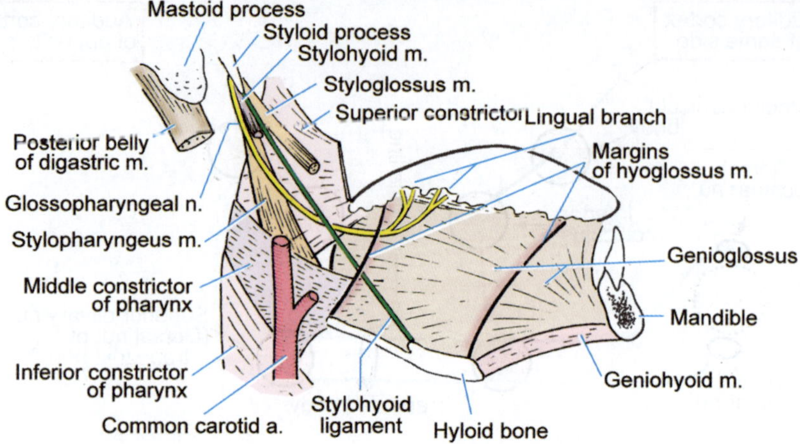

Fig. 9.76 Some relations of the glossopharyngeal nerve. Structures deep to the hyoglossus are shown as if the muscle was transparent.

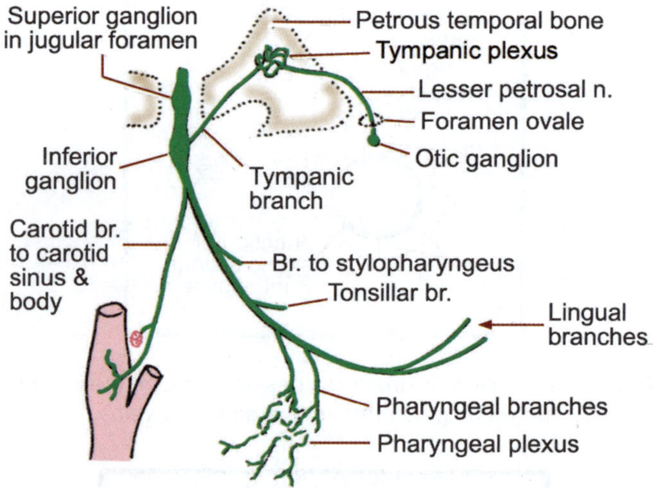

Fig. 9.77 Branches of the glossopharyngeal nerve.

5. As the glossopharyngeal nerve winds round the stylopharyngeus it supplies this muscle. (Note: This is the only motor branch of the nerve).
6. Some ***tonsilar branches*** supply the palatine tonsil and the soft palate.
7. The ***lingual branches*** supply the part of the tongue (mucous membrane) behind the sulcus terminalis. They also supply the vallate papillae (Fig. 9.80). As described below these branches carry fibres for both general sensation and taste.

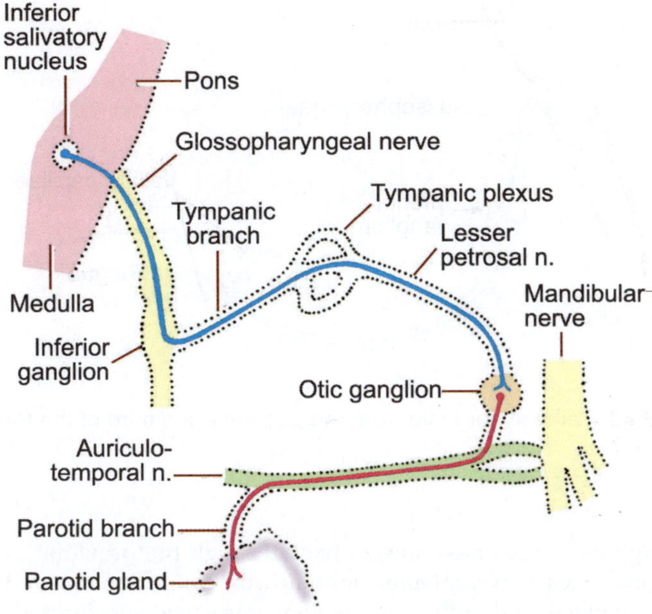

Fig. 9.78 Secretomotor pathway for the parotid gland.

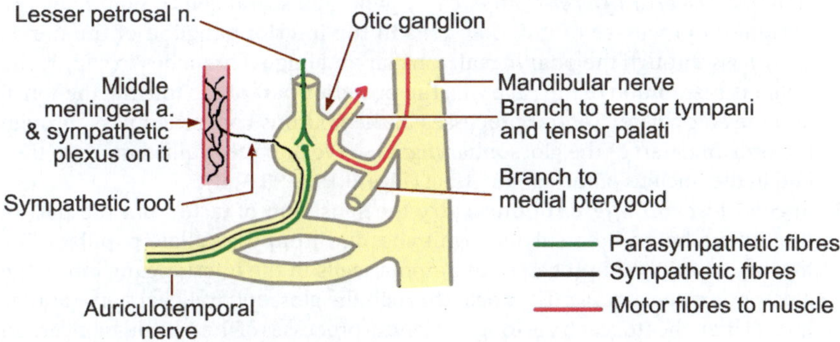

Fig. 9.79 Connections of the otic ganglion.

Functional Components of the Glossopharyngeal Nerve:

1. ***Special visceral efferent*** fibres arising in the nucleus ambiguus (Figs. 9.19, 9.20A, B) supply the stylopharyngeus muscle. This muscle develops from the mesoderm of the third branchial arch. The glossopharyngeal is the nerve of this arch.
2. ***General visceral efferent*** fibres supply the parotid gland. The pathway is shown in Fig. 9.78. The preganglionic neurons concerned are located in the inferior salivatory nucleus (Fig. 9.19) which lies at the junction of the pons and medulla just below the superior salivatory nucleus.

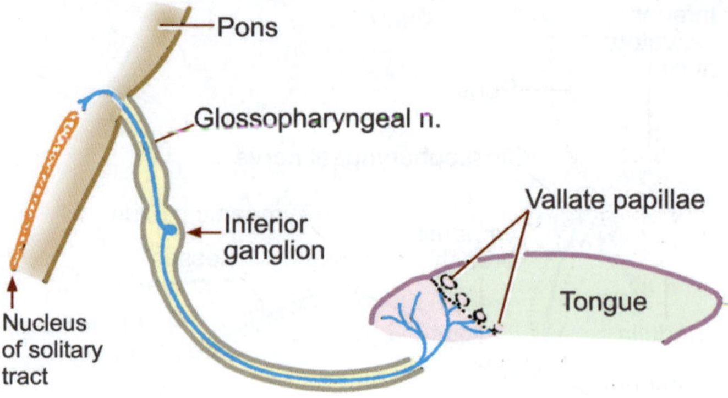

Fig. 9.80 Pathway for taste from the posterior one third of the tongue.

Preganglionic fibres pass successively through the proximal part of the glossopharyngeal nerve, its tympanic branch, the tympanic plexus and the lesser petrosal nerve to end in the otic ganglion. Postganglionic fibres arising from neurons located in the otic ganglion pass through a nerve connecting the otic ganglion to the auriculotemporal nerve, and then through the auriculotemporal nerve itself. They leave the latter through its parotid branch to reach the parotid gland.

3. ***General visceral afferent*** fibres carry general visceral sensations. They are peripheral processes of unipolar cells in the inferior ganglion of the nerve. They pass through the pharyngeal, tonsilar and lingual branches to supply the mucous membrane of the pharynx, the posterior part of the tongue, the tonsil and the soft palate. Central processes of the neurons concerned pass through the proximal part of the glossopharyngeal nerve into the brainstem. Here they end in the nucleus of the solitary tract (Figs. 9.19, 9.20 A, B).
4. ***Special visceral afferent*** fibres carry the sensation of taste from the part of the tongue behind the sulcus terminalis, and from the vallate papillae. The fibres are peripheral processes of unipolar cells in the inferior ganglion of the glossopharyngeal nerve. They pass through the glossopharyngeal nerve and its lingual branches to reach the tongue. Central processes of the neurons concerned pass through the proximal part of the glossopharyngeal nerve and enter the medulla where they end in the upper part of the nucleus of the solitary tract.
5. According to some authorities the glossopharyngeal nerve also contains some general somatic afferent fibres. These include some fibres from the skin of the auricle; and proprioceptive fibres from the stylopharyngeus. They are described as ending in the spinal nucleus of the trigeminal nerve.

The Otic Ganglion

The otic ganglion is situated just below the foramen ovale medial to the trunk of the mandibular nerve (Fig. 9.48). It is connected to the nerve to the medial pterygoid muscle. The middle meningeal artery and the roots of the auriculotemporal nerve lie close to it (see Fig. 9.78).

The fibres passing through the otic ganglion are as follows:

a Functionally the ganglion is autonomic and is a peripheral ganglion of the cranial parasympathetic outflow. It is the relay station for secretomotor fibres to the parotid gland.

b. Sympathetic fibres reach the ganglion from the plexus on the middle meningeal artery. They pass through the ganglion, without relay, and travel to the parotid gland through the auriculotemporal nerve.

c. Motor fibres reach the ganglion through the nerve to the medial pterygoid. These fibres are derived from the motor root of the mandibular nerve. They pass through the ganglion (without relay) and enter branches of the ganglion which supply the tensor tympani and the tensor palati muscles.

THE VAGUS NERVE

The vagus nerve arises from the lateral side of the medulla, by about ten rootlets which are attached to the groove between the olive and the inferior cerebellar peduncle, below the rootlets of the glossopharyngeal nerve (Fig. 9.29). Thus formed the nerve leaves the skull through the jugular foramen. Its position relative to other structures in the foramen is shown in Fig. 9.74. The part of the nerve within the jugular foramen shows an enlargement called the superior ganglion. Just below the foramen the nerve has a much larger enlargement called the inferior ganglion.

The vagus nerve descends vertically in the neck. It is enclosed within the carotid sheath. Here it lies in the interval between the posterior part of the internal or common carotid artery and the internal jugular vein. Some relations of this part of the nerve are shown in Figs. 8.3, 8.4. In the lower part of the neck the nerve crosses anterior to the first part of the subclavian artery, and enters the thorax. Passing through the thorax the vagus enters the abdomen where it has a wide distribution.

Branches of the Vagus Nerve in the Neck

The vagus nerve gives off numerous branches in the neck, in the thorax and in the abdomen. Branches arising in the thorax and the abdomen are considered in the appropriate sections. Here we will consider the branches that arise from the nerve in the neck.

1. A ***meningeal branch*** arises near the upper end of the nerve and supplies the duramater in the region.

2. The ***auricular branch*** arises from the superior ganglion. It is distributed to the skin of the auricle, the external acoustic meatus and the tympanic membrane.

Soon after its origin the nerve enters the mastoid canaliculus (which opens on the lateral wall of the jugular fossa: Fig. 9.82) and passes laterally through it within the temporal bone. The nerve emerges from the bone through the tympanomastoid fissure and divides into two branches. One of these supplies part of the skin of

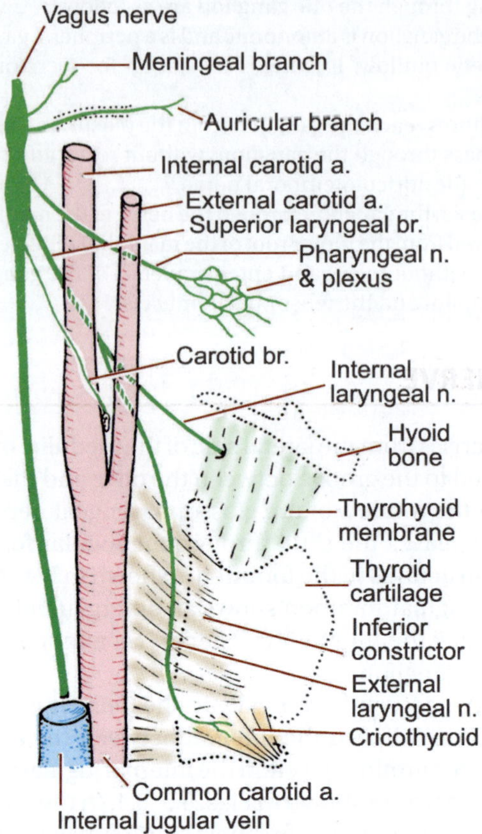

Fig. 9.81 Scheme to show some branches of the vagus nerve in the neck.

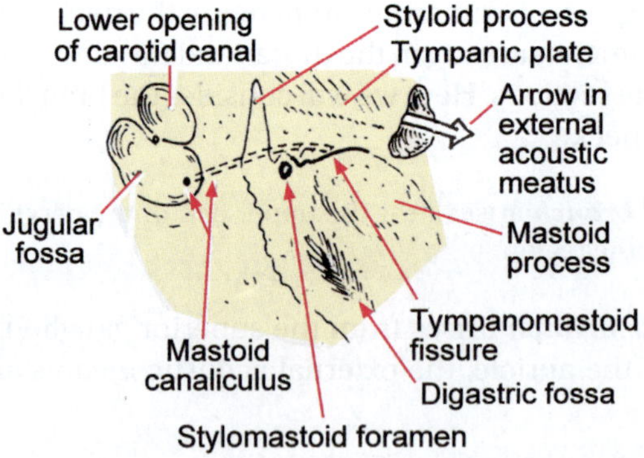

Fig. 9.82 Diagram of a part of the temporal bone seen from below to show the position of the mastoid canaliculus, and of the tympanomastoid fissure. The auricular branch of the vagus nerve passes through these passages.

the auricle: the part supplied is shown in Fig. 9.11. The other branch supplies the skin lining the posterior wall and floor of the external acoustic meatus, and the postero-inferior part of the outer layer of the tympanic membrane. (The rest of the meatus and of the membrane are supplied by the auriculo-temporal nerve).

3. The ***pharyngeal branch*** arises from the inferior ganglion. It passes forwards on the side wall of the pharynx crossing superficial to the internal carotid artery and deep to the external carotid artery. It divides into numerous branches which form the ***pharyngeal plexus***. Fibres continuing through the plexus supply the muscles of the pharynx and of the soft palate (except the tensor palati which is supplied by the mandibular nerve through the otic ganglion). The pharyngeal plexus is joined by branches from the glossopharyngeal nerve (sensory fibres) and by branches from the sympathetic trunk.

4. One or more branches are given off to the carotid body. They may arise from the inferior ganglion or from the pharyngeal branch.

5. The ***superior laryngeal nerve*** arises from the inferior ganglion. It descends on the side wall of the pharynx posterior to the internal carotid artery. It then curves forwards passing deep to the artery and ends by dividing into the internal and external laryngeal nerves.

   The ***internal laryngeal nerve*** is sensory. It enters the larynx by piercing the thyrohyoid membrane. It divides into branches which supply:
   a. The mucous membrane of the upper half of the larynx (up to the vocal folds); and
   b. The mucous membrane of part of the pharynx, the epiglottis, the vallecula, and the posteriormost part of the tongue.

   The ***external laryngeal nerve*** descends over the inferior constrictor muscle. It ends by supplying the cricothyroid muscle.
6. The course of the ***recurrent laryngeal nerve*** is different on the right and left sides.

   On the right side the nerve arises from the vagus as the latter passes in front of the subclavian artery. It passes backwards below the artery and then upwards behind the artery forming a loop. The nerve then runs upwards and medially deep to the common carotid artery to reach the side of the trachea.

   On the left side the recurrent laryngeal nerve arises from the vagus in the thorax, as the latter crosses lateral to the arch of the aorta. The nerve winds below the arch, immediately behind the ligamentum arteriosum and then passes upwards and medially to reach the side of the trachea. Having reached the trachea both the right and left nerves ascend in the groove between it and the oesophagus, deep to the medial surface of the thyroid gland. At the upper end of the trachea and oesophagus the nerve passes deep to the lower border of the inferior constrictor muscle and enters the larynx. It is distributed as follows.

a. The nerve provides the motor supply to all intrinsic muscles of the larynx (except the cricothyroid supplied by the external laryngeal nerve).
b. The nerve provides the sensory supply to the mucous membrane of the lower half of the larynx i.e., the part below the level of the vocal folds).
c. It gives sensory branches to the trachea, the oesophagus and to the inferior constrictor. It also gives branches to the cardiac plexus (See below).

At the lower pole of thyroid gland the recurrent laryngeal nerve is intimately related to the terminal branches of the inferior thyroid artery. Variations in the relationship are of surgical importance.

7. ***Cardiac branches***: Each vagus gives one (or more) superior cervical cardiac branch in the upper part of the neck; and an inferior cervical cardiac branch in its lower part. Additional cardiac branches arise from the nerve in the superior mediastinum; and also from the recurrent laryngeal branches. These branches end in the superficial and deep cardiac plexuses.

Functional Components of the Vagus Nerve

1. The vagus nerve is composed predominantly of parasympathetic fibres. We have seen that these are classified as ***general visceral efferent.*** These fibres are very widely distributed. The vagi are responsible for parasympathetic innervation of the thoracic viscera including the heart and bronchi and of the greater part of the gastrointestinal tract. Because of this fact the term 'vagal' is synonymous with parasympathetic while referring to these organs.

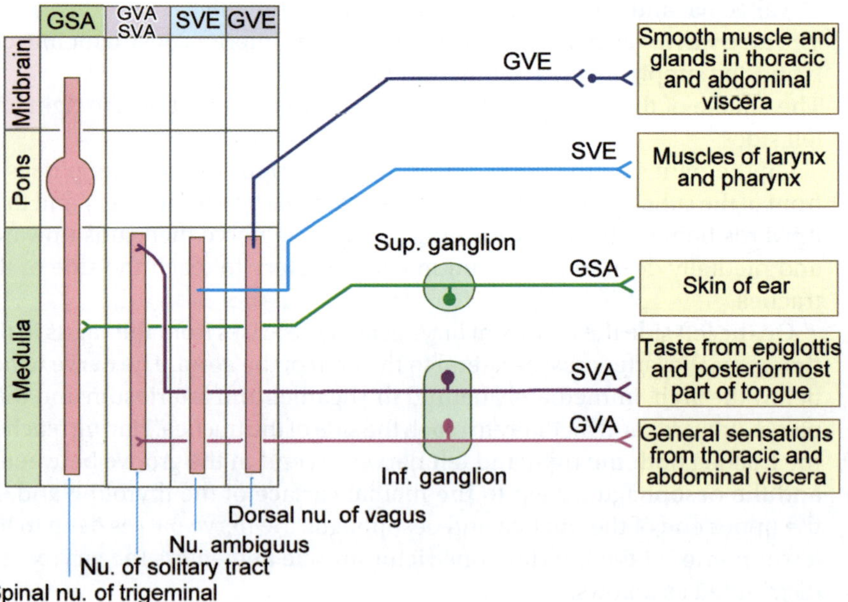

Fig. 9.83 Scheme to show the functional components of the vagus nerve.

The fibres in the vagus nerves are preganglionic. They arise from the dorsal nucleus of the vagus (Figs. 9.19, 9.20 E, F) and pass through the nerve and its ramifications to reach the viscera supplied. As a rule postganglionic neurons are located in plexuses situated close to the viscera, or in the walls of the viscera themselves. They innervate (i) smooth muscle and (ii) glands present in the walls of the viscera.

2. ***Special visceral efferent***: fibres arising from the nucleus ambiguus (Figs. 9.19, 9.20 E, F) pass through branches of vagus to innervate some of the musculature derived from the branchial arches. The superior laryngeal branch is the nerve of the fourth arch, and the recurrent laryngeal branch that of the sixth arch. Through these branches (and through the pharyngeal branches) the vagus supplies muscles of the pharynx, soft palate and larynx.
3. The vagus contains numerous ***general visceral afferent*** fibres. The neurons concerned are unipolar and are located in the inferior ganglion. The peripheral processes pass through the vagus and its branches to reach the pharynx, larynx, trachea, and oesophagus; and the thoracic and abdominal viscera. Central processes of these neurons end in the nucleus of the solitary tract. According to some authorities some of these fibres terminate in the dorsal nucleus of the vagus.
4. The vagus carries the sensation of taste from the posteriormost part of the tongue and from the epiglottis. These fibres are ***special visceral afferent.*** The neurons concerned lie in the inferior ganglion of the nerve. Their peripheral processes pass through the superior laryngeal nerve to reach the tongue and epiglottis. The central processes end in the nucleus of the solitary tract (Figs. 9.19, 9.20 E, F).
5. Finally the vagus also contains ***general somatic afferent*** fibres that supply skin. The neurons concerned lie in the superior ganglion of the nerve. Peripheral processes pass through the auricular branch to reach the skin of the auricle. The area supplied is shown in Fig. 9.11.

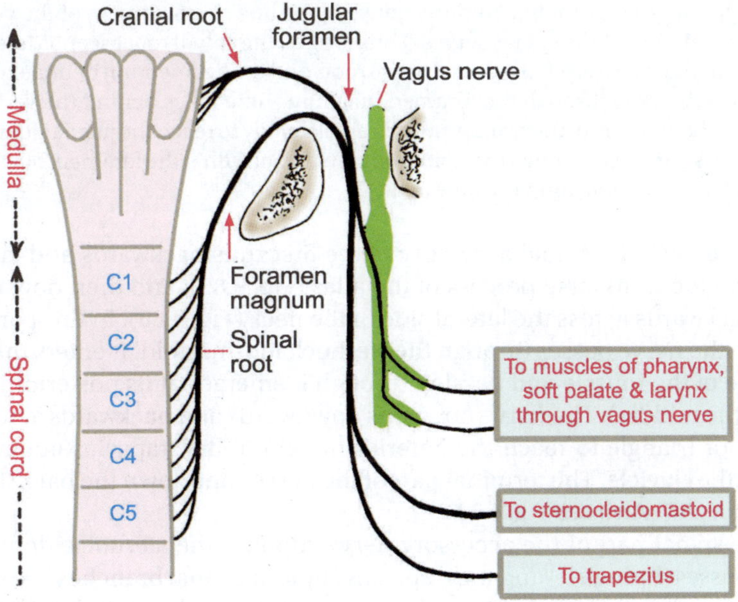

Fig. 9.84 Scheme to show the formation and distribution of the accessory nerve.

THE ACCESSORY NERVE

This is the eleventh cranial nerve. It consists of two distinct parts, cranial and spinal. both parts consist predominantly of efferent fibres as follows:

a. The fibres of the ***cranial part*** arise from the nucleus ambiguus. These fibres join the vagus nerve and are distributed through its pharyngeal and laryngeal branches to muscles of the pharynx, soft palate and larynx.
b. The fibres of the spinal part arise from the lateral part of the ventral grey column of the upper five or six cervical segments of the spinal cord. They supply the sternocleidomastoid and trapezius muscles.

Cranial Part of Accessory Nerve

The cranial part of the nerve is attached, by four or five rootlets, to the side of the medulla in the groove between the olive and the inferior cerebellar peduncle. The rootlets are attached in line with, but below, those of the vagus nerve (Fig. 9.29, 9.84). From here the nerve runs laterally to reach the jugular foramen where it is joined by the spinal root (see below). Its position in the jugular foramen is shown in Fig. 9.74. After passing through the jugular foramen the cranial root again separates from the spinal root and merges with the inferior ganglion of the vagus. The fibres of the cranial root of the accessory nerve pass into the pharyngeal and recurrent laryngeal branches of the vagus and contribute to the innervation of the muscles of the pharynx and larynx. It is believed that the muscles of the soft palate (except the tensor palati) are supplied exclusively by fibres derived from the accessory nerve.

Spinal Part of Accessory Nerve

The spinal part of the accessory nerve is formed by union of a number of rootlets that emerge from the upper five or six cervical segments of the spinal cord. The rootlets emerge along a vertical line midway between the line of attachment of the ventral and dorsal roots of the spinal nerves. Thus formed the spinal root ascends lateral to the spinal cord (between the dorsal nerve roots and the ligamentum denticulatum). It enters the skull through the foramen magnum, Here it lies behind the vertebral artery. The spinal root then runs upwards and laterally to reach the jugular foramen. We have seen that the spinal root joins the cranial root within the foramen, but leaves it again on emerging from the foramen.

In the neck the spinal accessory nerve first runs backwards and laterally to reach the transverse process of the atlas (Fig. 9.85); and then downwards and backwards across the lateral side of the neck (Fig. 9.86). In this part of its course the nerve passes through the sternocleido-mastoid. It enters the deep surface of the muscle and passing through it emerges at its posterior border (near the middle). The nerve now runs downwards and backwards across the posterior triangle to reach the anterior margin of the trapezius about 5 cm above the clavicle. The terminal part of the nerve runs down the back deep to the trapezius. Also see Fig. 1.11.

The spinal part of the accessory nerve supplies the sternocleidomastoid (as it passes through it) and the trapezius (by its terminal branches). Note that these muscles also receive branches from the cervical plexus, but these are generally regarded as having only proprioceptive fibres.

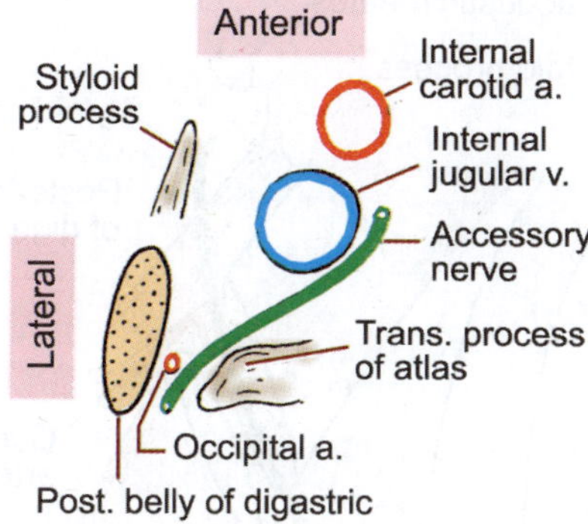

Fig. 9.85 Course of accessory nerve just below the base of the skull as seen from below.

Some important relations of the accessory nerve as it runs through the neck are as follows:

a. Between the jugular foramen and the transverse process of the atlas the nerve usually passes posterior to the internal jugular vein (Fig. 9.85), but may sometimes pass in front of it. In this part of its course the nerve lies deep to the styloid process and the posterior belly of the digastric muscle.
b. Over the transverse process of the atlas the nerve is crossed by the occipital artery (Figs. 9.85, 9.86).
c. While crossing the posterior triangle of the neck the nerve lies on the levator scapulae (Fig. 9.86).

The fibres of the accessory nerve are regarded as special visceral efferent as the muscles supplied are derived from branchial arches.

THE HYPOGLOSSAL NERVE

This is the twelfth cranial nerve. Its fibres are purely motor. They supply the muscles of the tongue. The neurons that give origin to these fibres are located in the hypoglossal nucleus which is shown in Figs. 9.19 and 9.20 E, F.

The hypoglossal nerve emerges from the medulla by ten to fifteen rootlets that are attached in the vertical groove separating the pyramid from the olive (Fig. 9.29). (It is of interest to note that the rootlets are in line with those of the ventral root of the first cervical nerve). The hypoglossal nerve leaves the cranial cavity through the hypoglossal canal (or anterior condylar canal).

On emerging at the base of the skull the nerve lies deep (medial) to the internal jugular vein and internal carotid artery (Fig. 9.88). It passes laterally and downwards to reach the interval between these vessels, and then runs vertically between them, up to the level of the angle of the mandible (Fig. 9.89). Here the nerve passes forwards crossing the internal and external carotid arteries, and enters the submandibular region. Also see Figs. 1.6, 1.7.

In the submandibular region the hypoglossal nerve at first lies superficial to the hyoglossus muscle and then to the genioglossus. It ends by dividing into its terminal branches. These supply all the intrinsic and extrinsic muscles of the

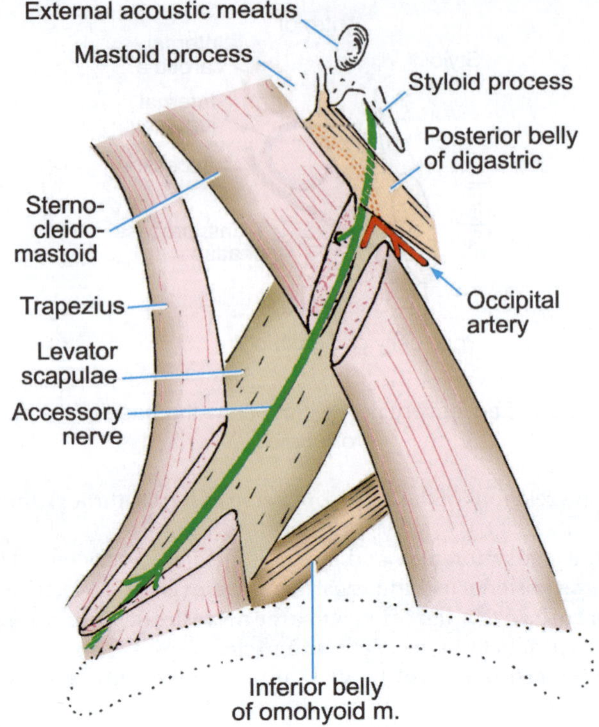

Fig. 9.86 Course and some relations of the accessory nerve.

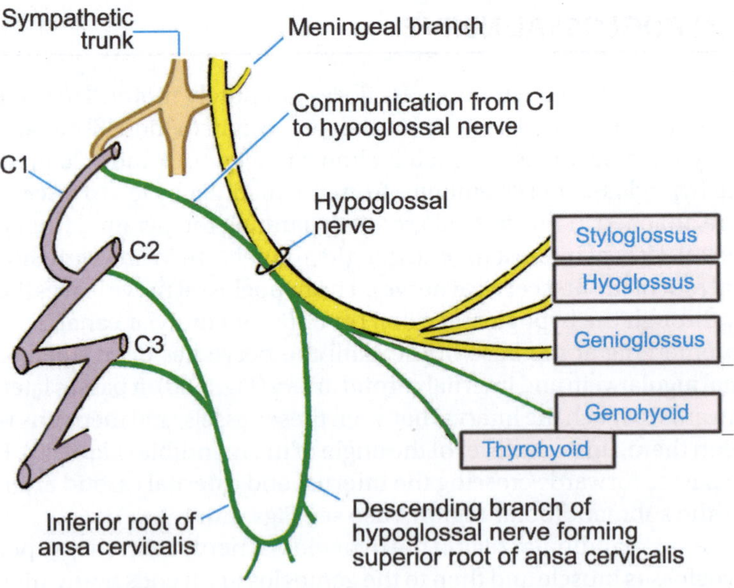

Fig. 9.87 Scheme to show the distribution of the hypoglossal nerve.

tongue (except the palatoglossus which is supplied, along with other muscles of the palate, by the cranial accessory nerve). (Also see below).

Some relations of the hypoglossal nerve are as follows:

1. In the initial part of its course the nerve passes laterally behind the internal carotid artery, the glossopharyngeal nerve and the vagus (Fig. 9.88). The nerve then winds round the lateral side of the inferior ganglion of the vagus to reach the front of the nerve.
2. Just before the nerve turns forwards (near the angle of the mandible) it lies deep to the posterior belly of the digastric muscle. Emerging from under this muscle the nerve loops round the inferior sternocleidomastoid branch of the occipital artery (Fig. 9.89).
3. As the nerve runs forwards in the neck it crosses the internal carotid artery, the external carotid artery and the loop formed by the lingual artery. The loop of the lingual artery is crossed just above the tip of the greater cornu of the hyoid bone.
4. As the nerve runs forwards above the greater cornu of the hyoid bone it is crossed by the digastric tendon and the stylohyoid.
5. The relations of the nerve as it crosses the hyoglossus are shown in Fig. 8.99 and in Fig. 1.7. The lingual nerve, the submandibular duct and the deep part of the submandibular gland lie above it. This part of the nerve is deep to the mylohyoid muscle.

Branches of the Hypoglossal Nerve

The branches of the hypoglossal nerve may be divided (a) into branches of the nerve proper and (b) branches that represent fibres which reach it from the first cervical nerve.

1. We have seen that the hypoglossal nerve itself supplies the muscles of the tongue (styloglossus, hyoglossus, genioglossus, and intrinsic muscles).

2. A ***meningeal branch*** arises from the nerve as it passes through the hypoglossal canal. It supplies the duramater of the posterior cranial fossa. The fibres of this branch are probably derived from the upper cervical nerves and from the superior cervical sympathetic ganglion.
3. The nerve gives a ***descending branch*** which forms the superior root of the ansa cervicalis. Its fibres are derived from the first cervical nerve (Figs. 9.13, 9.87).

4. Branches from the hypoglossal nerve also supply the thyrohyoid and geniohyoid muscles (Fig. 9.87). Like the fibres of the descending branch the fibres of these branches are also derived from the first cervical nerve.

The fibres of the hypoglossal nerve are classified as somatic efferent because the muscles of the tongue develop from somites (occipital somites).

CERVICAL PART OF SYMPATHETIC TRUNK

The cervical part of the sympathetic trunk bears three ganglia, superior, middle and cervicothoracic. The ***superior ganglion*** represents fused ganglia C1 to C4. The ***middle ganglion*** represents ganglia C5 and C6. The ***cervicothoracic ganglion*** represents ganglia C7, C8 and T1. This ganglion has numerous

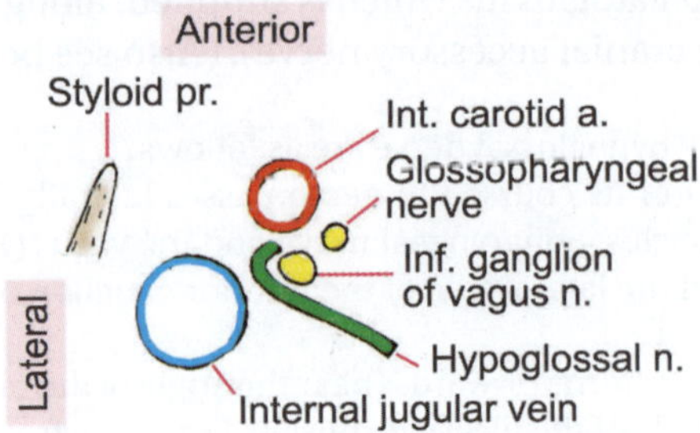

Fig. 9.88 Course of hypoglossal nerve just below the base of the skull.

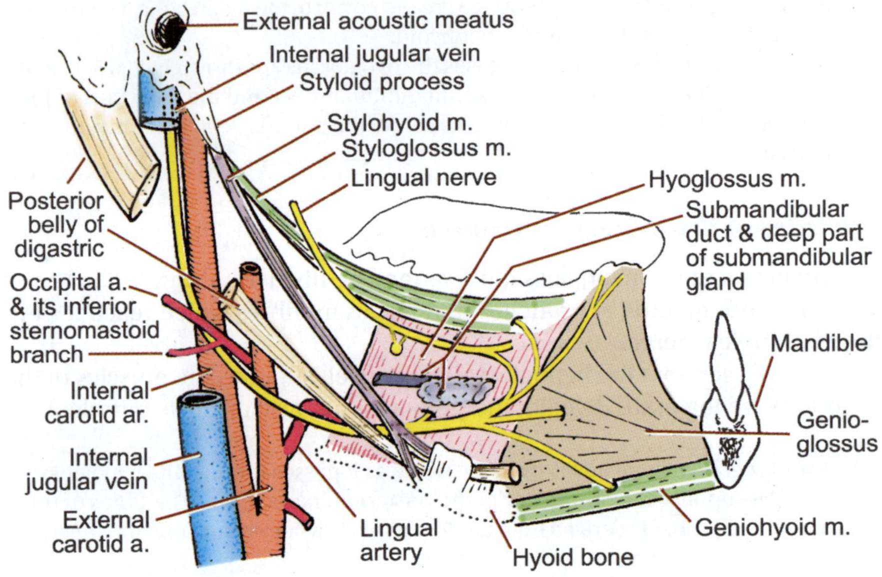

Fig. 9.89 Some relations of the hypoglossal nerve.

branches that give it a star like appearance and so it is also called the ***stellate ganglion***.

The superior cervical ganglion lies in front of the transverse processes of vertebrae C2 and C3; the middle ganglion in front of C6; and the cervicothoracic ganglion between the transverse process of C7 and the neck of the first rib.

Branches of Superior Cervical Ganglion

The branches of the superior cervical sympathetic ganglion are as follows (Fig. 9.91):

1. The ***internal carotid nerve*** arises from the upper pole of the ganglion. It is composed mainly of postganglionic fibres arising in the superior cervical

ganglion. The nerve ascends along the internal carotid artery and divides into branches that form a plexus over it. This plexus has numerous connections the more important of which are as follows (Fig. 9.90):

a. While in the carotid canal the plexus gives off the ***caroticotympanic nerves*** which enter the middle ear and join the tympanic plexus.
b. In the foramen lacerum the internal carotid plexus gives off the ***deep petrosal nerve***. This branch joins the greater petrosal nerve to form the nerve of the pterygoid canal through which the fibres reach the pterygopalatine ganglion. They pass through this ganglion, without relay, and travel through its orbital branches to supply the orbitalis muscle.
c. While the internal carotid nerve lies in the cavernous sinus it communicates with the ophthalmic division of the trigeminal nerve. These fibres pass into its nasociliary branch, and then into the long ciliary nerves to reach the eyeball where they supply the dilator pupillae muscle, and the blood vessels of the eyeball. Some fibres pass from the nasociliary nerve, or direct from the plexus round the internal carotid artery, to the ciliary ganglion. These fibres pass through this ganglion without relay and then pass into the short ciliary nerves to supply blood vessels of the eyeball. The fibres to the dilator pupillae sometimes follow the second route. It may be noted here that preganglionic sympathetic fibres for the eyeball begin in segment T1 of the spinal cord and ascend in the sympathetic trunk to the superior cervical ganglion in which the postganglionic neurons lie.

2. The ganglion gives grey rami to spinal nerves C1 to C4. It also communicates with the glossopharyngeal, vagus and hypoglossal nerves.
3. ***Laryngopharyngeal branches*** join the pharyngeal plexus. They also supply the carotid body.
4. The ***cardiac branch*** descends into the thorax along the common carotid artery. On the left side the nerve runs across the lateral side of the arch of the aorta and ends in the superficial cardiac plexus. On the right side it joins the deep cardiac plexus.

5 Branches are also given off to the common carotid and external carotid arteries and form plexuses over them. Branches of the plexus on the external carotid artery extend along its branches. The plexus on the middle meningeal artery gives a branch to the otic ganglion and that on the facial artery to the submandibular ganglion. Fibres running along the facial artery supply the sweat glands of the face.

Branches of Middle Cervical Ganglion

The branches of the middle cervical ganglion and its connections are as follows (Fig. 9.92):

1. The ganglion is connected superiorly to the superior cervical ganglion.
2. It is connected inferiorly to the cervicothoracic ganglion by an anterior and two posterior cords. The posterior cords enclose the vertebral artery. The anterior cord passes down across the subclavian artery, forms a loop below it and then passes up behind the artery to join the cervicothoracic ganglion. The loop formed is called the ***ansa subclavia***. Also see Fig. 51.13.
3. The middle cervical ganglion gives grey rami to nerves C5 and C6.
4. A cardiac branch descends into the thorax and ends in the deep cardiac plexus.

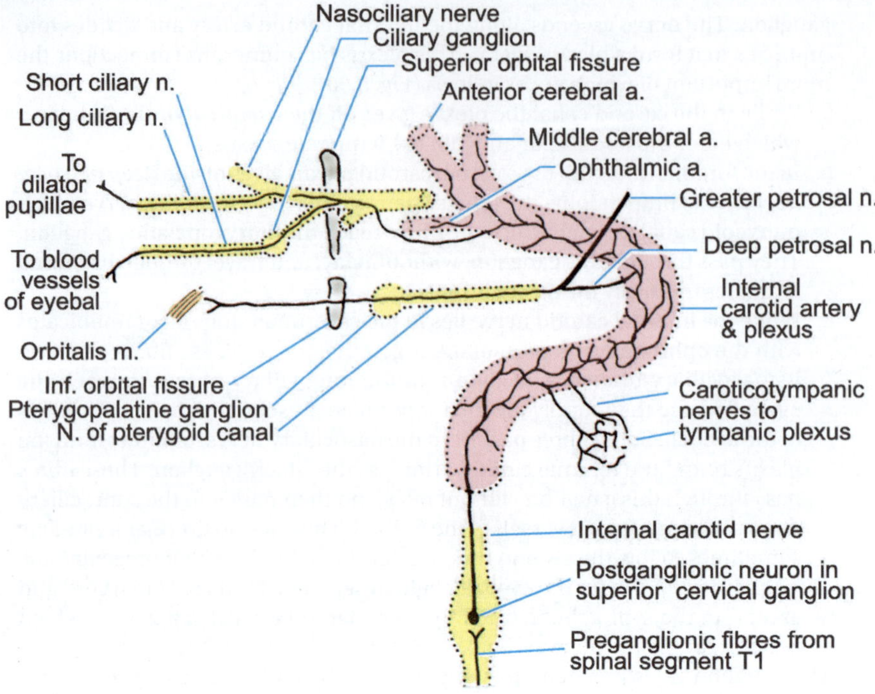

Fig. 9.90 Distribution of internal carotid nerve

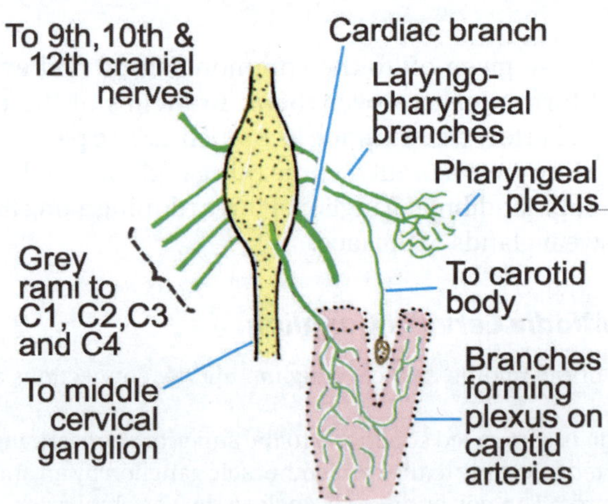

Fig. 9.91 Branches of superior cervical sympathetic ganglion.

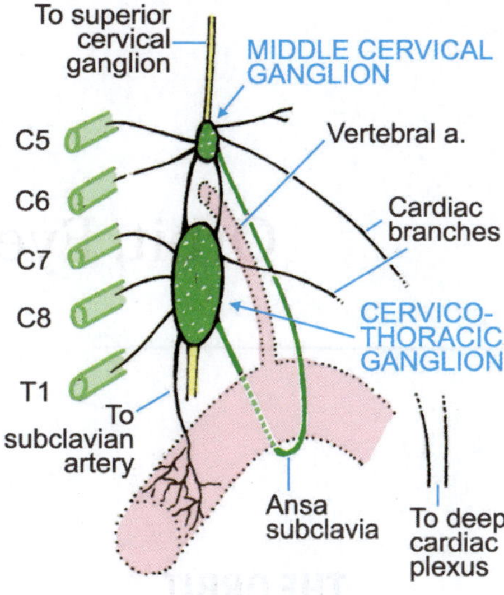

Fig. 9.92 Branches of the middle cervical sympathetic and cervicothoracic ganglia.

5. Branches are also given off to the thyroid and parathyroid glands. They pass along the inferior thyroid artery.

Branches of Cervicothoracic Ganglion

The branches of the cervicothoracic ganglion (or stellate ganglion) are as follows:

1. The connections of the ganglion to the middle cervical ganglion, including that through the ansa subclavia have been described above.
2. The ganglion gives grey rami to nerves C7, C8 and T1.
3. A cardiac branch arising from this ganglion ends in the deep cardiac plexus.
4. The cervicothoracic ganglion gives branches that form a plexus on the subclavian artery and extend on to the axillary artery; and on to branches of the subclavian artery including the vertebral and inferior thyroid arteries. The plexus on the vertebral artery extends along the artery into the cranial cavity and communicates with the internal carotid plexus. Branches from the vertebral plexus also pass to the cervical nerves.

The cervicothoracic ganglion is intimately concerned with the sympathetic innervation of the upper limb. The preganglionic neurons concerned lie in spinal segments T2 to T6 and emerge through the corresponding spinal nerves. These fibres ascend in the sympathetic trunk to reach the cervicothoracic ganglion in which they relay. Postganglionic fibres starting in the ganglion reach the blood vessels and sweat glands of the upper limb through the brachial plexus and its branches (mainly through nerves C8 and T1). The plexus on the subclavian artery was at one time considered to be the main pathway for sympathetic innervation of the upper limb, but it is now known that the fibres in the plexus do not extend much beyond the first part of the axillary artery.

CHAPTER

10

Orbit, Eye and Ear

THE ORBIT

General Review of Structures in the Orbit

Some Points about the Bony Orbit

The right and left orbits are bony depressions present on the anterior aspect of the skull, in which the eyeballs and some related structures are lodged. Before studying structures in the orbit it is important to have a knowledge of the bony orbit, and of the various apertures present in relation to it.

In the course of dissection, the orbits are usually approached from above, through the floor of the anterior cranial fossa (Fig. 1.16). The plate of bone that forms the floor of the anterior cranial fossa also forms the roof of the orbit. It is formed mainly by the orbital plate of the frontal bone, with a contribution, posteriorly, by the lesser wing of the sphenoid bone. Removal of this plate of bone, and the underlying periosteum (or ***periorbita***) brings the contents of the orbit into view. These are seen from above in Figs. 1.20 A and B; and from the lateral side in Figs. 1.19 A and B. The facts stated below should be verified in these figures.

The Eyeball

The most important structure in the orbit is the eyeball. It is considered in detail later in this Chapter. For the time being note that the eyeball is a (more or less) spherical structure placed in the anterior part of the orbit. The external surface of the eyeball is formed by a white coat called the ***sclera***. Some muscles are attached to the sclera. Over the anterior part of the eyeball, the sclera is replaced by the transparent ***cornea***, through which we see the ***iris*** and ***pupil***. When the eyes are viewed from the front we see the cornea and the anterior part of the sclera through the palpebral fissure.

The centre of the pupil can be regarded as the anterior pole of the eyeball; and the opposite end is the posterior pole. A line going round the eyeball midway between the anterior and posterior poles (in a coronal plane) is the equator of the eyeball.

Optic Nerve

Attached to the eyeball near the posterior pole we see the ***optic nerve*** (Figs. 1.19B, 1.20B). The optic nerve passes backwards and medially through the orbit to reach the optic canal. It passes through this canal to reach the middle cranial fossa (Fig. 1.16).

Extraocular Muscles

From Figs. 1.19 A and B we see that the posterior part of the eyeball, and the optic nerve, are surrounded by four muscles. Posteriorly, these muscles are attached to a tendinous ring, and lie close to the optic nerve which passes through the ring. Anteriorly, the muscles spread out and gain attachment to the eyeball a little in front of it's equator. As the muscles are ribbon like and follow a straight course they are called recti. In accordance with their position relative to the eyeball they are named the ***superior rectus,*** the ***inferior rectus,*** the ***medial rectus*** and the ***lateral rectus***. Identify these muscles in Fig. 1.20 A and B. In Fig. 1.20A the optic nerve is hidden from view by the superior rectus. It is seen in Fig. 1.20B in which the greater part of this muscle has been cut away.

The ***tendinous ring*** from which the four recti take origin is closely related to the optic canal and to the superior orbital fissure (Fig. 9.32). From this figure it will be clear how the optic nerve passes through the ring to reach the optic canal. It will also be clear that the ring divides the superior orbital fissure into upper, middle and lower parts. Structures passing into the orbit through the middle part of the fissure will come to lie within the space bounded by the four recti, while structures passing through the upper part of the fissure will lie 'outside' the recti.

In addition to the four rectus muscles, we see two muscles, the superior oblique and the inferior oblique. In Fig. 1.20A identify the ***superior oblique*** muscle running forwards along the (upper part of the) medial wall of the orbit. In the anterior part of the orbit the muscle ends in a tendon that passes through a pulley (or trochlea) and then turns backwards and laterally to reach the upper aspect of the eyeball. The course of the muscle and its tendon is seen from the lateral side in Figs. 1.19 A, B. Note that near its termination the tendon of the superior oblique muscle passes between the eyeball and the superior rectus muscle.

The ***inferior oblique*** muscle arises from the medial wall of the orbit near its anterior end. The muscle passes laterally and backwards below the eyeball, and then winds around its lateral side to be attached to the sclera deep to the lateral rectus muscle. Note that the attachments of the superior and inferior oblique muscles (to the eyeball) lie close to each other. Note also that the insertions lie posterior of the equator of the eyeball.

One more muscle of the orbit remains to be identified. This is the ***levator palpebrae superioris*** (Fig. 1.19A). Note that this muscle lies above the superior rectus, and that anteriorly it enters the upper eyelid. In Fig. 1.20A the greater part of this muscle has been removed (to expose deeper structures), but its anterior part can be seen spreading out to enter the upper eyelid in the form of a broad tendon.

In the preceding paragraphs we have identified seven muscles: four recti, two oblique muscles, and the levator palpebrae palpebrae superioris. These muscles are collectively referred to as ***extraocular muscles***. They are described in detail below.

Nerves of the Orbit

The nerves supplying the extraocular muscles are shown in Fig. 1.19B.

1. Observe the ***oculomotor nerve*** dividing into upper and lower rami both of which pass through the middle part of the superior oblique fissure and enter the space surrounded by the recti. The upper ramus ascends lateral to the optic nerve and supplies the superior rectus and the levator palpebrae superioris. The inferior ramus of the oculomotor nerve supplies the inferior rectus, the medial rectus, and the inferior oblique muscles. This division also gives a branch to the ***ciliary ganglion*** lying inferolateral to the optic nerve. A number of short ciliary nerves arising from the ganglion pass forwards to enter the eyeball (Fig. 1.20B).
2. The ***abducent nerve*** also enters the orbit through the middle part of the superior orbital fissure and supplies the lateral rectus. In Fig. 1.20A observe this nerve entering the muscle from its medial side.
3. The ***trochlear nerve*** (Figs. 1.19B, 1.20A) enters the orbit through the upper part of the superior orbital fissure. It passes medially above the superior rectus muscle to reach and supply the superior oblique muscle.

   Some other nerves to be seen in the orbit are as follows.

   a. The ophthalmic division of the trigeminal nerve (Fig. 1.20A) is seen dividing into three branches a short distance posterior to the superior orbital fissure. The three branches are the ***lacrimal nerve*** (most lateral), the ***frontal nerve***, and the ***nasociliary nerve*** (most medial). The lacrimal and frontal nerves enter the orbit by passing through the superior part of the superior orbital fissure. They, therefore, lie outside the ring formed by the rectus muscles. The nasociliary nerve enters the orbit by passing through the middle part of the superior orbital fissure (and through the tendinous ring that gives attachment to the rectus muscles). It is therefore seen within the ring formed by the recti.

      The ***lacrimal nerve*** runs forwards along the lateral wall of the orbit to reach the lacrimal gland. It is joined by a communicating branch from the zygomatic nerve (see below).

      The ***frontal nerve*** runs forwards above the superior rectus muscle and divides into supraorbital and supratrochlear nerves. These nerves pass out of the orbit and turn upwards into the scalp (where they are seen in Figs. 1.2 and 1.3).

The ***nasociliary nerve*** first lies deep to the superior rectus muscle, lateral to the optic nerve. It runs forwards and crosses superior to the optic nerve to reach the medial wall of the orbit. As the nasociliary nerve crosses the optic nerve it gives off a few ***long ciliary nerves*** that pass forwards to enter the eyeball. The terminal part of the nasociliary nerve becomes the ***infratrochlear nerve***.

b. The ***maxillary division of the trigeminal nerve*** passes from the middle cranial fossa into the pterygopalatine fossa (Fig. 1.19A). From here the nerve enters the orbit by passing through the inferior orbital fissure. The nerve is now called the ***inferior orbital nerve***. It runs forwards over the floor of the orbit. The distal part of the nerve enters the infraorbital canal, and emerges on the face through the infraorbital foramen.
c. The ***zygomatic nerve*** arises from the maxillary nerve while the latter is within the pterygopalatine fossa. It enters the orbit by passing through the inferior orbital fissure.

In the preceding paragraphs we have identified various nerves present in the orbit. These are described in detail in Chapter 9.

The orbit also contains some autonomic nerve fibres.

Blood Vessels

The main artery of the orbit is the ophthalmic branch of the internal carotid artery (Fig. 1.20). The artery enters the orbit through the optic canal. Within the canal the artery lies inferolateral to the optic nerve. After a short course the artery gives off a lacrimal branch that accompanies the lacrimal nerve. The ophthalmic artery then crosses above the optic nerve to reach the medial part of the orbit. In addition to the lacrimal branch the ophthalmic artery gives off several branches that accompany ramifications of the frontal and nasociliary nerves. It also gives off the ***central artery of the retina***. This artery runs forwards in the centre of the optic nerve and supplies the retina of the eyeball. The veins of the orbit end in ***superior and inferior ophthalmic veins***.

Lymph vessels from structures in the orbit drain into the parotid lymph nodes.

Lacrimal Gland

The lacrimal gland is an essential constituent of the lacrimal apparatus.

MUSCLES OF THE ORBIT

The muscles of the orbit include the ***extraocular muscles*** which are the four recti (superior, inferior, medial and lateral), two oblique muscles (superior and inferior), and the levator palpebrae superioris. In addition we have some muscles made up of smooth muscle fibres and supplied by autonomic nerves. These are the ***superior tarsal, inferior tarsal*** and ***orbitalis*** muscles. Some

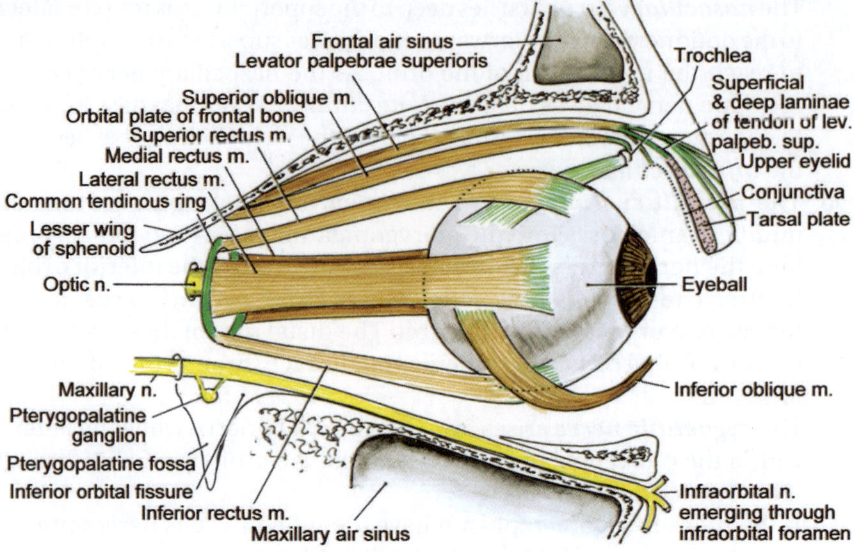

Fig. 10.1A Scheme to show extraocular muscles as seen from the lateral side.

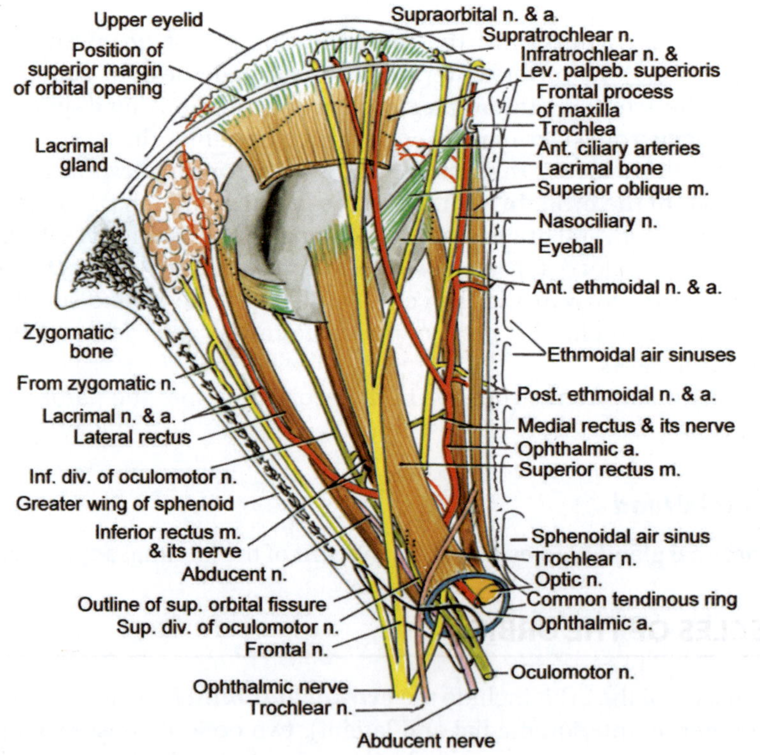

10.1B Scheme to show the arrangement of nerves supplying the extraocular muscles. The optic nerve is also shown.

muscles that lie within the eyeball (***sphincter and dilator pupillae, ciliaris***) will be considered when we study that organ.

THE FOUR RECTI

Origin

The superior rectus, the inferior rectus, the medial rectus and lateral rectus muscles all arise from the posterior part of the orbit through a common tendinous ring which surrounds the optic canal, and encloses a part of the superior orbital fissure (Fig. 10.2A). The superior, inferior, medial and lateral recti arise from the corresponding parts of the ring.

Insertion

The muscles run forwards (Figs. 1.19, 1.20) first around the optic nerve and then around the eyeball (in the positions indicated by their names) to be inserted into the sclera about 6 mm behind the junction of the sclera and cornea (Also see Fig. 10.3). Note that the insertions are in front of the equator of the eyeball.

The nerve supply and actions of the recti are considered below along with those of the oblique muscles.

THE OBLIQUE MUSCLES

Superior Oblique

The superior oblique muscle arises from the body of the sphenoid bone just above and medial to the optic canal (Fig. 10.2A). It runs forwards in the upper medial part of the orbit. Near the orbital margin the muscle ends in a tendon which passes through a tendinous pulley (trochlea). This pulley is attached to the wall of the orbit at the junction of its roof and medial wall (Figs. 10.2B, 10.3). (The wall of the orbit is formed here by the frontal bone). The tendon then runs backwards and laterally to be inserted into the upper lateral quadrant of the eyeball behind the equator (Fig. 10.3). Also see Figs. 1.19, and 1.20.

Inferior Oblique

The inferior oblique muscles arises from the anterior and medial part of the floor of the orbit (from the maxilla just lateral to the nasolacrimal groove: Fig. 10.2B). The muscle winds round the eyeball first passing laterally and backwards (below the inferior rectus) and then backwards and upwards (deep to the lateral rectus) to be inserted into the lateral part of the sclera behind the equator of the eyeball. The insertion is below and behind that of the superior oblique muscle (Figs. 1.19 A, B; 10.3).

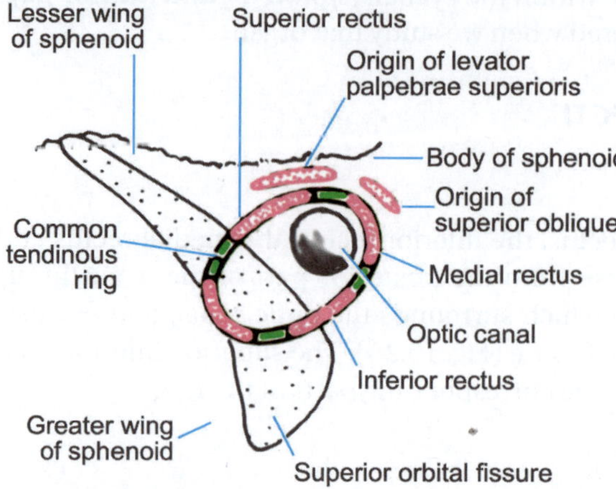

Fig. 10.2A Diagram showing the common tendinous ring for origin of the rectus muscles. Note its relationship to the optic canal and to the superior orbital fissure.

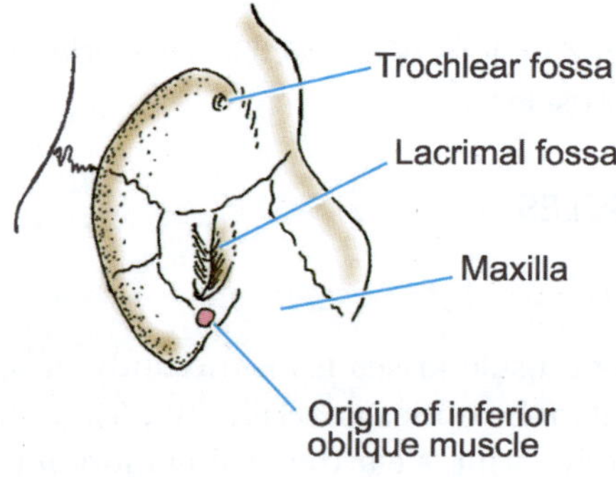

Fig. 10.2B Some features on the medial wall of the orbit, viewed from the anterolateral aspect.

ACTIONS OF RECTUS AND OBLIQUE MUSCLES: MOVEMENTS OF THE EYEBALL

As a convention movements of the eyeball are described with reference to its anterior end (or more simply, the cornea).

A. The cornea can move upwards or downwards, the movement occurring on an imaginary axis passing transversely through the equator of the eyeball. Upward movement can be produced (a) by pulling the anterior part of the eyeball upwards (superior rectus), or (b) by pulling the posterior part downwards (inferior oblique). Similarly, downward movement can be produced by (a) pulling the anterior part downwards (inferior rectus) or (b) pulling the posterior part upwards (superior oblique).

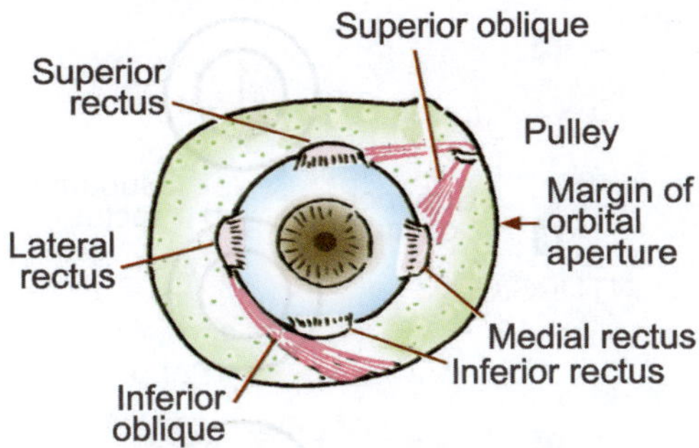

Fig. 10.3 Schematic anterior view of the orbit to show the attachment of extraocular muscles to the eyeball. In particular note the arrangement of the superior and inferior oblique muscles.

B. The cornea can move medially or laterally on an axis passing vertically through the equator of the eyeball. Medial movement can be produced by pulling the anterior part of the eyeball medially. This action is performed by the medial rectus. The superior and inferior recti can also move the cornea medially as they pass forwards and laterally from origin to insertion. Lateral movement can be produced (a) by pulling the anterior part of the eyeball laterally (lateral rectus) or (b) by pulling the posterior part medially (superior and inferior oblique).
C. The cornea can move obliquely by combination of the movements described above e.g., upwards and medially, downwards and laterally and so on.

D. The eyeball undergoes torsional movements on an anteroposterior axis. To understand these movements imagine a vertical line drawn through the middle of the cornea dividing it into medial and lateral halves (Fig. 10.4A). Torsion is described with reference to the ***upper*** end of this line (arrow). When the eyeball rotates so that the upper end of the line moves medially the movement is described as ***intorsion;*** and when it moves laterally the movement is called ***extorsion.*** From Fig. 10.4B it will be obvious that intorsion will be produced mainly by the superior oblique and partly by the superior rectus; while extorsion will be produced (Fig. 10.4C) mainly by the inferior oblique, and partly by the inferior rectus.

The movements produced by individual muscles, and the combinations of muscles producing a given movement, can now be summarised as shown in Fig. 10.5.

Levator Palpebrae Superioris

The levator palpebrae superioris arises from the posterior part of the orbit. The area of origin is on the lesser wing of the sphenoid bone (Fig. 10.2A) a little above the optic canal. The muscle passes forwards above the superior rectus and enters the upper eyelid. The muscle is responsible for keeping the palpebral fissure open.

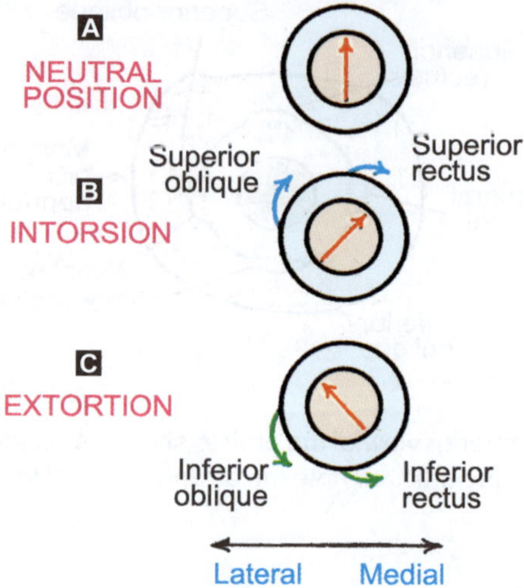

Fig. 10.4 Schematic diagram of the eye to explain the movements of intorsion and extorsion. The inner circle represents the cornea, and the outer circle represents the sclera.

It ends in an aponeurosis which divides into three layers. The superficial layer is inserted into the anterior surface of the tarsal plate of the upper eyelid; the middle layer into the upper margin of the tarsal plate; and the deep layer into the superior conjunctival fornix (Fig. 10.5). Also see Fig. 1.19A.

NERVE SUPPLY OF MUSCLES OF THE EYEBALL

The lateral rectus is supplied by the abducent nerve, and the superior oblique by the trochlear nerve. All other muscles are supplied by the oculomotor nerve: the superior rectus and the levator palpebrae superioris by its superior ramus; and the rectus medialis, rectus inferior and the inferior oblique by its inferior ramus.

Involuntary Muscles in the Orbit

1. The levator palpebrae superioris contains some smooth muscle fibres in its deeper part. These constitute the ***superior tarsal muscle***.
2. The ***inferior tarsal muscle*** connects the inferior tarsus to fascia around the inferior rectus and inferior oblique muscles.
   These smooth muscle fibres present in relation to the upper and lower eyelids can be responsible for involuntary, wide opening of the eyes under sympathetic stimulation associated with fear or anger.
3. The ***orbitalis*** bridges the inferior orbital fissure. The action of this muscle is uncertain. It could, theoretically, compress the inferior ophthalmic veins leading to their engorgement, thus pushing the eyeball forwards and making it more prominent.

These three involuntary muscles are supplied by sympathetic fibres. Destruction of sympathetic nerves supplying the head and neck results in Horner's syndrome two features of which are drooping of the upper eyelid (ptosis), and reduced prominence of the eyeball (enophthalmos). In addition there is constriction of the pupil because of paralysis of the dilator pupillae.

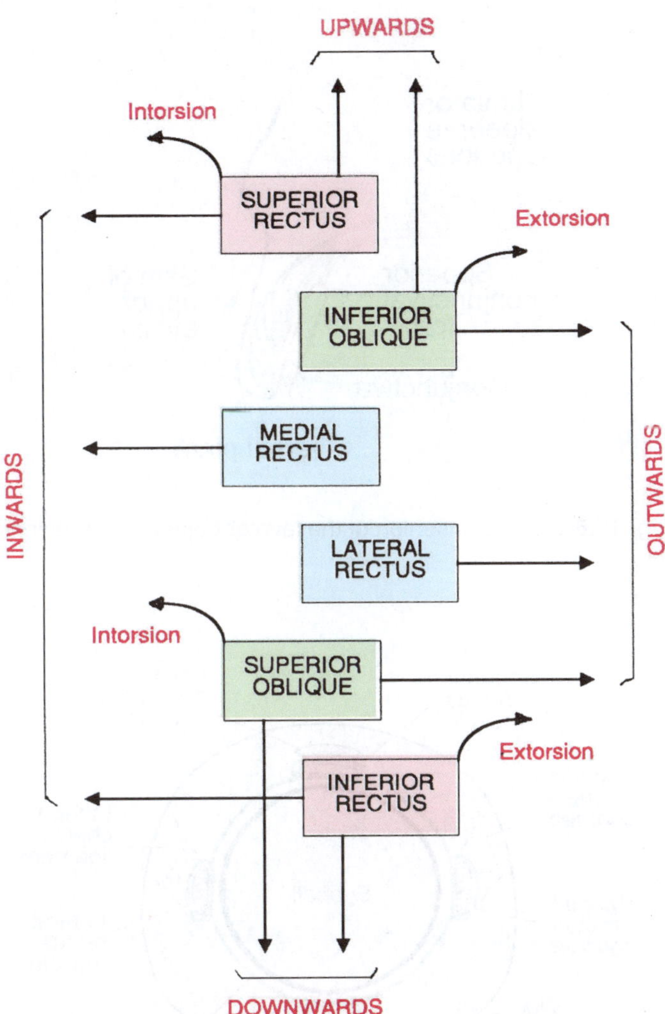

Fig. 10.5 Scheme showing the movements of the eyeball produced by individual extraocular muscles, and the muscles responsible for each movement.

ARRANGEMENT OF FASCIA IN THE ORBIT

Periorbita (Orbital Fascia)

The periosteum lining the inside of the bony orbit is called the orbital fascia or periorbita. At the anterior aperture of the orbit it becomes continuous with periosteum covering the bones around the aperture. At the superior orbital fissures, and at the optic canal, it becomes continuous with the endocranium of the middle cranial fossa. At the inferior orbital fissure it becomes continuous with periosteum lining the pterygopalatine fossa.

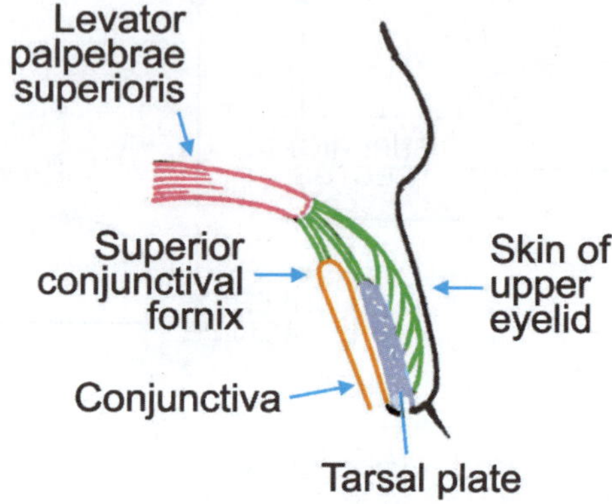

Fig. 10.6 Mode of insertion of the levator palpebrae superioris.

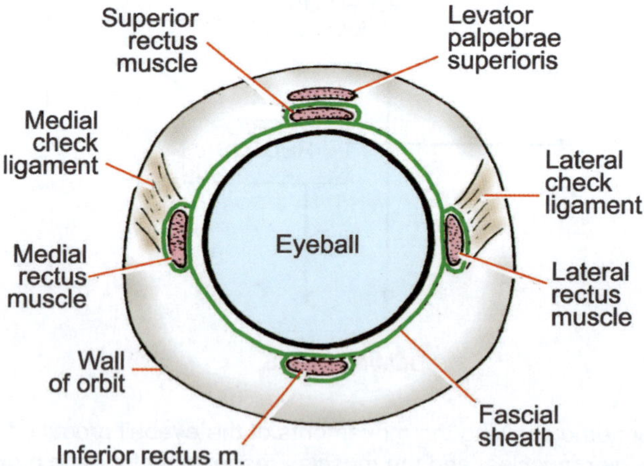

Fig. 10.7 Scheme to show some parts of the fascial sheath of the eyeball. Note the 'hammock' formed by the lower part of the sheath and the check ligaments.

The periorbita sends expansions into the eyelids. These extensions form the ***orbital septum***. The lacrimal fascia (Fig. 3.8), and the trochlea for the superior oblique tendon can be regarded as special regions of the periorbita.

Fascial Sheath of the Eyeball

The eyeball is surrounded by a fascial sheath which extends posteriorly up to the attachment of the optic nerve, where it fuses with the sheath of the nerve. Anteriorly, it extends up to the sclerocorneal junction. It is separated from the eyeball by the ***episcleral space*** (Fig. 10.11). The sheath is closely related to the ocular muscles which perforate it, and receive extensions from it. These extensions form tubular sheaths round the muscles: fibrous bands pass from them to the orbital wall. The most important of bands are the ***medial and lateral check ligaments***. The medial check ligament passes from the sheath around the medial rectus to the medial wall of the orbit. The lateral check ligament passes from the sheath over the lateral rectus to the lateral wall of the orbit. They are called check ligaments on the assumption that they limit the contraction of these muscles. The space between the fascial sheath of the eyeball and the orbital periosteum is filled mostly by fat. The sheath and the fat keep the eyeball in place. The sheath provides a smooth surface over which the surface of the eye ball can move freely. In this connection it is interesting to note that the fascial sheath has been compared to a hammock supporting the eyeball (Fig. 10.7).

THE LACRIMAL GLAND

The lacrimal gland lies in relation to the upper lateral part of the wall of the orbit (formed here by the zygomatic process of the frontal bone) (Fig. 1.20, 3.7). The gland is related inferiorly to the levator palpebrae superioris and to the lateral rectus muscle. An extension of the gland, that passes into the upper eyelid, is called its ***palpebral part*** (Fig. 3.7). The palpebral part is continuous with the ***main (or orbital) part*** around the lateral side of the aponeurosis of the levator palpebrae superioris. In other words the palpebral part lies deep to the aponeurosis of the levator (Fig. 3.4). The lacrimal gland drains into the superior conjunctival fornix through about twelve ducts. All ducts pass through the palpebral part of the gland. Accessory lacrimal glands may be present in relation to the superior conjunctival fornix, or less commonly in relation to the inferior fornix. The lacrimal gland is supplied by twigs from the lacrimal branch of the ophthalmic artery (Fig. 1.20). The secretomotor fibres to the gland follow a complicated course that is shown in Fig. 9.68.

NERVES AND VESSELS OF ORBIT

These are considered in detail in Chapters 8 and 9.

THE EYEBALL

Preliminary Remarks

It is common knowledge that the right and left eyes are the peripheral organs of vision. Each eyeball is like a camera. It has a ***lens*** which produces images of objects that we see. The images fall on a membrane called the ***retina***. Cells in the retina convert the light images into nervous impulses which pass through the optic nerves and other parts of the visual pathway to reach visual areas of the cerebral cortex. It is in the cortex that vision is actually perceived.

The structure of the eyeball has been studied in great detail, but many of the details are of interest only to the specialist. The account that follows is confined to the main facts that the undergraduate medical student should know.

The greater part of the eyeball (posterior five sixths) is shaped like a sphere and has a diameter of about 24 mm. The anterior one sixth is much more convex than the posterior part. It represents part of a sphere having a diameter of about 15 mm. The outer wall of the posterior five sixths of the eyeball is formed by a thick white opaque membrane called the ***sclera***. The wall of the anterior one sixth is transparent and is called the ***cornea***. When the 'eye' is viewed in the living person we see only a small part of the eyeball that appears in the interval between the upper and lower eyelids (i.e., in the palpebral fissure). The 'white' of the eye is formed by the sclera. The dark central part is formed by the cornea. The cornea itself is transparent: the dark appearance is because of the presence of a pigmented diaphragm, the ***iris***, deep to the cornea. In the centre of the iris there is an aperture called the ***pupil***. The pupil appears black as the interior of the eye is dark (like that of a camera).

A horizontal section across an eyeball is shown in Fig. 10.8. Note the following features:

The wall of the eyeball is made up of three main layers.

1. The outermost layer is called the ***fibrous coat***. It is formed posteriorly by the sclera; and anteriorly by the cornea.
2. The next layer is the ***vascular coat***. It has the following subdivisions. The part lining the inner surface of most of the sclera is thin and is called the ***choroid***. Near the junction of the sclera with the cornea the vascular coat is thick and forms the ***ciliary body***. The ciliary body is continuous with the ***iris*** which lies a short distance behind the cornea.
   The space between the iris and the cornea is called the ***anterior chamber***. The space between the iris and the front of the lens is called the ***posterior chamber***.
3. The innermost layer of the wall of the eyeball is called the ***retina.***

Light falling on the retina has to pass through a number of ***refracting media*** before reaching the retina and forming an image on it. These are (a) the cornea; (b) a fluid, the ***aqueous humour***, which fills the anterior and posterior chambers; (c) the lens; and (d) a jelly like ***vitreous body*** which fills the eyeball posterior to the lens.

The centre of the cornea is called the ***anterior pole*** of the eyeball. The opposite end is called the ***posterior pole***. The ***visual axis*** of the eye passes

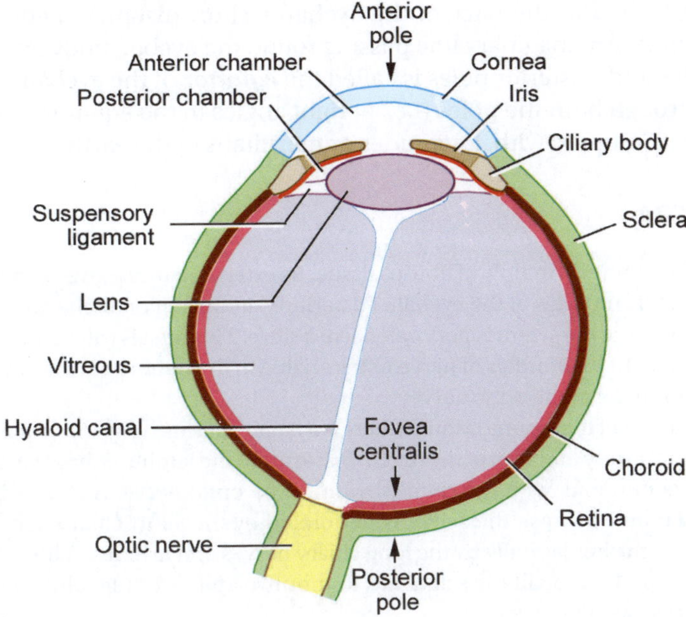

Fig. 10.8 Horizontal section across the eyeball to show the main features of its structure.

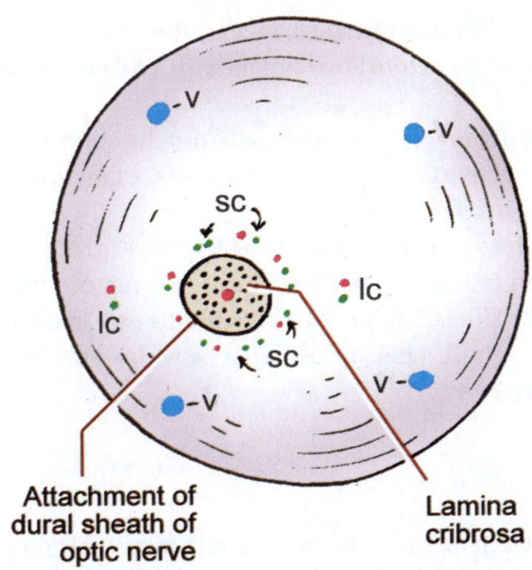

Fig. 10.9 Eyeball seen from behind to show the openings in the sclera. sc: foramina for short ciliary nerves and arteries; lc: foramina for long ciliary nerves and arteries; v: foramina for venae vorticosae.

from the anterior pole to the posterior pole. In Fig. 10.8 note that the optic nerve is attached to the back of the eyeball a short distance medial to the posterior pole. An imaginary line passing round the eyeball midway between the anterior and posterior poles is called the ***equator*** of the eyeball. Any line passing through both the poles (i.c., at right angles to the equator) is called a ***meridian***. (Compare with, longitudes or meridians of the earth).

THE SCLERA

The sclera is made up mainly of fibrous tissue. Its external surface gives attachment to the extrinsic muscles of the eyeball. Posteriorly, in the region of the attachment of the optic nerve the sclera is perforated like a sieve. This area is called the ***lamina cribrosa*** (Fig. 10.9). Bundles of nerve fibres arising in the retina pass through these perforations to form the optic nerve.

At the centre of the lamina cribrosa there is a larger aperture (Fig. 10.9) for passage of the central artery and vein of the retina. Just around the lamina cribrosa the sclera becomes continuous with the dural sheath of the optic nerve. A short distance from the lamina cribrosa the sclera is perforated by the short ciliary nerves and arteries, and further laterally by the long ciliary nerves and arteries. A little behind the equator of the eyeball the sclera has four or five apertures for veins called the venae vorticosae (Fig. 10.9).

Anteriorly, the sclera becomes continuous with the cornea at the ***sclerocorneal junction***. As this junction is circular it is also called the ***limbus***. A circular channel called the ***sinus venosus sclerae*** (or ***canal of Schlemm***) is located in the sclera just behind the sclerocorneal junction (Fig. 10.15). A triangular mass of scleral tissue projects into the cornea just medial to the sinus: this projection is called the ***scleral spur*** (Fig. 10.15).

The anterior part of the external surface of the sclera is covered by the ocular conjunctiva. The rest of the sclera is in contact with a ***fascial sheath*** which surrounds the eyeball.

The deep surface of the sclera is separated from the choroid by the ***perichoroidal space***. Delicate connective tissue present in this space constitutes the ***suprachoroid lamina*** (or ***lamina fusca***) (Fig. 10.11).

The contents of the eyeball are under positive pressure. This pressure is resisted by the sclera, which is not extensible. These two factors together maintain the shape of the eyeball. The sclera provides a smooth external surface that facilitates movements of the eyeball. This surface also provides attachment to the extrinsic muscles of the eyeball.

THE CORNEA

The cornea is not exactly circular. Its horizontal diameter is somewhat greater than 11 mm, but its vertical diameter is slightly less. As the cornea is more convex than the sclera the junction of the two is marked, on the exterior of the eyeball, by a groove called the ***sulcus sclerae***.

The cornea is made up of five layers that are shown in Fig. 10.10. For details of these layers consult the author's HUMAN HISTOLOGY.

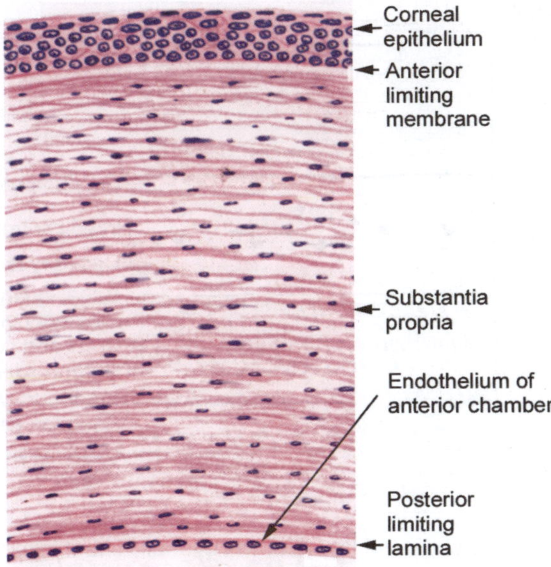

Fig. 10.10 Diagram of a section through the cornea to show its layers.

THE CHOROID

The choroid consists of a network of blood vessels supported by connective tissue containing many pigmented cells that give it a dark brown colour. It is the dark colour of the choroid that darkens the interior of the eyeball. It also prevents reflection of light within the eyeball. Both these factors are necessary for formation of sharp images on the retina.

Within the choroid there is an outer ***vascular layer*** made up of small arteries and veins; and an inner ***capillary layer*** (Fig. 10.11). The short ciliary arteries which pierce the posterior part of the sclera (Fig. 10.9) run forwards in the vascular lamina. However, most of the vascular lamina is filled by veins which converge on four or five ***venae vorticosae***. We have seen that these veins pierce the sclera a short distance behind the equator of the eyeball.

The choroid is separated from the sclera by a layer of delicate connective tissue called the ***suprachoroid lamina*** (or lamina fusca). The choroid is separated from the retina by a thin membrane called the ***basal lamina*** (or membrane of Bruch). Nutrients diffusing through this membrane, from capillaries in the choroid, provide nutrition to the outer part of the retina.

THE CILIARY BODY

The ciliary body represents an anterior continuation of the choroid. Anteromedially, it becomes continuous with the iris. It is made up of vascular tissue, muscle and connective tissue.

When the eyeball is cut coronally, some distance behind the lens, and is viewed from behind we see the appearance shown in Fig. 10.12. Identify the

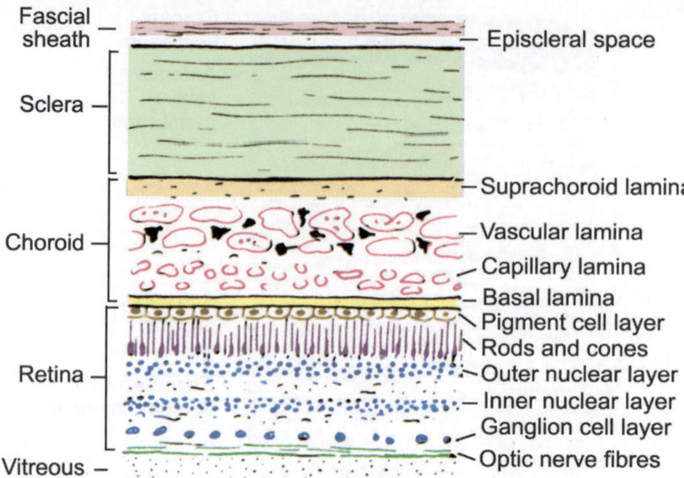

Fig. 10.11 Scheme to show the layers of the eyeball. The thickness of various layers is not drawn to scale. For some details of the retina see Fig. 10.17.

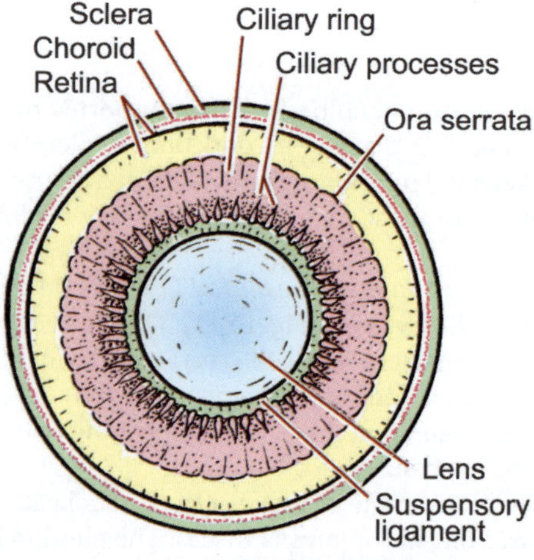

Fig. 10.12 Anterior part of the eyeball viewed from behind after cutting the eyeball in the coronal plane.

following in this figure. The retina proper ends anteriorly (a short distance behind the sclerocorneal junction) in a wavy line called the ***ora serrata***. This line also represents the junction of the choroid with the ciliary body. The ciliary body extends forwards (and medially) from the ora serrata to end near the periphery of the lens. Anterior to the ora serrata the retina is continued forwards as a double layer of simple epithelium which lines the inner surface of the ciliary body and the posterior surface of the iris.

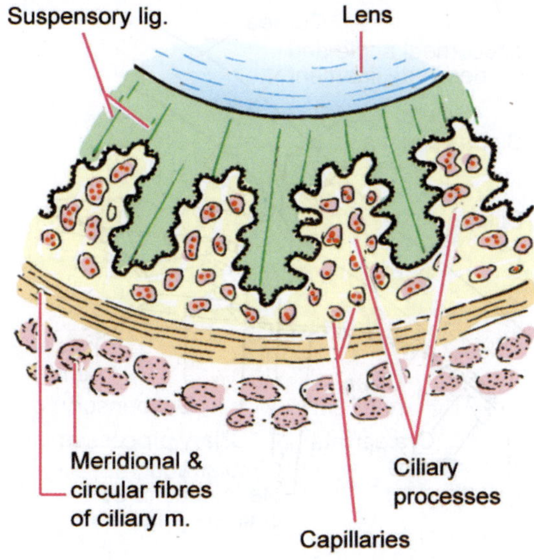

Fig. 10.13 Schematic coronal section through ciliary body.

The ciliary body can be divided into a posterior part called the ciliary ring, and an anterior part made of the ciliary processes.

The ***ciliary ring*** is about 3.5 mm wide. It has a relatively flat surface on which there are shallow radial grooves (Fig. 10.12).

The ***ciliary processes*** lie between the ciliary ring and the base of the iris (Fig. 10.12). The ciliary processes secrete the aqueous humour. They may also produce some components of the vitreous body

There are about 70 processes arranged radially (meriodonally). Each process may be regarded as an infolding of the surface of the ciliary body, and having a very irregular surface because of the presence of secondary folds. The substance of each process is made up of a plexus of blood vessels covered by the double layer of retinal epithelium mentioned above (Fig. 10.13).

The ciliary processes and the furrows between them give attachment to numerous delicate fibres that pass to them from the periphery of the lens (Fig. 10.13). Many of these fibres can run into the ciliary ring.

A meridional section (i.e., a section along a line joining the anterior and posterior poles of the eyeball) is shown in Fig. 10.14. In such a section the ciliary body appears to be triangular. Lateral to the ciliary processes (and medial to the anterior part of the sclera) there is a triangular mass of the ***ciliary muscle***. The fibres of the ciliary muscle are arranged in two main groups.

1. The ***circular fibres*** lie in the anterior and inner part of the ciliary body. They form a ring of muscle, contraction of which relaxes the fibres of the suspensory ligament. Release of tension on the lens makes it more convex.
2. The ***meriodonal fibres*** take origin from the scleral spur (Figs. 10.14, 10.15). They pass backwards and get attached to the ciliary processes and the ciliary ring. Some fibres extend into the choroid. When these fibres contract the ciliary ring

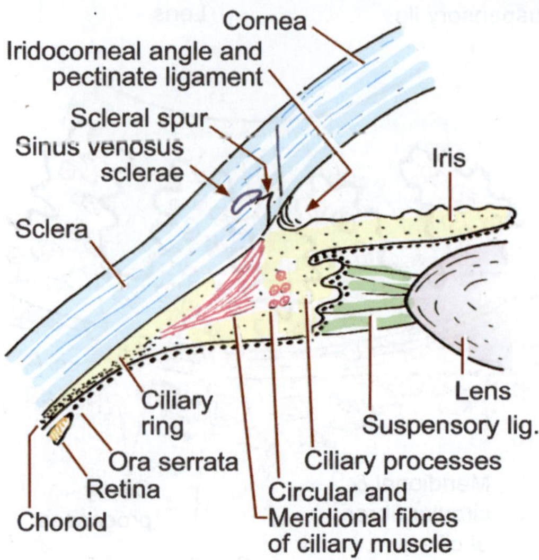

Fig. 10.14 Meridional section through the ciliary body and iris.

is drawn forwards (i.e., towards the lens). As a result the suspensory ligament is again relaxed. In this way the circular and meriodonal fibres act together to make the lens more convex; and enable it to focus images of near objects on the retina. This is called ***accommodation***.

The ciliary muscle (or ciliaris) is supplied by parasympathetic fibres that travel to it via the oculomotor nerve and the ciliary ganglion.

THE IRIS

The iris is the most anterior part of the vascular coat of the eyeball. It forms a diaphragm placed immediately in front of the lens. At its periphery it is continuous with the ciliary body. In its centre there is an aperture, the ***pupil***.

The iris is composed of a stroma of connective tissue containing numerous pigment cells, and in which are embedded blood vessels and smooth muscle (see below).

The posterior surface of the iris is lined by a double layer of epithelium which represents an anterior continuation of the retina: the cells of this epithelium are deeply pigmented. In the fetus the anterior surface of the iris is covered by a layer of flattened cells continuous with those lining the posterior surface of the cornea. However, this lining disappears after birth.

The pupil regulates the amount of light passing into the eye. In bright light the pupil contracts, and in dim light it dilates. In this way the optimum amount of light required for proper vision reaches the retina, within a considerable range in intensity of illumination. Changes in the size of the pupil are produced by the smooth muscle of the iris which consists of two parts.

i. The ***sphincter pupillae*** is a ring of circularly arranged muscle situated just around the pupil. Its contraction narrows the pupil.

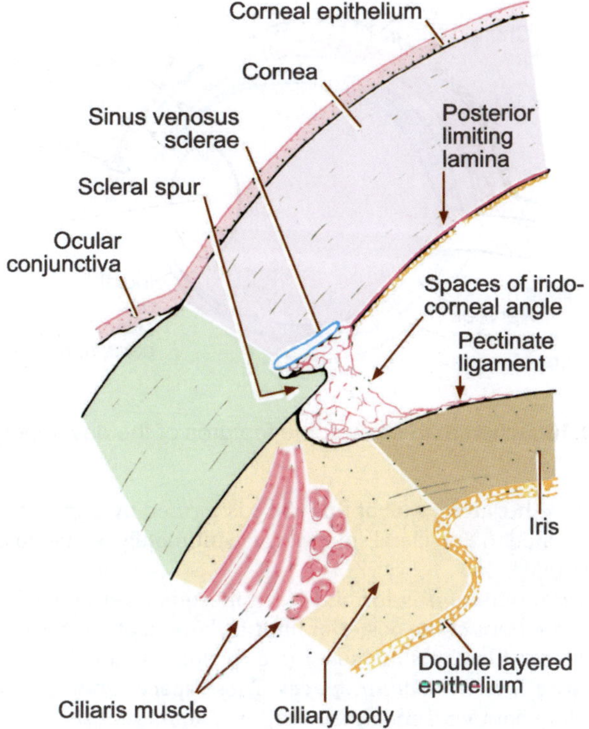

Fig. 60.15 Some features of the iridocorneal angle. Blood vessels in the ciliary body and iris are omitted.

ii. The ***dilator pupillae*** is in the form of muscle fibres that are arranged radially in the iris (Fig. 10.15). These fibres are intimately related to the anterior of the two layers of epithelium lining the posterior surface of the iris. Near the pupil these radial fibres merge with the sphincter pupillae.

Nerve Supply of the Sphincter and Dilator Pupillae

The sphincter pupillae has a parasympathetic nerve supply (similar to that of the ciliary muscle). Preganglionic neurons which are located in the Edinger Westphal nucleus (in the upper part of the midbrain) give off axons that pass through the oculomotor nerve and its branches to reach the ciliary ganglion. Postganglionic nerve fibres pass through the short ciliary nerves to reach the muscle.

The dilator pupillae is supplied by sympathetic nerves. The preganglionic neurons concerned are located in segment TI of the spinal cord. The postganglionic neurons lie in the superior cervical sympathetic ganglion.

THE IRIDOCORNEAL ANGLE

The angle between the peripheral margins of the iris and of the cornea is a region of importance. From Figs. 10.14 and 10.15 it will be seen that the most anterior part of the ciliary body appears in this angle. Laterally, the angle is related to the sinus

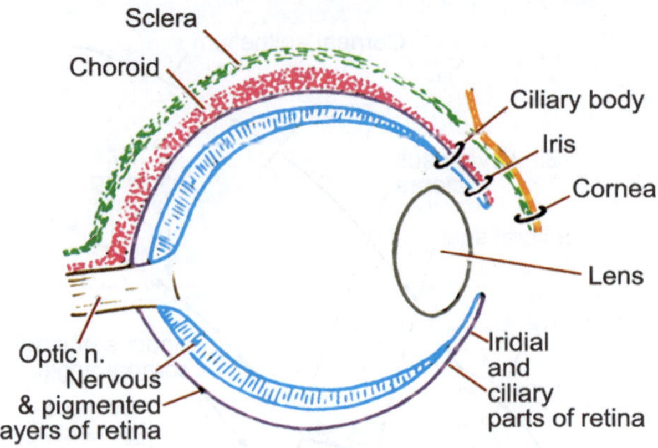

Fig. 10.16 Scheme to show some features of the developing eye.

venosus sclerae. The lateral wall of this sinus is formed by a groove in the sclera. Medially, it is related to the scleral spur. It is also intimately related to the pectinate ligament described below.

The ***pectinate ligament*** is formed by numerous interlacing filaments that represent continuations of the posterior limiting lamina of the cornea (Fig. 10.10), into the iris. These filaments are separated by spaces called the ***spaces of the iridocorneal angle***, or ***trabecular spaces***. These spaces communicate medially with the anterior chamber, and laterally with the sinus venosus sclerae. Aqueous humour secreted by the ciliary processes passes into the posterior chamber of the eye (i.e., the space between the posterior surface of the iris and the lens). It passes through the pupil into the anterior chamber. From here it filters through the spaces of the iridocorneal angle to enter the sinus venosus sclerae through which it is drained into the veins of the region. It will be easy to understand why the clinician often refers to the iridocorneal angle as the ***angle of filtration***. With advancing age these spaces may get blocked resulting in increased tension within the eyeball. This disease, called ***glaucoma,*** may have serious consequences.

THE RETINA

To understand the structure of the retina brief reference to its development is necessary. The retina develops as an outgrowth from the brain (diencephalon). The proximal part of the diverticulum remains narrow and is called the ***optic stalk***. It later becomes the optic nerve. The distal part of the diverticulum forms a rounded hollow structure called the ***optic vesicle***. This vesicle is invaginated by the developing lens (and other surrounding tissues) so that it gets converted into the two layered ***optic cup***. At first each layer of the cup is made up of a single layer of cells. The outer layer persists as a single layered epithelium which becomes pigmented and forms the ***pigment cell layer*** of the retina (Fig. 10.16). Over the greater part of the optic cup the cells of the inner layer multiply to form several layers of cells that become the ***nervous layer*** of the retina. The anterior limit of the region where this transformation takes place is later marked by the ora serrata. The part of the retina behind the ora serrata now consists of an outer pigmented layer, and an inner nervous layer. The two are separated by a cleft representing the original cavity of the optic cup. It is only

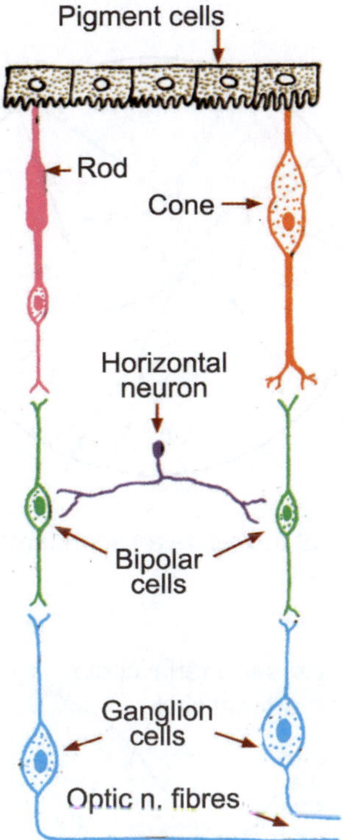

Fig. 10.17 Simplified scheme to show the main elements of the retina.

this part of the retina that is light sensitive and is referred to as the ***optical part*** of the retina, or the retina proper. Anterior to the ora serrata, both layers of the optic cup remain single layered. These two layers of epithelium line the inner surface of the ciliary body forming the ***ciliary part*** of the retina; and the posterior surface of the iris forming the ***iridial part*** of the retina. (For further details of development of the eyeball see the author's HUMAN EMBRYOLOGY).

The layer of pigment cells has greater adherence to the choroid than to the nervous layer of the retina. In some cases part of the retina may get detached from its normal position. In such detachment of the retina, it is only the nervous layer that gets detached, the pigment cells remaining attached to the choroid.

The essential features of the structure of the retina are shown in Fig. 10.17. It contains photoreceptors that convert the stimulus of light into nervous impulses. These receptors are of two kinds, ***rods*** and ***cones***. There are about seven million cones in each retina. The rods are far more numerous: they number more than 100 million. The cones respond best to bright light. They are responsible for sharp vision and for discrimination of colour.

Opposite the posterior pole of the eyeball the retina shows a ***central region*** about 6 mm in diameter. This region is responsible for sharp vision. In the centre of this region an area about 2 mm in diameter has a yellow colour and is called the ***macula lutea.*** The ***fovea centralis***, which is a depression in the centre of the macula is only 0.4 mm in diameter. Cones are most numerous in the central region. The fovea centralis is believed to contain cones only.

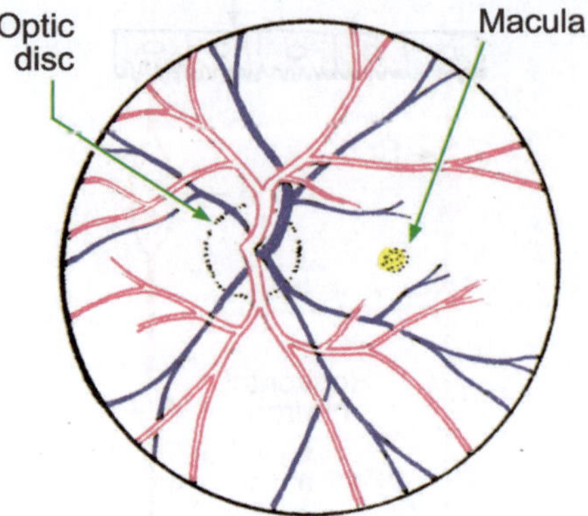

Fig. 10.18 Blood vessels of the retina as seen through an ophthalmoscope.

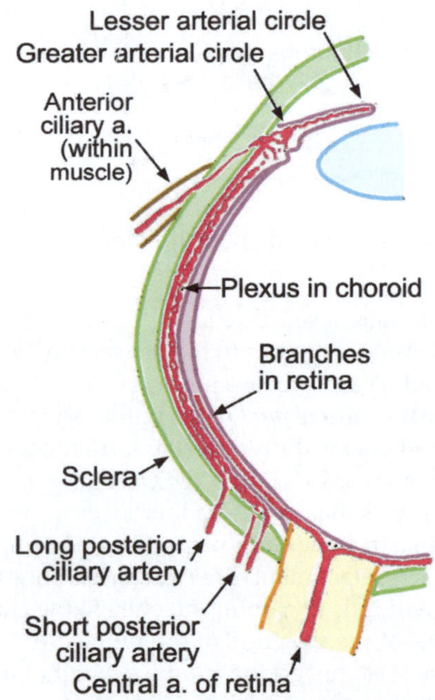

Fig. 10.19 Simplified scheme to show the arteries supplying the eyeball.

Rods can respond to poor light and specially to movement across the field of vision. They predominate in peripheral parts of the retina.

Each rod or cone can be regarded as a modified neuron. It consists of a cell body, a peripheral process and a central process. The cell body contains the nucleus. The peripheral process is rod-shaped in the case or rods, and cone-shaped in the case of cones (hence the names rods and cones). The ends of the peripheral processes are separated from one another by processes of pigment cells (Fig. 10.17). The central processes of rods and cones are like those of neurons: they end by synapsing with other neurons within the retina.

The basic neuronal arrangement within the retina is shown in Fig. 10.17. The central processes of rods and cones synapse with the peripheral processes of ***bipolar cells***. The central processes of bipolar cells synapse with dendrites of ***ganglion cells***. Axons arising from ganglion cells form the ***fibres of the optic nerve.*** The various elements mentioned above form a series of layers within the retina. The outermost layer (towards the choroid) is formed by the pigment cells, followed in sequence by the rods and cones, the bipolar cells, the ganglion cells, and a layer of optic nerve fibres. The layer of nerve fibres is apposed to the vitreous. It will be obvious that light has to pass through several layers of the retina to reach the rods and cones. At the fovea centralis the other layers are 'swept aside' to allow direct access of light to the cones here. For further details of the structure of the retina see the authors HUMAN HISTOLOGY.

We have seen that the optic nerve is attached to the eyeball a short distance medial to the posterior pole. The nerve fibres arising from the ganglion cells all over the retina converge to this region, where they pass through the lamina cribrosa to form the optic nerve. When viewed from the retinal side this region is seen as a circular area called the ***optic disc*** (Fig. 10.18). There are no photoreceptors here. The optic disc is, therefore, insensitive to light and is called the ***blind spot***. The optic disc is pierced, near its centre, by the central artery and vein of retina (see below).

THE LENS

We have seen that the lens lies in front of the vitreous body and behind the iris. It is surrounded by a capsule. It has convex anterior and posterior surfaces, and a peripheral margin (or equator) to which the suspensory ligament is attached. The anterior surface is less convex than the posterior surface. It comes into contact with the iris near the margin of the pupil. the posterior surface of the lens lies in a depression in the vitreous body called the ***hyaloid fossa***.

The lens has a maximum power of about 15 dioptres (A dioptre is the reciprocal of the focal length of a lens expressed in meters. A lens having a focal length of 1/2 meter has a power of 2 dioptres). However, the more important feature of the lens is its ability to alter its focal length (by action of the ciliary muscle). The range within which the power of the lens can be altered is greatest in children, and progressively decreases with age.

In connection with the dioptric power of the lens it may be noted that the cornea, the aqueous humour and the vitreous also have refractive power, and the total dioptric power of eye is as much as 58 dioptres. The greatest amount of refraction takes place at the surface of the cornea because of the great difference in refractive index of the cornea and that of air.

The Suspensory Ligament

The suspensory ligament of the lens is also called the ***zonule*** (Figs. 10.13, 10.14). We have seen that it is made up of fibres passing from the equator of the lens to the ciliary processes, and to the recesses between them.

The fibres of the ligament are said to be derived from the vitreous membrane which covers the vitreous body. Near the ciliary body the membrane extends into the spaces between the ciliary processes. This part of the membrane is called the ***ciliary zonule***. At the inner margin of the ciliary processes the membrane splits into anterior and posterior layers. The posterior layer which is very thin, lines the hyaloid fossa in which the lens lies. The anterior layer which is much thickened is made up fibres which form the suspensory ligament. The fibres of the ligament are separated from each other by ***zonular spaces.***

We have already seen that changes in the tension on the suspensory ligament, produced by contraction of the ciliary muscle, produce alterations in the convexity of the lens and enable it to focus objects at varying distances from the eye.

BLOOD VESSELS AND NERVES OF THE EYEBALL

The arteries supplying the retina are all branches of the ophthalmic artery.

The ***short ciliary arteries*** are several in number. They pierce the sclera near the lamina cribrosa (Fig. 10.9). They end in numerous branches that form a plexus in the choroid and supply it (Fig. 10.19). The capillary plexus in the choroid is also responsible for providing nutrition (by diffusion) to the outer part of the retina (i.e., the part nearer the choroid).

The long ciliary arteries are two in number (one medial and one lateral). They pierce the sclera a short distance to the corresponding side of the lamina cribrosa (Fig. 10.9). These arteries then run forward between the sclera and the choroid to reach the region of the ciliary body. Here each artery divides into one upper and one lower branch (Fig. 10.20). The upper branches of the medial and lateral sides anastomose with each other. Similarly the lower branches of the two sides anastomose to form the ***greater arterial circle*** at the periphery of the iris. This circle is joined by small anterior ciliary arteries that reach the region through the attachments of the rectus muscles to the eyeball. Branches pass radially into the iris from the greater circle, and join each other just round the pupil to form the ***lesser arterial circle***.

The veins draining the iris, the ciliary body and the choroid form a dense plexus deep to the sclera. The veins of this plexus converge on four or five ***venae vorticosae***. We have seen that these veins pierce the sclera a little behind the equator of the eyeball (Fig. 10.9) to end in the ophthalmic veins.

The main blood supply to the retina reaches it through the central artery of the retina. This artery runs forwards through the distal part of the optic nerve to enter the retina through the optic disc. It divides into upper and lower branches, each of which divides into medial (or nasal) and lateral (or temporal) branches. Further ramifications supply the entire retina. These arteries can be seen in the living subject by looking into the eye through the pupil using an instrument called an ophthalmoscope (Fig. 10.18). Branches of the central artery of the retina are end arteries i.e., they do not anastomose with each other. Blockage of any branch results in death of the part of the retina supplied by it, and to consequent loss of the part of the field of vision concerned. It may be noted that no large vessels are to be seen in the central region of the retina.

The blood from the retina is drained by tributaries that correspond to the branches of the central artery, but do not accompany them closely. These tributaries end in

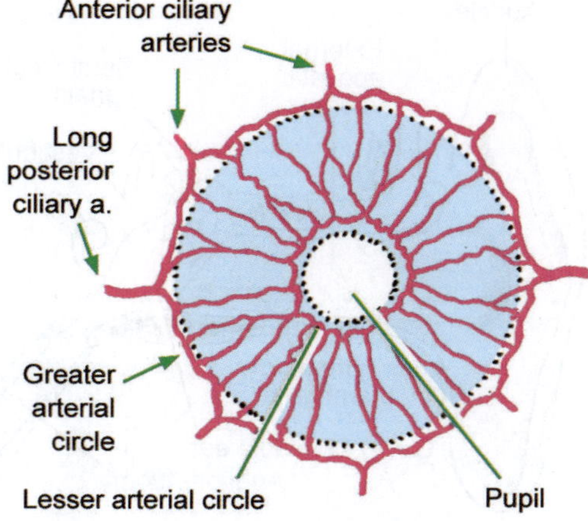

Fig. 10.20 Arteries of the iris.

two veins superior and inferior that pierce the lamina cribrosa and join each other to form the central vein of the retina.

The nerves (other than the optic nerve) that supply the eyeball are the long and short ciliary nerves . The long ciliary nerves are branches of the nasociliary nerve, while the short ciliary nerves arise from the ciliary ganglion. They enter the eyeball along with the corresponding arteries (Fig. 10.9). We have seen that the short ciliary nerves carry parasympathetic postganglionic fibres from the ciliary ganglion to the ciliary muscle and to the sphincter pupillae. They also carry sympathetic postganglionic fibres to blood vessels of the eyeball. Sympathetic postganglionic fibres meant for the dilator pupillae normally travel through the long ciliary nerves. Occasionally they may pass through the short ciliary nerves. In addition to autonomic efferents the long and short ciliary nerves carry sensory fibres from various structures in the eyeball including the ciliary body, the iris and the cornea.

Accessory Structures Related to The Eyeball

These are the extraocular muscles, the fascial sheath of the eyeball, the eyelids and conjunctiva; the lacrimal gland, and other parts of the lacrimal apparatus.

THE EAR AND SOME RELATED STRUCTURES

Preliminary Remarks About the Ear

Anatomically speaking, the ear is made up of three main parts called the ***external ear***, the ***middle ear*** and the ***internal ear***. The external ear and the middle ear are concerned exclusively with hearing. The internal ear has a ***cochlear part*** concerned with hearing; and a ***vestibular part*** which provides information to the brain regarding the position and movements of the head.

The main parts of the ear are shown in Fig. 10.21. The part of the ear that is seen on the surface of the body (i.e., the part that the lay person calls the

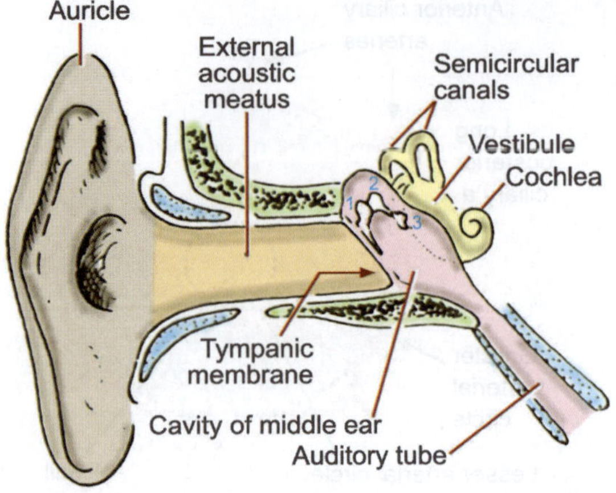

Fig. 10.21 Scheme to show the main parts of the ear. 1. Malleus; 2. Incus; 3. Stapes.

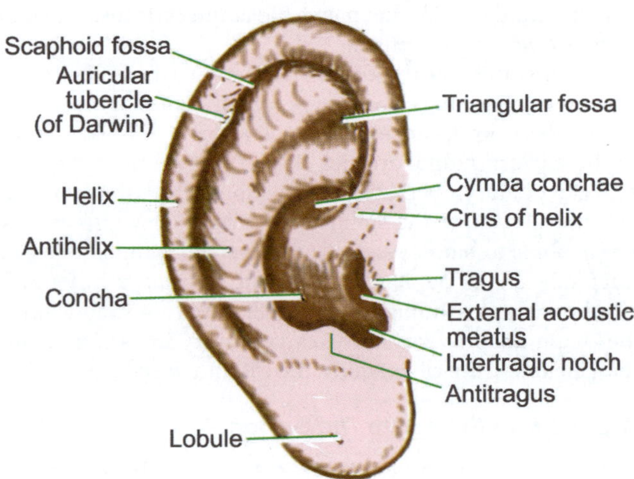

Fig. 10.22 Named features to be seen on the external aspect of the auricle.

ear) is anatomically speaking the ***auricle*** or ***pinna***. Leading inwards from the auricle there is a tube called the ***external acoustic meatus***. The auricle and external acoustic meatus together form the external ear. The inner end of the external acoustic meatus is closed by a thin membranous diaphragm called the ***tympanic membrane***. This membrane separates the external acoustic meatus from the middle ear.

The middle ear is a small space placed deep within the petrous part of the temporal bone. It is also called the ***tympanum*** (from which we get the adjective tympanic applied to structures connected with the middle ear). Medially the middle ear is closely related to parts of the internal ear. The cavity of the middle ear is continuous with that of the nasopharynx through a passage called the ***auditory tube***. Within the cavity of the middle ear there are three small bones that are collectively called the ***ossicles*** of the ear. The ossicles are called ***malleus*** (= like a hammer); the ***incus*** (= like an anvil, used by blacksmiths); and the ***stapes*** (= like a stirrup in which the foot of a horse rider fits). The three ossicles form a chain that is attached on one side to the tympanic membrane and at the other to a part of the internal ear.

The internal ear is in the form of a cavity within the petrous temporal bone having a very complex shape. This bony cavity (or ***bony labyrinth***) has a central part called the ***vestibule***. Continuous with the front of the vestibule there is a spiral shaped cavity, the bony ***cochlea***. Posteriorly, the vestibule is continuous with three ***semicircular canals***.

Sound waves travelling through air reach the ears. In many lower animals in which the auricle is large and mobile it may help in directing the sound waves into the external acoustic meatus. The auricle is of doubtful functional significance in man. Waves striking the tympanic membrane produce vibrations in it. These vibrations are transmitted through the chain of ossicles present in the middle ear to reach the internal ear. Specialised end organs in the cochlea act as transducers which convert the mechanical vibrations into nervous impulses. These impulses travel through the cochlear part of the vestibulocochlear nerve to reach the brain. Actual perception of sound takes place in the auditory (or acoustic) areas in the cerebral cortex.

We will now consider the different parts of the ear one by one. However, the descriptions that follow will be confined only to those facts that undergraduate students need to know.

THE AURICLE

The auricle is made up of a skeleton of elastic cartilage and fibrous tissue, which is covered on both sides by a layer of thin skin. The cartilage of the auricle is continuous with that of the external acoustic meatus. The auricle has an external surface facing laterally, and an inner or cranial surface that lies against the side of the head. The skin over the external surface is continuous with the skin lining the external acoustic meatus. Part of it passes forwards to become continuous with the skin over the parotid gland. The skin over the cranial surface passes backwards to become continuous with the skin lining the head behind the auricle. [These facts are emphasised because they help in understanding why the nerves and blood vessels that supply the cranial surface of the auricle reach it (mainly) from the back; and those supplying the external surface reach it from the front].

The cartilage of the auricle is curved on it self in a complicated manner so that a number of elevations and depressions are produced. Elevations on the external surface correspond to depressions on the cranial surface and vice versa. These elevations and depressions are given names that are shown in Fig. 10.22. In particular note that the lowest part of the auricle is soft. It does not contain cartilage and is composed only of a fold of skin with enclosed connective tissue. This part is called the ***lobule***. (It is through this part that perforations are made for wearing ear rings). At the centre of the external surface of the auricle there is a large depression called the ***concha***. Its anterior part is continued into the external acoustic meatus. On the cranial surface the position of the concha is marked by an elevation called the ***eminentia conchae***.

Auricular Muscles

A number of extrinsic auricular muscles pass from the skull to the auricle (Fig. 1.2). Some intrinsic muscles that are confined to the auricle are also present. In some lower animals, these muscles can move the auricle or can alter its shape to adapt it to receive sounds from a particular direction. In man the auricular muscles are to be regarded as vestigial structures of no importance. They, however, receive a nerve supply through branches of the facial nerve.

Blood Vessels, Lymphatics and Nerves of the Auricle

The auricle is supplied by the posterior auricular branch of the external carotid artery, the anterior auricular branch of the superficial temporal artery, and branches from the occipital artery (Fig. 8.11). The veins accompany the arteries.

The ***lymphatic drainage*** of the auricle is shown in Fig. 63.4.

The ***sensory nerves*** supplying the auricle are the auriculotemporal branch of the mandibular nerve; the great auricular nerve; and the auricular branch of the vagus nerve. The area supplied by each of these nerves is shown in Fig. 9.5.

EXTERNAL ACOUSTIC MEATUS

We have seen that the external acoustic meatus is a tube passing medially from the bottom of the concha of the auricle. It is closed medially by the tympanic membrane. The total length of the tube is approximately 24 mm. of this the wall of the outer 8 mm is cartilaginous, while that of the inner 16 mm is bony (Fig. 10.21).

The cartilage or bone is lined by a layer of thin skin which is continuous with that over the concha. The cartilage forming the wall of the outer part of the meatus is continuous with the cartilage of the auricle. The cartilage does not form a complete tube, but is deficient in its posterosuperior part (Fig. 10.23). Medially, the cartilage is firmly attached to the rough edge of the bony part of the tube. The wall of the bony part of the meatus is formed mainly by the tympanic plate of the temporal bone. The posterosuperior region of the wall is formed by the squamous part of the temporal bone (Fig. 10.24).

The medial end of the meatus is closed by the tympanic membrane. Here the bony wall is marked by a groove called the ***tympanic sulcus***. The tympanic membrane is placed obliquely both in the anteroposterior and vertical planes (Fig. 10.25). As a result the floor and anterior wall are longer than the roof and posterior wall. Further details of the tympanic membrane are considered with the middle ear.

The external acoustic meatus is not straight, but follows an S-shaped course. This is so because the cartilaginous part is not in line with the bony part, and is also bent on itself. The curves of the meatus are shown as seen from above in Fig. 10.25A, and as seen from behind in Fig. 10.25B. The cartilaginous part first

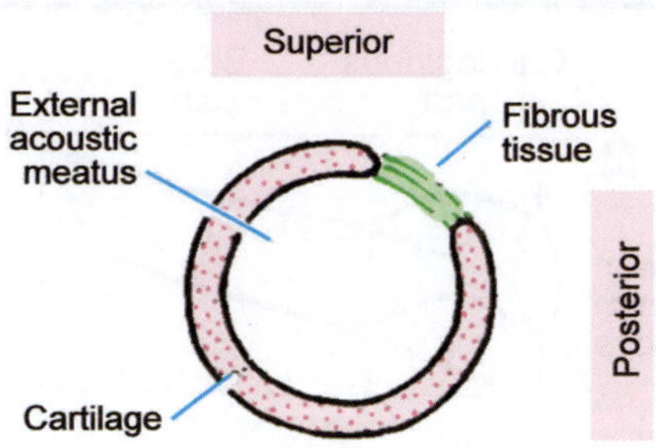

Fig. 10.23 Transverse section through the cartilage of the external acoustic meatus. Note the gap in the posterosuperior part. The gap is filled by fibrous tissue.

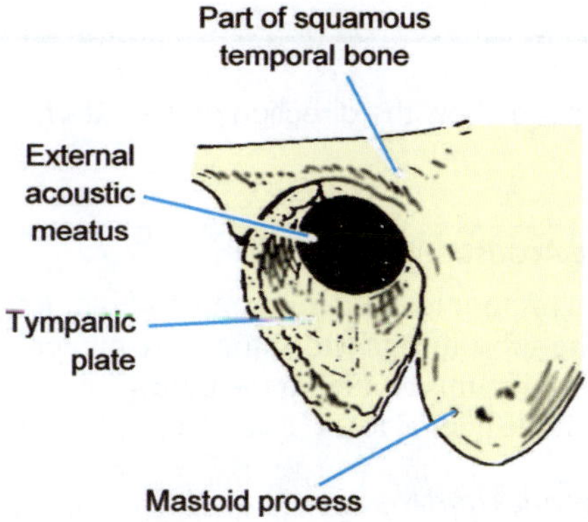

Fig. 10.24 Lateral end of the bony external acoustic meatus.

passes medially, forwards and upwards. It then passes medially, backwards and upwards. The bony part runs medially, forwards and downwards. In clinical examination of the meatus, and through it of the tympanic membrane, the auricle is pulled upwards, backwards and somewhat laterally. This renders the meatus straight (as shown in dotted lines in Figs. 10.25 A, B). It then has a uniform medial, forward and downward direction.

The meatus shows a narrowing at the junction of the cartilaginous and bony parts. It shows another narrowing called the ***isthmus*** about 4 mm from the tympanic membrane (i.e., 20 mm from the floor of the concha). The floor of the meatus shows a depression immediately lateral to the tympanic membrane. Foreign bodies entering the meatus can get stuck here.

The skin lining the external acoustic meatus contains numerous ***ceruminous glands***. These are modified sweat glands that produce the wax of the ear, or ***cerumen***.

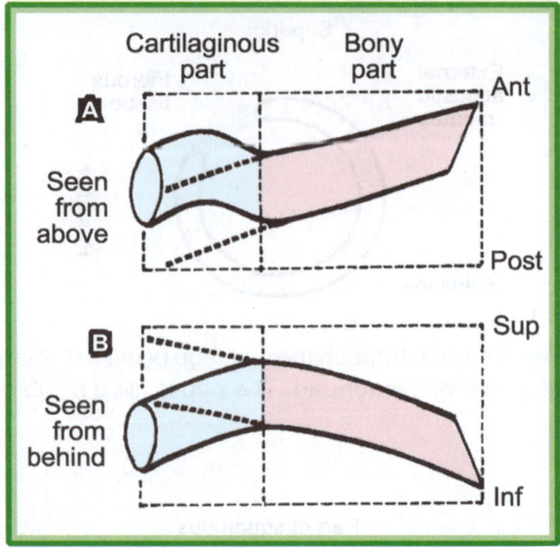

Fig. 10.25 Scheme to show the direction of the external acoustic meatus.

Relations of External Acoustic Meatus

The meatus is related in front to the temporomandibular joint, and behind to the mastoid process in the substance of which there are the mastoid air cells, and the mastoid antrum. Inferiorly, it is related to the parotid gland and superiorly (in its deeper part) to the middle cranial fossa (Figs. 1.4, 10.21, 10.24).

Blood Vessels, Lymphatics and Nerves

The external acoustic meatus is supplied by the posterior auricular branch of the external carotid artery, the auricular branches of the superficial temporal artery and by the deep auricular branch of the maxillary artery.

The veins of the meatus drain into the external jugular vein, the maxillary vein and veins of the pterygoid plexus.

The lymphatic drainage of the meatus is shown in Fig. 13.5.

The sensory nerve supply to the anterior wall and roof of the meatus is derived from the auriculotemporal nerve; and that to the posterior wall and floor from the auricular branch of the vagus nerve.

THE MIDDLE EAR

The middle ear is also called the ***tympanic cavity*** or ***tympanum*** (Fig. 10.21). It is a space lying in the petrous temporal bone. We have seen that the middle ear is separated from the external acoustic meatus by the tympanic membrane. From Fig. 10.21 it will be seen that part of the tympanic cavity lies above the level of the tympanic membrane: this part is called the ***epitympanic recess.*** We have also seen that three ossicles, the malleus, the incus and the stapes lie within the middle ear. The tympanic cavity communicates with the cavity of the nasopharynx through the ***auditory tube***. It also communicates with a large

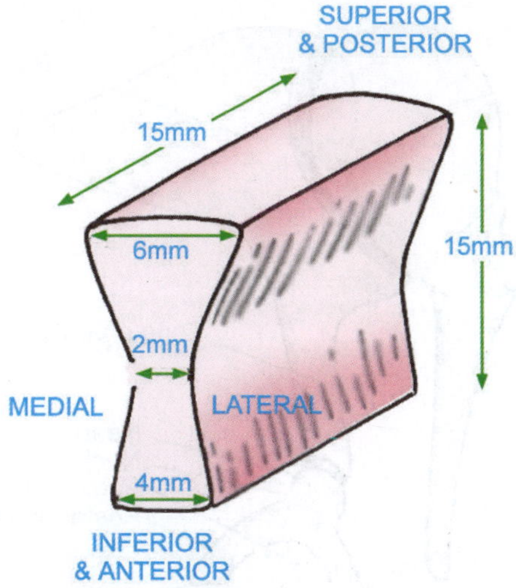

Fig. 10.26 Dimensions of the tympanic cavity.

space in the petrous part of the temporal bone, called the ***mastoid antrum;*** and with smaller spaces within the mastoid process called the ***mastoid air cells***. These spaces, the tympanic cavity itself, and the auditory tube are all lined by mucous membrane. Because of their communication with the nasopharynx these spaces are filled with air.

The tympanic cavity is shaped like a box (Fig. 10.26). It has six sides: a roof, a floor, and anterior, posterior, medial and lateral walls. The approximate dimensions of these walls are shown in Fig. 10.26. The anteroposterior and vertical diameters are each about 15 mm. The cavity is narrow from side to side. The distance between the medial and lateral wall is about 6 mm near the roof; about 4 mm near the floor; and only about 2 mm in the middle of the cavity.

OSSICLES OF THE EAR

In considering the walls of the middle ear reference has to be made to some features of the ossicles. The ossicles will, therefore, be considered first.

The Malleus:

The malleus is so called because it resembles a hammer (mallet = hammer) (Fig. 10.27). It has an upper rounded part called the ***head*** to which is attached a relatively long ***handle*** (or ***manubrium***). At the junction of the head with the handle there is a slight constriction called the ***neck***. Just below the neck the bone gives off two ***processes, anterior and lateral.***

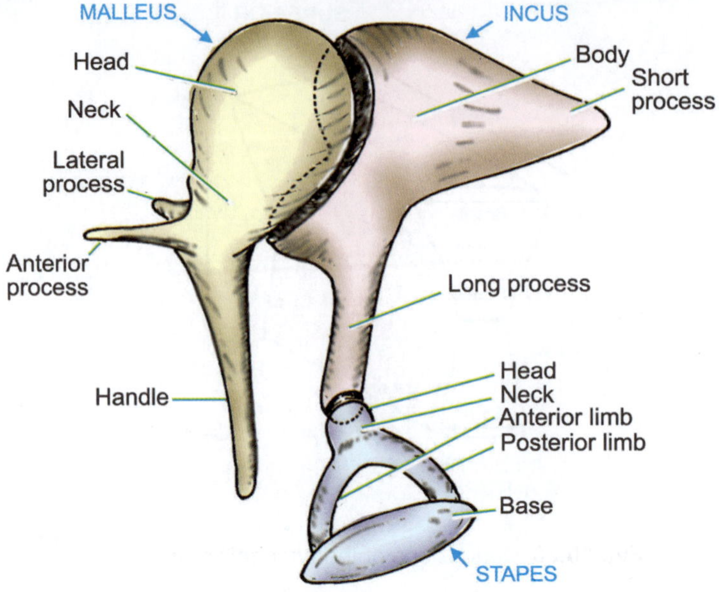

Fig. 10.27 Ossicles of the ear as seen from the medial side.

The Incus:

The incus (= anvil) has a main part or ***body*** and two ***processes, long and short***. The long process is directed downwards parallel to the handle of the malleus. The short process is directed backwards (Fig. 10.27).

The Stapes:

The stapes is shaped like a stirrup (Fig. 10.27). It has a ***head***, that is connected by two ***limbs***, or ***crura*** (anterior and posterior) to an oval plate called the ***base***. The constricted part adjoining the head is called the ***neck***.

Joints and Other Attachments of the Ossicles:

1. The handle of the malleus is intimately attached to the tympanic membrane (Fig. 10.28).
2. The posterior aspect of the head of the malleus, articulates with the anterior surface of the body of the incus. This incudo-malleolar joint is a saddle shaped synovial joint, surrounded by an articular capsule.
3. The lower end of the long process of the incus articulates with the head of the stapes to form the incudostapedial joint. This is a synovial joint of the ball and socket variety. It is surrounded by an articular capsule.
4. The base of the stapes is attached to the margins of an oval aperture (the fenestra vestibuli) in the medial wall of the middle ear, by the annular ligament.
5. The anterior process of the malleus is attached to the anterior wall of the tympanic cavity by the anterior ligament of the malleus (Fig. 10.32).

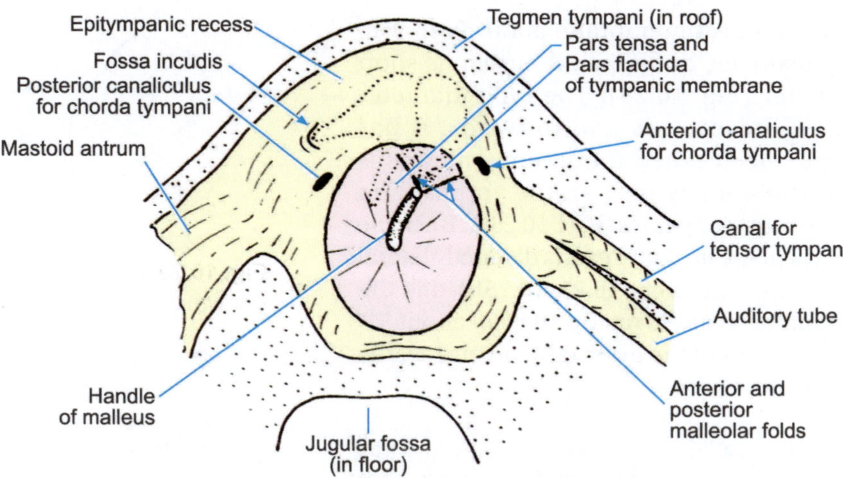

Fig. 10.28 Lateral wall of tympanic cavity. Parts of the roof, floor, anterior and posterior walls (adjoining the lateral wall) are also seen. The position of the upper part of the malleus, and of the incus is shown in dotted line.

6. The short process of the incus is attached to the posterior wall of the tympanic cavity by the posterior ligament of the incus (Fig. 10.32).
7. Finally, it may be noted that all the ossicles are covered by mucous membrane of the tympanic cavity which separates them from the lumen of the cavity.

Roof of the Middle Ear

The roof of the middle ear is formed by a plate of bone called the ***tegmen tympani***. (This plate forms the intracranial surface of the petrous temporal bone in the floor of the middle cranial fossa). The same plate of bone extends forwards to form the roof of the canal for the tensor tympani (see below), and backwards to form the roof of the mastoid antrum.

Floor of Middle Ear

The floor of the middle ear is formed by a thin plate of bone that separates it from the bulb of the internal jugular vein (Fig. 10.28).

Lateral Wall of Middle Ear

We have already seen that the greater part of the lateral wall of the middle ear is formed by the tympanic membrane. The part of the middle ear cavity lying above the level of the tympanic membrane is the epitympanic recess. The lateral wall of the epitympanic recess is formed by part of the temporal bone (Fig. 10.28).

The Tympanic Membrane:

This is an oval membrane about 9 mm in long diameter, and about 8 mm in its short diameter (Fig. 10.29). The long diameter passes downwards and forwards. It has already been noted that the membrane is placed obliquely both in the vertical and anteroposterior planes (Figs. 10.25 A, B). In the vertical plane its upper end is distinctly lateral to its lower end (Figs. 10.21, 10.25B), and the membrane forms an acute angle of about 55° with the floor of the external acoustic meatus (Fig. 10.30).

Fig. 10.29 Dimensions of the tympanic membrane.

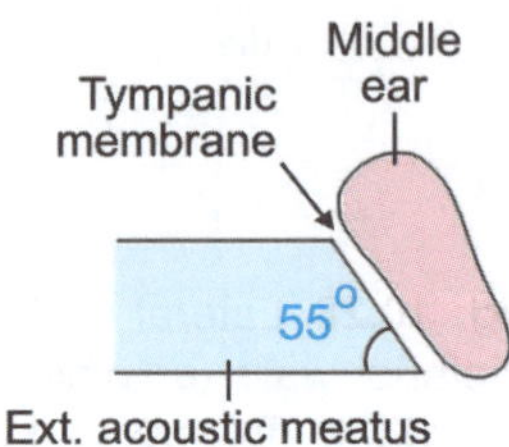

Fig. 10.30 Angle between the tympanic membrane and the floor of the external acoustic meatus.

Structurally, the tympanic membrane has three layers. The outer layer is continuous with the skin lining the external acoustic meatus. The inner layer is formed by the mucous membrane of the tympanic cavity. Between these two there is a layer of fibrous tissue. Some of the fibres in this tissue are arranged radially and some circularly (Fig. 10.31).

With the exception of a small area in its anterosuperior part, the circumference of the tympanic membrane is thickened because of the presence here of fibrocartilage. This ring of fibrocartilage fits into a groove, the ***tympanic sulcus***, present at the medial end of the external acoustic meatus (Fig. 10.31).

From Figs. 10.28 and 10.31 it will be seen that the handle of the malleus is closely attached to the medial side of the tympanic membrane. Its lower end lies approximately at the centre of the membrane. From here the handle passes upwards and forwards ending a little short of the circumference of the membrane. The lateral process of the malleus projects towards the membrane at this point. From Fig. 10.28 it will also be seen that a small area of the tympanic membrane, located in its anterosuperior region, is separated from the rest of the membrane by two small folds. This part of the membrane is not stretched like the rest of it; and is, therefore, called the ***pars flaccida***. In contrast the rest of the membrane is called the ***pars tensa***. The folds separating the pars flaccida from the pars tensa are called the ***anterior and posterior malleolar folds***. They pass from the lateral process of the malleus to the circumference of the tympanic membrane. It may be noted here that the part of the circumference of the tympanic membrane, formed by the pars flaccida is not thickened by fibrocartilage. Here the tympanic sulcus is replaced by a notch. In Fig. 10.31 note that on the whole the tympanic membrane is convex medially. The point

Fig. 10.31 Layers of the tympanic membrane.

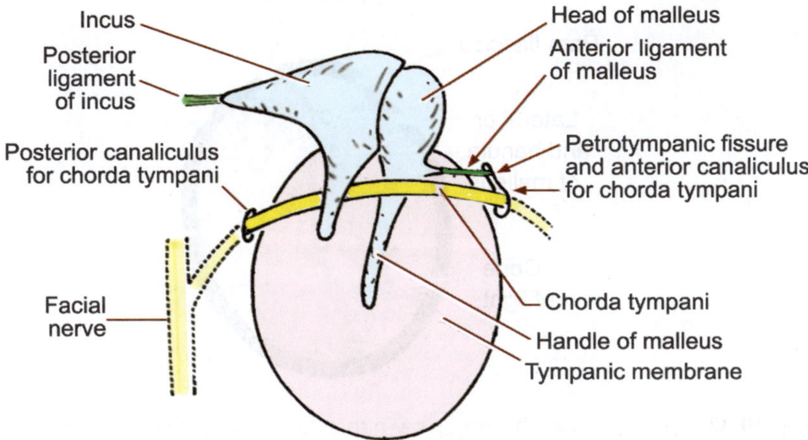

Fig. 10.32 Relationship of the chorda tympani to the lateral wall of the middle ear.

of greatest convexity corresponds to the lower end of the handle of the malleus and is called the ***umbo***. However, in passing from the umbo to the tympanic sulcus the layers of the membrane show a slight convexity outwards.

Relationship of Chorda Tympani to Lateral Wall:

The chorda tympani nerve has an intimate relationship to the tympanic membrane. To understand the relationship note the following points.

a. Just posterior to the upper part of the tympanic membrane there is a small aperture in the angle between the lateral and posterior walls of the middle ear. This aperture is called the ***posterior canaliculus*** for the chorda tympani (Fig. 10.28).
b. Just anterior to the upper part of the tympanic membrane there is a transverse slit (in the angle between the anterior and lateral walls of the middle ear). This slit is called the ***petrotympanic fissure*** (Fig. 10.32). At the medial end of this fissure there is an opening called the ***anterior canaliculus*** for the chorda tympani. In Fig. 10.32 note that the anterior ligament of the malleus passes into the petrotympanic fissure.
c. From Fig. 10.31 note that the handle of the malleus is actually embedded within the tympanic membrane and lies between the fibrous and mucosal layers.

The chorda tympani, which arises from the facial nerve within the substance of the temporal bone, enters the middle ear through the posterior canaliculus (Fig. 10.32). It passes forwards through the substance of the upper part of the tympanic membrane, lying between the fibrous and mucosal layers. As it does so it crosses medial to the handle of the malleus, near the upper end of the latter. The chorda tympani leaves the middle ear by passing through the anterior canaliculus to reach the infratemporal fossa.

Tympanic Membrane as Seen Through the External Acoustic Meatus:

Many of the features of the tympanic membrane described in the preceding paragraphs can be seen in the living through the external acoustic meatus (Fig.

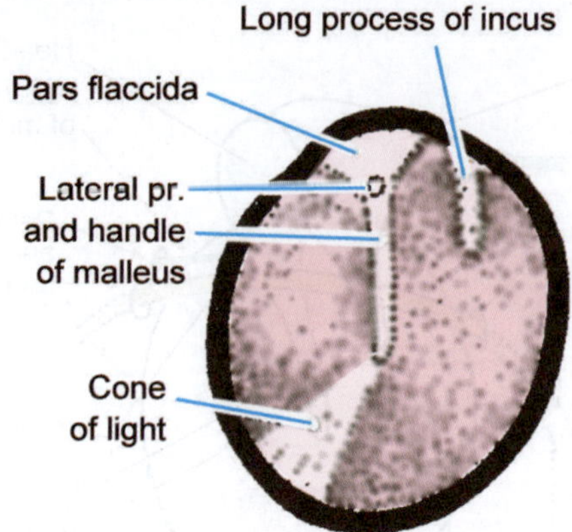

Fig. 10.33 Tympanic membrane as seen through the external acoustic meatus.

10.33). The pars flaccida can be seen in the anterosuperior corner of the membrane, and the anterior and posterior malleolar folds can also be distinguished. The lateral process of the malleus can be seen as a white dot where these folds meet. Running downwards and backwards from this dot to the centre of the membrane there is the handle of the malleus. A little behind and parallel to the upper part of the handle of the malleus the long process of the incus may be visible as a faint white streak.

The anteroinferior part of the membrane (between the lower end of the handle of the malleus and the circumference of the membrane) reflects light more than the rest of the membrane and is referred to as the ***cone of light***.

It is sometimes necessary to incise the tympanic membrane to let out pus from the middle ear. Such an incision is always made in the lower part to avoid damage to the chorda tympani. Another advantage of such an incision is that the lower part of the membrane is less vascular.

Blood Vessels and Nerves of Tympanic Membrane:

The blood vessels and nerves to the external surface of the tympanic membrane are derived from those supplying the external acoustic meatus. Those to its internal surface are derived from vessels and nerves that supply the middle ear.

The external surface is supplied by the deep auricular branch of the maxillary artery, and drains into the external jugular vein. It is supplied by the auriculotemporal nerve, and the auricular branch of the vagus (Compare with external acoustic meatus).

The internal surface of the tympanic membrane is supplied by the tympanic branches of the maxillary artery; and by the stylomastoid branch which arises either from the posterior auricular artery or from the occipital artery. The nerves to the internal surface are derived from the tympanic branch of the glossopharyngeal nerve.

Anterior Wall of Middle Ear

We have noted that the medial and lateral walls of the middle ear are fairly close to each other. It follows that the anterior and posterior walls are narrow.

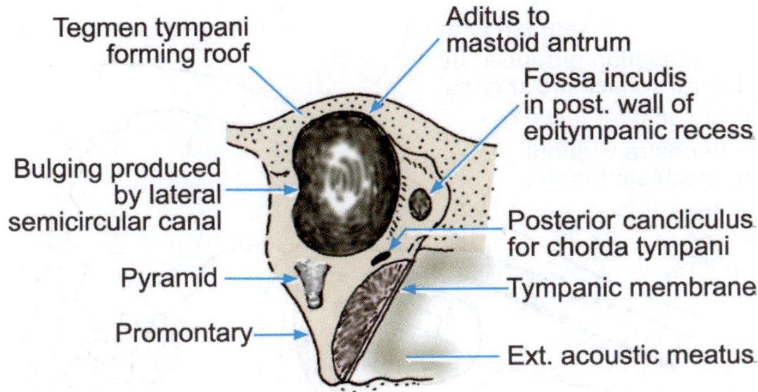

Fig. 10.34 Features to be seen on the posterior wall of the middle ear.

The various structures to be seen on the anterior wall are shown in Fig. 10.28. In the upper part of the wall there are two openings. The upper opening leads into a canal in which the tensor tympani muscle lies. The lower opening is that of the auditory tube.

The two openings are separated by a thin bony septum. This septum extends onto the medial wall of the middle ear where it curves on itself to form a pulley ***(processus trochleariformis)*** around which the tendon of the tensor tympani winds (to change from a backward direction to a lateral one) (See Figs. 10.35, 10.36). Below the opening for the auditory tube the anterior wall of the middle ear is formed by a plate of bone which separates the middle ear from the carotid canal (through which the internal carotid artery passes). Minute apertures in this plate give passage to branches from the internal carotid artery to the middle ear; and also to ***caroticotympanic nerves*** which arise from the sympathetic plexus surrounding the artery to reach the middle ear.

The petrotympanic fissure and the canaliculus for the chorda tympani (already described) lie in the angle between the anterior and lateral walls of the middle ear.

Posterior Wall of Middle Ear

The features to be seen on the posterior wall of the middle ear are shown in Fig. 10.34. The upper part of the wall is relatively broad. It shows a large round aperture through which the middle ear communicates with the mastoid antrum. This aperture is called the ***aditus to the mastoid antrum***. On the medial wall of the aditus there is a bulging produced by the lateral semicircular canal.

Anterior to the aditus there is the posterior wall of the epitympanic recess. On it we see a depression, the ***fossa incudis***. The tip of the short process of the incus extends into this depression; and is attached to the fossa by fibres of the posterior ligament of the incus. The aditus to the mastoid antrum and the fossa incudis are also seen in Fig. 10.28.

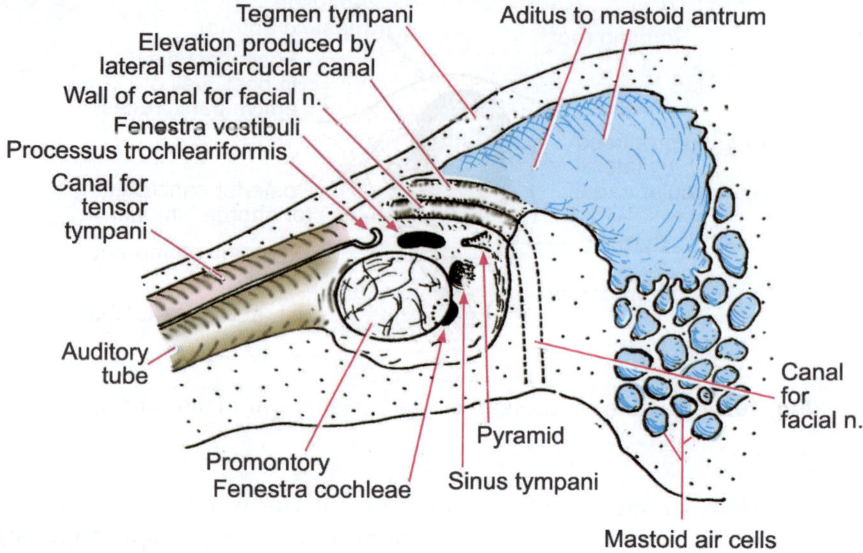

Fig. 10.35 Medial wall of middle ear. Parts of the anterior and posterior walls, and of the mastoid antrum and mastoid air cells, are also seen. Compare with Fig. 10.34.

Inferior to the aditus, the medial end of the posterior wall of the middle ear bears a conical elevation called the ***pyramid***. The tip of the pyramid projects forwards, and has an opening which leads into a canal in which the stapedius muscle is lodged. The tendon of the stapedius emerges from the opening at the tip of the pyramid and runs forwards to be inserted into the posterior surface of the neck of the stapes (Fig. 9.64).

The facial nerve is closely related to the internal ear and to the medial and posterior walls of the middle ear. Part of it runs vertically downwards in a bony canal placed along the junction of the medial and posterior walls (See Fig. 9.60).

Medial Wall of Middle Ear

The medial wall of the middle ear is also the lateral wall of the internal ear. It can be properly understood only after examining some features of the internal ear as follows:

We have noted that the bony internal ear consists of a central part called the vestibule, which is connected anteriorly to the cochlea, and posteriorly to three semicircular canals. Some further details should be noted by examining Fig. 10.43 in which the internal ear is seen from the lateral side. Note that the cochlea is in the form of a spiral and that its 'turns' are narrow in the centre and become wider as we proceed outwards. The lowest (or basal) turn of the cochlea is large and is continuous posteriorly with the vestibule. If we look into the interior of the basal turn of the cochlea (Fig. 10.45) we find that its cavity consists of two parts, upper and lower. The upper part, which is called the ***scala vestibuli***, becomes continuous with the cavity of the vestibule. [The vestibule communicates with the middle ear through a large oval aperture called the ***fenestra vestibuli***. Thus the scala vestibuli is in indirect communication with the middle ear]. The lower part of the cavity of the cochlea (or ***scala tympani***) opens independently into the middle ear through a round opening called the ***fenestra cochleae***. This fenestra is situated inferior to the vestibule. Also note in Fig. 10.43 that the three semicircular canals are named anterior, posterior and lateral. Note further that the lateral canal bulges in a lateral direction and is, therefore, closest to the middle ear.

With this brief introduction we can now proceed to study the features to be seen on the medial wall of the middle ear as shown in Fig. 10.35. In the anterior and posterior parts of this figure we see some features of the anterior and posterior walls of the middle ear already described. Anteriorly, identify the canal for the tensor tympani, and below it the auditory tube. In particular note that the septum between these tubes reaches the medial wall and curves on itself to form the processus trochleariformis (or cochleariformis). Posteriorly, note the aditus to the tympanic antrum and below it the pyramid. Also note that superiorly the medial wall meets the roof, formed by the tegmen tympani; and inferiorly it meets the floor.

The most prominent feature to be seen on the medial wall is the ***promontory***. This is a large circular bulging produced by the basal turn of the cochlea. Its surface bears a number of grooves. The apex of the cochlea comes in contact with the medial wall of the middle ear just in front of the promontory.

Posterosuperior to the promontory we see the ***fenestra vestibuli*** which is also called the ***oval window***. Note its shape in Fig. 10.35. We have seen that the base of the stapes fits into this opening and is attached to its margins by the annular ligament. Posteroinferior to the promontory there is a round aperture called the ***fenestra cochleae*** (also called the ***round window***). This aperture is only partially seen (or not seen at all) because it is overlapped by the lower edge of the promontory which overhangs it. We have seen that this opening is continuous with part of the cavity of the cochlea. It is closed by the ***secondary tympanic membrane***. Posterior to the promontory there is a depression called the ***sinus tympani***, which lies between the fenestra vestibuli and the fenestra cochleae. A part of the posterior semicircular canal (ampulla) lies deep to the sinus tympani.

The part of the medial wall above the promontory, and the fenestra vestibuli, is marked by two rounded ridges that run anteroposteriorly. The upper of these is produced by the lateral semicircular canal. The lower ridge is the wall of a canal through which the facial nerve runs backwards. Only a thin layer of bone separates the nerve from the cavity of the middle ear. Occasionally, this bone may be missing and the nerve may lie just under the mucosa. Running backwards across the medial wall of the middle ear the facial canal reaches the aditus to the mastoid antrum. Here it bends downwards and runs through bone just behind the angle between the medial and posterior walls of the middle ear to reach the stylomastoid foramen (See Fig. 9.60).

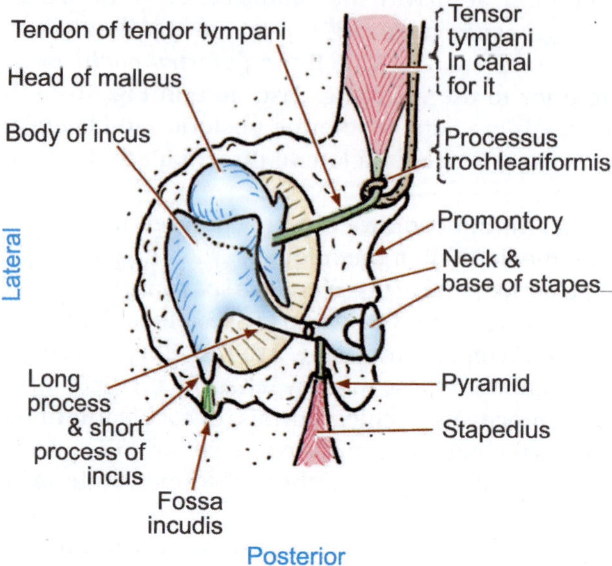

Fig. 10.36 Scheme to show the muscles of the middle ear. They are viewed from above after removing the roof of the middle ear.

Muscles of the Middle Ear

These are the stapedius and the tensor tympani.

The ***stapedius*** is a small muscle lying in a bony canal that is related to the posterior wall of the middle ear. Posteriorly and below, this canal is continuous with the vertical part of the canal for the facial nerve. Anteriorly, the canal opens into the middle ear at the apex of the pyramid.

The fibres of the stapedius arise from the walls of this canal. They end in a tendon which enters the middle ear through the pyramid and runs forwards to be inserted into the posterior surface of the neck of the stapes. The muscle is supplied by a branch from the facial nerve (Figs. 9.64, 10.36).

The ***tensor tympani*** lies in a canal that opens into the anterior wall of the middle ear. At its other end this canal opens on the base of the skull (in the interval between the anterior margin of the petrous temporal bone, and the posterior margin of the greater wing of sphenoid). Muscle fibres arise from the wall of this canal. Some fibres arise from the cartilaginous part of the auditory tube and some from the base of the skull formed here by the greater wing of the sphenoid. The muscle ends in a tendon which reaches the middle ear cavity near its medial wall. Here it bends sharply to the lateral side by passing around the processus trochleariformis. It is inserted into the upper end of the handle of the malleus.

Both the tensor tympani and the stapedius protect the ear against very loud sounds by restricting the vibrations of the tympanic membrane and the ossicles. Paralysis of the muscles (specially of the stapedius) gives rise to a condition called ***hyperacusis*** in which even normal sounds appear too loud.

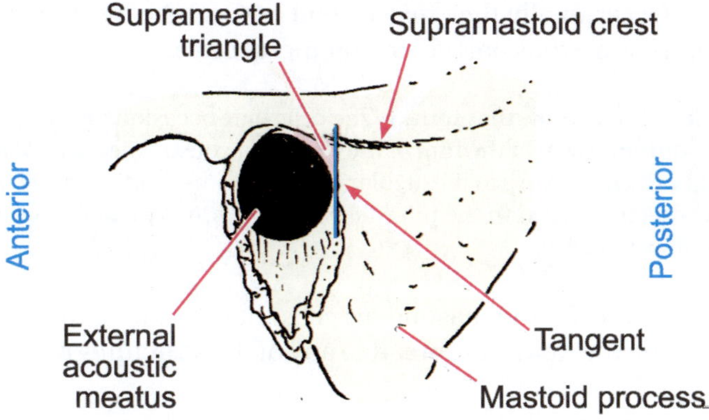

Fig. 10.37 Boundaries of the suprameatal triangle.

The Mastoid Antrum

The mastoid antrum is of considerable importance as it is a frequent site of infection, which may be difficult to eradicate. Furthermore, infection may spread from it to neighbouring structures with serious consequences.

Although it is called the 'mastoid' antrum this space lies in the ***petrous*** part of the temporal bone. Anteriorly the antrum opens, through its aditus, into the epitympanic recess. We have seen that the medial side of the aditus is related to the lateral semicircular canal (Figs. 10.34, 10.35).

The following additional relationships are obvious from Fig. 10.35. Superiorly, the roof of the antrum is formed by the tegmen tympani which separates it from the middle cranial fossa; and from the temporal lobe of the cerebral hemisphere. Inferiorly, the mastoid antrum is continuous with the mastoid air cells (see below). Anteriorly, below the aditus, the antrum is related to the facial nerve as it descends within its bony canal. Posteriorly, the antrum is close to the posterior surface of the temporal bone (i.e., to the posterior cranial fossa) and here it may be separated only by a thin plate of bone from the sigmoid sinus. Medially, behind the aditus, the antrum is related to the posterior semicircular canal. The lateral wall of the mastoid antrum is related to the suprameatal triangle (Fig. 10.37). This triangle is bounded above by the supramastoid crest; antero-inferiorly by the posterosuperior margin of the (bony) external acoustic meatus; and posteriorly by a vertical line drawn as a tangent to the posterior margin of the meatus. The thickness of bone separating the mastoid antrum from the surface of the skull is only about 2 mm at birth, but it increases by about 1 mm for every year of age until it is about 13 to 14 mm thick. (In other words it attains its full thickness by puberty).

The Mastoid Air Cells

These are a series of intercommunicating spaces of variable size present within the mastoid process. They communicate above with the mastoid antrum. Their number varies considerably. Sometimes there are just a few, and are confined to the upper part of the mastoid process. In other case they may extend throughout the process. Occasionally they may extend beyond the mastoid process into the squamous or petrous parts of the temporal bone.

It is of interest to know that some of the cells may occasionally lie (1) very close to the sigmoid sinus; (2) in the roof of the external acoustic meatus; (3) in the floor of the tympanic cavity close to the jugular bulb; (4) in the medial part of the petrous temporal bone in relation to the internal ear, the carotid canal, the auditory tube, and the abducent nerve.

Infection can reach the mastoid air cells though the tympanic cavity and the mastoid antrum, and can spread to any of the structures related to them.

The Auditory Tube

The auditory tube is also called the ***pharyngotympanic tube***, or the ***Eustachian tube***. It provides a communication between the nasopharynx and the middle ear (Fig. 10.21). Because of this communication air passes into the tympanic cavity (and into the mastoid antrum and air cells). As a result, air pressure on both sides of the tympanic membrane is the same: this is important for proper vibration of the tympanic membrane. However, the auditory tube is not patent all the time. It opens during deglutition, or even during the swallowing of saliva. When we suddenly ascend to a higher altitude (as in going up a hill in a car) the air pressure on the outside of the tympanic membrane falls, but that on its inner side remains the same as before. This inequality in pressure gives rise to a change in the quality of sound perceived. However, on swallowing of saliva, and the consequent equalisation of pressure, the sound suddenly returns to normal. The same phenomenon takes place much more acutely during the take off of an aircraft, and can give rise to distress in the ear; more so in persons who have a mild infection. [The sweets handed out by air hostesses just before take off are meant to keep passengers swallowing so that discomfort is avoided or lessened].

The communication between the pharynx and the middle ear is also a path along which infection frequently reaches the middle ear. This occurs more commonly in children, in whom the auditory tube is shorter and wider than in the adult. In the presence of infection the tube is easily blocked. When this happens air within the tympanic cavity is gradually absorbed and pressure on the outside of the tympanic membrane becomes greater than on the inside. This can give rise to discomfort which can be relieved by introducing air into the auditory tube through a catheter. If obstruction to the auditory tube is prolonged pus can accumulate in middle ear resulting in severe pain. The pus may burst through the tympanic membrane leading to discharge from the ear, and to the formation of a perforation in the membrane. It is for these reasons that the anatomy of the auditory tube is of much practical importance.

The auditory tube is about 36 mm long. It consists of an outer bony part, which is about 12 mm long; and of an inner cartilaginous part which is about 24 mm long. Both these parts are directed downwards, forwards and medially (Fig. 10.38). The lateral end of the bony part opens on the anterior wall of the middle ear (Figs. 10.28, 10.35). The medial end of the bony part opens on the base of the skull (at the lateral

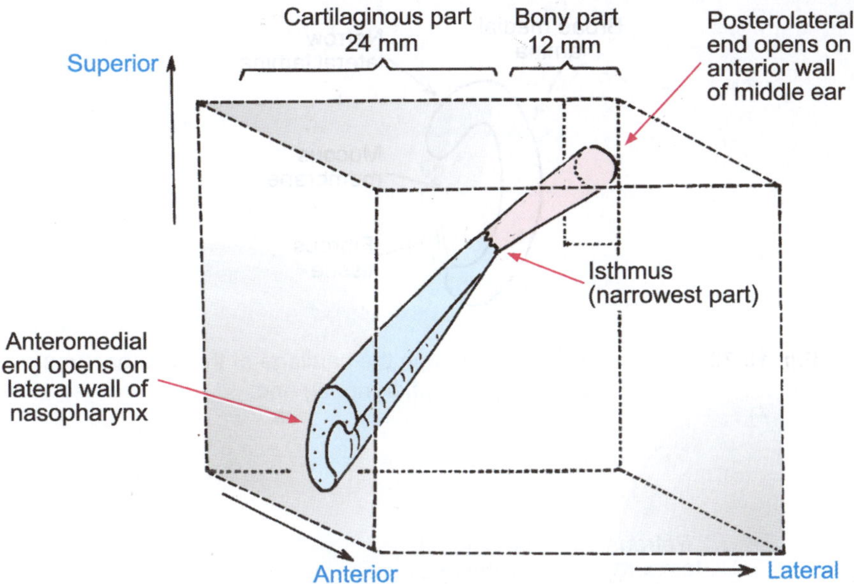

Fig. 10.38 Scheme to show the direction of the bony and cartilaginous parts of the auditory tube.

end of the groove between the anterior margin of the petrous temporal bone and the posterior margin of the greater wing of the sphenoid bone). The cartilaginous part extends from the medial end of the bony part to the lateral wall of the nasopharynx. The auditory tube is narrowest at the junction of the bony and cartilaginous parts: this part is called the ***isthmus***.

The cartilage forming the wall of the auditory tube is not tubular, but consists of a triangular plate that is bent on itself. Its lateral end (which joins the bony part) is narrow (Fig. 10.38). Its medial end is broad and lies just under the mucous membrane of the lateral wall of the nasopharynx where it forms the tubal elevation (Fig. 1.18). The cartilage consists of a larger medial lamina (facing backwards and medially) and of a smaller lateral lamina (facing forwards and laterally). There is a gap in the cartilage in the inferolateral wall of the tube. This gap is filled by fibrous tissue.

The cartilaginous part of the auditory tube lies in close relation to the base of the skull in the groove between the anterior margin of the petrous temporal bone and the posterior margin of the greater wing of the sphenoid bone. The interior of the auditory tube is lined by mucous membrane continuous with that of the nasopharynx and of the middle ear.

The cartilaginous part of the auditory tube lies in close relationship to the roof of the infratemporal fossa (Fig. 10.40). The tensor palati muscle lies immediately to its lateral side, and the levator palati lies immediately medial to it. Both the muscles partially arise from the wall of the tube. The part of the tensor palati arising from the tube is believed to be responsible for opening the auditory tube during swallowing. It is, therefore, called the ***dilator tubae***. The salpingopharyngeus (Fig. 10.40) takes origin from the lower part of the tube near its medial end. The tensor palati separates the tube from several structures in the infratemporal fossa including the mandibular nerve, the chorda tympani, the middle meningeal artery and the otic ganglion.

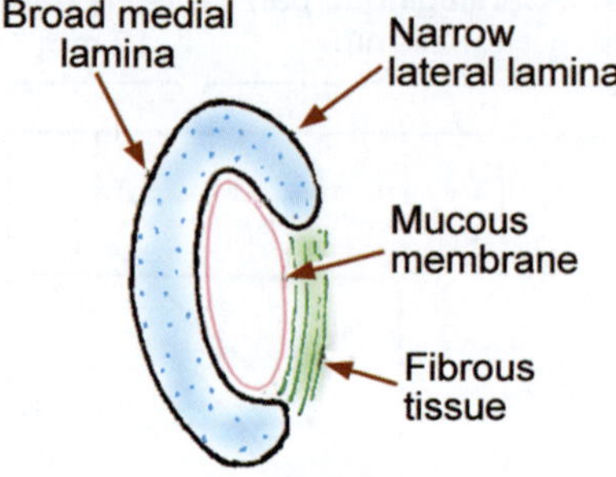

Fig. 10.39 Transverse section through the cartilage of the auditory tube, near its medial (pharyngeal) end.

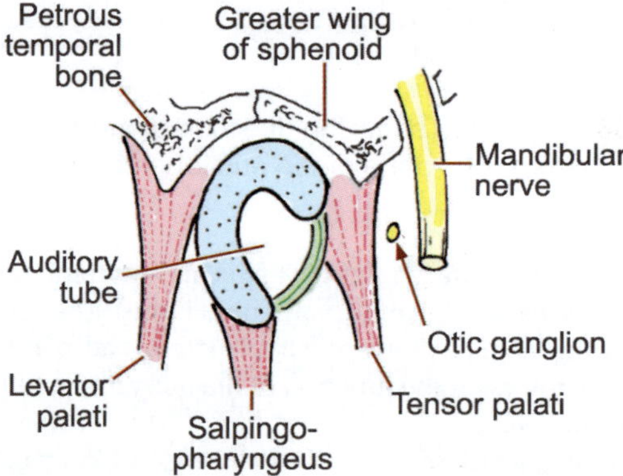

Fig. 10.40 Some relations of the cartilaginous part of the auditory tube.

Blood Vessels, Lymphatics and Nerves of Middle Ear:

The middle ear receives several small branches that arise from arteries that lie in its neighbourhood. These are shown in Fig. 10.41. The veins of the middle ear drain downward (along the auditory tube) towards the infratemporal fossa where they end in the pterygoid plexus. Some veins drain through apertures in the petrous temporal bone to end in the superior petrosal sinus.

The lymphatics from the middle ear and the mastoid air cells end in the parotid lymph nodes while those from the auditory tube reach the deep cervical nodes.

The nerves supplying the mucous membrane of the middle ear, the mastoid antrum and air cells and the auditory tube are derived from the tympanic plexus which lies over the promontory. It is formed mainly by the tympanic branch of the glossopharyngeal nerve. It also receives some fibres from the sympathetic plexus around the internal carotid artery (caroticotympanic nerves). The tympanic plexus gives off the lesser petrosal nerve, which ends in the otic ganglion.

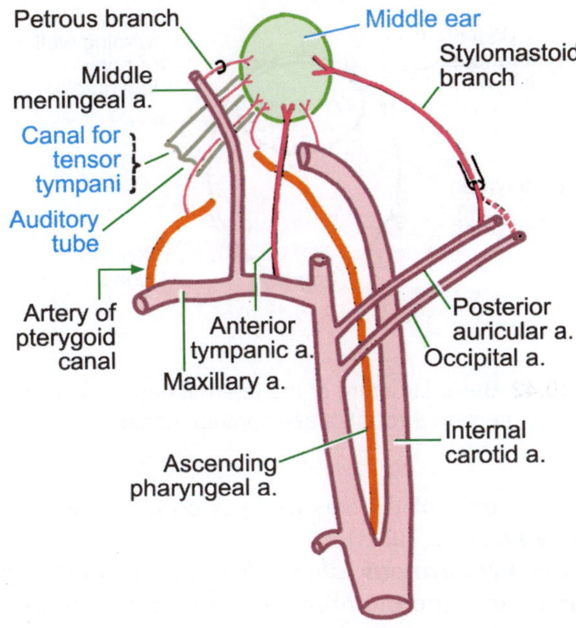

Fig. 10.41 Scheme to show the arteries supplying the middle ear.

THE INTERNAL EAR

Preliminary Remarks

We have seen that the internal ear is in the form of a complex system of cavities within the petrous temporal bone. Because of the complex shape of these intercommunicating cavities the internal ear is referred to as the ***labyrinth***.

The basic arrangement of the labyrinth is best understood by looking at a transverse section through a relatively simple part of it like a semicircular canal (Fig. 10.42). The wall of the ***bony labyrinth*** is made up of dense bone. Its inner surface is lined by periosteum. Lying within the bony labyrinth there is a system of ducts which constitute the ***membranous labyrinth***. The space within the membranous labyrinth is filled by a fluid called the ***endolymph.*** The space between the membranous labyrinth and the bony labyrinth is filled by another fluid called the ***perilymph.***

The ***parts of the bony labyrinth*** are shown in Fig. 10.43. These are as follows.

a. In the central part of the bony labyrinth there is a cavity called the ***vestibule***.
b. Anterior to the vestibule we see the ***bony cochlea***. The cavity of the bony cochlea is divided into two parts. One part, called the ***scala vestibuli*** (Fig. 10.45), is continuous posteriorly with the cavity of the vestibule. The second part is called the ***scala tympani***. The scala tympani opens into the middle ear at the fenestra cochleae (Fig. 10.45).

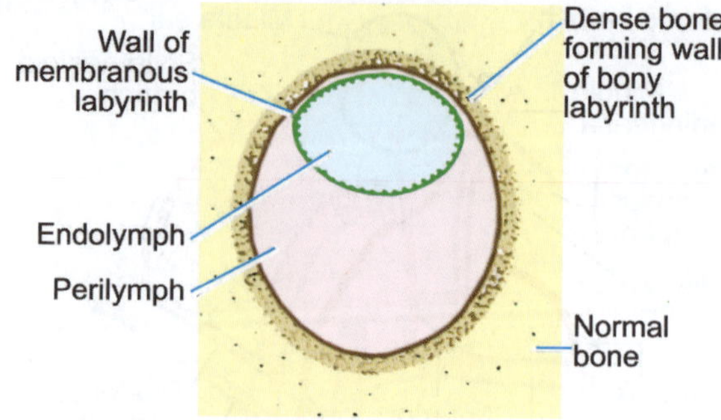

Fig. 10.42 Basic structure of the internal ear as seen in a section through a semicircular canal.

c. Posteriorly, the cavity of the vestibule is continuous with the three ***semicircular canals*** (Fig. 10.43).

The ***parts of the membranous labyrinth*** are shown in Fig. 10.44. Within each semicircular canal the membranous labyrinth is represented by a ***semicircular duct*** [It is important to distinguish carefully between the terms semicircular canal, and semicircular duct]. The part of the membranous labyrinth in the cochlea is called the ***duct of the cochlea***. In the vestibule the membranous labyrinth is represented by two distinct membranous sacs called the ***saccule*** and the ***utricle.***

The saccule communicates with the duct of the cochlea through a narrow duct called the ***ductus reunions***. The semicircular ducts open into the utricle. The utricle and the saccule communicate with each other through the ***utriculosaccular duct*** which also gives attachment to a diverticulum called the ***saccus endolymphaticus***.

We will now consider the parts of the bony and membranous labyrinth one by one.

The Vestibule

The vestibule is an oval space about 5 mm in diameter. We have seen that anteriorly it is continuous with the scala vestibuli of the cochlea. Posterosuperiorly, the vestibule has five openings for the semicircular canals. Its lateral wall is formed by the part of the same plate of bone which forms the medial wall of the middle ear. We have seen that in this wall there is an aperture, the fenestra vestibuli, through which the vestibule and middle ear communicate. This aperture is closed by the base of the stapes and by the annular ligament. The plate of bone that forms the medial wall of the vestibule closes the inner end of the internal acoustic meatus.

The medial wall of the vestibule shows a number of features that are shown in Fig. 10.45. In the anterior part of the medial wall there is a depression called the spherical recess in which the saccule is lodged. Posterosuperior to the spherical recess there is another depression called the elliptical recess in which the utricle lies. These two

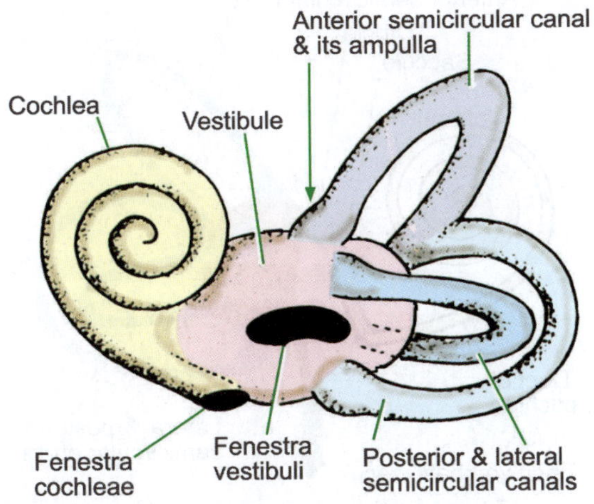

Fig. 10.43 Bony labyrinth seen from the lateral side.

recesses are separated by an elevation called the vestibular crest (the anterior part of which is also called the pyramid). The elliptical recess extends on to the roof and lateral wall of the vestibule also. Just below the elliptical recess there is an aperture leading into a canal called the aqueduct of the vestibule. This aqueduct descends through the petrous temporal bone to open on its posterior surface. It contains the endolymphatic duct (Fig. 10.44).

The Semicircular Canals

There are three semicircular canals, ***anterior*** (or superior), ***posterior,*** and ***lateral*** (Fig. 10.43). One end of each canal is dilated, and the dilatation is called an ***ampulla***. The non-ampullated ends of the anterior and posterior canals join to form a common channel, the ***crus commune***. As a result the semicircular canals open into the vestibule through five (not six) openings.

Each canal is about 0.8 mm in diameter. The lengths of the canals are variable, the posterior canal being the longest (about 20 mm) and the lateral canal being the shortest (about 13 mm).

The most important facts about the semicircular canals concern their orientation. The three canals lie in planes at right angles to one another (Fig. 10.46). The anterior and posterior canals are both vertical, while the lateral canal is horizontal. The plane of the posterior canal is parallel to the long axis of the petrous temporal bone. The plane of the anterior canal is at right angles to this axis. The plane of the lateral canal is transverse. From Fig. 10.46 it will be clear that the right and left lateral semicircular canals lie in the same plane. The anterior canal of one side lies in the same plane as the posterior canal of the opposite side.

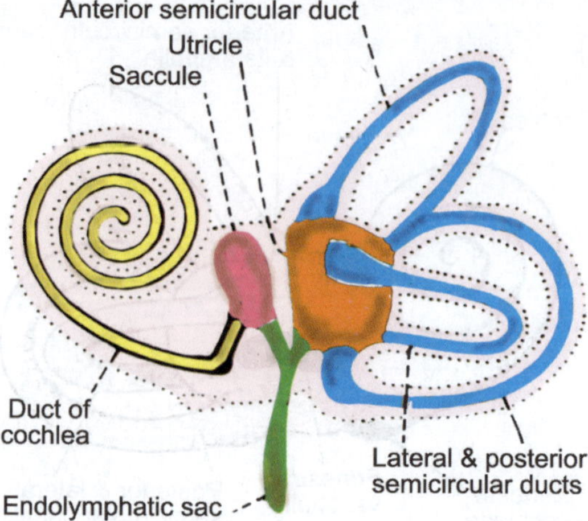

Fig. 10.44 Scheme to show the parts of the membranous labyrinth. Note the ampullated ends of the semicircular ducts.

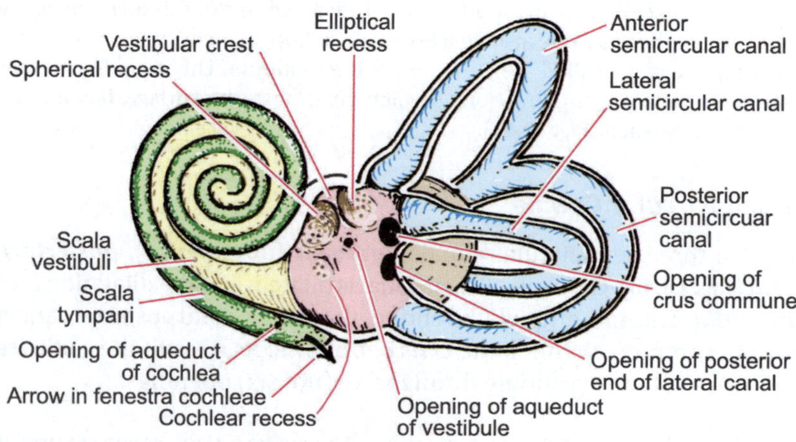

Fig. 10.45 Interior of the bony labyrinth as seen from the lateral side.

The convexity of the lateral canal points laterally. That of the posterior canal points backwards and laterally. The convexity of the anterior canal points upwards. Its position corresponds to an elevation, the arcuate eminence, seen on the anterior surface of the petrous temporal bone.

Finally, we may note the position of the ends of each canal in relation to the vestibule (Figs. 10.45, 10.46).

The anterior canal has anterolateral and posteromedial ends. The anterolateral end is ampullated and opens into the upper part of the vestibule. The posteromedial end joins the crus commune and opens through it on the medial wall of the vestibule.

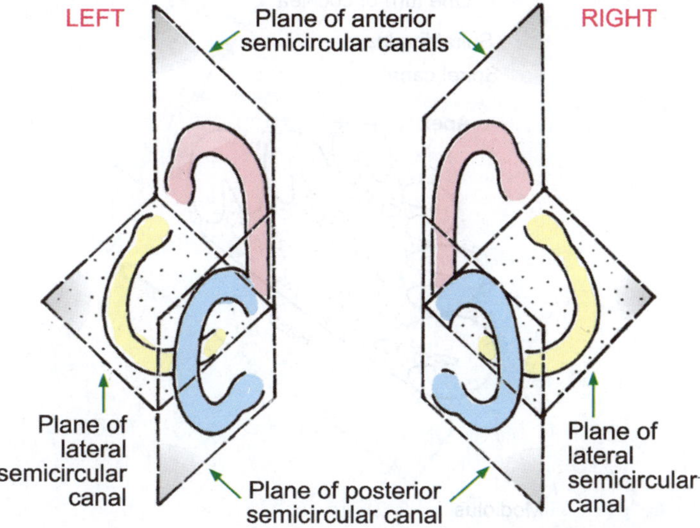

Fig. 10.46 Planes in which the semicircular canals lie as seen from behind.

The lateral canal also has anterolateral and posteromedial ends. The anterolateral end is ampullated and opens into the upper part of the vestibule near the ampullated end of the anterior canal. Its posteromedial end opens into the vestibule just below the opening of the crus commune.

The posterior canal has upper and lower ends. The upper end joins the crus commune. The lower end, which is ampullated, opens into the lower part of the vestibule.

The Bony Cochlea

The cochlea is continuous with the anterior part of the vestibule. From Fig. 10.43 it is seen that the cochlea is basically a tube that is coiled on itself for two and three quarter turns. The diameter of the tube is greatest at its junction with the vestibule, and this part is called the ***basal turn*** of the cochlea. The tube becomes progressively narrower towards the centre or ***apex*** of the cochlea. We have seen that basal turn of the cochlea produces an elevation, the promontory, on the medial wall of the middle ear, and that the apex of the cochlea is related to this wall of the middle ear just in front of the promontory.

The use of the terms base and apex with reference to the cochlea can be understood if we see a transverse section through it (Fig. 10.47). Note that the overall configuration is conical (and, therefore, appears triangular on section). The base is directed medially and backwards, while the apex is directed laterally and forwards. It is also seen that the turns of the cochlea rest on a solid core of bone called the modiolus. The base of the cochlea lies in relation to the blind end of the internal acoustic meatus.

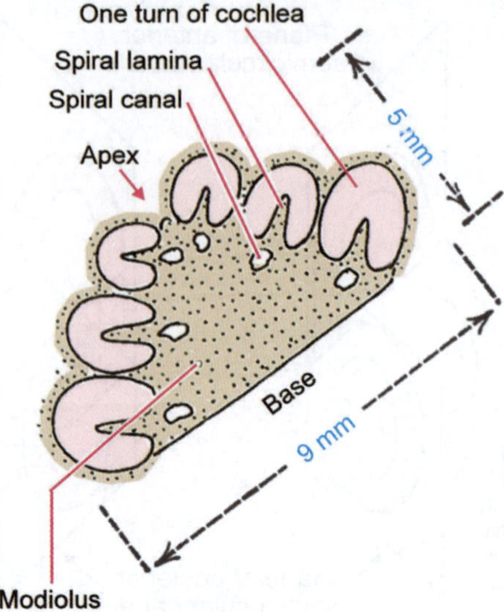

Fig. 10.47 Transverse section through the cochlea to show its general configuration.

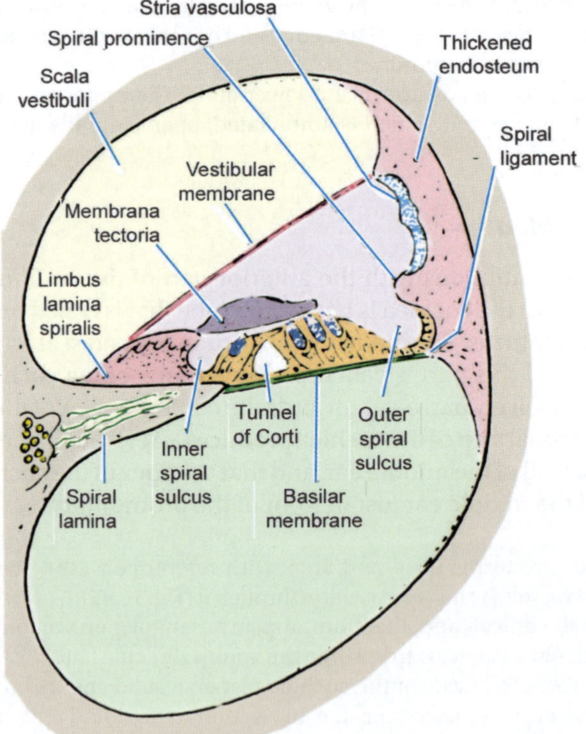

Fig. 10.48 Transverse section through one turn of the cochlea.

If we examine the basal turn of the cochlea shown in Fig. 10.45 we find that it is made up of an upper channel the scala vestibuli which is continuous with the vestibule; and of a lower channel, the scala tympani, which opens into the middle ear through the fenestra cochleae. The fenestra cochleae is closed by the ***secondary tympanic membrane.***

The scala vestibuli and the scala tympani are partially separated from each other by a shelf of bone. The shelf follows the coiling of the cochlea and is, therefore, called the ***spiral lamina***. From Fig. 10.47 it will be seen that the spiral lamina is a projection from the modiolus. Further details of the cochlea can be appreciated if we study a transverse section through one turn of the cochlea (Fig. 10.48). In this figure we see that the spiral lamina extends only partially into the canal of the cochlea. The division of the canal into the scala vestibuli and the scala tympani is completed by the ***basilar membrane*** which stretches from the 'free' edge of the spiral lamina to the outer wall of the cochlear canal.

The spiral lamina ends just short of the apex of the cochlea so that the scala vestibuli becomes continuous with the scala tympani at the apex (Fig. 10.45). This communication is called the ***helicotrema***.

We have seen that the part of the membranous labyrinth in the cochlea is called the ***duct of the cochlea***. This duct lies just above the basilar membrane. It is separated from the scala vestibuli by a thin ***vestibular membrane.***

Near the attached margin of the spiral lamina there is a canal. This canal is also shaped like a spiral and is called the ***spiral canal***. This canal contains a collection of neurons that constitute the ***spiral ganglion***. Fibres arising from the ganglion pass through the spiral lamina to supply the spiral organ (See below).

In Fig. 10.45 we see a small opening on the medial wall of the scala tympani just near the fenestra cochleae. This opening leads into a canal called the aqueduct of the cochlea (or perilymphatic duct, or cochlear canaliculus). This canal descends through the substance of the petrous temporal bone to open on the upper part of the jugular fossa. The importance of this canal is that it represents a communication between the perilymph and the subarachnoid fluid.

The Membranous Labyrinth

The parts of the membranous labyrinth are shown in Fig. 10.44.

The Utricle

The utricle lies in the elliptical recess of the vestibule. The semicircular ducts open into it through five openings that correspond in position with the openings of the semicircular canals into the vestibule. The utricle is connected to the saccule by the ***utriculo-saccular duct***. (Also see below).

The Saccule

The saccule lies in the spherical recess on the medial wall of the vestibule. It is connected to the utricle by the utriculo-saccular duct, and to the duct of the cochlea by the ductus reunions.

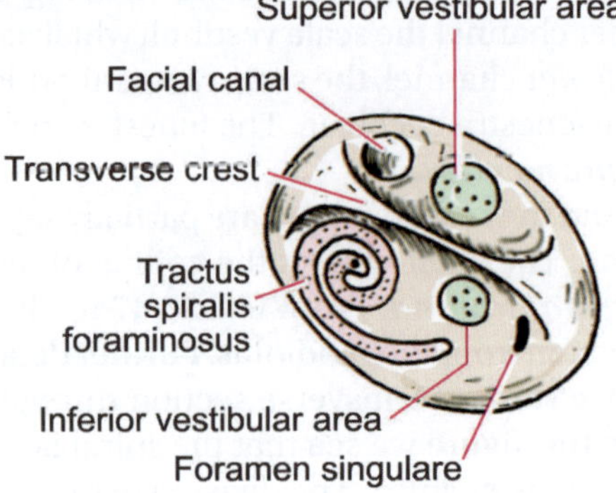

Fig. 10.49 Blind end (fundus) of the right internal acoustic meatus.

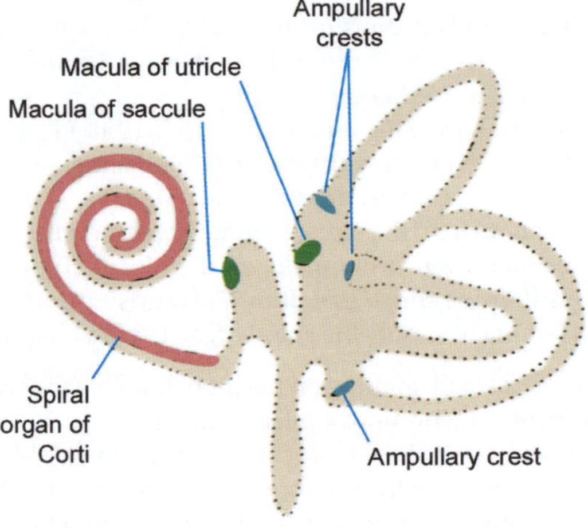

Fig. 10.50 End organs in the membranous labyrinth.

Saccus Endolymphaticus

The saccus endolymphaticus is a blind pouch-like extension of the membranous labyrinth. It lies outside the bony labyrinth, on the posterior surface of the petrous temporal bone, between the bone and the endocranium covering it. The sac is connected to the utriculosaccular duct through the ductus endolymphaticus. The ductus endolymphaticus lies in a narrow canal, the aqueduct of the vestibule. We have seen that this aqueduct opens on the medial wall of the vestibule just below the elliptical recess. The utriculosaccular duct and the ductus endolymphaticus together form a Y-shaped structure.

Semicircular Ducts

The semicircular ducts correspond in names and orientation to the corresponding semicircular canals. They open into the utricle, the positions of the openings corresponding to those of the canals into the vestibule.

Duct of the Cochlea

The duct of the cochlea is shown in Fig. 10.44. From this figure it will be seen that the duct is coiled on itself just like the bony cochlea. Its basal end becomes continuous with the saccule through the ductus reunions, while its apical end (which lies near the helicotrema) is blind and is called the ***lagena***. A cross section through the duct of the cochlea is shown in Fig. 10.48. It will be seen that the duct is triangular. In the basal turn of the cochlea it is bounded below by the vestibular membrane; and towards the 'outer' wall of the cochlea by a thickening of the endosteum that is called the ***spiral ligament***. (Also see below).

Specialized End Organs in the Membranous Labyrinth

We have seen that the internal ear is a highly specialised end organ that performs the dual functions of hearing and of providing information about the position and movements of the head. The names, positions and nervous connections of the end organs concerned with these functions are given below. The structure of these end organs is complex, and is described in the author's HUMAN HISTOLOGY.

In describing the nerves supplying the various end organs reference has to be made to a series of foramina present in the medial wall of the vestibule and on the fundus of the internal acoustic meatus.

The features to be seen on the fundus of the internal acoustic meatus (right side) are shown in 10.49. We see that the floor is divided into upper and lower parts by a transverse crest. The area above the crest shows an opening into the facial canal anteriorly; and the superior vestibular area, posteriorly. The latter is perforated by a number of small foramina. Below the transverse crest we see an area perforated by several foramina arranged in the form of a spiral. This area is, therefore, called the tractus spiralis foraminosus. The centre of this area shows a larger central foramen. Behind the tractus spiralis foraminosus there is the inferior vestibular area (showing a number of foramina), and still further back there is a single aperture called the foramen singulare.

These features should now be compared with Fig. 10.45 in which the medial wall of the left internal ear can be seen. (Note that if we examine the medial wall of the internal ear, and the fundus of the internal acoustic meatus, of the same side, the two do not correspond as the former has to be viewed from the lateral side and the latter from the medial side, resulting in lateral inversion. Visualisation is facilitated by examining the internal ear of one side, and the meatus of the opposite side).

The tractus spiralis foraminosus corresponds in position to base of the cochlea. The part of the spiral tract corresponding to the basal turn of the cochlea lies opposite the cochlear recess in the medial wall of the vestibule. The foramina seen in the superior vestibular area correspond to those seen in the floor of the elliptical recess, while those in the inferior vestibular area correspond to those seen on the floor of the spherical recess.

The end organ for hearing is the ***spiral organ (of Corti).*** It lies in the duct of the cochlea, just above the basilar membrane (Fig. 10.48). We have seen that sound waves travelling through air produce vibrations in the tympanic membrane. These are transmitted through the malleus and incus to the stapes. The base of the stapes (which fits into the fenestra vestibuli) transmits these vibrations to the perilymph of the vestibule. From there the vibrations pass into the scala vestibuli. Each time the base of the stapes moves inwards into the vestibule it creates a pressure wave which extends along the perilymph filling the entire length of the scala vestibuli. Reaching the helicotrema the pressure wave passes into the perilymph filling the scala tympani. Traversing the entire length of the scala tympani it reaches the secondary tympanic membrane (which closes the fenestra cochleae) causing it to bulge into the middle ear. The process is reversed when the base of the stapes moves outwards. These changes take place almost instantaneously. In this way vibrations are set up in the perilymph. These in turn produce vibrations of the basilar membrane and of the spiral organ. The spiral organ contains highly specialised ***hair cells***. Distortions produced in these cells as a result of vibrations generate nervous impulses. These impulses travel along nerve fibres that are peripheral processes of neurons located in the spiral ganglia. These processes reach the hair cells through canals in the spiral lamina.

Central processes arising from neurons of the spiral ganglion constitute the cochlear nerve.

Small bundles of these fibres pass through canals in the modiolus to reach its base. Here they pass through the foramina of the tractus foraminosus spiralis to enter the internal acoustic meatus. Corresponding fibres from the basal turn of the cochlea reach the posterior end of this tract by passing through foramina in the cochlear recess (in the medial wall of the vestibule).

Information about changes in the position of the head are provided by end organs called ***maculae*** (singular = macula) present in he utricle and saccule.

The macula of the saccule is present on its anterior wall. The macula of the utricle is present on its floor and the adjoining part of its lateral wall. The maculae of the utricle and saccule are placed at right angles to each other.

Each macula consists essentially of hair cells, surrounded by supporting cells. The 'hair' of the hair cells are covered by a membrane which contains crystals of calcium carbonate (***otoliths***). With changes in the position of the head the otoliths are displaced leading to distortion of hair cells. Nervous impulses are generated as a result of this distortion.

Information about angular movements (acceleration) of the head is provided by end organs called the ***ampullary crests*** (or ***cristae ampullae***) one of which is present in the ampulla of each semicircular duct. Each crista consists of hair cells (and supporting cells) that are surmounted by a gelatinous covering that forms a partition (***cupola***) within the ampulla. Movements of the head produce currents in the endolymph within the semicircular ducts. These cause the cupolae to move resulting in deformation of hair cells and production of nerve impulses.

The nerve fibres innervating the cristae of the semicircular ducts and the maculae of the utricle and saccule are peripheral processes of neurons located in the vestibular ganglion. This ganglion lies in the internal acoustic meatus. The central processes of cells of the ganglion form the vestibular nerve.

The peripheral processes arising from neurons in the ganglion form three branches, superior, inferior and posterior. The fibres of the superior branch pass through foramina in the superior vestibular area; and enter the vestibule through foramina in the elliptical recess. They supply the macula of the utricle and the cristae in the ampullae of the anterior, superior and lateral semicircular ducts. The fibres of the inferior branch pass through the inferior vestibular area. They appear in the vestibule through foramina present in the spherical recess and supply the macula of the saccule. The fibres of the posterior branch pass through the foramen singulare to reach the crista in the posterior semicircular duct.

Blood Vessels of the Internal Ear:

The internal ear is supplied by the labyrinthine artery which usually arises from the anterior inferior cerebellar artery. It sometimes arises from the basilar artery. The internal ear also receives some twigs from the stylomastoid artery which supplies the middle ear (Fig. 10.41). The internal ear is drained by veins which end in the superior petrosal sinus or in the transverse sinus.

CHAPTER

11

Oral Cavity, Nasal Cavity, Pharynx, Larynx, Trachea, Oesophagus

THE ORAL CAVITY AND SOME RELATED STRUCTURES

The anatomy of the oral cavity is considered below. In addition to the oral cavity proper we will also consider the palate, and the teeth. Other important structures present in relation to the oral cavity are tongue and the salivary glands. Three pairs of salivary glands are present in relation to the oral cavity. These are the parotid glands, the submandibular glands, and the sublingual glands. The tongue and salivary glands have already been described in Chapters 3 and 5.

THE ORAL CAVITY

The lay person uses the word 'mouth' loosely both for the external opening and for the cavity it leads to. Strictly speaking, the term mouth should be applied only to the external opening which is also called the ***oral fissure.*** The cavity (containing the tongue and teeth) is the mouth cavity or ***oral cavity***.

A basic idea of the boundaries of the oral cavity can be had from Fig. 11.1 which is a coronal section through it. Laterally the cavity is bounded by the cheeks; above by the palate (which separates it from the nasal cavity); and below it has a floor to which the tongue is attached. Projecting into the cavity from above and below, just medial to the each cheek, there are the alveolar processes of the upper and lower jaws which bear the teeth. When the mouth is closed bringing the upper and lower teeth into apposition, the oral cavity is seen to consist of a part between the teeth of the two sides (the ***oral cavity proper***); and a part between the alveolar processes and the cheeks. The latter is called the ***vestibule***. In Fig. 11.1 the vestibule is seen in two halves right and left, but when traced anteriorly the two halves become continuous in the middle line in front of the teeth. Here the vestibule communicates with the exterior; and its external walls are formed by the upper and lower lips. When the teeth are

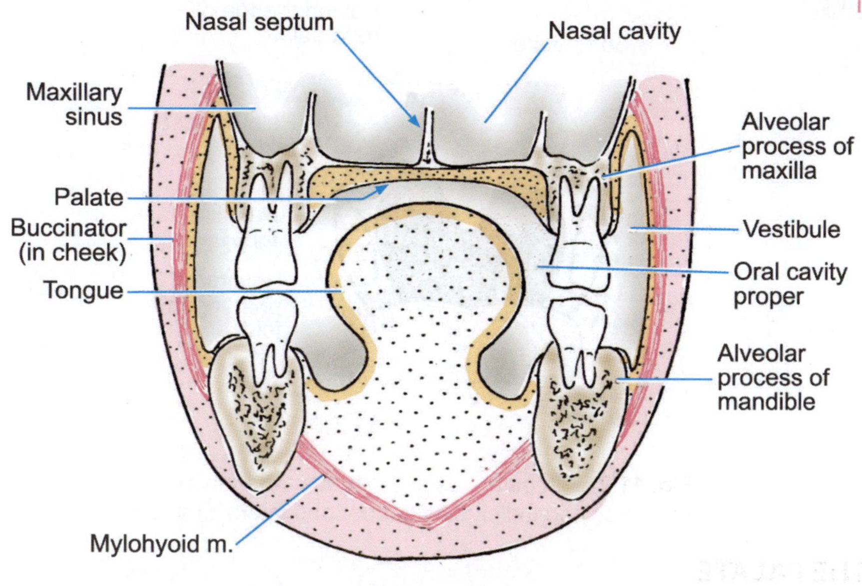

Fig. 11.1 Schematic coronal section through the oral cavity.

in apposition the vestibule communicates with the oral cavity proper through a space behind the last tooth. (This is a point of practical importance. It means that any liquid put into the vestibule will find its way into the mouth even if the jaws are kept closed).

With the exception of the teeth all structures in the oral cavity are covered by mucous membrane. That over the alveolar processes of the jaws is firmly attached to underlying bone and is referred to as the gum. The reflections of mucosa between the different walls of the mouth are obvious from Fig. 11.1.

The oral cavity proper communicates posteriorly with the oral part of the pharynx. The communication between the two is called the ***oropharyngeal isthmus*** (Fig. 11.2). The roof of the cavity is formed by the palate (described below). The chief structure in the floor is the tongue. The rest of the floor is formed by mucous membrane passing from the sides of the tongue to the gum. The anterior part of the tongue is not attached to the floor and that is why it can be protruded out of the mouth. This part of the tongue is attached to the floor by a median fold of mucosa called the ***frenulum linguae***.

Three pairs of salivary glands are present near the oral cavity and pour their secretions into it. These are the parotid, submandibular and sublingual glands. The secretions of the parotid glands are poured into mouth through the right and left parotid ducts which open into the corresponding half of the vestibule, on the inner side of the cheek, opposite the crown of the second upper molar tooth. The duct for each submandibular gland opens on the ***sublingual papilla*** located just lateral to the frenulum linguae (Fig. 5.12). The sublingual glands lie just below the mucosa on the floor of the mouth. Each gland raises a ridge of mucosa which starts at the sublingual papilla and runs laterally and backwards. This ridge is called the ***sublingual fold***.

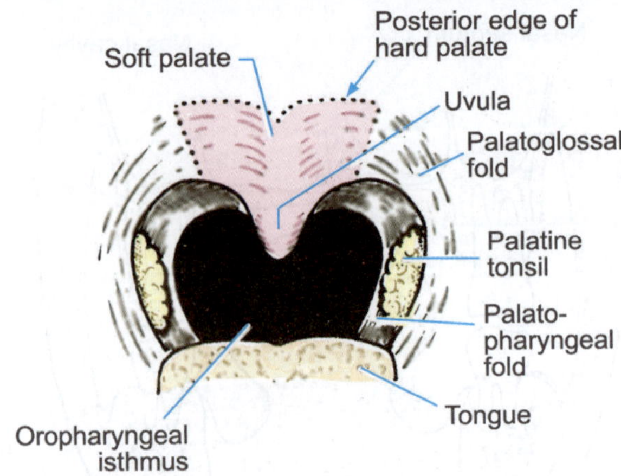

Fig. 11.2 Soft palate as seen through the mouth. The dotted line indicates its upper and lateral limits.

THE PALATE

The palate separates the oral cavity from the nasal cavity. It is divisible into an anterior, larger, part the ***hard palate***, and a posterior part the ***soft palate***.

The hard palate has a skeletal basis formed by the palatal processes of the right and left maxillae, and the horizontal plates of the palatine bones. This bony basis is covered by periosteum. The lower surface of the palate is lined by mucous membrane of the mouth and its upper surface by mucous membrane of the nasal cavity.

The soft palate is shown as seen from the front (i.e., through the mouth) in Fig. 11.2, and as seen from behind in Fig. 11.25. It is shown in median section in Fig. 11.9. The soft palate is attached to the posterior margin of the hard palate. In its normal relaxed position it has one surface directed upwards and backwards, and another surface directed forwards and downwards (Fig. 11.9). Its median part is prolonged downwards as a conical projection called the ***uvula*** (Fig. 11.2). Its lateral margins are continuous with two folds of mucous membrane. The anterior of these connects the palate to the lateral margin of the posterior part of the tongue and is called the ***palatoglossal fold.*** The posterior fold connects the palate to the wall of the pharynx and is called the ***palatopharyngeal fold***. (Also see Fig. 5.11).

The soft palate consists of two layers of mucous membrane (continuous with those lining the upper and lower surfaces of the hard palate). Between these layers of mucosa there is a fibrous basis called the ***palatine aponeurosis*** (See below). Several muscles are present in the soft palate and are described below.

MUSCLES OF THE SOFT PALATE

These are the tensor palati, the levator palati, the musculus uvulae, the palatoglossus and the palatopharyngeus (Fig. 11.3).

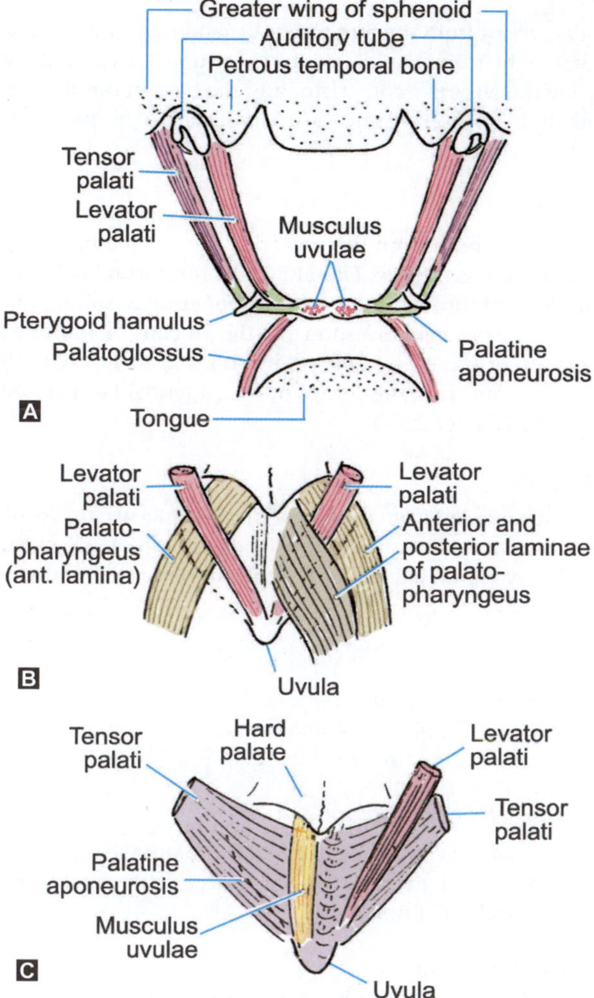

Fig. 11.3 Muscles of the palate. A. Schematic coronal section to show arrangement of muscles. B. Muscles seen from behind and above after removal of mucosa. C. The palatopharyngeus has been removed on both sides, and the levator palati on one side to expose the palatine aponeurosis and the musculus uvulae,

Tensor Palati

The tensor palati arises from the lateral wall of the auditory tube and part of the base of the skull adjoining it (sphenoid: greater wing and scaphoid fossa) (Fig. 11.3A). It descends and ends in a tendon which winds round the pterygoid hamulus and expands into a wide fibrous band called the ***palatine aponeurosis***. This aponeurosis is attached anteriorly, to the posterior edge of the hard palate (formed by the palatine bones). In the middle line the aponeuroses of the two sides fuse with each other. The palatine aponeurosis forms the fibrous basis of the soft palate and gives attachment to other muscles of the palate.

Levator Palati

The levator palati arises from the auditory tube, and part of the petrous temporal bone just medial to the tube (Fig. 11.3A). It passes downwards in the gap between the upper edge of the superior constrictor and the base of the skull (Fig. 1.8), and then turns medially to be inserted into the upper surface of the palatine aponeurosis near the uvula (Fig. 11.3B).

Musculus Uvulae

The musculus uvulae arises from the posterior edge of the hard palate near the middle line (posterior nasal spine: Fig. 11.3C). Its fibres run backwards (on either side of the middle line) through the palatine aponeurosis, splitting it up into two lamellae (Fig. 11.3A). They gain insertion into the mucous membrane of the uvula. (The muscle is seen in transverse section in 11.3A; in surface view in Fig. 11.3C right half; and after removing the posterior (or superior) lamella of the palatine aponeurosis in Fig. 11.3C left half).

Palatopharyngeus

The palatopharyngeus arises from the posterior (pharyngeal) surface of the palatine aponeurosis by two laminae, anterior and posterior which are separated by the levator palati. The two lamellae join and descend to the wall of the pharynx (Fig. 11.14).

Palatoglossus

The palatoglossus arises from the oral (anterior) surface of the palatine aponeurosis. It passes downwards and forwards to reach the side of the tongue (Figs. 11.3A, 5.14). The muscle lies within the palatoglossal fold (Fig. 5.11).

Nerve Supply of Muscles of the Palate:

All muscles of the palate, except the tensor palati, are supplied by the cranial part of the accessory nerve through the pharyngeal branch of the vagus. The tensor palati is supplied by the mandibular nerve.

Actions of Palatine Muscle:

The palatine muscles are responsible for movements of the palate associated with deglutition and with speech. The levator palati helps to close the pharyngeal isthmus (communication between nasopharynx and oropharynx) by elevating the palate and bringing it into contact with the posterior wall of the pharynx.

In this action it is helped by the palatopharyngeal sphincter that produces a ridge on the pharyngeal wall which comes in contact with the palate. The tensor palati helps in deglutition by pressing the bolus between the palate and the tongue. The palatopharyngeus also helps in deglutition by pulling the pharynx up thus shortening its length. The palatoglossus closes the oropharyngeal isthmus.

Nerve Supply and Blood Supply of the Palate

The palate is supplied by the greater palatine branch of the maxillary artery (Fig. 8.24), the ascending palatine branch of the facial artery (Fig. 8.18), and by the palatine branch of the ascending pharyngeal artery (Fig. 8.14). The veins from the palate end in the pterygoid and tonsilar plexuses. The lymph vessels drain into the deep cervical lymph nodes.

The nerves supplying the palate are the greater and lesser palatine nerves and the nasopalatine nerves (Fig. 9.46).

For clinical correlations of the palate see Chapter 65. For development of the palate see the author's HUMAN EMBRYOLOGY.

THE TEETH

As the teeth can be seen and felt some facts about them are commonly known. We know that the new born have no teeth; that the first tooth appears when the infant is about six months old; that the teeth in young children gradually fall off and are replaced by new ones that can last throughout life. The teeth that appear in children and fall off with time are called ***deciduous*** (or milk) teeth. The teeth of the second set that gradually replace the deciduous teeth constitute the ***permanent*** teeth.

The teeth, both deciduous and permanent, have varying shapes. Some have sharp cutting edges and are, therefore, called ***incisors***. Others are sharp and pointed: these are called ***canines*** as they form the most prominent teeth in canine species (e.g., dogs). Still others have edges suitable for a grinding function: these are called ***molars***. In the permanent set we also have grinding teeth that are some what smaller than the molars and are called the ***premolars*** (as they lie in front of the molars).

A set of deciduous teeth consists of the following. Beginning from the middle line (in front) there is a central incisor, a lateral incisor (i.e., two incisors); one canine; and two molars (distinguished from each other by being called the first and second molars). There are, thus, five teeth in each half of each jaw i.e., twenty in all.

A set of permanent teeth consists of the following. Beginning from the middle line there is a central incisor, a lateral incisor, a canine, two premolars (first and second, that replace the deciduous molars), and three molars (first, second and third). Thus in each half of each jaw there are eight teeth, or thirty two in all.

There is considerable variation in the ages at which the various teeth erupt. The following scheme gives the approximate ages of appearance in a form easy to remember.

Deciduous teeth

Central incisor.................. = ...6 months
Lateral incisor.................. = (+2)....................8 months
First molar........................ = (+4)....................12 months
Canine.............................. = (+4)....................16 months
Second molar.................... = (+4)....................20 months
Note that the first deciduous molar appears before the canine.

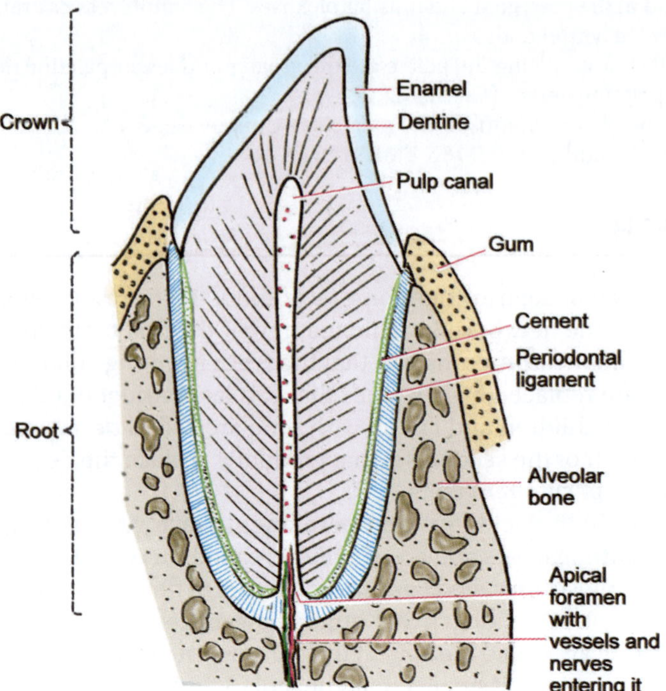

Fig. 11.4 Vertical section through a typical tooth.

Permanent teeth

First	=	6 years
Central incisor	=	(+1)....................7 years
Lateral incisor	=	(+1)....................8 years
Canine	=	(+1)....................9 years
Premolars	=	(+1)....................10 years
Second molar	=	(+1)....................11 years
Third molar	=	..........................17 years +

Note that the first permanent tooth to appear is the first molar. Approximately one tooth appears every year from the 6th to 11th years.

The third molar teeth appear at the age of 17 years or later and are, therefore, called the ***wisdom teeth***. Not infrequently one or more third molars may fail to erupt.

STRUCTURE OF A TYPICAL TOOTH

A tooth consists of an upper part, the ***crown***, which is seen in the mouth; and of one or more ***roots*** which are embedded in sockets in the jaw bone (mandible or maxilla). The greater part of the tooth is formed by a bone like material called ***dentine***. In the region of the crown the dentine is covered by a much harder white material called the ***enamel***. Over the root the dentine is covered by a thin layer of ***cement***. The cement is united to the wall of the bony socket in the jaw through a layer of fibrous tissue called the ***periodontal ligament***. The external surface of the alveolar process is covered by the gum which normally overlaps the lower edge of the crown. Within the dentine there is a ***pulp canal*** which contains a mass of cells, blood vessels and nerves which constitute the pulp. The blood vessels and nerves enter the pulp canal at the apex of the root through an ***apical foramen***.

Differences in Structure of Different Teeth

Details of the anatomy of individual teeth are beyond the scope of this book. The following information is, however, sufficient for medical students.

In describing teeth the dentist uses certain terms that the medical student should be familiar with. As the teeth are arranged in an arch, terms like anterior, posterior, medial or lateral are confusing. The surface of the tooth facing the lip or cheek is the ***buccal*** (or ***labial***) surface; while that towards the tongue is the ***lingual*** (or ***palatal***) surface. The surface nearest to the middle line is the ***mesial*** surface: this term corresponds to 'medial' in case of the anterior teeth, and to 'anterior' for the posterior teeth. The surface opposite to the mesial surface is called the ***distal*** surface. The upper surfaces of the lower teeth, and the lower surfaces of the upper teeth are referred to as the ***occlusal*** surfaces. In the case of the incisors the occlusal surface forms a sharp cutting edge. In the canines it is pointed. In the molars and premolars the occlusal surface bears rounded elevations or ***cusps***: typically two on each premolar and four or five in each molar. The incisors and canines have one root each. The premolars may have one or two roots. The molars have two or three roots, but the last molar may have only one.

The meeting of the upper and lower teeth is called ***occlusion***. In the relaxed mouth the upper and lower teeth are a short distance apart. In proper occlusion there is minimal space between the upper and lower teeth, the cusps of one set fitting into the depressions on the occlusal surface of the other set. The upper incisors lie slightly in front of the lower. In fact all lower teeth lie slightly anterior (and mesial) to their upper counterparts.

Blood Supply and Nerve Supply of Teeth

The lower teeth are supplied by branches from the inferior alveolar artery (branch of maxillary artery); and by the inferior alveolar nerve (branch of mandibular nerve, Fig. 9.57).

The upper teeth are supplied by the anterior and posterior superior alveolar branches of the maxillary artery; and by the anterior, middle and posterior superior alveolar nerves (branches of the maxillary nerve and its infraorbital continuation).

For development of teeth and their anomalies see the author's HUMAN EMBRYOLOGY. Some clinical correlations of the teeth and gums are discussed in Chapter 15.

THE NASAL CAVITY AND PARANASAL SINUSES

Preliminary Remarks

The nasal cavity is divided by a median septum into right and left halves. Each half of the nasal cavity opens to the exterior through the external (or anterior) nares; and posteriorly it opens into the nasopharynx. A schematic coronal section through the nasal cavity is shown in Fig. 11.5. It is seen that each half of the cavity is triangular. It has a vertical medial wall formed by the nasal

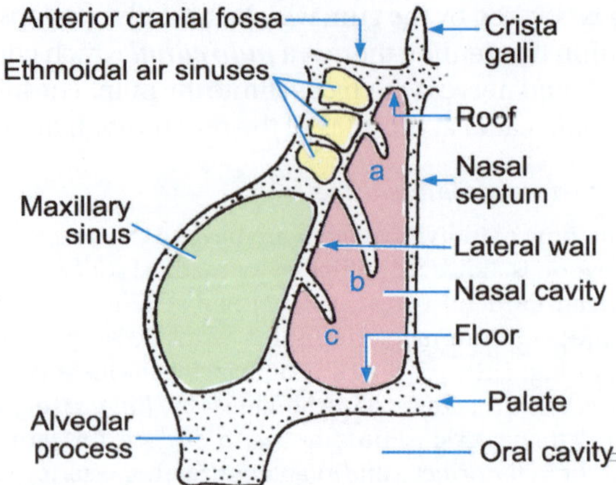

Fig. 11.5 Highly simplified coronal section through the nasal cavity. **a, b, c**: superior, middle and inferior conchae respectively.

septum; a sloping lateral wall; a relatively broad floor formed by the palate (which separates it from the oral cavity); and a narrow roof which lies at the junction of the medial and lateral walls.

These walls have a skeletal basis that is made up predominantly of bone, but is cartilaginous at some places. The skeletal basis is covered (over most of the nasal cavity) by mucous membrane. Typically the mucosa is moist and highly vascular. It serves to warm inspired air and also helps to remove dust (which sticks to the moist wall). For these reasons the mucosa is referred to as ***respiratory***. The mucosa lining the uppermost part of the septum and the adjoining part of the lateral wall differs from that present elsewhere in the nasal cavity. It is characterized by the presence of receptor cells that are sensitive to smell: the mucosa in this region is, therefore, called the ***olfactory mucosa.*** Olfactory nerves arise from this mucosa. A small area of the nasal cavity (near the anterior nares) is lined not by mucous membrane, but by skin. This skin bears hair which serve to trap dust present in inspired air.

Medial Wall of Nasal Cavity: Nasal Septum

The skeletal basis of the medial wall of the nasal cavity (formed by the nasal septum) is shown in Fig. 11.1. It is formed mainly by the perpendicular plate of the ethmoid bone (posterosuperior part); the vomer (posteroinferior part); and the septal cartilage (anterior part).

Around the edges of the septum there are small contributions from the nasal, frontal, sphenoid, maxillary and palatine bones.

As a point of practical importance it may be remembered that the septum is fairly often deflected to one side so that one half of the nasal cavity may be larger than the other.

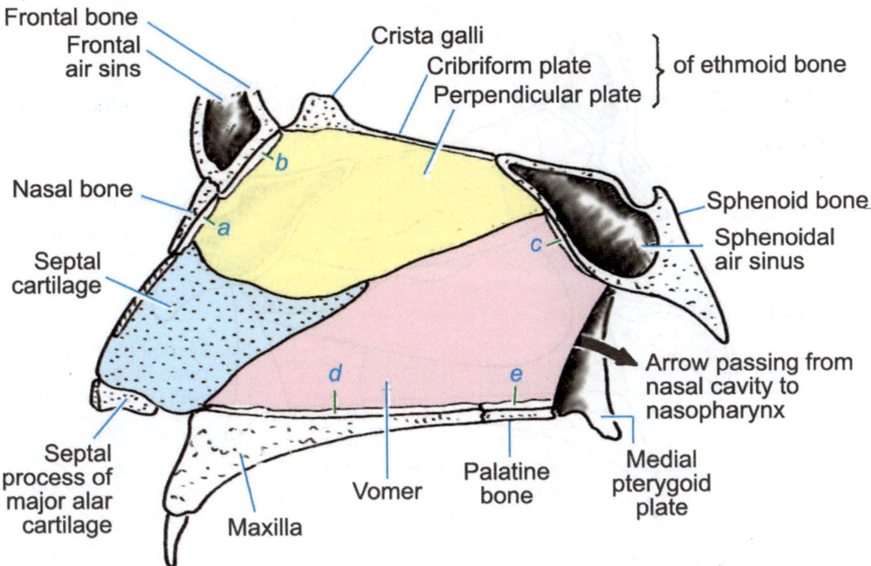

Fig. 11.6 Skeletal basis of the nasal septum.

The nasal cartilages have been considered in Chapter 3 while describing the external nose and are shown in Fig. 3.1. At this stage some details about the septal cartilage may be noted. As implied by its name this cartilage lies mainly in the nasal septum. Posteriorly it is attached to the perpendicular plate of the ethmoid bone and to the vomer (Fig. 11.6). In front it is attached in its uppermost part to the suture between the two nasal bones (Fig. 3.1B); lower down it is continuous with the right and left lateral nasal cartilages (Fig. 3.1C); and still lower down its anterior edge is free (See part labelled septal cartilage in Fig. 3.1A). From Fig. 3.1D note that the right and left major alar cartilages have ***septal processes*** which form the part of the nasal septum just above the anterior nares (Also see Fig. 11.6).

Lateral Wall of Nasal Cavity

The skeletal basis of the lateral wall of the nasal cavity is shown in Figs. 11.7 and 11.8. The bones taking part are the maxilla (medial surface), the ethmoid bone, the palatine bone, the inferior nasal concha and the lacrimal bone.

Note that the lateral wall of the external nose also forms the anterior part of the lateral wall of the nasal cavity. The medial surfaces of the lateral nasal cartilage, and the major and minor alar cartilages appear in the lateral wall of the nasal cavity (Fig. 11.7).

The lateral wall of the nasal cavity as seen with the mucous membrane intact is shown in Fig. 11.9. The following points may be noted. There are three anteroposterior elevations on the lateral wall. These are the superior, middle and inferior nasal ***conchae.*** Each concha has a core of bone covered by mucous membrane. The bony core of the superior and middle conchae is formed by parts of the ethmoid bone, while that of the inferior concha is independent (Fig.

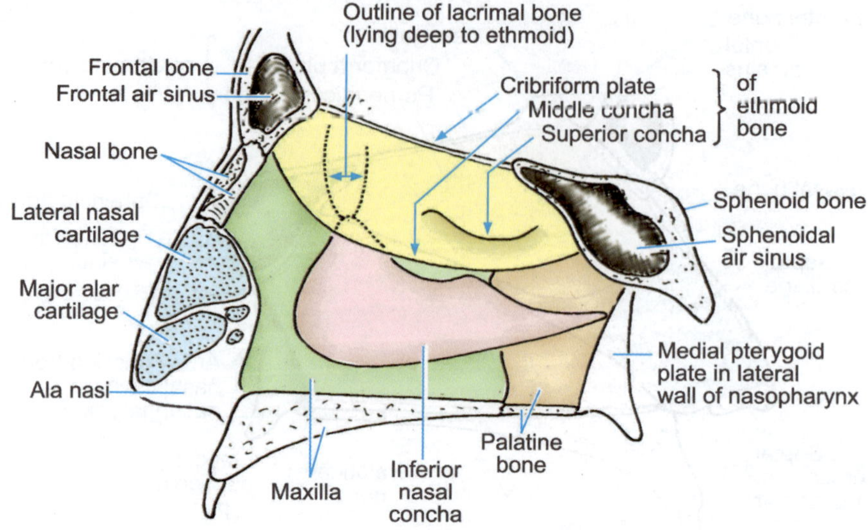

Fig. 11.7 Skeletal basis of the lateral wall of the nasal cavity.

11.8). Each concha has an upper border attached to the rest of the lateral wall and a free lower margin. The spaces deep to the superior, middle and inferior conchae are called the superior, middle and inferior ***meatuses*** respectively (2, 3, 4 in Fig. 11.8). There is a triangular space above the superior concha (1 in Fig. 11.8). This is the ***sphenoethmoidal recess*** (Also see Fig. 11.9). Occasionally an additional concha (called the highest nasal concha) may be present on the lateral wall of the sphenoethmoidal recess.

The part of the nasal cavity just above the anterior nares is called the ***vestibule.*** It is bounded laterally by the ala and the major alar cartilage (Fig. 11.7). The vestibule is lined by skin. At the upper limit of the vestibule (where skin meets mucous membrane) there is a curved elevation called the ***limen nasi*** (Fig. 11.9). Above the limen nasi there is a depression called the ***atrium.*** The atrium represents a forward continuation of the middle meatus beyond the anterior end of the middle concha. The upper limit of the atrium is marked by another curved ridge called the ***aggar nasi.***

Some structures in the lateral wall of the nose can be seen only when the conchae are cut away (Fig. 11.10). In the middle meatus we see a rounded elevation called the ***bulla ethmoidalis.*** Below and in front of the bulla there is a curved groove called the ***hiatus semilunaris***. The lower curved margin of the hiatus is sharp: it is produced by a process of the ethmoid bone called the uncinate process. The anterior end of the hiatus is continuous with a depression called the ***ethmoidal infundibulum.*** The upper end of the infundibulum is usually continuous with the ***frontonasal duct*** which connects the frontal sinus to the nasal cavity.

There are a number of openings in the meatuses of the nose (Fig. 11.10). They are described in connection with paranasal sinuses below.

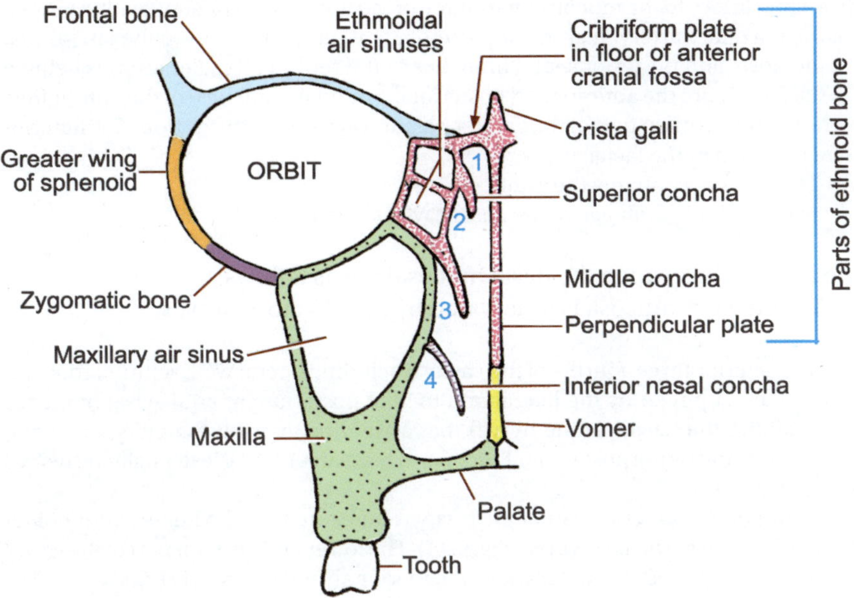

Fig. 11.8 Schematic coronal section through the nasal cavity to show some bones forming its walls. The orbit is also shown.

The presence of conchae in the lateral wall of the nasal cavity greatly increases the surface area of the nasal mucosa. This factor combined with the presence of a highly vascular and moist mucous membrane enables the nose to effectively warm inspired air and to make it moist.

Roof of Nasal Cavity

We have already seen that the roof of the nasal cavity lies at the junction of the medial and lateral walls (Fig. 11.5). From Figs. 11.6 and 11.7 it will be seen that, when traced anteroposteriorly, the roof is divisible into three parts. The middle part is formed by the mucous membrane covering the ethmoid bone and is almost horizontal. The anterior part slopes downwards and forwards. It is formed by the mucous membrane covering the frontal bone above, and the nasal bone below. The posterior part slopes downwards and backwards. It is formed by the mucous membrane covering the sphenoid bone.

Floor of Nasal Cavity

The floor of the nasal cavity is formed by the mucous membrane covering the upper surface of the hard palate. Each half of the hard palate is formed in its anterior three-fourths by the maxilla (palatine process); and in its posterior one-fourth by the palatine bone (horizontal plate).

Blood Supply and Nerve Supply of the Nasal Cavity

The chief artery to the mucous membrane of the nose is the sphenopalatine branch of the maxillary artery. It gives off posterolateral nasal branches to the lateral wall of the nose, and posterior septal branches to the septum. Smaller arteries helping in the supply are the anterior and posterior ethmoidal branches (of the ophthalmic artery); the terminal part of the greater palatine artery; and twigs from the superior labial branch of the facial artery.

The veins accompany the arteries.

For lymphatic drainage of the nasal cavity see Chapter 13

The nerves innervating the nasal mucosal are as follows:

1. The olfactory mucosa is innervated by the olfactory nerves.
2. The posterior three-fourths of the cavity (including lateral wall, septum, roof and floor) are supplied by the lateral and medial posterior superior nasal branches (including the nasopalatine nerve) that arise directly from the pterygopalatine ganglion; and by the posterior inferior nasal branches of the greater palatine nerves (See Fig. 9.46).
3. The upper and anterior part of the cavity is innervated by the anterior ethmoidal branch of the nasociliary nerve (Fig. 9.44). The lower and anterior part of the cavity is supplied by twigs from the anterior superior alveolar nerve (Fig. 9.47).

Clinical Correlations

Some clinical correlations of the nasal cavity are described in Chapter 15.

THE PARANASAL SINUSES

These are spaces present in the substance of bones related to the nasal cavities. Each sinus opens into the nasal cavity, and is lined by mucous membrane continuous with that of the latter. Because of this communication each sinus is normally filled with air.

Frontal Sinuses

The right and left frontal sinuses are present in the part of the frontal bone deep to the superciliary arches. Each sinus lies deep to a triangular area the angles of which lie:

(a) at the nasion (point where the frontonasal suture meets the internasal suture), (b) at a point about 3 cm above the nasion, and (c) at a point on the supraorbital margin at the junction of the medial one third with the lateral two thirds.

The cavity of the frontal sinus extends for some distance into the orbital plate of the frontal bone between the roof of the orbit and the floor of the anterior cranial fossa.

Each frontal sinus usually opens into the middle meatus through the frontonasal duct. This duct is usually continuous, below, with a funnel like space the ethmoidal infundibulum (Fig. 11.10) which is continuous with the upper end of the hiatus semilunaris.

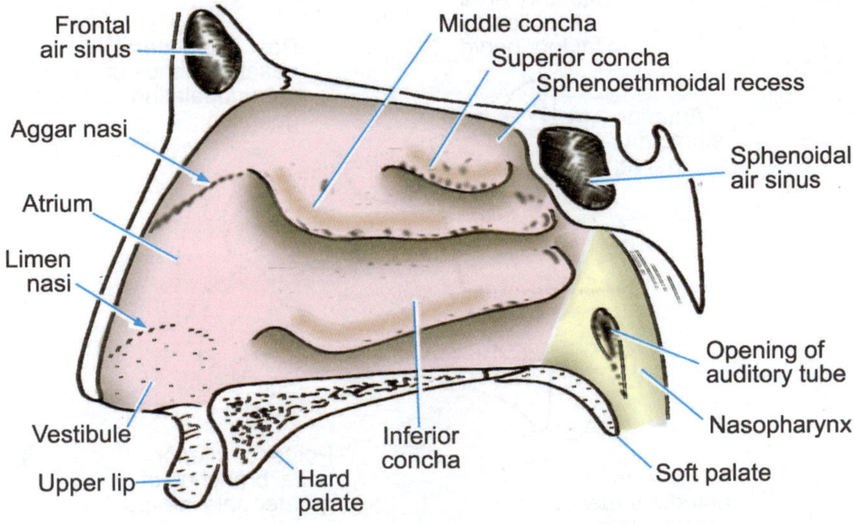

Fig. 11.9 Lateral wall of the nasal cavity with the mucous membrane intact.

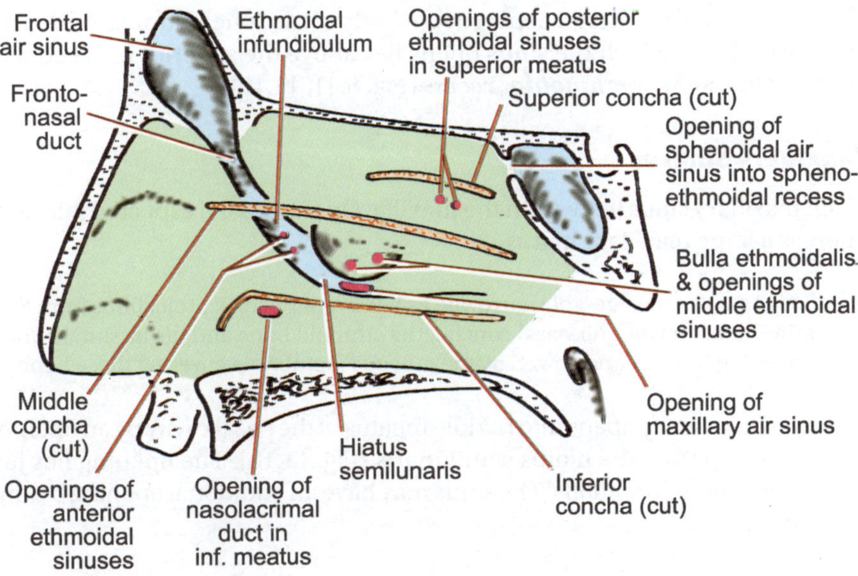

Fig. 11.10 Lateral wall of the nasal cavity after cutting the conchae to reveal structures deep to them.

Sphenoidal Sinuses

The right and left sphenoidal sinuses are present in the body of the sphenoid bone. Each sinus opens into the corresponding half of the nasal cavity through

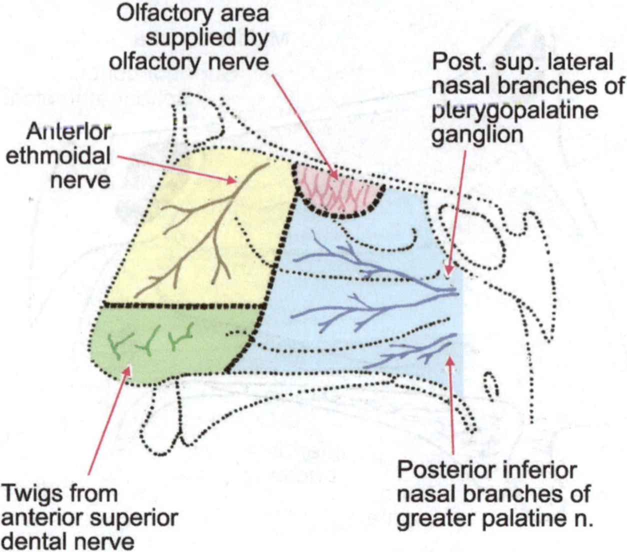

Fig. 11.11 Nerves supplying the lateral wall of the nasal cavity, and their areas of distribution. Compare with Fig. 11.8.

an aperture on the anterior aspect of the body of the sphenoid. The part of the nasal cavity into which the sinus opens lies above the superior nasal concha and is called ***sphenoethmoidal recess*** (Fig. 8.41, 11.10).

Maxillary Sinuses

Each maxillary sinus lies within the maxilla. On the medial aspect of this bone there is a large maxillary hiatus.

This hiatus is considerably narrowed as it is overlapped by projections from the palatine bone, the inferior nasal concha, the ethmoid bone and the lacrimal bone. The opening is further narrowed by the mucous membrane covering these bones.

The sinus usually opens into middle meatus of the nasal cavity by an opening in the lower part of the hiatus semilunaris (Fig. 11.10). The opening lies just below the bulla ethmoidalis. The sinus may have an additional opening behind the main one.

Ethmoidal Air Sinuses

The ethmoidal air sinuses are located within the lateral part (or labyrinth) of the ethmoid bone. They can be divided into anterior, middle and posterior groups.

Each labyrinth (right or left) is bounded medially by the medial plate and laterally by the orbital plate of the bone. The ethmoidal air sinuses lie between these plates. they are seen from the medial side after removing the superior and middle nasal conchae, and the medial plate. They are seen in coronal section in Fig. 11.8 in which their close relationship to the orbit can be appreciated.

The walls of some of the ethmoidal sinuses are incomplete. In the intact skull they are completed by parts of the frontal, maxillary, lacrimal, sphenoidal and palatine bones.

The anterior ethmoidal sinuses open into the ethmoidal infundibulum, or into the upper part of the hiatus semilunaris. The middle ethmoidal sinuses open on or near the bulla ethmoidalis. The posterior ethmoidal sinuses open into the superior meatus.

Important clinical correlations of the paranasal sinuses are discussed in Chapter 15.

Other Openings in the Nasal Cavity

In addition to the openings of the paranasal sinuses, the lateral wall of the nose shows the opening of the ***nasolacrimal duct.*** This duct conveys lacrimal fluid from the conjunctival sac, via the lacrimal sac. It opens into the anterior part of the inferior meatus (Fig. 11.10). The nasolacrimal duct is described in Chapter 3.

THE PHARYNX

Preliminary Remarks

The pharynx is a median passage that is common to the alimentary and respiratory systems (Fig. 11.12). It is divisible (from above downwards) into a ***nasal part*** (or ***nasopharynx***) into which the nasal cavities open; an ***oral part*** (or ***oropharynx***) which is continuous with the posterior end of the oral cavity; and a ***laryngeal part*** (or ***laryngopharynx***) which is continuous in front with the larynx, and below with oesophagus.

The communication between the nasopharynx and the oropharynx is called the ***pharyngeal isthmus***. This isthmus can be closed (e.g., during swallowing) by elevation of the soft palate.

Closure is helped by contraction of muscle fibres in the pharyngeal wall that constitute the ***palatopharyngeal sphincter***. Contraction of this sphincter produces a ridge (of Passavant) on the posterior pharyngeal wall with which the soft palate comes in contact.

The communication between the oral cavity and the pharynx is called the ***oropharyngeal isthmus*** (Fig. 11.2). It is bounded above by the soft palate, below by the posterior part of the tongue, and on either side by the palatoglossal arches. The oropharyngeal isthmus can be closed by contraction of the palatoglossus muscles. This closure plays an important part in deglutition.

The relationship of the laryngopharynx to the inlet of the larynx is shown in Fig. 11.25. This figure also shows the anterior wall of the nasopharynx and oropharynx. We may now proceed to consider some further details about the features to be seen in the three parts of the pharynx (Fig. 11.12).

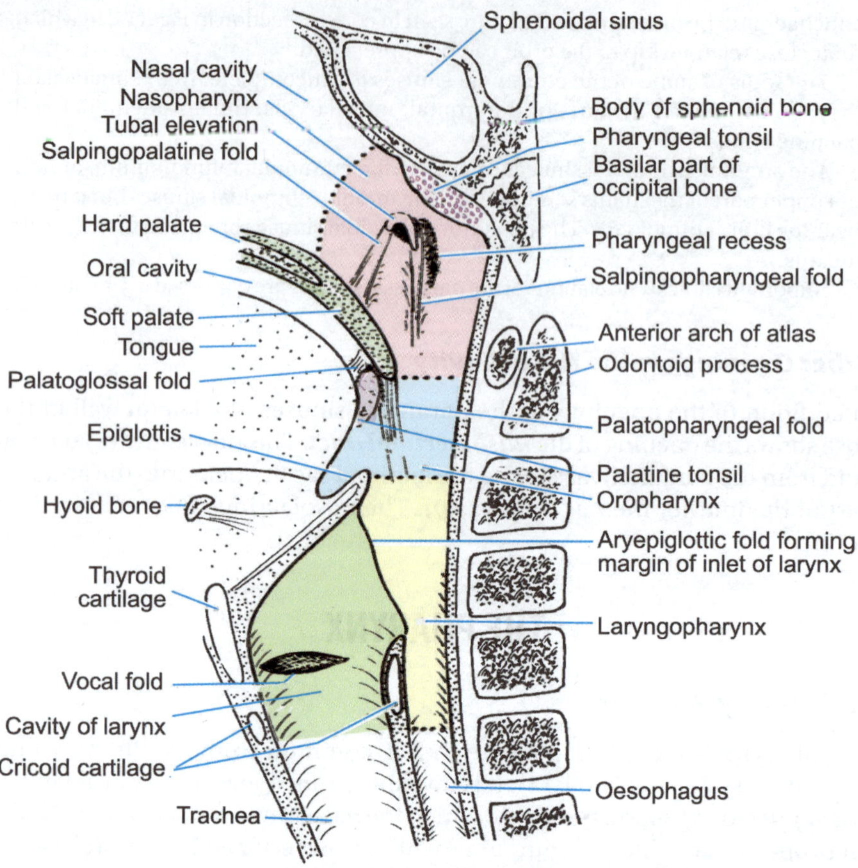

Fig. 11.12 Schematic median section through the pharynx (and neighbouring structures to show its lateral wall. The limits of the subdivisions of the pharynx are indicated in dotted lines.

The Nasal Part of the Pharynx

On each lateral wall of the nasopharynx there is an opening which leads into the auditory tube. This tube connects the nasopharynx to the middle ear. Above and behind the opening of the auditory tube the wall of the nasopharynx shows a bulging called the ***tubal elevation***. This elevation is produced by the projecting end of a cartilage which forms part of the wall of the auditory tube. A fold of mucous membrane starting at the tubal elevation passes down the pharyngeal wall. This is the ***salpingopharyngeal fold*** and is produced by a muscle called the salpingopharyngeus. Another mucosal fold passes from the tubal elevation to the soft palate. This is the ***salpingopalatine fold***. Behind the tubal elevation the wall of the nasopharynx shows a depression called the ***pharyngeal recess***. The nasopharynx has a roof congruous with the posterior end of the roof of the nasal cavity. The roof and posterior wall of the nasopharynx form a continuous curve which rests on the posterior part of the body of the sphenoid, the basilar part of the occipital bone, and the anterior arch of the atlas.

The mucosa of the median part of the roof shows a bulging produced by a mass of lymphoid tissue. This lymphoid tissue constitutes the ***pharyngeal tonsil***. (When enlarged, the pharyngeal tonsils are referred to as ***adenoids***). Some lymphoid tissue is also present behind the opening of the auditory tube. This collection of lymphoid tissue is called the ***tubal tonsil***.

The Oral Part of the Pharynx

The oropharynx lies in front of the second cervical vertebra and the upper part of the third. The only features to be noted on its lateral walls are the ***palatopharyngeal folds*** (or arches). These stretch from the uvula to the lateral wall of the pharynx and enclose the palatopharyngeus muscle. The palatine tonsil lies between the palatoglossal and palatopharngeal folds. The depression in which the palatine tonsil lies is called the ***tonsilar sinus***. The palatine tonsil is considered later in this Chapter.

Laryngeal Part of Pharynx

The laryngeal part of the pharynx lies in front of the third to sixth cervical vertebrae. Its relationships can be properly appreciated after the larynx has been studied. They are given here for sake of completeness].

In terms of laryngeal cartilages the upper end of the laryngeal part of the pharynx corresponds to the upper end of the epiglottis; and its lower end lies at the caudal border of the cricoid cartilage. In other words it is coextensive with the larynx. The anterior wall of the laryngeal part of the pharynx is shown in Fig. 11.25. Its upper part is formed by the inlet of the larynx; and below by the posterior surfaces of the arytenoid and cricoid cartilages. Lateral to the inlet of the larynx the mucosa shows a depression called the ***piriform recess*** or fossa (Fig. 11.25).

Walls of the Pharynx

The walls of the pharynx are constituted mainly by muscles. The muscles of the pharynx are considered below. The layer of muscle is covered on the outside by a layer of fascia called the ***buccopharyngeal fascia*** (Fig. 11.13). This

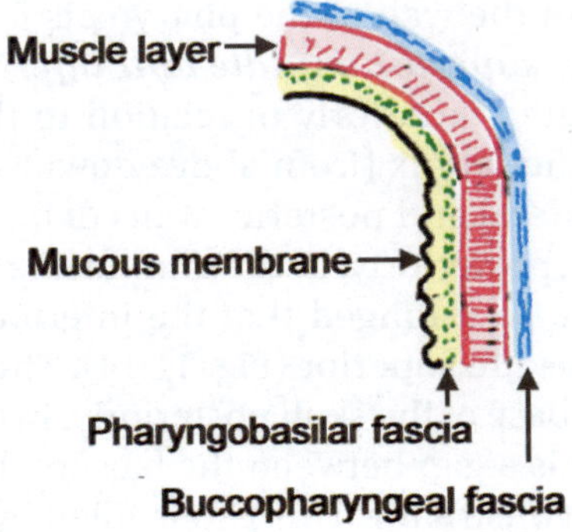

Fig. 11.13 Layers in the wall of the pharynx.

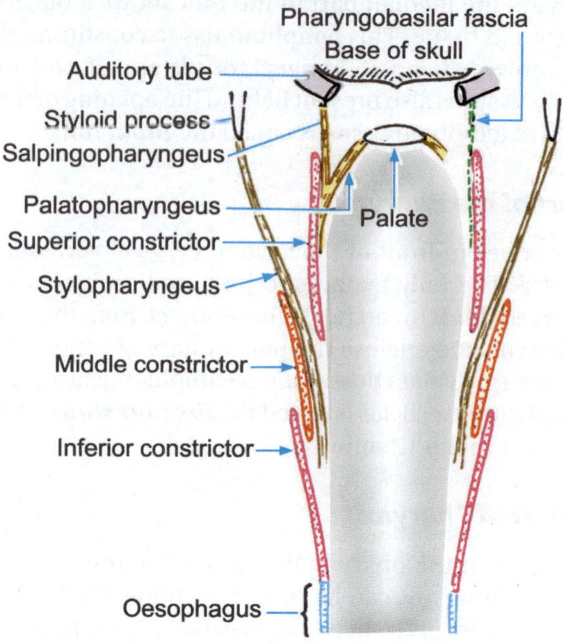

Fig. 11.14 Schematic coronal section to show the arrangement of muscles of the pharynx.

fascia extends forwards on to the buccinator (and hence its name). Between the mucous membrane and the layer of muscle there is a thicker fascia called the ***pharyngobasilar*** fascia. This fascia is so called because it is thickest in its upper part where it bridges across a gap between the muscle layer of the pharynx and the base of the skull (Figs. 11.14, 11.15).

MUSCLES OF THE PHARYNX

Preliminary Remarks

The muscular basis of the wall of the pharynx is formed mainly by three pairs of ***constrictors, superior, middle and inferior***. The origins of the constrictors are situated anteriorly in relation to the posterior openings of the nose, mouth and larynx (from above downwards). From here their fibres pass into the lateral and posterior walls of the pharynx, the fibres of the two sides meeting posteriorly, in the middle line in a fibrous raphe. The three constrictors are so arranged that the inferior overlaps the middle, which in turn overlaps the superior (Fig. 11.14). The fibres of the superior constrictor reach the base of the skull posteriorly, in the middle line. On the sides, however, there is a gap between the base of the skull and the upper edge of the superior constrictor. This gap is filled by the upper part of the pharyngobasilar fascia which is thickened in this situation. The lower edge of

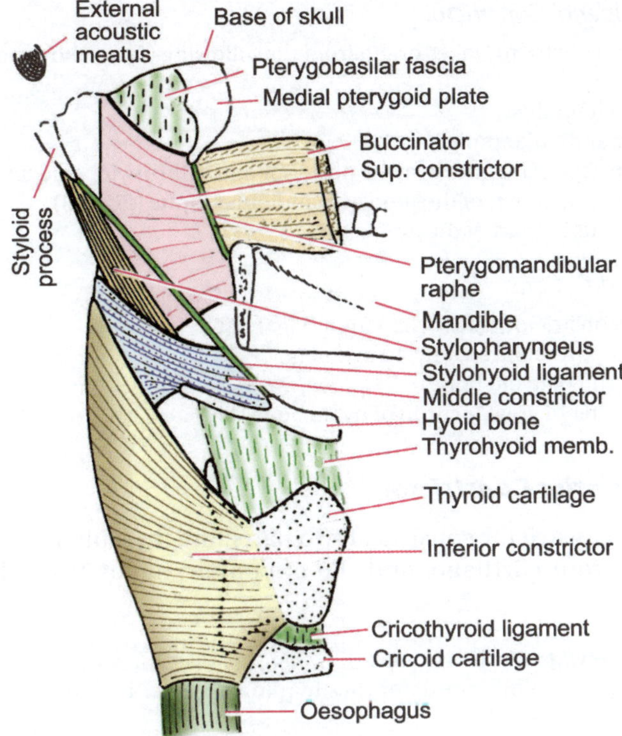

Fig. 11.15 Muscles of the pharynx seen from the lateral side.

the inferior constrictor becomes continuous with the circular muscle of the oesophagus. The constrictors of the pharynx are considered in detail below.

In addition to the constrictors, the pharynx has three muscles the fibres of which run longitudinally. These are the ***stylopharyngeus,*** the ***palatopharyngeus*** and the ***salpingopharyngeus***.

1. The ***stylopharyngeus*** arises from the styloid process. It passes through the gap between the superior and middle constrictors to run downwards on the inner surface of the middle and inferior constrictors.
2. The fibres of the ***palatopharyngeus*** descend from the sides of the palate and run longitudinally on the inner aspect of the constrictors.
3. The ***salpingopharyngeus*** descends from the auditory tube to merge with the palatopharyngeus.

CONSTRICTORS OF THE PHARYNX

Origin of Constrictors of the Pharynx

As stated above the origin of the constrictors is situated anteriorly. We will first consider the origin of each constrictor and then consider the insertion which is common to all three of them.

Origin of Superior Constrictor

The superior constrictor takes origin from the following (from above downwards) (Fig. 11.16):

1. Pterygoid hamulus.
2. Pterygomandibular raphe.
3. Medial surface of mandible, at the posterior end of the mylohyoid line (i.e., near the lower attachment of the pterygomandibular raphe (Fig. 5.5).
4. Side of posterior part of the tongue.

Origin of Middle Constrictor

The middle constrictor takes origin from (Fig. 11.16):

1. The lower part of the stylohyoid ligament.
2. Lesser cornu of hyoid bone,
3. Upper border of greater cornu of hyoid bone (Fig. 5.8).

Origin of Inferior Constrictor

The inferior constrictor consists of two parts: the thyropharyngeus arising from the thyroid cartilage, and the cricopharyngeus from the cricoid cartilage.

The ***thyropharyngeus*** arises from:

1. The oblique line on lamina of the thyroid cartilage, including the inferior tubercle.
2. A tendinous band that crosses the cricothyroid muscle (and is attached above to the inferior tubercle of the thyroid cartilage and below to the cricoid cartilage).
3. The inferior cornu of the thyroid cartilage.

The ***cricopharyngeus*** arises from the cricoid cartilage behind the origin of the cricothyroid muscle.

Insertion of Constrictors of Pharynx

All the constrictors of the pharynx are inserted into a median raphe on the posterior wall of the pharynx. The upper end of the raphe reaches the base of the skull where it is attached to the pharyngeal tubercle on the basilar part of the occipital bone.

There is a gap between the upper edge of the superior constrictor and the base of the skull. It gives passage to the auditory tube and is closed by the pharyngobasilar fascia. Two small muscles, the tensor palati and the levator palati are seen in relation to the gap (1.8, 11.17).

Actions of Muscles of the Pharynx

The muscles of the pharynx play an important part in deglutition.

Food entering the oropharynx is carried downwards by successive contraction of the superior, middle and inferior constrictors. The stylopharyngeus,

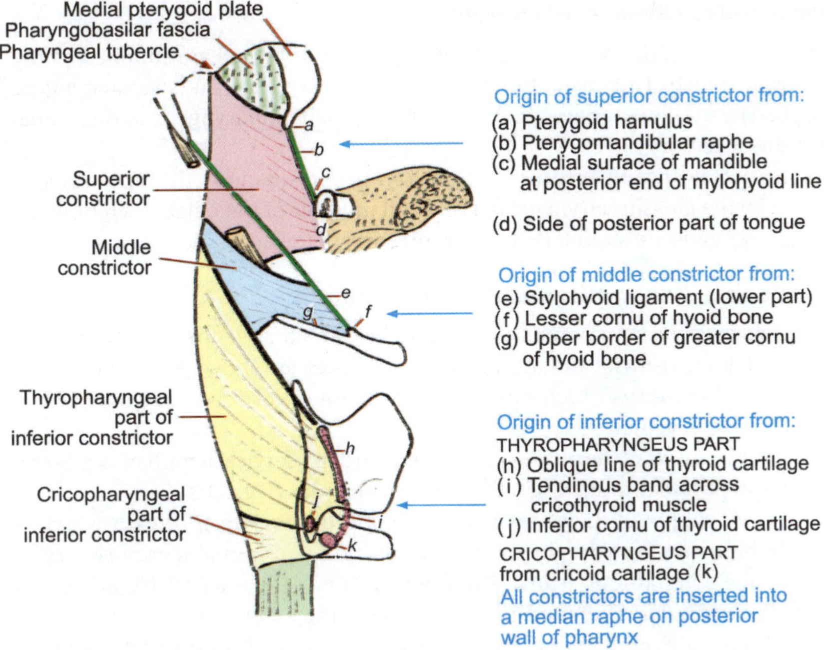

Fig. 11.16 Diagram showing details of origin of the constrictors of the pharynx.

salpingopharyngeus and the palatopharyngeus help by pulling the pharynx upwards and by shortening it. It is usually said that the cricopharyngeal part of the inferior constrictor is 'sphincteric' in contrast to the thyropharyngeal part which is 'propulsive'. Incoordination in the action of the two parts may result in the formation of a diverticulum on the posterior wall of the pharynx at the junction of the two parts.

The inner surface of the superior constrictor is lined by a band of muscle fibres arising from the sides of the palate. These fibres form the ***palatopharyngeal sphinc-ter*** which produces a ridge (of Passavant) on the pharyngeal wall at the junction of nasopharynx with the oropharynx. Acting along with the soft palate the palatopharyngeal sphincter closes the pharyngeal isthmus pre-venting food from entering the nasopharynx.

Relations of Constrictors of Pharynx

The constrictors of the pharynx are related to numerous structures. These are shown in Fig. 11.17. Also see Fig. 1.8.

Other relations not shown in the figures cited are as follows. The constrictors are related posteriorly to the vertebral column, the prevertebral muscles and fascia. Their external surface is covered by the buccopharyngeal fascia, by the pharyngeal plexus of nerves and some lymph nodes. The carotid sheath and its contents lie lateral to the constrictors. The internal surface of the constrictors is lined by the pharyngobasilar fascia, and by longitudinal fibres of the stylopharyngeus and the palatopharyngeus.

Nerve Supply of Muscles of Pharynx

The constrictors of the pharynx, and the salpingopharyngeus are supplied by the pharyngeal branch of the vagus, through the pharyngeal plexus. The stylopharyngeus is supplied by the glossopharyngeal nerve, and the palatopharyngeus by the cranial part of the accessory nerve.

[Note two points of interest. 1. The stylopharyngeus is the only muscle supplied by the glossopharyngeal nerve. 2. All muscles of the palate including the palatopharyngeus are supplied by the cranial part of the accessory nerve.]

Blood Vessels, Lymphatics and Nerves of Pharynx

The pharynx receives numerous small branches which arise from the ascending pharyngeal, lingual, facial and maxillary arteries. They are shown in Fig. 11.18. The veins drain into a plexus which surrounds the pharynx and drains into the internal jugular and facial veins.

The lymph vessels of the pharynx drain into the deep cervical lymph nodes. Some of the lymph passes through the retropharyngeal nodes (Fig. 63.3).

The nerve supply of the pharynx is through the ***pharyngeal plexus*** which is formed by branches from the glossopharyngeal, vagus and cranial accessory nerves; and from the sympathetic trunk. The fibres of the cranial accessory nerve run through the vagus and (as stated above) constitute the main supply of the muscles of the pharynx, including that of the soft palate. Sensory fibres travel through the glossopharyngeal and vagus nerves. Some sensory fibres also travel through the lesser palatine branch of the pterygopalatine ganglion.

Clinical correlations of the pharynx are discussed in Chapter 15.

THE PALATINE TONSILS

The palatine tonsils are masses of lymphoid tissue. Each palatine tonsil (right or left) lies in the tonsilar sinus on the lateral wall of the oropharynx (Figs. 11.2, 11.12). This sinus is bounded by the palatoglossal fold in front and the palatopharyngeal fold behind. Relative to the surface of the body the palatine tonsils lies just in front of and above the angle of the mandible.

The medial surface of the palatine tonsil is covered by mucous membrane which is continuous with that of the palatoglossal folds; and below with the mucous membrane on the tongue. Deep to the mucosa the lymphoid tissue of the tonsil extends upwards into the soft palate and downwards into the tongue. The mucosa over the upper part of the tonsil dips into the substance of the tonsil forming a deep ***intratonsillar cleft*** (Fig. 11.19). A number of smaller recesses called the ***tonsilar crypts*** are also present. The lateral surface of the tonsil is covered by fascia which forms a ***capsule*** for it and separates it from the superior constrictor of the pharynx.

The right and left palatine tonsils form the most conspicuous parts of a ring of lymphoid tissue ***(Waldeyer's ring)*** present near the oropharyngeal isthmus (Fig. 11.20). The ring is completed below by the lingual tonsil and above by the pharyngeal and tubal tonsils.

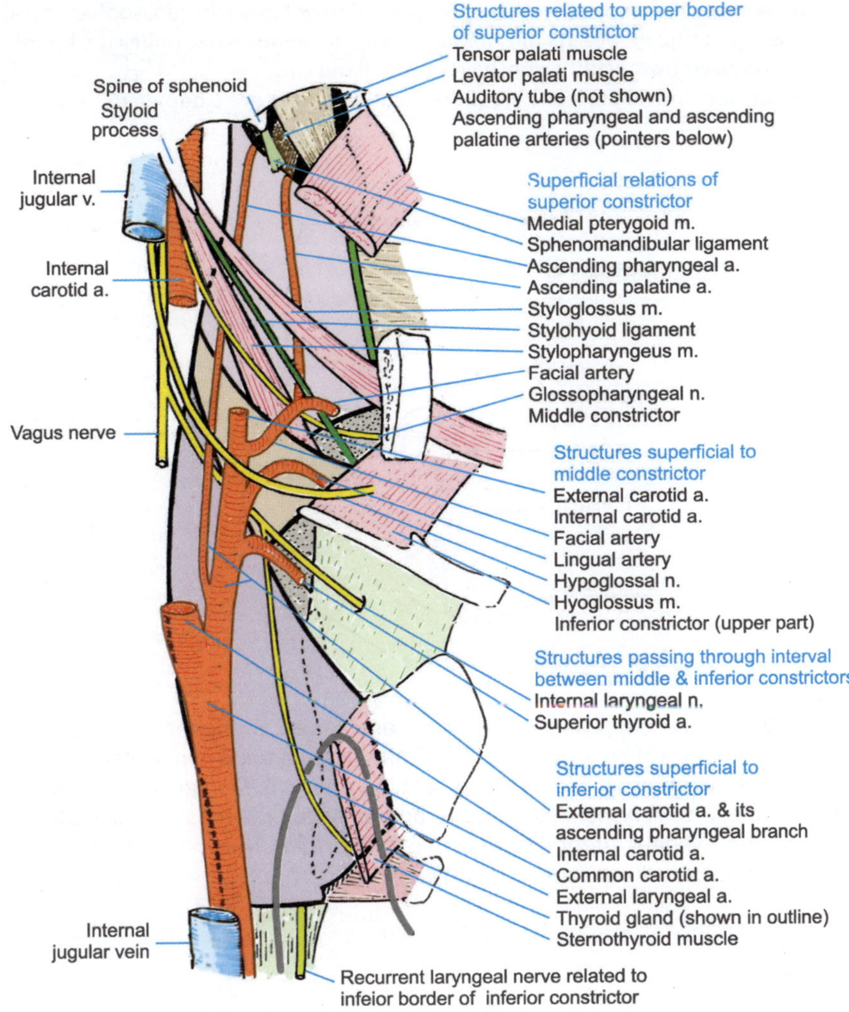

Fig. 11.17 Diagram showing the relations of the contrictors of the pharynx.

The arteries supplying the tonsil are shown in Fig. 11.18. The chief supply is through the tonsilar branch of the facial artery. This artery reaches the lower part of the tonsil by piercing the superior constrictor of the pharynx. Note that the ascending palatine branch of the facial artery (and sometimes the facial artery itself) is separated from the tonsil only by the superior constrictor muscle. It can be injured in operations for removal of the tonsil ***(tonsillectomy)***.

Veins from the tonsil may join a vein descending from the soft palate across its lateral side (between the capsule and the superior constrictor). This is the external palatine or paratonsilar vein (Fig. 11.19). It can be injured during tonsillectomy and can cause troublesome bleeding. Some veins from the tonsil may pierce the superior constrictor muscle to end in the facial vein or in the pharyngeal plexus of veins.

The sensory nerves supplying the tonsil are derived from the glossopharyngeal and lesser palatine nerves. As the glossopharyngeal nerve also supplies the middle ear, pain caused by tonsillitis may be referred to the ear.

For further clinical correlations of the palatine tonsils see Chapter 15.

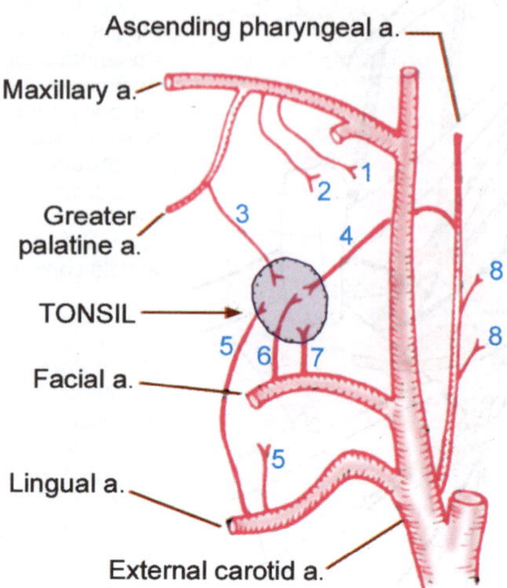

Fig. 11.18 Arteries supplying the pharynx and tonsil. Branches to the pharynx arise from: 1. Artery of pterygoid canal. 2. Pharyngeal branch of maxillary artery. 3. Greater palatine artery. 4. Descending palatine artery. 5. Dorsal lingual branches of lingual artery. 6, 7. Ascending palatine and tonsillar branches of facial artery. 8. Ascending pharyngeal artery. The outline of the tonsil is shown in dotted line, and branches to the tonsil are seen entering it.

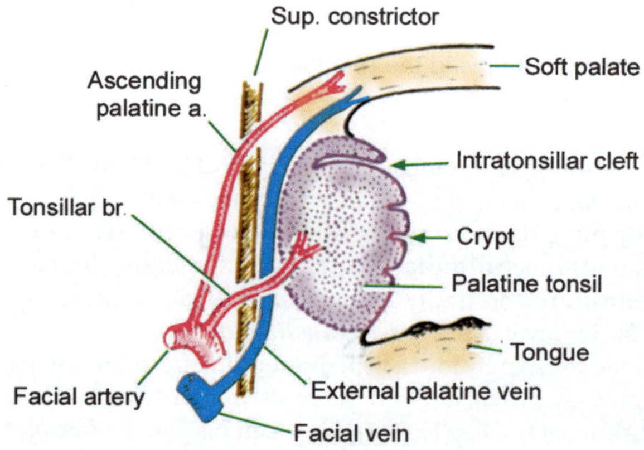

Fig. 11.19 Coronal section through the palatine tonsil. For a transverse section see Fig. 5.11.

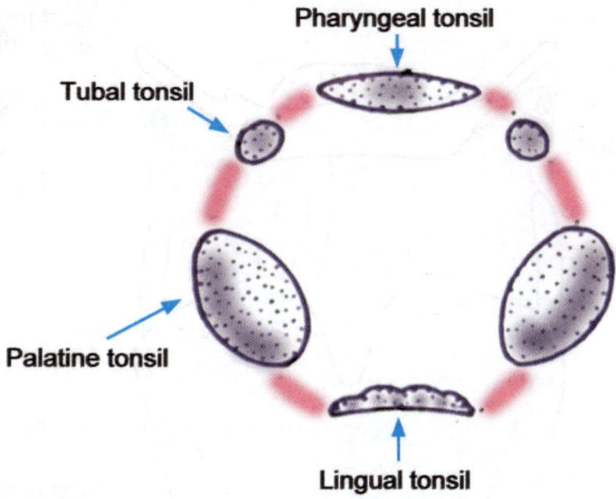

Fig. 11.20 Waldeyer's ring of lymphoid tissue.

THE LARYNX

Introductory Remarks about The Larynx

The larynx is a space that communicates above with the laryngeal part of the pharynx, and below with the trachea. Apart from being a respiratory passage the larynx is the organ where voice is produced. Near the middle of the larynx there are a pair of ***vocal folds*** (one right and one left) that project into the laryngeal cavity. Between these folds there is an interval called the ***rima glottidis.*** The rima is fairly wide in ordinary breathing. When we wish to speak the two vocal folds come close together narrowing the rima glottidis. Expired air passing through the narrow gap causes the vocal folds to vibrate resulting in the production of sound. Variation in the loudness of sound is produced by the force with which air is expelled through the rima glottidis. Variation in pitch is achieved by stretching of the vocal folds to different degrees. The difference in the voice of a man and that of a woman (or of a child) is due to the fact that the vocal folds are considerably longer in the male adult. The structure of the larynx has to be studied keeping these facts in view.

The larynx has a rigid framework made up of cartilages. The cartilages are joined to one another by ligaments. A number of muscles are attached to the cartilages. They produce movements of the vocal folds that are necessary for speech. The cartilages, ligaments and muscles are covered on the inside by mucous membrane that is continuous above with that of the laryngeal part of the pharynx and below with that of the trachea.

Cartilages of The Larynx

These are seen from the front in Fig. 11.21; from the lateral side in Fig. 11.22A; from above in Fig. 11.22B and from behind in Fig. 11.23A. There are three

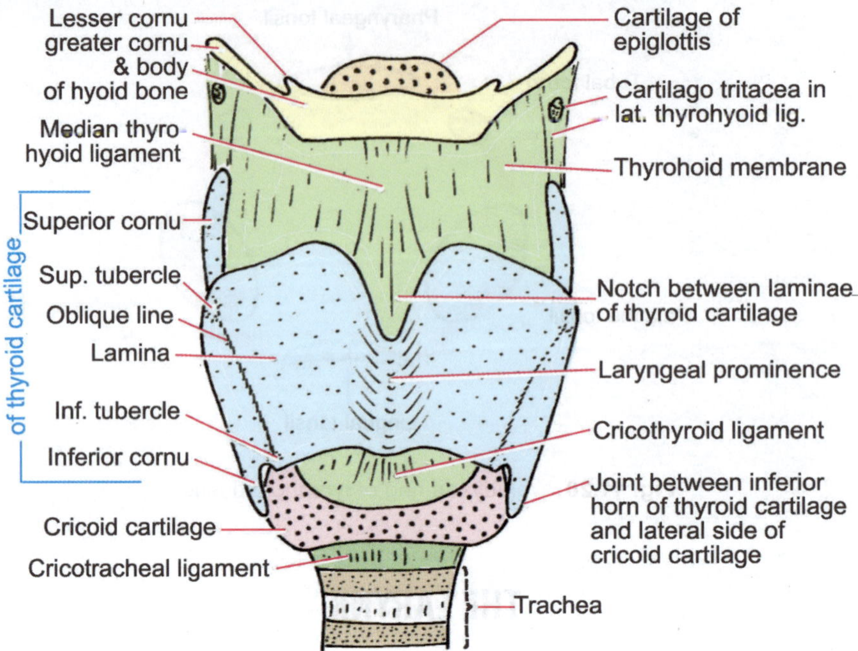

Fig. 11.21 Cartilages of the larynx as seen from the front.

unpaired cartilages: these are the thyroid cartilage, the cricoid cartilage, and the cartilage of the epiglottis. The paired cartilages are the right and left arytenoid cartilages; and the corniculate and cuneiform cartilages which are small nodules.

Thyroid Cartilage

The thyroid cartilage consists of right and left ***laminae.*** Each lamina is roughly quadrilateral (Fig. 11.22A). As seen in Fig. 11.22B the laminae are placed obliquely relative to the midline: their posterior borders are far apart but the anterior borders approach each other at an angle that is about 90° in the male and about 120 degrees in in the female. The lower parts of the anterior borders of the right and left laminae fuse and form a median projection called the ***laryngeal prominence*** (Fig. 11.21). The upper parts of the anterior borders (of the laminae) do not meet: they are separated by a ***notch.*** The posterior margins of the laminae are prolonged upwards to form a projection called the ***superior cornu***; and downwards to form a smaller projection called the ***inferior cornu***. The medial side of each inferior cornu articulates with the corresponding lateral aspect of the cricoid cartilage. The lateral surface of each lamina is marked by an ***oblique line*** that runs downwards and forwards. At its upper and lower ends the oblique line ends in projections called the ***superior*** and ***inferior tubercles***, respectively (Figs. 11.21, 11.22A).

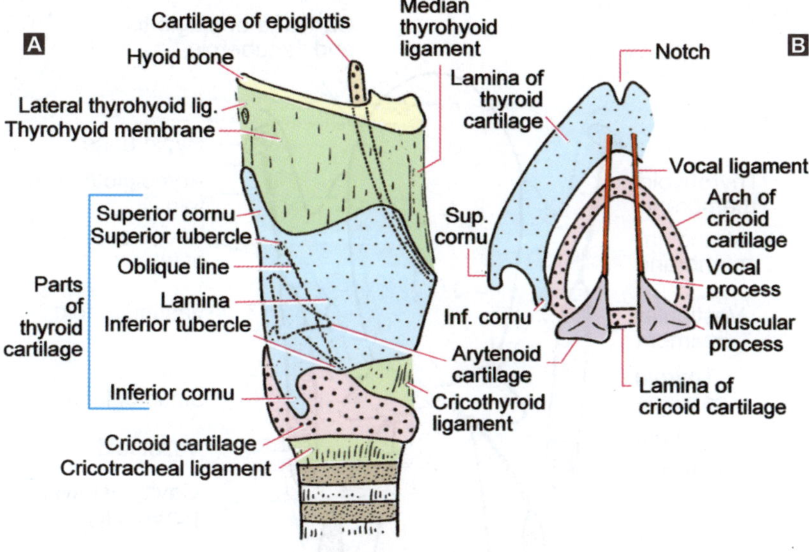

Fig. 11.22 Cartilages of the larynx. A. Seen from the lateral side. B. Seen from above.

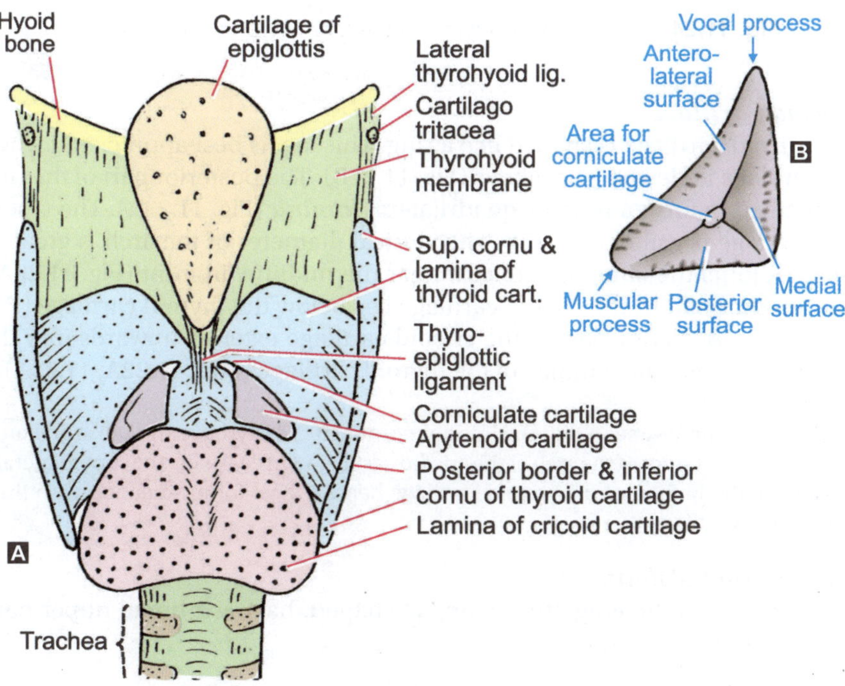

Fig. 11.23 A. Cartilages of the larynx seen from behind. B. Arytenoid cartilage of the left side seen from above.

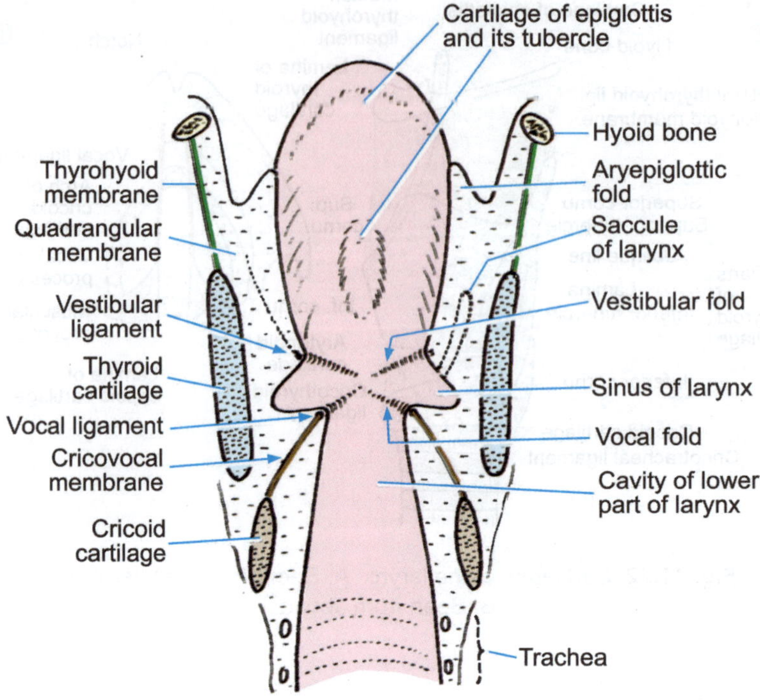

Fig. 11.24 Coronal section through the larynx viewed from behind.

Cricoid Cartilage

The cricoid cartilage is shaped like a ring. This fact is best appreciated when the cartilage is viewed from above (Fig. 11.22B). The posterior part of the ring is enlarged to form a roughly quadrilateral ***lamina*** (Fig. 11.23A). The rest of the cartilage is called the ***arch.*** The vertical diameter of the arch is greatest where it joins the lamina, and least near the midline, in front (Fig. 11.22A). The anterior part of the cricoid cartilage lies below the thyroid cartilage (Fig. 11.21). The posterior part of the cricoid cartilage extends upwards into the interval between the laminae of the thyroid cartilage (Figs. 11.22A, 11.23A).

We have already seen that the inferior cornua of the thyroid cartilage articulate with the lateral sides of the arch of the cricoid cartilage. On each side the superolateral aspect of the lamina of the cricoid cartilage bears a facet for articulation with the arytenoid cartilage.

Cartilage of Epiglottis

The cartilage of the epiglottis is tongue shaped, having a broad upper part, and a narrow lower end.

The upper broad part lies just behind the tongue. The lower end is attached to the angle formed by the anterior margins of the laminae of the thyroid cartilage, just below the notch.

The lower part of the epiglottis shows a backward projection in the midline. This projection is called the ***tubercle*** of the epiglottis.

Arytenoid Cartilage

Each arytenoid cartilage (right or left) is pyramidal (Fig. 11.23B). It has a ***base*** (below) which articulates with the cricoid cartilage; an ***apex*** which is directed upwards and to which the corniculate cartilage is attached; and three ***surfaces, medial, posterior*** and ***anterolateral.*** The anteroinferior angle of the cartilage is prolonged forwards to form the ***vocal process.*** The inferolateral angle is enlarged to form the ***muscular process.***

Corniculate and Cuneiform Cartilages

The ***corniculate cartilage*** is small and conical; it is present near the apex of the corresponding arytenoid cartilage to which it is attached.

The ***cuneiform cartilages*** are small nodules present near the corniculate cartilages, within the aryepiglottic folds.

Ligaments and Membranes of Larynx

1. The thyroid cartilage (upper border) is connected to the hyoid bone (body and greater cornu) by the ***thyrohyoid membrane*** (Figs. 11.21, 11.22A). The membrane is thickened near the midline to form the ***median thyrohyoid ligament***; and along its lateral edges to form the ***lateral thyrohyoid ligaments.*** On each side the lateral thyrohyoid ligament is attached, below, to the tip of the greater cornu of the thyroid cartilage; and, above, to the posterior end of the greater cornu of the hyoid bone. A small nodule of cartilage, called the ***cartilago triticea*** is frequently seen in the lateral thyrohyoid ligament.
2. Near the middle line, in front, the lower border of the thyroid cartilage is attached to the arch of the cricoid cartilage by the ***anterior cricothyroid ligament*** (Fig. 11.21).
3. The lower margin of the cricoid cartilage is attached to the trachea through the ***cricotracheal ligament*** (Fig. 11.21).
4. The cartilage of the epiglottis is attached to the thyroid cartilage by the ***thyroepiglottic ligament*** (Fig. 11.23A). This attachment is on the posterior aspect of the thyroid cartilage, on the angle, just below the notch. The cartilage of the epiglottis is attached to the hyoid bone by the ***hyoepiglottic ligament*** (Fig. 11.26A).
5. The joints between the arytenoid cartilages and the cricoid cartilage; and the joints between the inferior cornuae of the thyroid cartilage and the lateral sides of the cricoid cartilage, are synovial. They are surrounded by joint capsules.
6. The cricovocal membranes and the vocal ligaments are described below.

INTERIOR OF THE LARYNX

The essential features to be seen in the interior of the larynx are best appreciated by examining a coronal section (Fig. 11.24). Almost midway between the upper and lower ends of the larynx, two pairs of mucosal folds project into its cavity. The upper pair are the right and left ***vestibular folds.*** The lower pair are the right and left ***vocal folds.*** The part of the laryngeal cavity lying above the vestibular folds is called the ***vestibule.*** The narrow recess between the levels of the vestibular and vocal folds (on either side) is called the ***sinus*** or

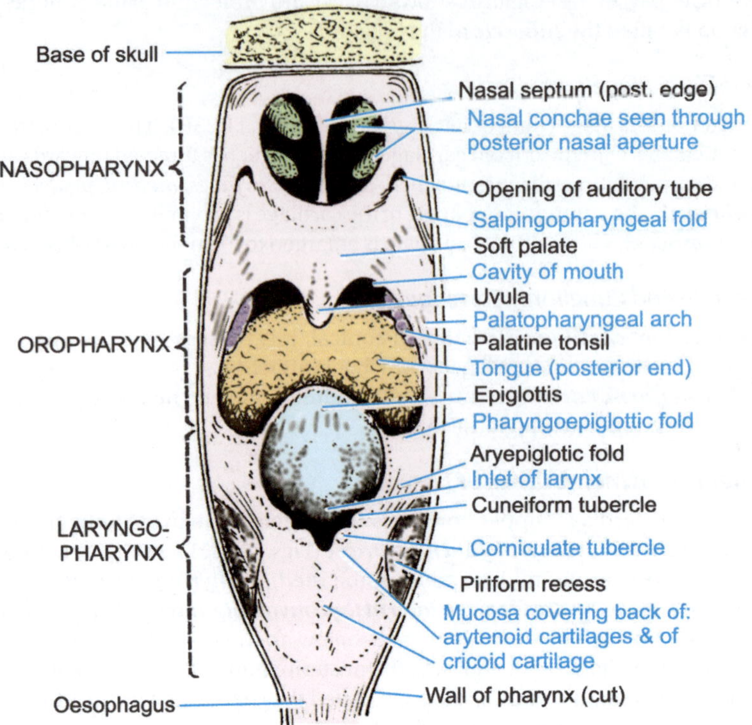

Fig. 11.25 Openings in the anterior wall of the larynx seen from behind.

ventricle of the larynx. The lower part of the cavity, below the vocal folds is not given any special name.

The upper aperture of the larynx is called its ***inlet***, or ***aditus.*** The aperture is directed backwards and a little upwards (so that its anterior margin lies distinctly higher than the posterior margin). It is bounded (Fig. 11.25) in front by the mucous membrane covering the epiglottis; behind by a fold of mucous membrane that covers the two arytenoid cartilages; and on either side by the ***aryepiglottic folds.*** These folds are made of mucous membrane that pass from the sides of the epiglottis (in front) to the arytenoid cartilages. The corniculate and cuneiform cartilages lie within the aryepiglottic folds.

Each vestibular fold encloses a bundle of fibres that constitute the ***vestibular ligament*** (Figs. 11.24, 11.26).

The ligament is attached, in front, to the angle of the thyroid cartilage; and, behind, to the anterolateral surface of the arytenoid cartilage. The fissure separating the right and left vestibular folds is called the ***rima vestibuli*** (shown but not labelled in Fig. 11.28).

Each vocal fold contains a bundle of elastic fibres that constitute the ***vocal ligament*** (Figs. 11.24, 11.26). The ligament is attached in front to the angle of

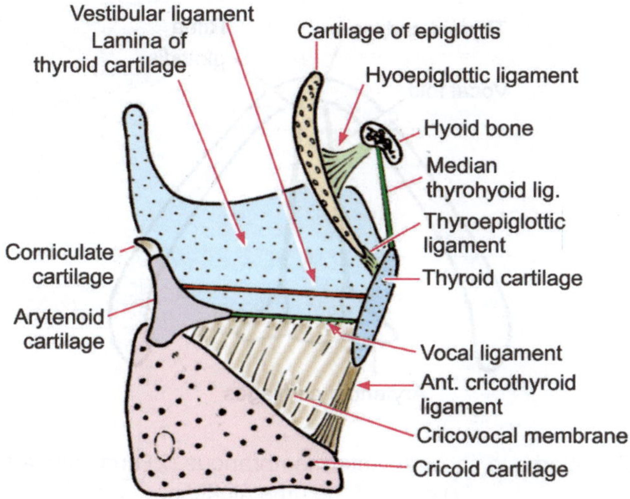

Fig. 11.26 Lateral view of cartilages and ligaments of the larynx. One lamina of the thyroid cartilage has been removed.

the thyroid cartilage (below the attachment of the vestibular ligament); and behind to the vocal process of the arytenoid cartilage (Figs. 11.22B, 11.26).

Each vocal ligament is really the free upper edge of the ***cricovocal membrane.*** This membrane is attached below to the arch of the cricoid cartilage. From here the membrane passes upwards and medially (Fig. 11.24) to be attached (in front) to the thyroid cartilage, and (behind) to the arytenoid cartilage (Fig. 11.26). Because of the attachment to the thyroid cartilage the membrane is also referred to as the ***lateral cricothyroid ligament.*** The right and left cricovocal membranes are continuous (by their anterior edges) with the anterior cricothyroid ligament (Fig. 11.24). The cricovocal membranes constitute the lower parts of a fibroelastic membrane that lies deep to the mucous membrane of the larynx. The upper part of this membrane lies in the aryepiglottic fold: this part is called the ***quadrangular membrane*** (Fig. 11.24).

The function of voice production (by vibration) demands that the vocal folds be firm and of uniform thickness. This aim is achieved by close adherence of the lining epithelium to the vocal ligaments, and by the absence of blood vessels. As a result the vocal foldswithstand the stress of repeated and intense vibration.

The right and left vocal folds are separated by the anterior or ***intermembranous*** part of a fissure called the ***rima glottidis.*** The posterior part of the fissure lies between the two arytenoid cartilages and is, therefore, called the ***intercartilaginous*** part (Fig. 11.27).

The shape of the rima varies in different phases of respiration and of phonation (see below).

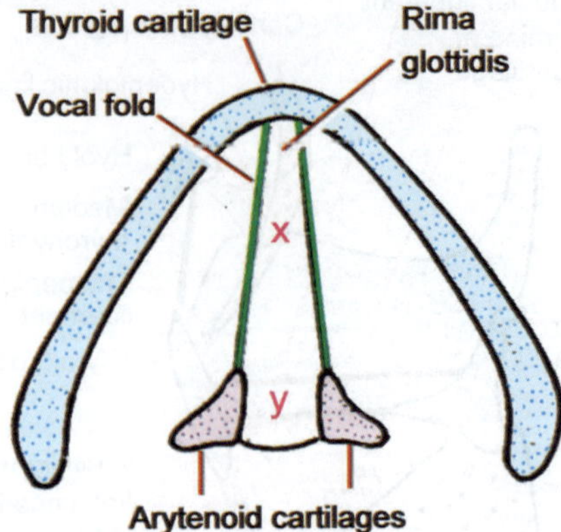

Fig. 11.27 Scheme to show the intermembranous (**x**) and intercartilaginous (**y**) parts of the rima glottidis.

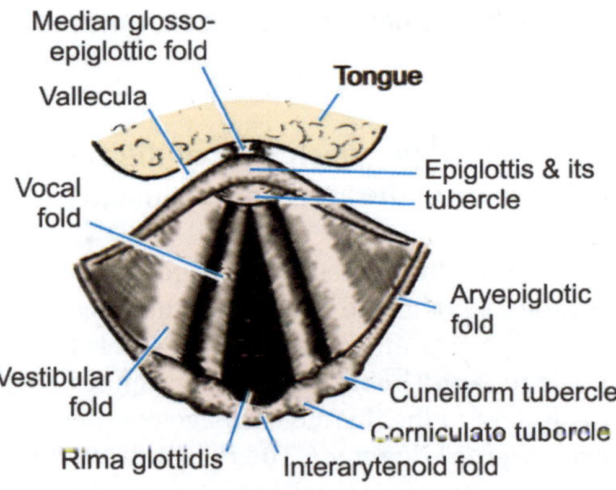

Fig. 11.28 Some features of the larynx as seen through a laryngoscope (i.e., from above). The gap between the two vestibular folds is the rima vestibuli.

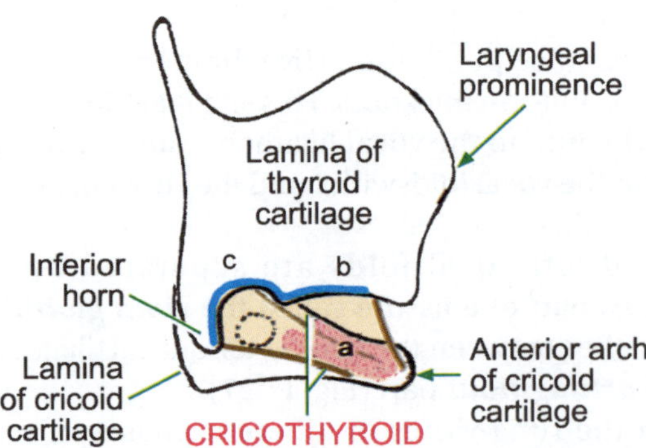

Fig. 11.29 Scheme to show attachments of the cricothyroid muscle.

We have seen that the part of the cavity of the larynx lying between the vocal and vestibular folds of each side is called the sinus or ventricle of the larynx. A pouch like diverticulum arises from the anterior part of each sinus. This pouch is called the ***saccule*** of the larynx (Fig. 11.24). It passes upwards lateral to the vestibular fold, and medial to the lamina of the thyroid cartilage. The size of the saccule is variable.

(As a point of interest it may be noted that the saccule is large in apes. In them it extends through the thyrohyoid membrane into the superficial tissues of the neck which may, therefore, balloon out during phonation).

MUSCLES OF THE LARYNX

The muscles of the larynx are extrinsic and intrinsic.

The ***extrinsic muscles*** are those in which one end of the muscle is attached to a cartilage of the larynx whereas the other end is attached elsewhere. These muscles raise or lower the larynx as a whole during deglutition. The extrinsic muscles include the sternothyroid and thyrohyoid muscles and the inferior constrictor of the pharynx. Some muscles attached to the hyoid bone can raise the larynx indirectly.

The ***intrinsic muscles*** are confined to the larynx. They may be classified in accordance with their actions as follows.

a. ***Muscles that increase or decrease tension of the vocal folds***:
   These are the cricothyroid, the thyroarytenoid and the vocalis.
b. ***Muscles that open or close the glottis***:
   These are the posterior cricoarytenoid, the lateral cricoarytenoid and the transverse arytenoid.
c. ***Muscles that open or close the inlet of the larynx***.
   These are the oblique arytenoids, the aryepiglottic and thyroepiglottic muscles.

Cricothyroid Muscle

The cricothyroid is the only intrinsic muscle of the larynx that is seen on its outer aspect (Fig. 11.29). It arises from the anterior part of the outer surface of the cricoid cartilage (a). Its fibres run upwards and backwards to be inserted into the thyroid cartilage (on the lower border of the posterior part of the lamina) (b); and into the inferior cornu (c). It is subdivided into so called straight (anterior) and oblique (posterior) parts but the direction of fibres in both parts is oblique. The action of this muscle is described along with that of the thyroarytenoid muscle below.

Thyroarytenoid Muscle

The thyroarytenoid arises from the thyroid cartilage (Fig. 11.30) from the posterior aspect of the angle between the laminae (d). The fibres pass backwards to be inserted into the anterolateral surface of the arytenoid cartilage (e). The deeper fibres of the thyroarytenoid muscle form a band that runs along the vocal ligament, just lateral to it. This band is called the ***vocalis***. All its fibres are attached behind to the arytenoid cartilage (anterolateral surface), but anteriorly they are attached to the vocal ligament at varying distances along its length.

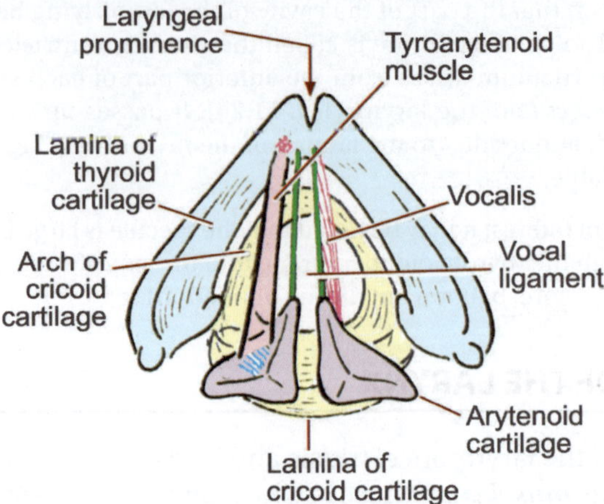

Fig. 11.30 Scheme showing attachments of the thyroarytenoid muscle.

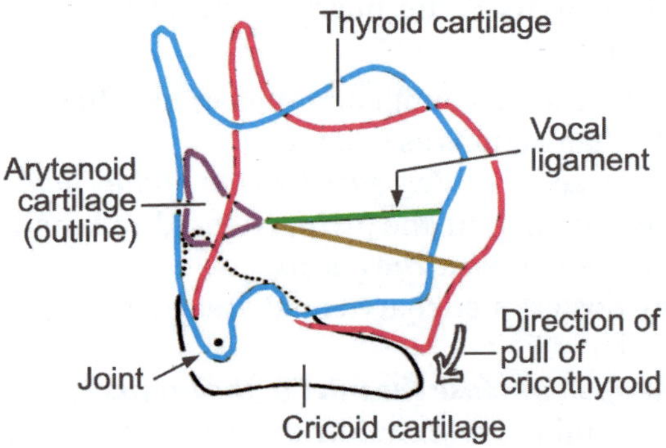

Fig. 11.31 Diagram to illustrate the action of the cricothyroid muscle.

Actions of Cricothyroid and Thyroarytenoid

The cricothyroid muscles lengthen the vocal folds and make them tense. The thyroarytenoids have the opposite action.

To understand how they do so the following facts may be considered. The vocal folds stretch between the vocal process of the arytenoid cartilage (behind) and the angle of the thyroid cartilage (in front) (Fig. 11.31).

The arytenoid cartilages are fixed to the cricoid cartilage and move with the latter. The cricoid and thyroid cartilages can move on each other at the joints between the inferior cornua of the thyroid cartilage and the sides of the cricoid cartilage, the axis of movement being transverse and passing through both the joints. When the cricothyroids of the two sides contract, the anterior parts of the thyroid and cricoid cartilages come together as shown in Fig. 11.31. This increases the distance between the two ends of the vocal ligaments thus stretching them and increasing their tension. The thyroarytenoid reverses this movement by directly pulling the arytenoid and thyroid cartilages towards each other.

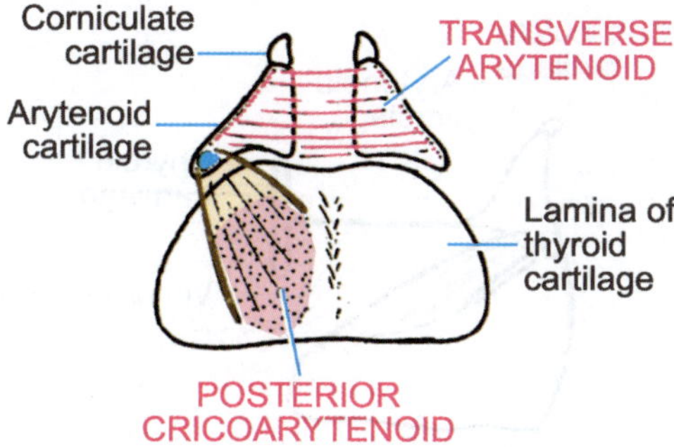

Fig. 11.32 Attachments of the posterior cricoarytenoid muscle.

Action of vocalis: We have seen that the fibres of the vocalis are attached, posteriorly, to the arytenoid cartilage and anteriorly at various distances along the vocal ligament. By contraction of different fibres of the muscle different lengths of the (anterior part of the) vocal ligament can be made tense, thus varying the pitch of the voice. The vocalis has, therefore, been called the 'tuning fork' of the larynx; but its action can be compared, more aptly, to that of a finger placed on a wire of a 'sitar' to vary the length of the vibrating segment.

Posterior Cricoarytenoid Muscle

The posterior cricoarytenoid muscle arises from the (corresponding half) of the posterior aspect of the lamina of the cricoid cartilage (Fig. 11.32). Its fibres pass upwards and laterally to be inserted on the back of the muscular process of the arytenoid cartilage of that side. The muscle is concerned with movements of the vocal folds as described below.

Transverse Arytenoid

The fibres of the transverse arytenoid pass transversely from one arytenoid cartilage to the other, being attached to the muscular process and the lateral border of each cartilage. (See Fig. 11.32, in which the cricoid and arytenoid cartilages are seen from behind). Note that while all the other intrinsic muscles of the larynx are paired the transverse arytenoid is unpaired.

Lateral Cricoarytenoid muscle

The lateral cricoarytenoid muscle arises from the upper border of the arch of the cricoid cartilage. Its fibres pass upwards and backwards to be inserted on the front of the muscular process of the arytenoid cartilage. (See Fig. 11.33. In this figure the cricoid and arytenoid cartilages are seen from the lateral side after removing the lamina of the thyroid cartilage).

The lateral cricoarytenoid muscle is concerned with movements of the vocal folds as described below.

Actions of Posterior and Lateral Cricoarytenoid muscles and of Transverse arytenoid: Movements of the vocal folds aperture called the ***glottis*** (or ***rima glottidis***). The glottis has an anterior (membranous) part placed between the two vocal folds, and a posterior (cartilaginous) part placed between the medial

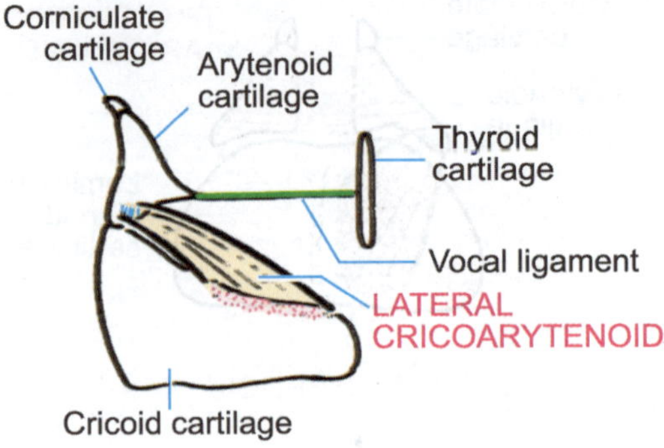

Fig. 11.33 Attachments of the lateral cricoarytenoid muscle.

surfaces of the two arytenoid cartilages (Fig. 11.34A). The size and shape of the glottis undergoes changes during different phases of respiration and of speech. The changes are produced by movements at the joints between the arytenoid and cricoid cartilages. The movements are of two types. One is a rotation of the arytenoid cartilage on a vertical axis. When the muscular process is pulled backwards (and medially) by the posterior cricoarytenoid, the vocal process moves laterally (lateral rotation) abducting the vocal folds. The reverse movement (medial rotation) is brought about by the lateral cricoarytenoid which pulls the muscular process forwards.

The other movement is one in which the arytenoid cartilages glide medially (by action of the transverse arytenoid) or laterally. The movements of rotation and gliding usually take place simultaneously, lateral rotation being associated with lateral gliding and medial rotation with medial gliding.

During quiet respiration (and after death) the glottis is moderately wide, the anterior part being triangular and the posterior part rectangular (Fig. 11.34A). In this position the laryngeal muscles are relaxed. The glottis is narrowest during speech (Fig. 11.34B), both the vocal folds and the arytenoid cartilages being close together. This position is produced mainly by contraction of the transverse arytenoid which pulls the cartilages towards each other. In whispering (Fig. 11.34C) the glottis is closed in its anterior part, because of medial rotation of the arytenoid cartilages by the lateral cricoarytenoid, but the posterior part is wide open. The glottis is widely opened in forced respiration, both the anterior and posterior parts becoming triangular (Fig. 11.34D). This is produced by lateral rotation and lateral gliding of the arytenoid cartilages by contraction of the posterior cricoarytenoid.

Other Muscles of the Larynx

The ***oblique arytenoids*** pass from one arytenoid cartilage to the other (Fig. 11.35), superficial to the transverse arytenoid. The muscles of the two sides cross each other. Each muscle arises from the muscular process of one cartilage and is inserted into the apex of the opposite arytenoid cartilage.

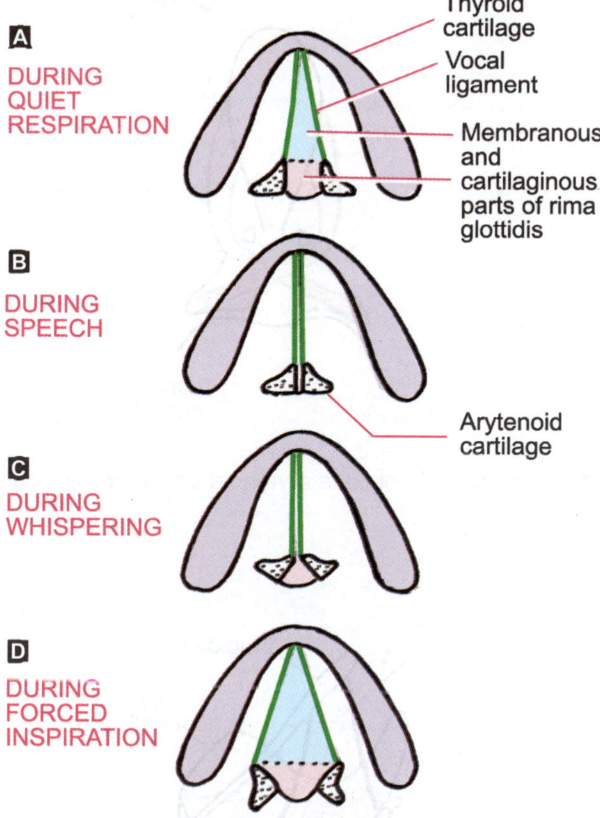

Fig. 11.34 Alterations in shape of the rima glottidis during respiration and during speech.

The ***aryepiglotticus*** is made of some fibres of the oblique arytenoid that pass through the aryepiglottic fold (Fig. 11.35) to the epiglottis. The ***thyroepiglotticus*** is made up of some fibres of the thyroarytenoid which enter the aryepiglottic fold to reach the lateral margin of the epiglottis.

The oblique arytenoids and the aryepiglottic muscles close the inlet of the larynx by drawing the two aryepiglottic folds together. The thyroepiglottic muscles pull the aryepiglottic folds apart to open the inlet.

Vessels and Nerves of Larynx

The ***arteries*** supplying the larynx are branches from the superior and inferior thyroid arteries. The ***veins*** accompany the arteries.

The ***lymphatic drainage*** of the larynx is described in Chapter 13.

The sensory ***innervation*** of the part of the larynx above the vocal folds is by the internal laryngeal nerve. Sensations of taste from the epiglottis also travel through this nerve. The part of the larynx below the vocal folds receives it's sensory innervation through branches of the recurrent laryngeal nerve. Most of the intrinsic muscles of the larynx are supplied by the recurrent laryngeal

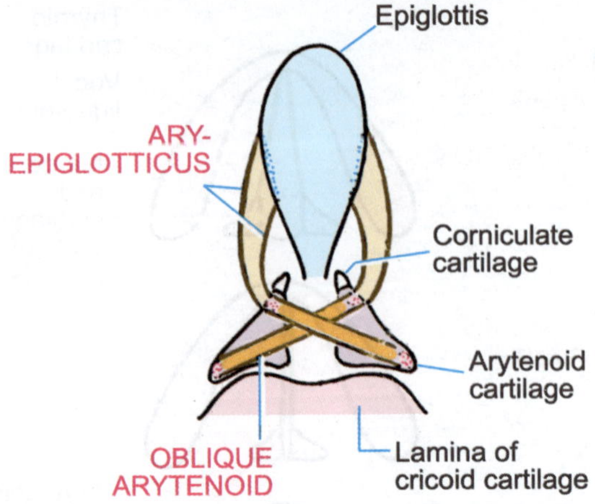

Fig. 11.35 Attachments of oblique arytenoid and aryepiglotticus muscles.

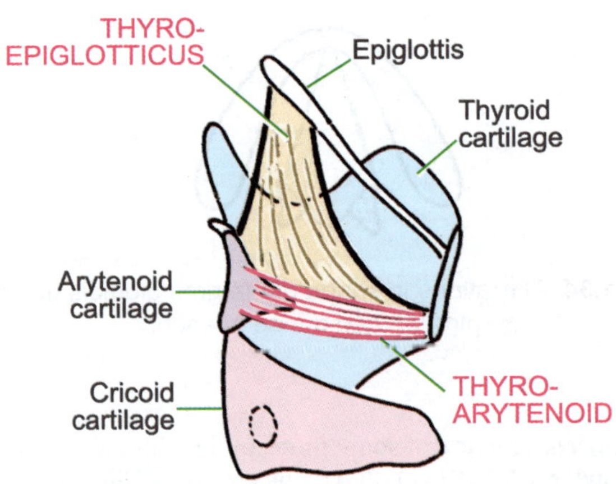

Fig. 11.36 Attachments of the thyroepiglotticus and thyroarytenoid muscles.

nerve. The only exception is the cricothyroid which is supplied by the external laryngeal nerve.

For ***clinical correlations*** of larynx see Chapter 15.

THE TRACHEA

The trachea is a wide tube lying on the front of the neck more or less in the middle line. The upper end of the trachea is continuous with the lower end of the larynx. The junction lies opposite the lower part of the body of the sixth cervical vertebra. At the root of the neck the trachea passes into the superior

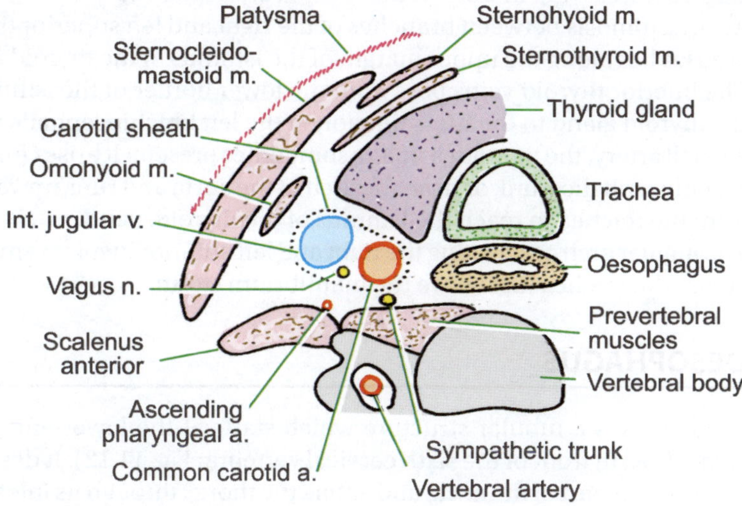

Fig. 11.37 Transverse section through the upper part of the trachea to show some of its relations in the neck.

mediastinum of the thorax. Here we will consider the relations of the trachea in the neck.

Relations of the Trachea in the Neck

The trachea is related to a large number of structures in the neck as follows.

1. Posteriorly the trachea is related to the oesophagus which runs vertically behind it, and separates it from the bodies of vertebrae C6 and C7 (Fig. 11.37).
2. Anteriorly, over its entire length, the trachea is covered by skin, superficial and deep fascia. The deep fascia is represented by a superficial part, the investing layer; and a deeper part, the pretracheal fascia. The right and left sternohyoid and sternothyroid muscles overlap the part of the trachea near the inlet of the thorax.
3. Near its upper end (over the 2nd, 3rd and 4th rings) the trachea is covered anteriorly by the isthmus of the thyroid gland. The right and left lobes of the gland overlap the corresponding sides of the trachea (Fig. 11.23).
4. The right and left common carotid arteries ascend along the corresponding side of the cervical part of the trachea.
5. On either side the inferior thyroid artery is closely related to the trachea (Fig. 8.1).
6. On either side the recurrent laryngeal nerve lies in the groove between the trachea and the oesophagus. (On the left side the nerve is related to both the thoracic and cervical parts of trachea, but on the right side it is related to the cervical part only).

7. Small structures lying in front of the trachea are as follows:
   a. An anastomosis between branches of the right and left superior thyroid arteries lies along the upper margin of the isthmus of the thyroid gland.
   b. The inferior thyroid veins pass from the lower border of the isthmus of the thyroid gland to their termination in the left brachiocephalic vein.
   c. A small artery, the thyroidea ima, is sometimes present. It arises from the brachiocephalic trunk or from the arch of the aorta and runs upwards in from the trachea to reach the isthmus of the thyroid gland.
   d. The jugular arch connecting the right and left anterior jugular veins runs across the trachea just above the manubrium sterni.

THE OESOPHAGUS

The oesophagus is a tubular structure which starts at the lower end of the oropharynx (i.e., in front of the sixth cervical vertebra: Fig. 11.12). It descends through the lower part of the neck, and enters the thorax through its inlet. After passing through the thorax the oesophagus enters the abdomen and ends by joining the cardiac end of the stomach.

Relations of Oesophagus in the Neck

These are shown in Fig. 11.23. Posteriorly, the oesophagus is related to the sixth and seventh cervical vertebrae (covered by prevertebral muscles and fascia). Anteriorly it is related to the trachea. Laterally the oesophagus is related to the corresponding common carotid artery.

The upper part of the oesophagus is overlapped laterally by the corresponding lobe of the thyroid gland. The thoracic duct ascends along the left side of the oesophagus in the lower part of the neck. The right and left recurrent laryngeal nerves lie anterolateral to the oesophagus in the corresponding grooves between it and the trachea.

CHAPTER

12

Endocrine Glands of the Head and Neck, Carotid Sinus and Carotid Body

The endocrine glands that lie in the head and neck are the hypophysis cerebri, the pineal gland, the thyroid gland, and the parathyroid glands.

Some endocrine functions are also ascribed to the carotid body. The carotid body, and the carotid sinus, will also be considered.

THE HYPOPHYSIS CEREBRI

The hypophysis cerebri is also called the pituitary gland. It is placed in the cranial cavity, in the floor of the middle cranial fossa. It lies in a depression on the superior surface of the body of the sphenoid bone called the ***hypophyseal fossa*** or ***sella turcica***. The hypophysis is suspended from the floor of the third ventricle of the brain by a narrow funnel shaped stalk called the ***infundibulum.***

The hypophysis cerebri is a small ovoid structure measuring about 13 mm from side to side, about 10 mm front to back, and about 8 mm in vertical diameter.

The relations of the hypophysis cerebri are shown in Fig. 12.1 which is a coronal section; and in Fig. 12.2 which is a sagittal section. The hypophyseal fossa is lined by duramater which is adherent to the lower part of the hypophysis. Superior to the hypophysis the duramater is folded on itself to form the ***diaphragma sellae***. The infundibulum passes through an aperture in the diaphragma to join the inferior wall of the third ventricle. The optic chiasma lies anterosuperior to the hypophysis cerebri being separated from it by the anterior part of the diaphragma. It lies anterior to the infundibulum. Inferiorly, the hypophysis cerebri is related to the sphenoidal air sinuses and beyond them to the nasopharynx. On the right and left sides the hypophysis cerebri is related to the corresponding cavernous sinus (and to structures in its wall). The cavernous sinuses are connected across the midline by anterior and posterior intercavernous sinuses which are located within the layers of the diaphragma sellae.

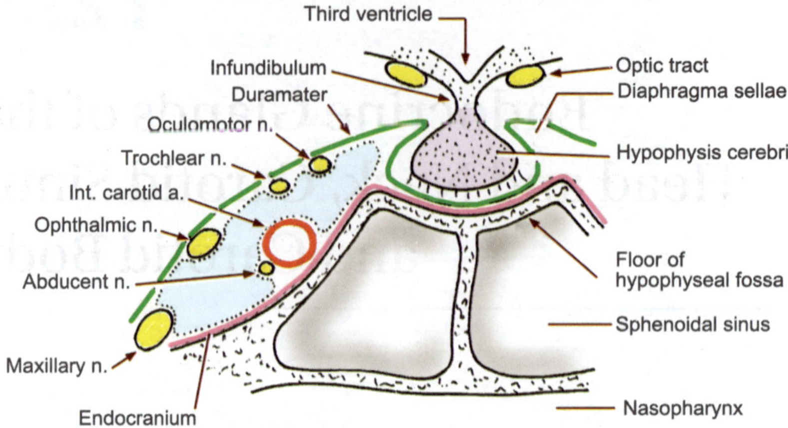

Fig. 12.1 Coronal section through hypophysis cerebri to show some of its relations.

The relations of the hypophysis cerebri help us to understand the effects of pressure by a tumour of the organ. Pressure on the optic chiasma leads to loss of both temporal halves of the fields of vision (bitemporal hemianopia). Lateral pressure may lead to paralysis of muscles supplied by the oculomotor nerve. The trochlear and abducent nerves are rarely affected (as they are too low down). Downward pressure of an enlarging hypophysis leads to 'ballooning' of the hypophyseal fossa; and backward pressure can cause erosion of the dorsum sellae. These features can be recognised on a skiagram.

Subdivisions of the Hypophysis Cerebri

The hypophysis cerebri has, in the past, been usually divided into an anterior part, the ***pars anterior***; an intermediate part, the ***pars intermedia***; and a posterior part, the ***pars posterior*** (or ***pars nervosa***) (Fig. 12.3). The pars posterior contains numerous nerve fibres. It is directly continuous with the central core of the infun-dibulum, which is made up of nervous tissue. These two parts are together referred to as the ***neurohypophysis***. The area of the floor of the third ventricle (tuber cinerium) immediately adjoining the attachment to it of the infundibulum is referred to as the ***median eminence***. Some authorities include the median eminence in the neurohypophysis.

The pars anterior (which is also called the ***pars distalis***) and the pars intermedia are both made up of cells having a direct secretory function and are collectively referred to as the ***adeno-hypophysis***. An extension of the pars anterior surrounds the central nervous core of the infundibulum. Because of the tubular shape of this extension (Fig. 12.3B) it is called the ***pars tubularis***. The pars tubularis is part of the adenohypophysis.

A distinction between the adenohypophysis and the neurohypophysis can also be made on the basis of their development. The neurohypophysis is formed as a downgrowth from the floor of the third ventricle. In contrast the adenohypophysis

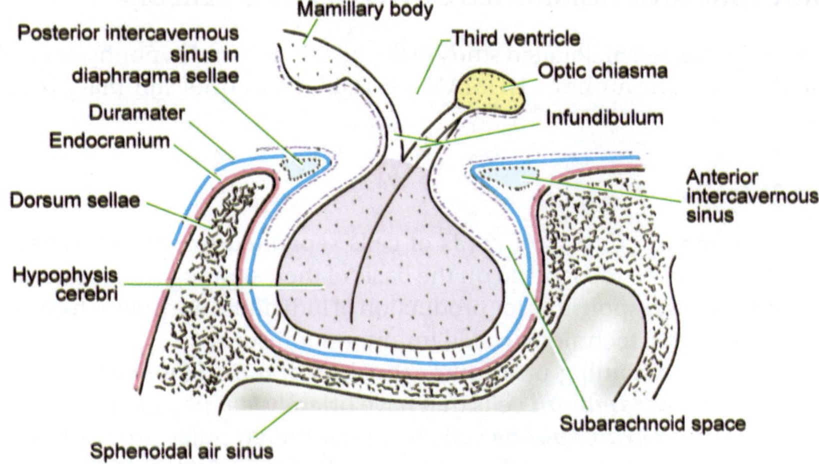

Fig. 12.2 Sagittal section through the hypophysis cerebri to show its relations.

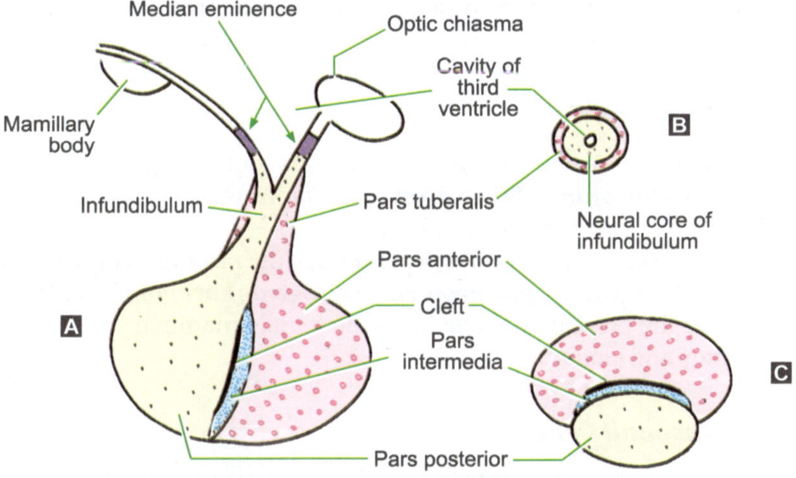

Fig. 12.3 Schemes to show the subdivisions of the hypophysis cerebri. A. Sagittal section. B. T.S. through infundibulum. C. T.S. through the hypophysis cerebri.

is derived from ***Rathke's pouch*** which arises from the ectoderm lining the roof of the primitive mouth (stomodaeum). This pouch has a cavity. The pars anterior develops in the anterior wall of the pouch and the pars intermedia in its posterior wall. The original cavity of Rathke's pouch may persist as a cleft separating the pars anterior and intermedia. For further details of development see the author's HUMAN EMBRYOLOGY.

STRUCTURE AND HORMONES OF HYPOPHYSIS CEREBRI

Students interested in detailed study of the histology of the hypophysis cerebri should consult the author's HUMAN HISTOLOGY. A brief summary is given below.

Pars Anterior

The pars anterior consists of cords of cells separated by sinusoids. Several types of cells can be recognised on the basis of their staining characters. More recently the cells responsible for production of individual hormones have been distinguished by a technique called immunofluorescence.

Using routine staining procedures the cells of the adenohypophysis can be divided into ***chromophil*** cells that have brightly staining granules in their cytoplasm; and ***chromophobe*** cells in which the granules are not present. Chromophil cells are further classified as ***acidophil*** when they stain with acid dyes (like eosin or orange G); or ***basophil*** when they stain with basic dyes (like haematoxylin). The acidophil cells are often called alpha cells, and the basophils are called beta cells.

Both acidophils and basophils can be divided into subtypes on the basis of structural details and on the basis of the hormones produced by them. The following types are described.

Types of Acidophil Cells

1. ***Somatotrophs (or somatotropes)*** produce the somatotropic hormone (also called ***somatotropin***, ***STH*** or ***growth hormone***). This hormone controls body growth, specially before puberty.
2. ***Mammotrophs*** (or ***mammotropes***) produce the ***mammotropic hormone*** (also called ***mammotropin***, ***prolactin***, ***lactogenic hormone***, or ***LTH***) which stimulates the growth and activity of the female mammary gland, during pregnancy and lactation.

Types of Basophil Cells

1. ***Corticotrophs*** (or ***corticotropes***) produce the ***corticotropic hormone*** (also called ***adrenocorticotropin*** or ***ACTH***). This hormone stimulates the secretion of some hormones of the adrenal cortex. [Note: The staining characters of these cells are intermediate between acidophils and basophils; and they are sometimes classified amongst acidophils].
2. ***Thyrotrophs*** (or ***thyrotropes***) produce the ***thyrotropic hormone*** (***thyrotropin*** or ***TSH***)) which stimulates the activity of the thyroid gland.
3. ***Gonadotrophs*** (***gonadotropes*** or delta basophils) produce two types of hormones each type having a separate action in the male and female.
   a. In the female the first of these hormones stimulates the growth of ovarian follicles. It is, therefore, called the ***follicle stimulating hormone (FSH)***. It also stimulates the secretion of oestrogens by the ovaries. In the male the same hormone stimulates spermatogenesis.

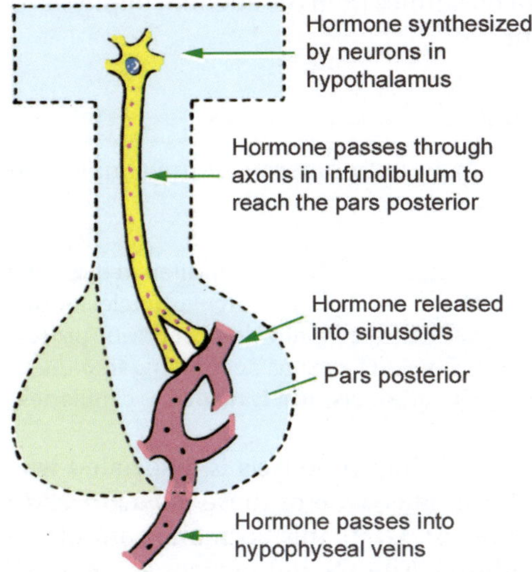

Fig. 12.4 Scheme to show the relationship of the hypothalamus and the pars posterior of the hypophysis cerebri.

b. In the female the second hormone stimulates the maturation of the corpus luteum and the secretion by it of progesterone. It is called the ***luteinizing hormone (LH)***. In the male the same hormone stimulates the production of androgens by interstitial cells of the testes, and is called the ***interstitial cell stimulating hormone (ICSH)***.

Chromophobe Cells

The chromophobe cells probably represent alpha or beta cells that have been depleted of their granules. Some of them are stem cells that give rise to new chromophil cells.

Pars Tubularis

The pars tubularis contains undifferentiated cells and some cells similar to those of the pars anterior. Numerous blood vessels are present (see below).

Pars Intermedia

This is poorly developed in the human hypophysis. In ordinary preparations the most conspicuous features are colloid filled vesicles: these are remnants of the pouch of Rathke. Beta cells and other secretory cells are also present. Some cells of the pars intermedia produce the ***melanocyte stimulating hormone*** (MSH) which causes increased pigmentation of the skin. Other cells may produce ACTH.

The secretion of hormones from the adenohypophysis is under the control of the hypothalamus.

The Pars Posterior

The pars posterior consists of numerous unmyelinated nerve fibres, and of cells called pituicytes.

The nerve fibres are the axons of neurons located in the hypothalamus. Most of them arise in the supraoptic and paraventricular nuclei. Situated between these axons there are pituicytes. These cells have long dendritic processes many of which lie parallel to the nerve fibres. The axons descending into the pars posterior from the hypothalamus end in terminals closely related to capillaries.

The pars posterior of the hypophysis is associated with the release into the blood of two hormones. One of these is ***vasopressin*** (also called the ***antidiuretic hormone*** or ***ADH***): this hormone controls the reabsorption of water by kidney tubules. The second hormone is ***oxytocin***: this hormone controls the contraction of smooth muscle of the uterus and also of the mammary gland. It is now known that these two hormones are not produced in the hypophysis at all. They are synthesised in neurons located mainly in the supraoptic and paraventricular nuclei of the hypothalamus. Vasopressin is produced mainly in the supraoptic nucleus; and oxytocin in the paraventricular nucleus. These secretions (which are bound with other proteins) pass down the axons of the neurons concerned, through the infundibulum into the pars posterior. Here they are released into the capillaries of the region and enter the general circulation (Fig. 12.4).

Blood Supply of The Hypophysis Cerebri

The hypophysis cerebri is supplied by superior and inferior branches arising from the internal carotid arteries (Fig. 8.9). Some branches also arise from the anterior and posterior cerebral arteries. The inferior hypophyseal arteries are distributed mainly to the pars posterior. Branches from the superior set of arteries supply the median eminence and infundibulum. Here they end in capillary plexuses from which portal vessels arise (Fig. 12.5). These portal vessels descend through the infundibulum and end in the sinusoids of the pars anterior. The sinusoids are drained by veins that end in neighbouring venous sinuses.

It will be noticed that the above arrangement is unusual in that two sets of capillaries intervene between the arteries and veins. One of these is in the median eminence and the upper infundibulum. The second set of capillaries is represented by the sinusoids of the pars anterior. This arrangement is referred to as the ***hypothalamohypophyseal portal system***. (Compare with ***the*** portal system). The functional significance of this system is described below.

Control of Secretion of Hormones of Adenohypophysis

The secretion of hormones by the adenohypophysis takes place under higher control of neurons in the hypothalamus, notably those in the median eminence and in the infundibular nucleus. The axons of these neurons end in relation to capillaries in

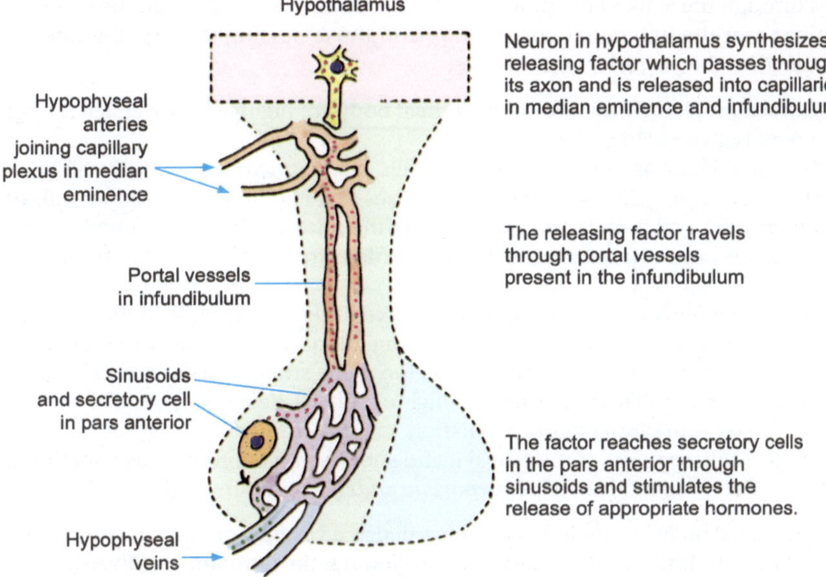

Fig. 12.5 Scheme to show the hypothalamo-hypophyseal portal circulation, and the control of secretions of the adenohypophysis by the hypothalamus.

the median eminence and in the upper part of the infundibulum. Different neurons produce specific ***releasing factors*** (or releasing hormones) for each hormone of the adenohypophysis. These factors are released into the capillaries mentioned above. Portal vessels arising from the capillaries carry these factors to the pars anterior of the hypophysis. Here they stimulate the release of appropriate hormones. Some factors inhibit the release of hormones.

THE PINEAL BODY

The pineal body is a small piriform structure present in relation to the posterior wall of the third ventricle of the brain. It is also called the ***epiphysis cerebri***. It is about 8 mm in length, and about 4 cm in width and in thickness. It is situated in the median plane just below the splenium of the corpus callosum, and just above the superior colliculi of the midbrain (Fig. 12.6).

The following details will be understood after the brain is studied. They are included here for completeness. The pineal body is separated from the splenium by a double layered fold of piamater, the tela choroidea, which contains the great cerebral vein. The lower layer of the piamater forming the tela choroidea intimately covers the pineal body and passes from it to the colliculi.

The posterior end of the pineal body is rounded and is called the apex. The anterior end, or base, is attached to the wall of the third ventricle by a stalk which divides into superior and inferior laminae. A part of the cavity of the third ventricle extends into the interval between these laminae forming the pineal recess of the ventricle. Some commissural fibres passing from one side of the brain to the other pass through the stalk of the pineal body. The fibres passing through the superior lamina form the habenular commissure and those passing through the inferior lamina form the posterior commissure.

The structure and functions of the pineal body are highly controversial. A brief summary is given below.

The pineal body is made up mainly of cells called ***pinealocytes***. Each cell has a polyhedral body which gives off long processes that end in relation to the walls of capillaries, or in relation to the ependyma of the third ventricle. The pinealocytes are separated by neuroglial cells that resemble astrocytes. The organ has a rich network of capillaries.

The pineal body receives sympathetic nerve fibres. These arise in the superior cervical sympathetic ganglion and travel along blood vessels. Many of them pass through the tentorium cerebelli (in the region of the straight sinus) and constitute the ***nervus conarii.*** (This nerve may be single or paired). Release of pineal secretions appears to require sympathetic stimulation.

In the adult, sections of the pineal gland show aggregations of salts containing calcium. These are referred to as ***corpora arenacea***, or 'brain sand'.

The pineal body has for long been regarded as a vestigial organ of no functional importance. From an evolutionary point of view it is the remnant of a diverticulum that formed a median eye. In many species the pinealocytes show similarities in ultrastructure to those of rods in the retina, even though the organ is no longer exposed to light. In terms of embryology the pineal body is formed as an outgrowth from the third ventricle and is the main part of what is called the epiphysis (in contrast to hypophysis).

Recent investigations have shown that the pineal body is an endocrine gland of great importance. It produces hormones that may have an important regulatory influence on many other endocrine organs (including the adenohypophysis, the neurohypophysis, the thyroid, the parathyroids, the adrenal cortex and medulla, and the gonads).

The hormones of the pineal body reach the hypophysis both through the CSF and through blood. The other organs can, obviously, be influenced only through the blood.

The best known hormone of the pineal body is the amino acid ***melatonin*** (so called because it causes changes in skin colour in amphibia). Large concentrations of melatonin are present in the pineal body. Considerable amounts of 5-hydroxytrptamine (serotonin), which is a precursor of melatonin, are also present. Related enzymes are also present. The synthesis and discharge of melatonin is remarkably influenced by exposure of the animal to light: the release is stimulated by darkness and is inhibited by light.

The neurological pathway for this effect is as follows. Some nerve fibres arising in the retina end directly in the suprachiasmatic nucleus (of the hypothalamus). This nucleus gives origin to fibres that relay in nuclei in the brainstem to reach the intermediolateral grey column of the spinal cord in the upper thoracic segments. Preganglionic sympathetic neurons starting here carry these impulses to the superior cervical sympathetic ganglion. Postganglionic fibres arising in this ganglion reach the pineal body along blood vessels and along the nervus conarii. Some fibres may relay in the habenular nuclei and travel to the pineal along a habenulopineal tract.

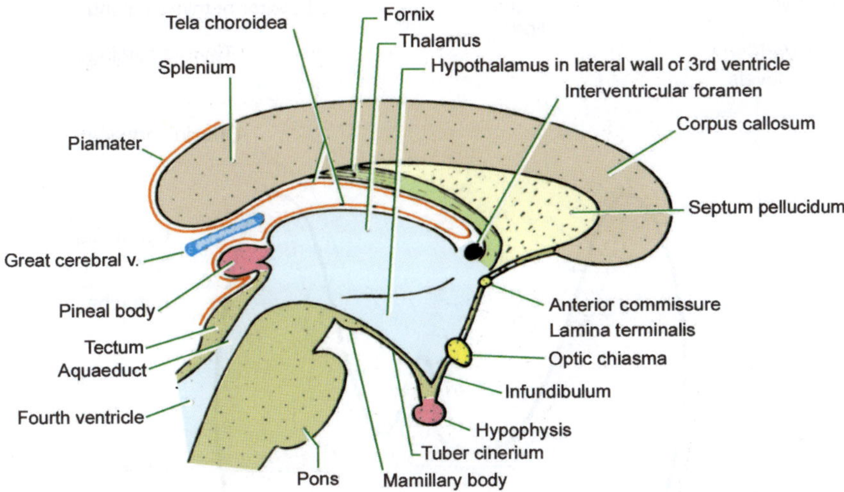

Fig. 12.6 Diagram to show the position of the hypophysis cerebri and of the pineal body relative to the third ventricle of the brain.

Because of this light mediated response the pineal body may act as a kind of biological clock which may produce circadian rhythms (variations following a 24 hour cycle) in various parameters.

The corpora arenacea have been regarded in the past as signs of atrophy and ageing of the pineal body. Recent work has shown that they are bye products of active secretory activity.

For further details about the pineal gland see the author's HUMAN HISTOLOGY.

THE THYROID GLAND

The thyroid gland lies in the front of the neck, in front of the lower part of the larynx and the upper part of the trachea (Figs. 1.11, 1.13). It consists of right and left ***lobes*** that are joined, across the midline, by an ***isthmus*** (Fig. 12.7). The vertical diameter of each lobe is about 5 cm (2 inches) and that of the isthmus is about 1 cm (1/2 inch). The anteroposterior diameter of each lobe is about 2 cm. The transverse diameter of the entire thyroid is about 8 cm. (As there is no sharp line of demarcation between the isthmus and the lobes, different authorities give very different figures for width of the lobes and of the isthmus, but under the circumstances these figures have no value).

When seen in cross section each lobe of the thyroid is seen to have three surfaces, lateral (or superficial); medial and posterior. The ***lateral surface*** is directed forwards and laterally (Figs. 1.21, 12.8)). It is covered by skin and fascia; by the sternothyroid and sternohyoid muscles; by the superior belly of the omohyoid muscle; and by the anterior part of the sternocleidomastoid muscle. The ***medial surface*** lies over the thyroid and cricoid cartilages of the larynx, and the uppermost parts of the trachea and oesophagus. Parts of two muscles, the inferior constrictor of the pharynx, and the cricothyroid, are

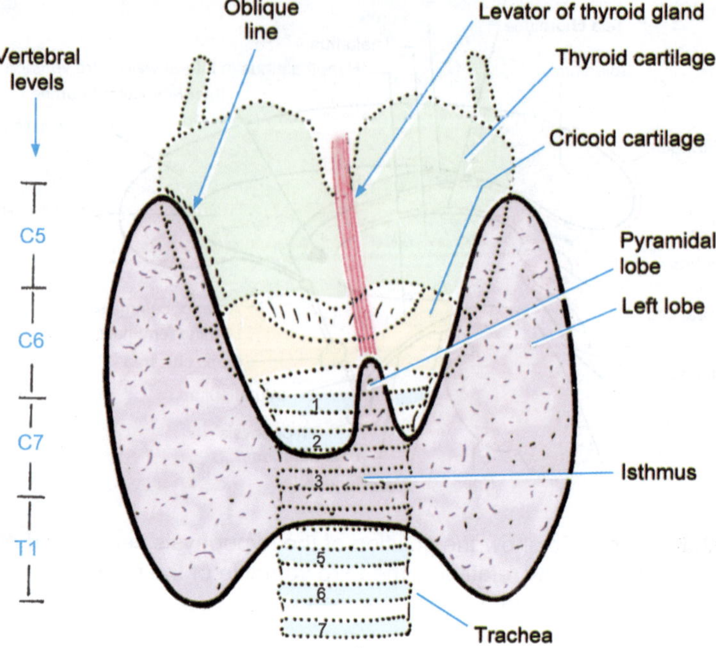

Fig. 12.7 Outline of the thyroid gland as seen from the front, and its relationship to the larynx and trachea.

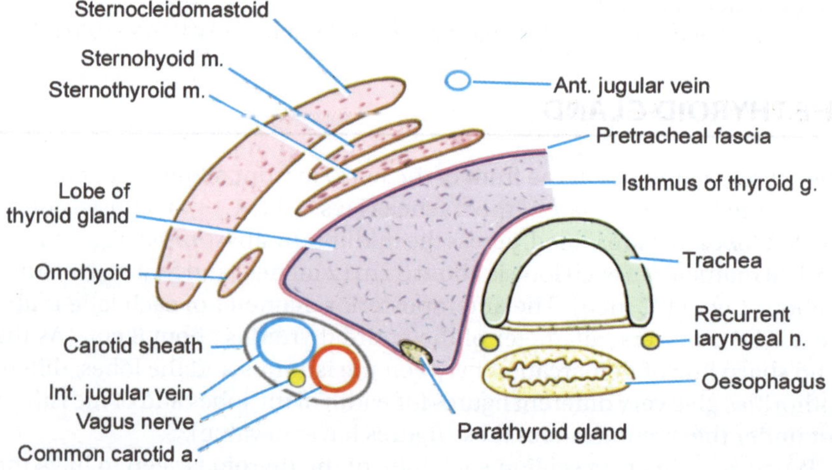

Fig. 12.8 Transverse section across the thyroid gland and related structures.

deep to it. Two important nerves lie deep to the medial surface. These are recurrent laryngeal nerve as it ascends in the groove between the trachea and oesophagus; and the external laryngeal nerve as it descends to reach the cricothyroid (Fig. 12.9).

The ***posterior surface*** of the lobe is directed posterolaterally. It is in contact with the carotid sheath and its contents.

The lateral and medial surfaces are separated by a sharp ***anterior border.*** A branch of the superior thyroid artery descends along this border (Fig. 1.14). The posterior and medial surfaces are separated by the ***posterior border*** which is rounded. It is related to the inferior thyroid artery, and to the parathyroid glands. On the left side the posterior border is related to the thoracic duct (Fig. 12.10).

The ***upper end*** of each lobe extends up to the oblique line of the thyroid cartilage (Fig. 12.7). [It is prevented from extending further upwards by the insertion of the sternothyroid muscle to the oblique line]. The upper end lies opposite vertebra C5. The ***lower end*** of the lobe lies at the level of the fifth or sixth tracheal ring (corresponding to vertebra T1). The level of the lower end is variable. An enlarging thyroid usually extends downwards.

The isthmus of the thyroid glands lies in front of the second, third and fourth rings of the trachea. It is covered in front by skin and fascia; and by the sternothyroid and sternohyoid muscles and by the anterior jugular veins.

A finger like projection of thyroid tissue frequently arises from the upper border of the isthmus. This is called the ***pyramidal lobe*** (Fig. 12.7). Its upper end is attached to the hyoid bone by fibrous tissue or muscle (***levator of the thyroid gland***).

The thyroid is surrounded by a ***capsule*** of connective tissue. Outside this capsule the thyroid has another sheath (or ***false capsule***) formed by the pretracheal fascia. On each side this fascia is thickened posteromedially to form a band connecting the lobe of the thyroid gland to the side of the cricoid cartilage. This band is called the ***lateral ligament*** or the ligament of Berry.

The thyroid has a rich blood supply. The arteries supplying it are the superior thyroid branch of the external carotid artery; the inferior thyroid branch of the thyrocervical trunk; a small artery the thyroidea ima arising from the brachiocephalic trunk; and accessory thyroid arteries derived from those supplying the trachea and oesophagus. The superior thyroid artery gives an anterior branch that runs down along the anterior border of the lobe, and along the upper border of the isthmus, to anastomose with the corresponding artery of the opposite side. An anastomotic branch joining the superior and inferior thyroid arteries runs along the posterior border of the lobe. It is important to note that the superior thyroid artery is relatively superficial, whereas the inferior artery is very deep. The superior artery is closely related to the external laryngeal nerve. In operations for removal of the thyroid gland the surgeon has to carefully separate these nerves from the arteries before ligating the latter to avoid injury to the nerves.

The thyroid gland is drained by three veins, superior, middle and inferior. The veins form a plexus deep to the capsule of the gland. In order to avoid injury to them the surgeon removes the thyroid along with its true capsule.

The lymphatic drainage of the thyroid gland is described in Chapter 13.

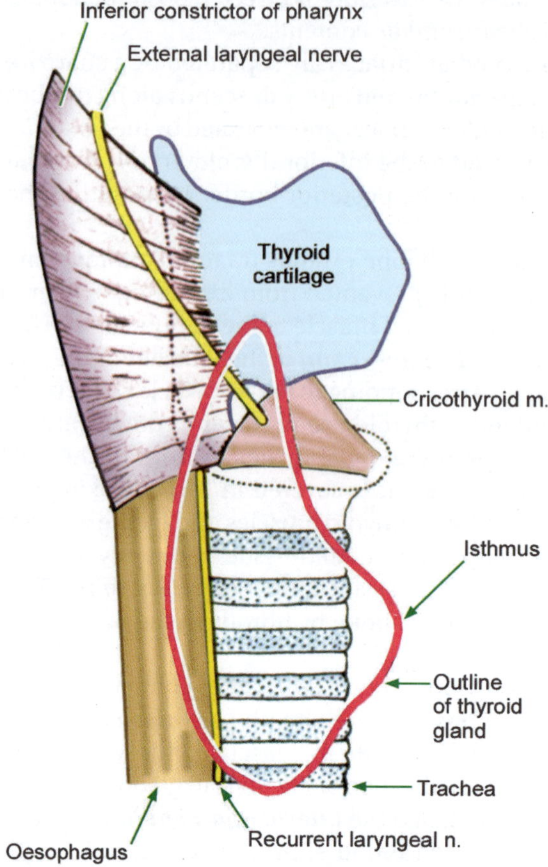

Fig. 12.9 Modial rclations of the thyroid gland. The outline of the gland is shown in pink line.

A brief note on Structure and Function of the Thyroid Gland

We have seen that the thyroid gland is covered by a fibrous ***capsule***. Septa extending into the gland from the capsule divide it into ***lobules***. On microscopic examination each lobule is seen to be made up of an aggregation of ***follicles***. Each follicle is lined by ***follicular cells*** that are typically cubical. It has a cavity which is filled by a homogeneous material called ***colloid*** (which appears pink in haematoxylin and eosin stained preparations). The follicular cells rest on a basement membrane. At some places cells of a different type intervene between the follicular cells and the basement membrane. These are called the ***parafollicular cells***.

The follicular cells secrete hormones that influence the rate of metabolism. Iodine is an essential constituent of these hormones. One hormone containing three atoms of iodine in each molecule is called ***triiodothyronine*** or T3. Another hormone containing four atoms of iodine is called ***tetraiodothyronine*** or T4. Colloid present in the follicles is an intermediate product (iodinated thyroglobulin).

During moderate activity of the thyroid gland the follicular cells are cubical, and a moderate amount of colloid is present in the follicles. When the gland is inactive, the follicles get distended with stored colloid and the cells are flattened.

In highly active states there is little colloid in the follicles and the cells become columnar.

The parafollicular cells are completely different in function from the follicular cells. They produce a hormone called ***calcitonin***, the significance of which is considered below, along with that of the parathyroid hormone.

The development and anomalies of the thyroid gland are important. They are described in the author's HUMAN EMBRYOLOGY. Some clinical correlations of the thyroid gland are described on Chapter 65.

THE PARATHYROID GLANDS

The parathyroid glands are so called because they lie in close relationship to the thyroid gland. Normally there are two glands, one superior and one inferior, on either side, there being four glands in all. However, the number can be more or less. Each gland is roughly oval and weighs about 50 mg.

On each side, the ***superior parathyroid gland*** lies near the middle of the posterior border of the thyroid gland. It is relatively constant in position.

The ***inferior parathyroid gland*** lies near the lower end of the posterior border of the thyroid gland. Its position is variable. It may lie above or below the inferior thyroid artery. It may lie outside the false capsule of the thyroid, between the false and true capsules; or deep to the true capsule within the substance of the thyroid. Occasionally the inferior parathyroid gland may lie below the level of the thyroid gland, and may even descend into the superior or posterior mediastinum.

The superior parathyroid gland receives a branch from the anastomotic channel connecting the superior and inferior thyroid arteries. The inferior gland receives a branch from the inferior thyroid artery.

A brief note on Parathyroid Structure and Function

The parathyroid glands consist essentially of columns of cells separated by sinusoids. The cells are of two types. The large majority of cells are called ***chief cells*** or ***principal cells.*** The second type of cells are called ***oxyphil or eosinophil cells*** as they contain granular structures that stain with eosin.

The parathyroid glands produce a hormone called the ***parathyroid hormone*** (PTH) or ***parathormone.*** This hormone helps to maintain a suitable level of calcium ions in blood. When there is a tendency for serum calcium levels to fall calcium is removed from stores in bone bringing serum levels back to normal. Simultaneously the excretion of calcium by the kidney is decreased, and calcium absorption by the intestines is increased.

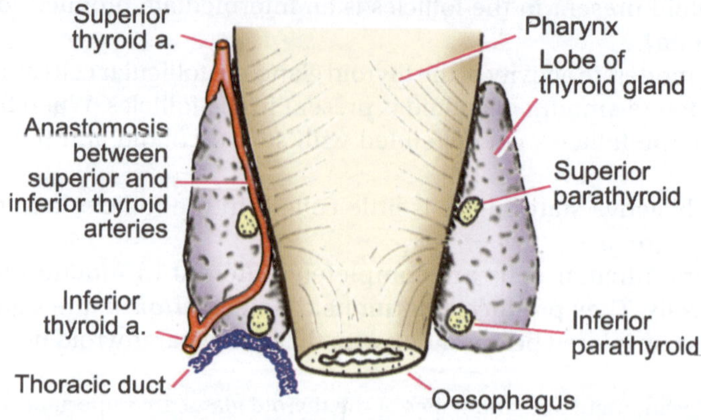

Fig. 12.10 Thyroid and parathyroid glands seen from behind.

Calcitonin secreted by the parafollicular cells of the thyroid gland has effects opposite to those of the parathyroid hormone. A decrease in serum calcium levels stimulates the secretion of parathyroid hormone, while an increase stimulates the secretion of calcitonin.

For development and anomalies of the parathyroid glands see the author's HUMAN EMBRYOLOGY. For details of histology see the author's HUMAN HISTOLOGY.

Some clinical correlations of the parathyroid glands are given in Chapter 15.

THE CAROTID SINUS

The term carotid sinus is applied to a dilated segment of the common carotid body at its bifurcation. The dilatation usually extends on to the initial part of the internal carotid artery, and may be confined to it.

In the region of the dilatation, the tunica media in the arterial wall is thin, but the adventitia is thick. Numerous nerve endings are seen in the adventitia.

The region of the carotid sinus is surrounded by a nerve plexus. The main contribution to this plexus is by the carotid branch of the glossopharyngeal nerve. The plexus also receives fibres from the superior cervical sympathetic ganglion, and from the vagus nerve.

The afferent nerve terminals present over the carotid sinus are stimulated by alterations in blood pressure. Afferent impulses arising from the sinus play an important role in reflex control of blood pressure.

THE CAROTID BODIES

These are small oval structures, present one on each side of the neck, at the bifurcation of the common carotid artery (i.e., near the carotid sinus). The main function of the carotid bodies is that they act as chemoreceptors that monitor the oxygen and carbon dioxide levels in blood. They reflexly control the rate and depth of respiration through respiratory centres located in the brainstem. In addition to this function the carotid bodies are also believed to have an endocrine function.

The carotid bodies contain a network of capillaries in the intervals between which there are several types of cells. The carotid bodies have a rich innervation (see below).

The most conspicuous cells of the carotid body are called ***glomus cells*** (or type I cells). These are large cells that have several similarities to neurons.

Because of the similarities to neurons, and because of the possibility that the cells release peptides they are described as neuroendocrine cells. Enkephalins have been identified in the human carotid body. In other species VIP, substance P and catecholamines have been found. The exact significance of the glomus cells, and of their nervous connections, is not understood at present. They could possibly be sensory receptors sensitive to oxygen and carbon dioxide tension. Peptides released by them may influence the sensitivity of chemoreceptor nerve endings.

Apart from the glomus cells various other cells present in the carotid bodies. They include a few sympathetic and parasympathetic postganglionic neurons.

The carotid body is richly innervated as follows.

1. Afferent nerve terminals from the glossopharyngeal nerve form synapses with glomus cells.
2. Preganglionic sympathetic and parasympathetic fibres end on the corresponding ganglion cells. Some preganglionic sympathetic fibres end by synapsing with glomus cells.
3. Postganglionic fibres arising from the sympathetic and parasympathetic nerve cells within the carotid body innervate muscle in the walls of arterioles present within the carotid body.

The precise mechanism by which the carotid bodies respond to changes in oxygen and carbon dioxide tension is not understood. It is not certain as to which cells, or nerve terminals are responsible for this function.

Carotid bodies are best formed in children, and normally retrogress with age. However, in persons with chronic hypoxia (caused by lung disease, or by residence at high altitudes) the carotid bodies may increase in size.

The carotid bodies are included under the general heading of ***paraganglia***. This term is used to describe small collections of neuroendocrine cells present in association with autonomic nerves. Structures similar to the carotid bodies, present in relation to the inferior aspect of the arch of the aorta are also included in paraganglia. They are called the ***aortic bodies***, or ***aorticopulmonary paraganglia***.

CHAPTER

13

Lymphatics of the Head and Neck

We have seen that lymph from the head and neck is ultimately collected by the right and left jugular lymph trunks. On the left side this trunk drains into the thoracic duct, while on the left side it ends in the right lymphatic duct. These ducts have been described in Chapter 34.

LYMPH NODES OF HEAD AND NECK

Superficial Lymph Nodes

The lymph nodes that drain the superficial tissues of the head and neck are shown in Fig. 13.1. They are as follows.

1. The nodes of the ***occipital group*** lie along the attachment of the trapezius to the occipital bone.
2. The nodes of the ***retroauricular group*** (or mastoid group) lie superficial to the upper attachment of the sternocleidomastoid muscle.
3. The parotid lymph nodes nodes are in two groups, superficial and deep. The nodes of the ***superficial parotid group*** lie over the parotid gland. Those of the ***deep parotid group*** (shown in dots in Fig. 13.1) are embedded in the gland.
4. The nodes of the ***submandibular group*** lie over the submandibular gland. Some of them are embedded within the gland.
5. The ***submental nodes*** lie below the chin overlying the mylohyoid muscle, between the anterior bellies of the right and left digastric muscles.
6. The ***buccal nodes*** lie along the facial vein.
7. The ***superficial cervical nodes*** lie along the external jugular vein, superficial to the sternocleidomastoid muscle.
8. The ***anterior cervical nodes*** lie along the anterior jugular vein.

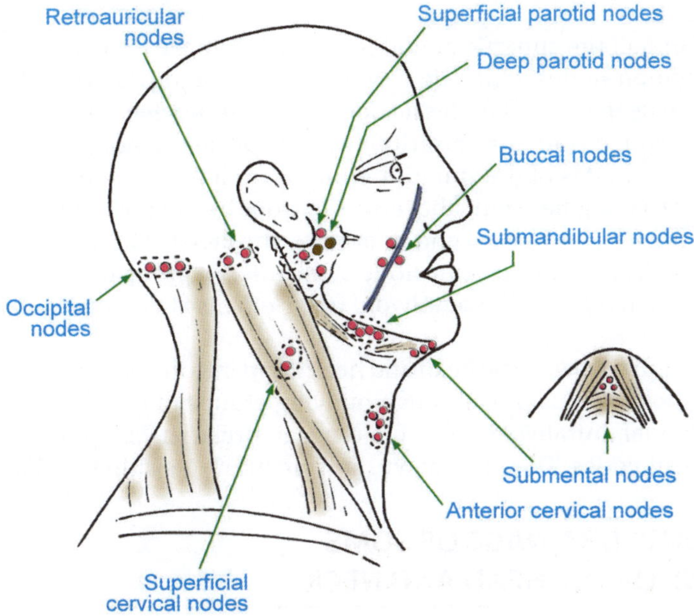

Fig. 13.1 Lymph nodes draining superficial tissues of the head and neck.

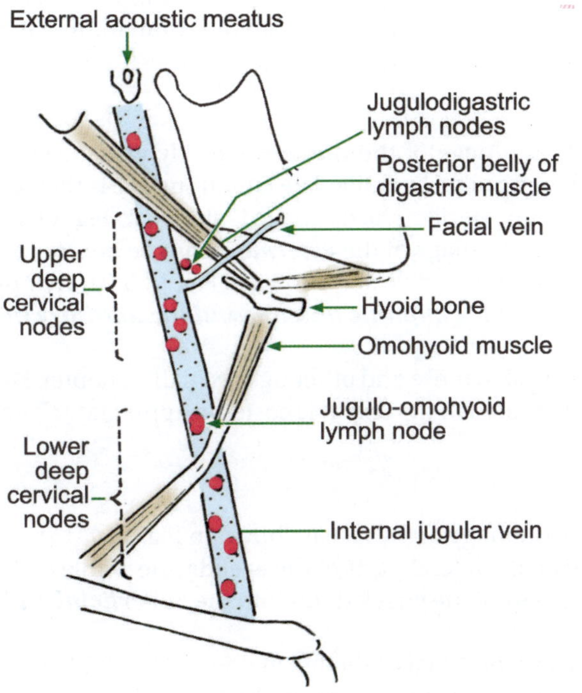

Fig. 13.2 Scheme to show the deep cervical lymph nodes.

Deep Cervical Nodes

Lymph from all the superficial nodes described above drains into the deep cervical lymph nodes which lie along the internal jugular vein (Fig. 13.2). Most of the deep cervical nodes lie deep to the sternocleidomastoid muscle. They are divided (rather arbitrarily) into a ***superior group*** and an ***inferior group.*** Some nodes of the superior group lie in a triangle bounded behind by the internal jugular vein, above and in front by the posterior belly of the digastric muscle, and below and in front by the facial vein. These are called the ***jugulodigastric nodes***. One node of the inferior group lies just above the intermediate tendon of the omohyoid muscle. This is the ***jugulo-omohyoid node.***

The deeper tissues of the head and neck drain into the deep cervical nodes. Some of these vessels pass through outlying groups of lymph nodes. These are the lingual, infrahyoid, retro-pharyngeal, prelaryngeal, pretracheal and paratracheal nodes. They are shown, and are briefly described in Fig. 13.3.

LYMPHATIC DRAINAGE OF SOME REGIONS OF THE HEAD AND NECK

The Scalp

From behind forwards lymph vessels from the scalp end in the occipital, retroauricular and superficial parotid nodes (Fig. 13.1). The part of the forehead just above the root of the nose drains into the submandibular nodes.

The Ear

The lymphatic drainage of the ***auricle*** is easily visualized if the auricle is imagined as being pulled laterally. The lateral surface is then anterior and the medial surface is posterior. The drainage is shown in Fig. 13.4.

The lymphatic drainage of the ***external acoustic meatus*** is similar to that of the upper half of the auricle. It is shown in Fig. 13.5. The lymphatic drainage of the ***middle ear, the tympanic antrum and the auditory tube*** is shown in Fig. 13.6.

(Please do not skip these and other figures in this chapter. Details shown in them are not repeated in the text. It is easier to appreciate them in diagrams).

The Face

The lymphatic drainage of the face is shown in Fig. 13.7.

The forehead, the lateral parts of the eyelids, the whole of the conjunctiva, and the lateral part of the cheek drain into the ***superficial and deep parotid*** lymph nodes.

The central part of the face (shaded in dots in Fig. 13.7) including the lower part of the forehead, the medial parts of the eyelids, the nose, the medial parts of the cheeks, the upper lip and the lateral parts of the lower lip drain into the

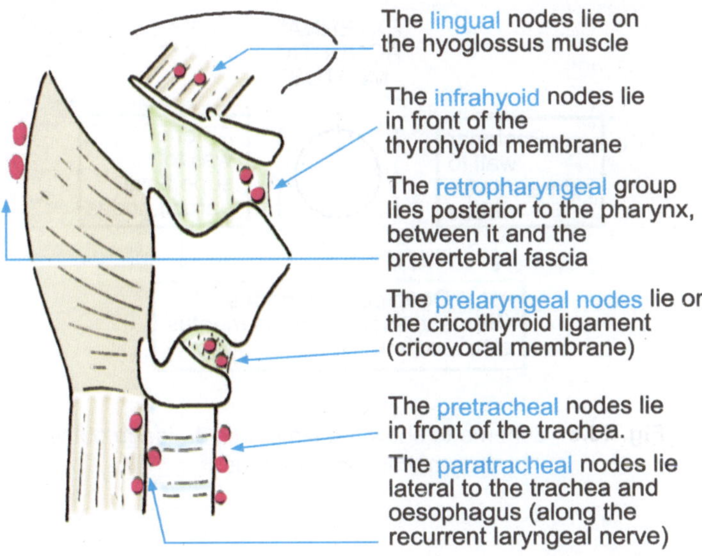

Fig. 13.3 Outlying members of the deep cervical group of lymph nodes.

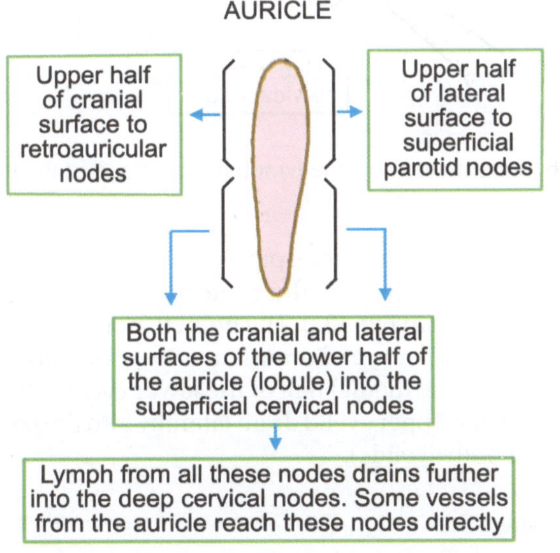

Fig. 13.4 Lymphatic drainage of the auricle.

submandibular lymph nodes. Some of these vessels pass through the ***buccal*** nodes.

The median part of the lower lip, the chin (and the floor of the mouth) drain into the ***submental*** nodes, and through them into the ***submandibular*** nodes.

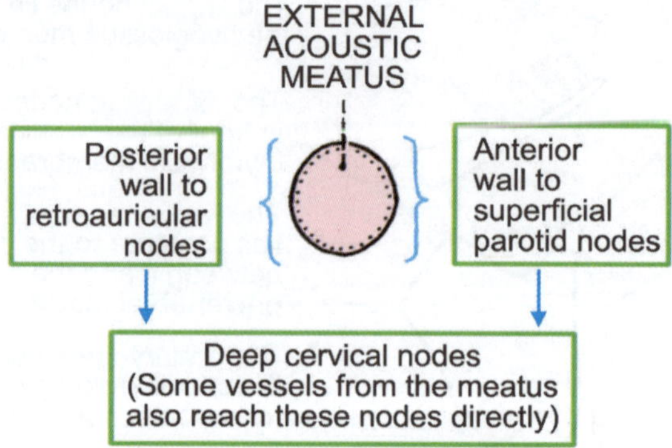

Fig. 13.5 Scheme to show the lymphatic drainage of the external acoustic meatus.

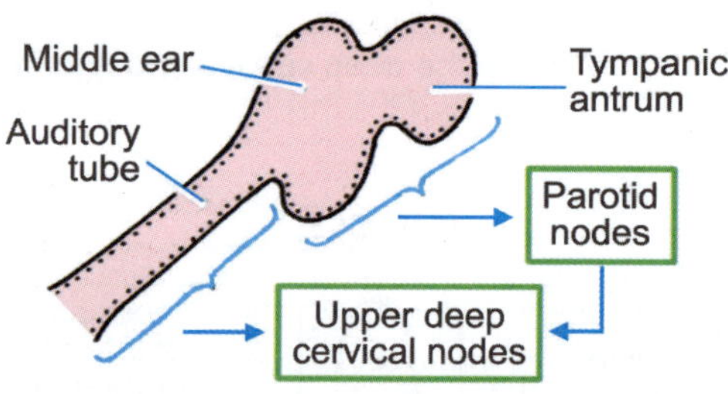

Fig. 13.6 Scheme to show the lymphatic drainage of the middle ear.

We have seen above that the lateral parts of the eyelids drain into the parotid lymph nodes, while the medial parts drain into the submandibular nodes. Some further details are shown in Fig. 13.8. The point to note is that while the skin of the medial half of the upper eyelid drains into the submandibular nodes (like the entire thickness of the medial half of the lower eyelid), the deeper tissues of the medial half of the upper eyelid drain laterally into the parotid nodes (like the lateral parts of both eyelids).

The Nasal Cavity

The lymphatic drainage of the nasal cavity is shown in Fig. 13.9. Most of the nasal cavity, the paranasal sinuses and the nasopharynx drain directly into the deep cervical lymph nodes.

Some lymphatics from the upper part of the nasal cavity reach the skin covering the nose and drain (as shown in Fig. 13.7) to the submandibular nodes.

Some lymphatics of the nasopharynx drain into the retropharyngeal nodes.

Lymphatics of the nasal cavity may communicate with the subarachnoid space by passing along the olfactory nerves.

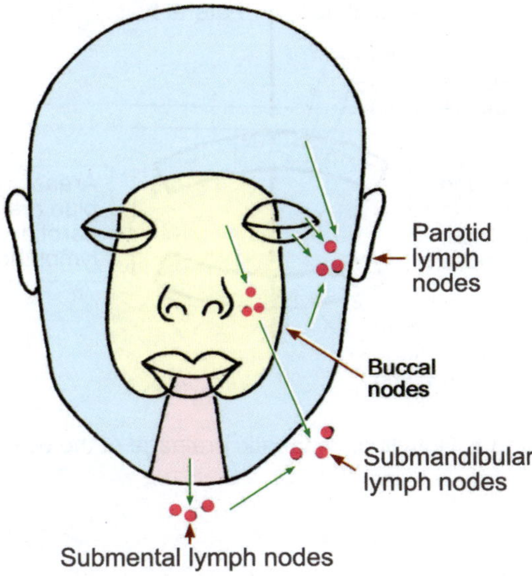

Fig. 13.7 Scheme to show the lymphatic drainage of the face.

The Palate

Lymph from the hard palate, the soft palate and the nasopharynx drains into the retro-pharyngeal nodes, and through them, or directly, to the deep cervical lymph nodes (Fig. 13.10).

Floor of Mouth

Lymphatic vessels from the floor of the mouth, gums and teeth drain into the submandibular nodes, and through them into the deep cervical nodes. Some vessels from the anterior part of the floor of the mouth pass to the submental nodes. Some lymph vessels from the mouth go directly to the deep cervical lymph nodes.

The Tonsil

The lymphatic drainage of the palatine tonsil is shown in Fig. 13.11. Lymph vessels pass through the superior constrictor of the pharynx to reach the jugulodigastric nodes and some other nodes of the upper deep cervical group.

Lymphatic Drainage of the Tongue

The tongue is a frequent site of carcinoma and hence a knowledge of its lymphatic drainage is of special importance. From this point of view the tongue may be divided into a part behind the vallate papillae (***a*** in Fig. 13.12); and a

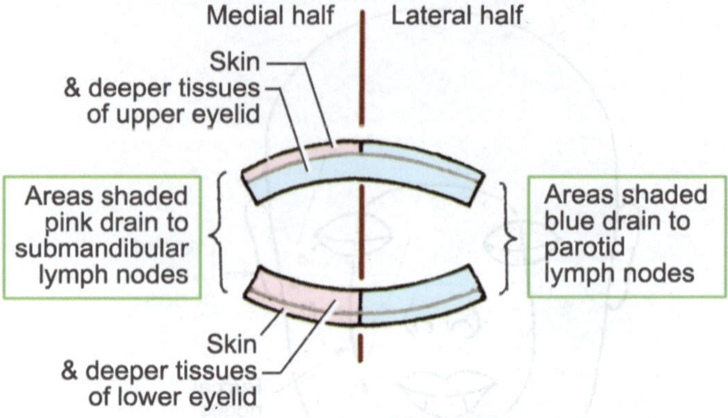

Fig. 13.8 Details of lymphatic drainage of the eyelids.

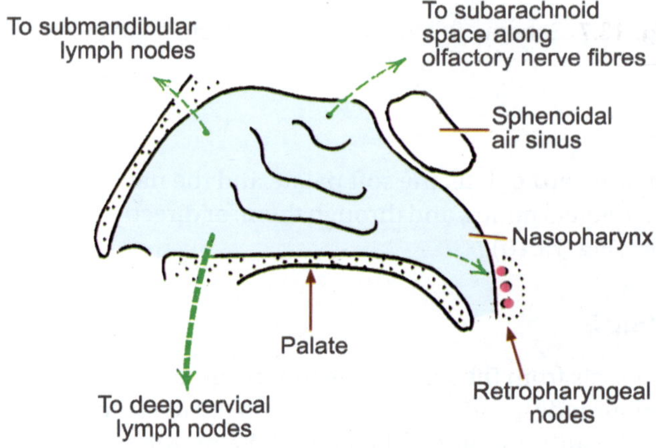

Fig. 13.9 Lymphatic drainage of the nasal cavity.

part in front of them. The latter is further divided into a central area (***b***) and a marginal area (***c***) which includes the tip (***d***). Lymph from area ***a***, area ***b***, and the posterior part of area ***c*** drains directly into the jugulodigastric, jugulo-omohyoid and other deep cervical nodes. Lymph from the anterior part of area ***c*** and from the tip of the tongue (area ***d***) reaches the same nodes after passing through the submandibular nodes. Lymph from the tip of the tongue also passes into the submental nodes, and from there into the submandibular and deep cervical nodes. In Fig. 13.12 note particularly that lymph from areas of the tongue near the middle line can pass to lymph nodes of either the right or left side.

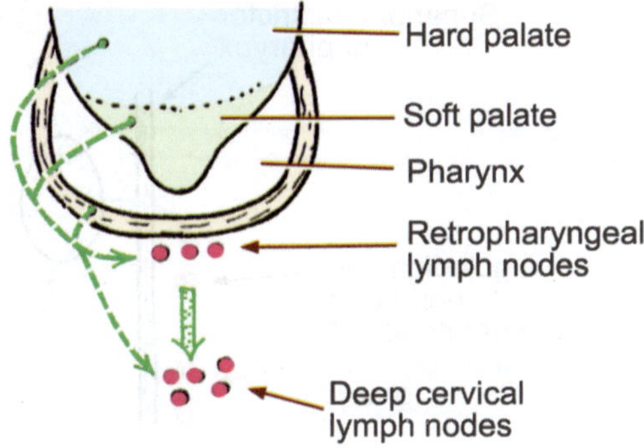

Fig. 13.10 Lymphatic drainage of the palate.

Some of the routes followed by lymph vessels draining the tongue are shown in Figs. 13.13 A, B and C.

1. Lymph vessels passing to the jugulodigastric nodes from the tip of the tongue (***c*** in Figs. 13.13 A, C) and from the lateral margin of the anterior part of the tongue (***b*** in Figs. 13.13 A, C) follow the course of the hypoglossal nerve. They run deep to the sublingual gland and to the mylohyoid muscle (Fig. 13.13 C). Some of these vessels descend along the internal jugular vein to the jugulo-omohyoid node (***e*** in Fig. 13.13 A).
2. Lymph vessels from the posterior part of the marginal area and from the part of the tongue behind the vallate papillae (***a*** in Figs. 13.13 A, C) reach the jugulodigastric nodes by piercing the wall of the pharynx (Fig. 13.13 C).
3. Lymph vessels from the central part of the tongue pass vertically downwards in the midline between the two genioglossus muscles (***g*** in Figs. 13.13 B, C), and turn either to the left or right. They then travel along the lingual vessels (i.e., deep to the hyoglossus) to reach the jugulodigastric and jugulo-omohyoid nodes and other nodes of the deep cervical group.
4. Vessels travelling to the submandibular lymph nodes (from the marginal areas and from the tip) reach them by piercing the mylohyoid muscle. Some of these vessels pass over the sublingual gland (***h*** in Fig. 13.13B).
5. Some vessels from the tip of the tongue reach the submental nodes by piercing the mylohyoid (***d*** in Fig. 13.13A). Some of these vessels may descend over the hyoid bone to reach the jugulo-omohyoid node.

It is important to note that vessels from a fairly wide area of the tongue near the midline (including the tip) can pass either to the right or the left and end in lymph nodes of that side. Lymph vessels passing from the submental nodes to the deep cervical nodes behave in the same way (Fig. 13.12). Cancer, of the tongue in this region can, therefore, spread to nodes of both sides. Lymph vessels piercing through the mylohyoid are often closely related to the periosteum of the mandible accounting for early spread of cancer to the bone.

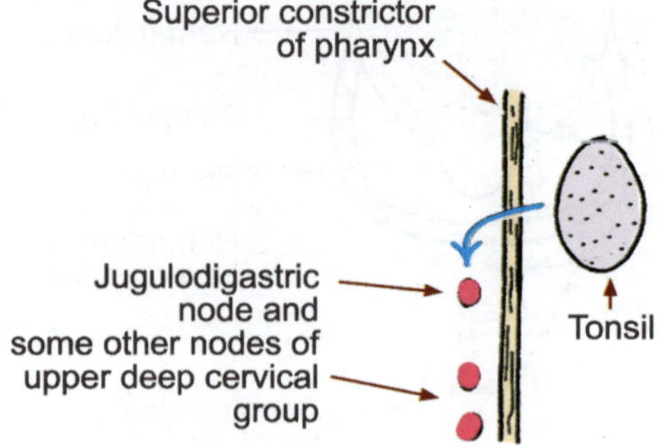

Fig. 13.11 Lymphatic drainage of the palatine tonsil.

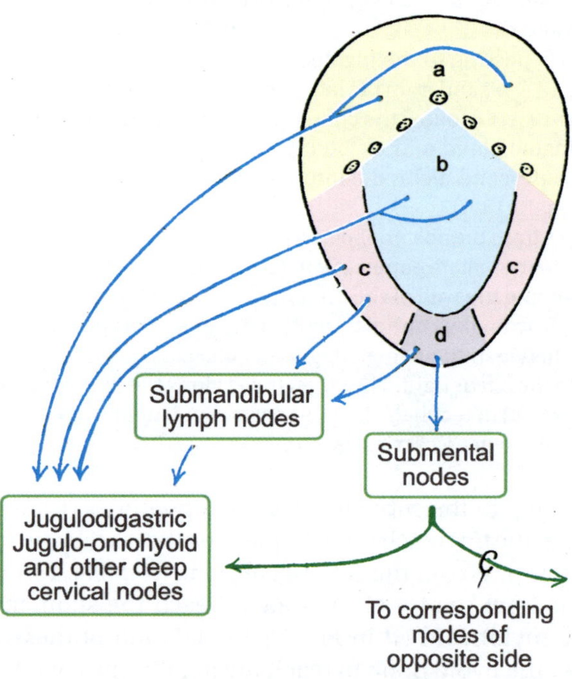

Fig. 13.12 Scheme to show the lymph nodes receiving lymph from different areas of the tongue.

Lymphatic Drainage of The Neck

Some of the superficial tissues of the neck drain directly into the deep cervical lymph nodes. Lymph from areas near the occipital nodes, the superficial cervical nodes, the submandibular nodes and the anterior cervical nodes drains first into these nodes and through them to the deep cervical nodes. Lymph

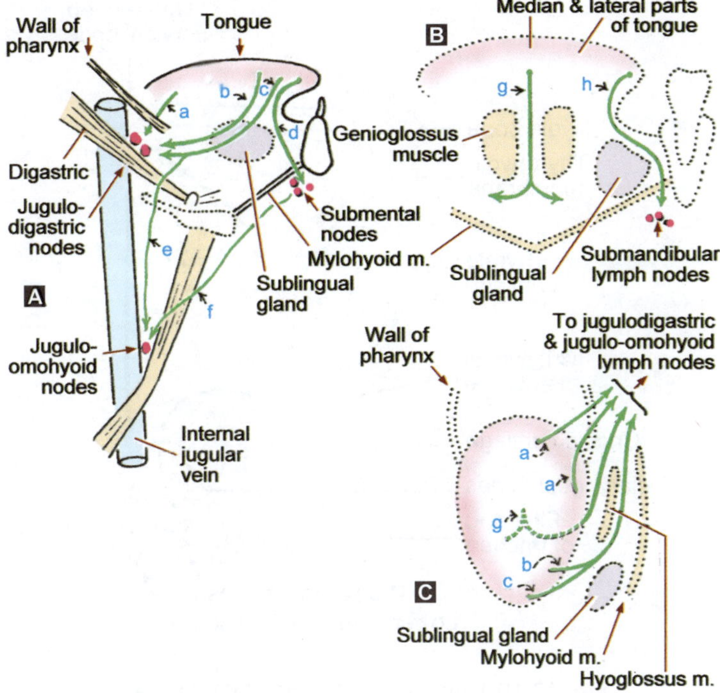

Fig. 13.13 Schemes to show pathways followed by lymph vessels from the tongue. A. Lateral view. B. Coronal section C.Transverse section. All figures are highly schematic.

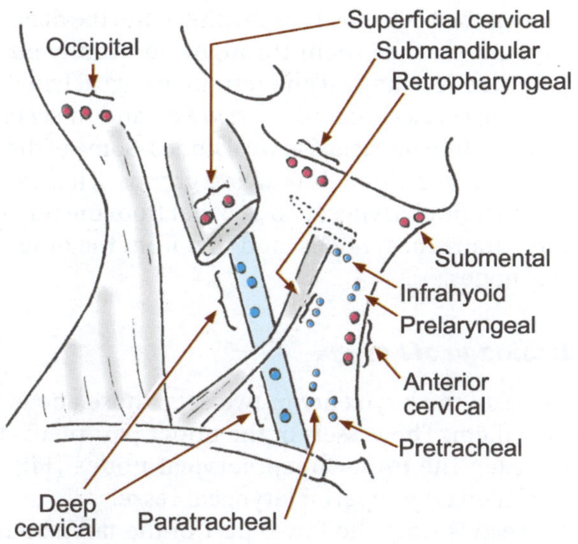

Fig. 13.14 Lymph nodes draining the tissues of the neck. The superficial nodes are shown in red and the deep nodes in blue.

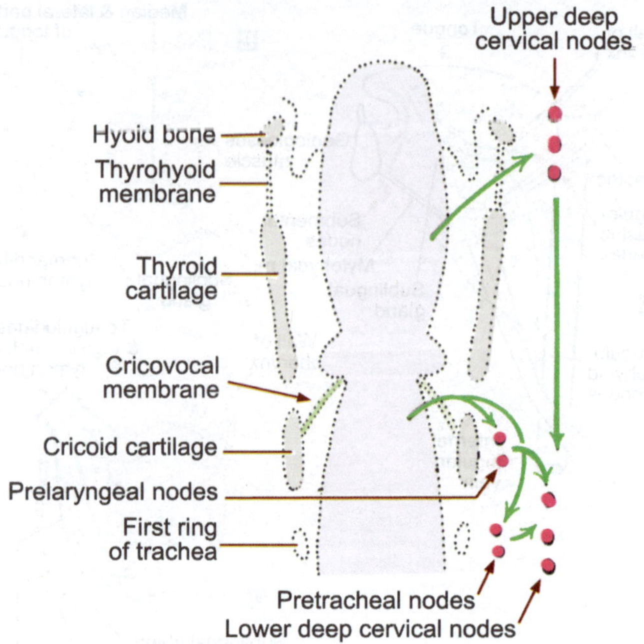

Fig. 13.15 Lymphatic drainage of the larynx.

from the anterior cervical nodes passes to the infrahyoid, prelaryngeal and pretracheal nodes (See Fig.13.14 and also Figs. 13.3, 13.15 and 13.16).

Deeper tissues in the neck mostly drain direct into the deep cervical nodes. Some of this lymph reaches them through the infrahyoid, prelaryngeal, pretracheal, para-tracheal, lingual and retropharyngeal lymph nodes.

The ***pharynx***, the cervical part of the ***trachea*** and the cervical part of the ***oesophagus*** all drain into the deep cervical nodes. Some of the lymph reaches these nodes after passing through outlying groups. That from the pharynx passes through the retropharyngeal nodes; that from the trachea through the pretracheal and paratracheal nodes; and that from the oesophagus through the paratracheal nodes.

Lymphatic Drainage of Larynx

The lymph vessels of the larynx are in two sets: those above the vocal folds and those below them. The vessels of the upper part pierce the thyrohyoid membrane to reach the upper deep cervical nodes (Fig. 13.15). These lymphatics travel along the superior laryngeal vessels.

Some of the vessels from the lower part of the larynx pass through the cricovocal membrane to reach the prelaryngeal and pretracheal nodes. From here they pass to the deep cervical nodes. Some vessels pass below the cricoid cartilage and reach the lower deep cervical nodes directly.

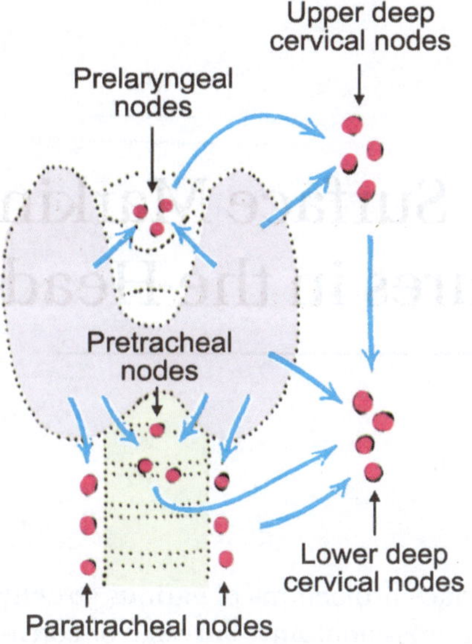

Fig. 13.16 Lymphatic drainage of the thyroid gland.

Lymphatic Drainage of Thyroid Gland

The lymph vessels draining the thyroid gland are shown in Fig. 13.16. The thyroid is sometimes described as being divided into distinct parts draining in different directions. However, it must be noted that in the thyroid (and for that matter in most other organs) the lymphatics form a plexus through which lymph may pass in any direction. Such divisions are, therefore, artificial and misleading. The arrows in the figure only indicate the predominant direction of flow.

Lymph from the upper part of the gland reaches the upper deep cervical nodes either directly or through the prelaryngeal nodes. Lymph from the lower part of the gland drains to the lower deep cervical nodes directly, and also through the pretracheal and paratracheal nodes.

CHAPTER

14

Surface Marking of Some Structures in the Head and Neck

The study of the surface projections of various structures is best undertaken while studying their gross anatomy. For sake of convenience in revision the descriptions are grouped together in this chapter.

SURFACE MARKING OF SOME VISCERA

Parotid Gland

The parotid gland has been described on page 65. Its projection on the surface can be marked as follows.

1. To mark the ***anterior border***, begin at the upper border of the head of the mandible. Draw a line downwards and forwards to reach the centre of the masseter muscle. Now carry the line downwards and backwards to reach a point just posteroinferior to the angle of the mandible.
2. To mark the ***posterior border*** begin at the lower end of the anterior border. Draw a line upwards to the reach the anterior border of the mastoid process, near its upper end.
3. To mark the ***superior border*** join the upper ends of the posterior and anterior borders by a line that is convex downwards. This line corresponds to the lower part of the margin of the external acoustic meatus. It can be marked on the lobule of the ear, but it is more useful to mark it by lifting the lobule upwards.

Parotid Duct

Draw a line running forwards from the lower border of the tragus to a point midway between the ala of the nose and the upper lip. Divide this line into three parts. The position of the parotid duct corresponds to the middle one third of this line.

Thyroid Gland

The thyroid gland has been described on page 381. Before marking the gland you must have an idea of its shape and of its division into the isthmus and the right and left lobes.

1. To mark the isthmus of the gland begin by feeling the lower border of the arch of the cricoid cartilage. Take one point half an inch below this border, and another point one inch below the border. (Remember that one inch is equal to 2.5 cm approximately). At each of these levels draw transverse lines, half an inch long. These lines represent the upper and lower borders of the isthmus.
2. Each lobe of the thyroid gland is marked as follows.

To mark the anterior border start at the lateral end of the upper border of the isthmus (marked above). Carry the line upwards and slightly backwards to reach the anterior border of the sternocleidomastoid muscle, at the level of the middle of the thyroid cartilage.

To mark the posterior border begin at the upper end of the anterior border. Draw a line running downwards (with a slight backward convexity) to reach the clavicle.

To complete the marking of the lobe, join the lower end of the posterior border to the lateral end of the lower border of the isthmus by a broad line convex downwards.

Submandibular Gland

The submandibular gland has been described on page 87. The outline of this gland is oval. To mark it feel the angle of the mandible. To draw the upper margin of the gland draw a line convex upwards, starting at the angle and reaching the middle of the base of the mandible. To mark the lower margin of the gland join the two ends of the upper margin (drawn as described above) by a line convex downwards. The curve should extend below to the level of the greater cornu of the hyoid bone.

Palatine Tonsil

The palatine tonsil is described on page 354.

To mark it draw a small oval just in front of, and above, the angle of the mandible. The marking will lie over the masseter muscle.

PARANASAL SINUSES

The paranasal sinuses have been described on page 344. We will consider the surface marking only of the frontal and maxillary sinuses (as these are large and lie near the surface).

Frontal Air Sinus

The projection of this sinus lies above the medial part of the orbit. It is triangular.

To mark the medial border of the sinus draw a vertical line one inch (2.5 cm) long over the lower part of the forehead, in the middle line. The lower end of the line should be just above the depression between the forehead and the upper end of the nose. (The point corresponds to the ***nasion*** which is the point at which the internasal and frontonasal sutures meet).

To mark the lower border of the sinus draw a line starting at the lower end of the medial border, and passing laterally and slightly upwards to reach the upper margin of the orbit. The line should lie just above the medial one third of the superior orbital margin.

The third border (above and laterally) is drawn by joining the upper end of the medial border with the lateral end of the lower border.

Maxillary Sinus

The outline of this sinus is irregular. It can be marked on the face following the outline of the maxilla. Above, the line is just below the orbit. Below, the line lies just above the alveolar process of the maxilla. Medially it reaches the lateral wall of the nose. Laterally it reaches the zygomatic process of the maxilla

ARTERIES

Common Carotid Artery

The common carotid artery has been described on page 153. The left artery runs part of its course in the thorax. In the neck the position of the artery is similar on both sides.

To mark the artery draw a broad line starting over the sternoclavicular joint, passing upwards along the anterior border of the sternocleidomastoid muscle, and ending at the level of the upper border of the thyroid cartilage.

Internal Carotid Artery

The internal carotid artery has been described on page 155. The lower end of this artery corresponds to the termination of the common carotid artery. It lies over the anterior border of the sternocleidomastoid muscle at the level of the upper border of the thyroid cartilage. From this level draw a broad line running upwards and ending just behind the condyle of the mandible.

External Carotid Artery

The external carotid artery has been described on page 161. The lower end of this artery corresponds to the termination of the common carotid artery. It lies over the anterior border of the sternocleidomastoid muscle at the level of the thyroid cartilage. From here draw a line upwards to end just behind the neck of the mandible. The line should be slightly convex forwards in its lower half, and slightly convex backwards in its upper half.

Subclavian Artery

The subclavian artery has been described on page 172. The left subclavian artery runs part of its course in the thorax. The course of the right and left arteries is similar in the neck.

The artery can be marked by drawing a broad line beginning over the sternoclavicular joint, and passing laterally with an upward convexity to a point over the middle of the clavicle. The highest point of the upward convexity rises 2 cm above the clavicle.

Facial Artery

The facial artery has been described on page 165. We have seen that the artery runs part of its course in the neck, and passes through the submandibular region before entering the face. Its course in the face can be marked as follows.

Ask the subject to clench his teeth. This makes the masseter prominent and its anterior border can be felt. The facial artery enters the face where the anterior border of the masseter cuts the lower border of the mandible. The pulsations of the artery can be felt here.

From here the artery runs upwards and forwards to reach a point half an inch (1.2 cm) lateral to the angle of the mouth. It then bends more sharply upwards to reach the medial angle of the eye.

Middle Meningeal Artery

This artery has been described on page 168. Its relationship to the surface of the skull is shown in Fig. 8.23. The artery can be marked as follows.

1. Feel the zygomatic arch (zygoma) and take its midpoint. This is the level at which the artery enters the skull.
2. Draw a line vertically upwards from this point for 2 cm. This line represents the stem of the artery. The artery divides into frontal and parietal branches at the upper end of this line.
3. The frontal branch is marked as follows. Draw a line starting at the upper end of the mainstem (see above) and running upwards with a forwards convexity (Fig. 8.23). The upper end of the line ends over the centre of pterion which lies 3.5 cm behind and 1.5 cm above the frontozygomatic suture. From here the frontal branch runs upwards and backwards to end approximately midway between the root of the nose and the external occipital protuberance.
4. The parietal branch begins at the upper end of the main stem of the middle meningeal artery (see above). It runs backwards to a point about 6 cm above the external occipital protuberance.

VEINS

Internal Jugular Vein

The internal jugular vein has been described on page 183.

The upper end of the vein lies on the neck just deep to the lobule of the ear. Its lower end lies deep to the medial end of the clavicle. The vein can be marked by drawing a broad line joining these points.

Subclavian Vein

The subclavian vein has been described on page 186. Its lateral end lies behind the clavicle a little medial to its midpoint. Its medial end lies behind the medial end of the clavicle. The vein can be marked by a broad line over the clavicle joining these points. Note that the vein lies at a lower level than the subclavian artery.

External Jugular Vein

This vein has been described on page 197. Its upper end lies a little behind and below the angle of the mandible. The vein runs downwards across the sternocleido-mastoid and ends deep to the clavicle immediately behind the sternocleidomastoid muscle. The vein can be marked by drawing a line joining these points. The vein can often be seen in the living subject.

INTRACRANIAL VENOUS SINUSES

The intracranial venous sinuses have been described on page 187.

Superior Sagittal Sinus

The relationship of this sinus to the surface of the body is simple. It lies in the midline of the vault of the skull. Its anterior end reaches the raised area between the right and left eyebrows (glabella). Its posterior end reaches the external occipital protuberance. The sinus is narrow at its anterior end. At the posterior end it is about 1 cm broad.

Transverse Sinus

The sinus is about 1 cm broad. Its posterior end (beginning) lies deep to the external occipital protuberance. Its anterior end lies deep to the mastoid process. The sinus is marked by a line joining these points. The line should be drawn with an upward convexity.

Sigmoid Sinus

This sinus is also about 1 cm broad. It begins where the transverse sinus ends i.e., deep to the upper part of the mastoid process. Its lower end lies about 1 cm above the tip of the mastoid process. The line joining the two points is short because of foreshortening of the projection.

NERVES

Of the many nerves to be seen in the head and neck the surface projection of only a few is considered below. The nerves considered are those than can be approached surgically from the surface. (It is always useful to read the course of the nerve before trying to understand surface marking).

SOME BRANCHES OF TRIGEMINAL NERVE

The ***mandibular nerve*** is described on page 238. The *main stem* of the mandibular nerve can be marked on the surface as a short vertical line just in front of the head of the mandible.

The ***auriculotemporal nerve*** is described on page 238. It can be marked by a line that runs backwards from the mainstem of the mandibular nerve, across the neck of the mandible. The nerve then turns upwards passing immediately in front of the tragus (preauricular point).

The ***lingual nerve*** is described on page 240. To mark it draw a line continuous with the main stem of the mandibular nerve (see above). It is represented by a line that runs downwards and forwards to reach opposite the lower third molar tooth. It then runs forwards in relation to the mandible up to the level of the first molar tooth.

Facial Nerve

The facial nerve is described on page 242. It is useful only to mark the extracranial part of the nerve, before it divides into several branches. Remember that the nerve emerges from the skull through the stylomastoid foramen. This foramen lies deep to the middle of the anterior border of the mastoid process. (In the adult the nerve lies at a depth of 2 cm, but the depth is much less in children). From here draw a horizontal line that runs forwards to end just behind the neck of the mandible.

Glossopharyngeal Nerve

The glossopharyngeal nerve is described on page 258. This nerve is marked by a line that runs downwards and forwards with a downward convexity. The line begins over the tragus and runs to the angle of the mandible. It then runs for a short distance along the lower border of the mandible.

Vagus Nerve

The vagus nerve is described on page 263. It can be represented by a straight line running down the entire length of the neck. The upper end of the line should lie over the anterior part of the tragus. The lower end should lie over the medial end of the clavicle.

Spinal Accessory Nerve

This nerve is described on page 268. Its upper end lies over the same point as for the vagus (i.e., over the anterior part of the tragus). From here draw a line downwards and backwards to reach a point midway between the mastoid process and the angle of the mandible. (Deep pressure here will show that the point lies over the transverse process of the atlas). From this point carry the line further downwards and backwards to reach the middle of the posterior border of the sternocleidomastoid muscle. The nerve then runs across the posterior triangle to reach the anterior border of the trapezius about two inches above the clavicle.

Phrenic Nerve

This nerve is described on page 206.

To mark this nerve first feel for the upper border of the thyroid cartilage. At this level take a point 3.5 cm from the anterior midline of the neck. This is the upper end of the nerve. From here draw a line downwards and medially to reach the medial end of the clavicle.

Sympathetic Chain in the Neck

This is described on page 271. To mark this chain remember that it runs vertically immediately behind the carotid sheath. Its upper end lies just behind the condyle of the mandible. Its lower end lies over the sternoclavicular joint.

CHAPTER 15

Clinical Correlations of Head and Neck

CLINICAL CORRELATIONS OF BONES AND JOINTS OF THE HEAD AND NECK

THE SKULL

Congenital Malformations

1. Anencephaly is a malformation in which the greater part of the vault of the skull is missing. It is caused by failure of the neural tube to close in the region where the brain is to be formed. Neural tissue, which is exposed to the surface degenerates. The condition is fairly frequent and is not compatible with life.
2. Establishment of the normal shape of the skull depends on orderly closure of sutures. Premature union of the sagittal suture gives rise to a boat shaped skull (***scaphocephaly***). Early union of the coronal suture results in a skull that is pointed upwards (***acrocephaly***). Asymmetrical union of sutures (on the right and left sides) results in a twisted skull (***plagiocephaly***).
3. ***Congenital hydrocephalus*** is a condition in which there is obstruction to the flow of cerebrospinal fluid. As a result pressure in the ventricular system of the brain increases and leads to its dilatation. In turn this leads to enlargement of the head, and wide separation of the bones of the skull.
4. The maxilla, the mandible and the zygomatic bone are derived from the first branchial arch. Occasionally growth of this arch is defective so that the bones concerned remain underdeveloped, and the face is deformed. The condition is called ***mandibulofacial dysostosis***.
5. Many bones of the skull are formed by intramembranous ossification. The clavicle is also formed in membrane. In the condition called ***cleidocranial dysostosis*** formation of membrane bones is interfered with. Deformities of the skull are seen in association with absence of the clavicle.

Fractures of the Skull

Fractures of the skull are serious because of the likelihood of damage to the brain. Some facts of interest regarding these fractures are as follows.

1. The skull of a child is highly elastic and is seldom fractured. A localized blow on the skull of a child produces a depression on the area struck (***pond***

fracture), the rest of the skull remaining unaffected. In contrast a blow on the skull of an adult can shatter it, with cracks running in various directions from the area that is hit. The fractures run along lines that are weak. Injury on the vault of the skull can thus result in fractures of the base of the skull (cranial fossae). A blow over the parietal bone can lead to a fracture that extends into the squamous part of the temporal bone and into the middle cranial fossa. In the cranial fossae the fracture line often runs across foramina (which represent sites of weakness).

The inner table of the skull is more brittle than the outer table, and so a fracture may involve the inner table more extensively than the outer. Sometimes injury to the head may fracture the inner table leaving the outside of the skull intact.

2. Apart from its elasticity (in the young) other factors that tend to protect the skull from fractures are its rounded shape, and the presence of muscles over the temporal fossa and the occipital region (where the skull wall is thin).
3. **Fractures of middle cranial fossa**: The body and greater wing of the sphenoid are closely related to the middle cranial fossa. A fracture involving the body of the sphenoid bone can lead to leakage of blood and CSF into the sphenoidal air sinuses, and through them into the nose and mouth.
   The 3rd, 4th and 6th cranial nerves lie in relation to the cavernous sinus (which lies against the body of the sphenoid bone). These nerves can be involved in fractures of the middle cranial fossa.
   Posteriorly, the middle cranial fossa is bounded by the petrous temporal bone. Involvement of this bone can lead to bleeding and discharge of CSF into the middle ear and external acoustic meatus. The 7th and 8th cranial nerves (which pass through the internal acoustic meatus) can also be injured in a fracture through the petrous temporal bone.
4. **Fractures of the anterior cranial fossa**: This fossa is closely related to the nasal cavity and to the orbits. Fracture through the fossa can lead to bleeding or leakage of CSF through the nose (the blood flowing directly into nose through its roof, or through the frontal air sinus). Bleeding into the orbit can push the eyeball forwards (exophthalmos). Blood in the orbit can seep into the eyelids resulting in a 'black eye'
5. **Fractures of the posterior cranial fossa**: Fractures through this fossa can lead to bleeding, the blood seeping into the muscles of the back of the neck. The blood often appears superficially over the mastoid process and the sternomastoid muscle. If the fracture passes through the jugular foramen there can be injury to the 9th, 10th and 11th cranial nerves. The walls of the hypoglossal canal are strong and so the 12th cranial nerve usually escapes injury.
6. Injuries (e.g., blows) on the face can lead to fracture of the mandible, the zygomatic bone, the maxilla or the nasal bones.
   The mandible is commonly fractured. The fracture can involve the neck, the body, the angle, the symphysis menti or the ramus of the bone. The fracture can be bilateral. A fracture through the body of the bone often takes place at the level of the canine socket (the deep socket making the bone weak here). Such a fracture can involve the inferior alveolar nerve.
   A fracture of the maxilla can deform the floor of the orbit causing ocular displacement. Involvement of the infraorbital nerve can produce anaesthesia over the cheek and upper lip. Fractures of the maxilla, or of the mandible, can cause malocclusion of teeth.

Injuries to the Brain Following Injury to the Skull

Fractures of the skull often lead to injury to the brain. An impact on the head can damage the brain even in the absence of a fracture. In this connection it is to be remembered that the brain is a very delicate tissue. However, it is not damaged by normal bodily movements because (a) it is surrounded by a cushion of CSF, and (b) its displacement is prevented by folds of duramater (falx cerebri, tentorium cerebelli, falx cerebelli). Veins passing from the brain to the dural venous sinuses (specially the superior cerebral veins passing to the superior sagittal sinus) also help to keep the brain in position.

The importance of the cushion of CSF can be demonstrated by removing a fresh brain (unfixed) from the cranial cavity and putting it in a tray. It is then seen that brain substance loses its shape and spreads into the tray like a semisolid mass. However, if the same brain is suspended in any fluid it resumes its normal shape. In life, the cushion of CSF prevents the brain from striking against the inner wall of the skull].

A strong impact on the head can shake up the brain. When this shaking up leaves no apparent physical damage the condition is called ***cerebral concussion***. It is usually followed by a variable period of unconsciousness. On regaining consciousness the patient may suffer from headaches and loss of memory.

An injury in which there is superficial injury to brain tissue (but without any break on its surface) is called ***cerebral contusion***; and when there is tearing of brain tissue it is a ***cerebral laceration***. Severe damage to be brain, specially the brain stem, can lead to prolonged periods of deep unconsciousness (coma) and to death. Patients who come out of coma may show various neurological symptoms depending on the part of the brain injured.

Apart from direct injury to the brain, injury to the skull can affect the brain by causing haemorrhage. Such bleeding can be of various types.

a. **Extradural haemorrhage**: Injury to meningeal vessels can cause bleeding into the potential space between the inner (meningeal) layer of duramater and the skull. The haematoma can press upon the brain surface and produce symptoms. Extradural haemorrhage is often caused by injury to the anterior division of the middle meningeal artery, resulting in pressure over the motor area of the brain.
b. **Subdural haemorrhage**: Blood accumulates in the space between the dura and arachnoid. It is often caused by rupture of superior cerebral veins at their entry into the superior sagittal sinus. Such injury is most likely to be caused by a blow on the front or back of the head (as such injury causes anteroposterior displacement of the brain stretching the veins).
c. **Subarachnoid haemorrhage**: Blood flows into the subarachnoid space and mixes with CSF. Such haemorrhage can be caused by rupture of aneurysms that are not uncommon on arteries forming the circulus arteriosus.

Fracture of the Hyoid Bone

The hyoid bone can be fractured when the neck is forcibly pressed upon as in strangulation, or in hanging. Such a fracture is of considerably medicolegal significance.

CERVICAL SPINE

Congenital Malformations

1. ***Spina bifida*** can be present in the cervical region.
2. Two or more cervical vertebrae may be fused to one another resulting in a short neck (***Klippel Feil syndrome***). The atlas vertebra may be fused to the occipital bone (***occipitalization of atlas***).

The dens may not be fused to the body of the axis vertebra. See cervical spondylolisthesis, below.

3. ***Congenital torticolis***: See infantile torticolis, below.

Other Correlations

1. In the condition called ***infantile torticolis*** the mastoid process of one side is pulled towards the sternoclavicular joint of the same side (i.e., the two attachments of the sternocleidomastoid are pulled towards each other). As a result the head is tilted to one side and rotated to the opposite side. The condition (previously regarded as congenital) is now believed to be a result of injury to the sternocleidomastoid muscle during birth, and its gradual fibrosis. The altered position of the neck leads to deformity of cervical vertebrae which may become wedge shaped. The face can also become asymmetrical. The torticolis is often preceeded by a swelling (tumour) on the sternocleidomastoid.
2. Degenerative changes taking place in the cervical spine, with age, often lead to stiffness and pain in the neck (***cervical spondylosis***). The intervertebral joints undergo inflammation which is associated with the formation of bony outgrowth (osteophytes). The outgrowths can encroach on intervertebral foramina narrowing them so that cervical nerves may be pressed upon. Such pressure (accentuated by the presence of oedema) can lead to pain which often radiates into the upper limb.
3. Prolapse of an intervertebral disc can occur in the cervical region. The symptoms are similar to those of cervical spondylosis.
4. Cervical vertebrae can be dislocated or fractured by falls on the head. This is because such falls cause acute flexion of the neck.
   In the thoracic and lumbar regions of the vertebral column adjoining vertebrae are maintained in position by close interlocking of the articular processes. Dislocation of the vertebral column can take place only after fracture of the articular processes. However, in the cervical region the articular surfaces are flat and almost horizontal, so that dislocation is possible without fracture.
   Dislocation and fracture of the vertebral column are very serious because of damage to the spinal cord.
   In death by hanging, the dens (of the axis) dislocates backwards (by tearing through the transverse ligament of the atlas), and crushes the lower medulla and the spinal cord. Sometimes there is fracture of the axis vertebra.
5. A cervical vertebra (usually the atlas) may slip forwards over the next vertebra even in the absence of injury (***cervical spondylolisthesis***). This may be caused (a) by failure of the dens to fuse with the body of the axis, or (b) by weakness of the transverse ligament of the atlas caused by inflammation.

TEMPOROMANDIBULAR JOINT

The movements at the temporomandibular joint have been described on page 761. We have seen that when the mouth is closed, or is slightly open, the head of the mandible lies in the articular fossa. In this position the joint is stable, and a blow on the chin causes fracture of the mandible rather than dislocation. Backwards dislocation (towards the external acoustic meatus) is also prevented by the strong lateral temporomandibular ligament.

When the mouth is opened wide the head of the mandible moves forwards and comes to lie just below the articular tubercle. In this position the temporomandibular joint is highly unstable. A blow on the chin, or even sudden opening of the mouth as in yawning (involving sudden contraction of the lateral pterygoid muscle) can cause the head of the mandible to slip forwards to the front of the articular tubercle. Once the joint is thus dislocated the mouth cannot be closed. To reduce the dislocation the surgeon inserts both his thumbs into the mouth and exerts downward pressure over the lower molar teeth. Simultaneously, the mandible is pressed backwards.

The term derangement of the temporomandibular joint is applied to a condition in which part of the articular disc gets detached from the joint capsule. This happens after injury. Movements of the jaw become painful, and clicking sounds may be produced while opening and closing the mouth.

CLINICAL CORRELATIONS OF BLOOD VESSELS OF HEAD AND NECK

THE ARTERIES

In considering the arteries of the head and neck it must always be remembered that the common and internal carotid arteries, and the vertebral arteries, convey blood to the brain. Similarly, although the subclavian arteries lie in the neck they are the main channels of supply to the upper extremities. Therefore, any form of obstruction to these arteries of the neck can produce symptoms referable to the brain, and to the upper limb.

Congenital Anomalies

The large arteries of the head and neck develop from a series of aortic arch arteries that lie in the embryonic pharyngeal arches. For understanding their interesting mode of formation see the author's HUMAN EMBRYOLOGY. Some anomalies that can be produced by maldevelopment are given below.

1. Normally, the left common carotid artery is a direct branch of the arch of the aorta. Sometimes it may arise as a branch of the brachiocephalic trunk. [The brachiocephalic trunk then divides into three branches viz., right subclavian, right common carotid, and left common carotid]. Sometimes the left common carotid and left subclavian arteries may arise from the arch of the aorta by a common stem (which is then called the left brachiocephalic trunk).
2. The right subclavian artery may arise as the last branch of the arch of the aorta (or of the descending thoracic aorta). To reach the neck the artery has to run upwards behind the oesophagus. Along with the arch of the aorta the artery forms an arterial ring enclosing the trachea and oesophagus. The ring may obstruct the oesophagus leading to dysphagia (***dysphagia lusoria***). The ring can also be a cause of obstruction of the trachea.
3. The left vertebral artery may arise as a direct branch of the arch of the aorta (instead of arising from the subclavian artery).

Other Correlations

1. During surgical operations the anaesthetist sits at the head end of the patient and often feels for the pulse in the superficial temporal artery near the zygomatic arch, or in the facial artery as it crosses the lower border of the mandible (near the anterior border of the masseter). Pulsation of the common carotid artery (carotid pulse) can be felt at the level of the superior border of the thyroid cartilage, beneath the anterior border of the sternocleidomastoid muscle.

2. Weakening of the wall of any artery can lead to dilatation of the artery (***aneurysm***) at that site.

   Aneurysms on any intracranial artery can burst and can be a cause of bleeding into the subarachnoid space (see above). An aneurysm of the third part of the subclavian artery can press on the brachial plexus leading to motor and sensory symptoms in the upper extremity.
3. With age any artery of the body can undergo degenerative changes associated with deposition of fatty substances in the arterial wall (***atheromatosis***). Blockage of the common carotid or internal carotid arteries in this way can interfere with blood supply of the brain and of the eyeball. In suspected cases of blockage the carotid system of arteries is investigated by ***carotid angiography***. A radioopaque dye is injected into the common carotid artery either directly or through a catheter (passed up through the femoral artery to reach the arch of the aorta). Skiagrams taken after the injection reveal the site of blockage. In such skiagrams the petrous, cavernous and cerebral parts of the internal carotid artery cast a typical S-shaped shadow to which the term ***carotid syphon*** is applied.

   Atheroma may affect the vertebral arteries, specially their first and fourth parts. These arteries may also be pressed upon by osteophytes in cervical spondylosis. Inadequacy in blood flow through the vertebral and basilar arteries can give rise to attacks of transient ischaemia in which the patient complains of dizziness.

   Obstruction of one vertebral artery usually does not produce symptoms because of blood flow through the contralateral vertebral artery. Collateral anastomoses also exist through the ascending cervical, thyrocervical and occipital arteries.

   One cause of possible obstruction to flow of blood in the subclavian artery is the presence of a cervical rib. The artery has to loop over the cervical rib to enter the axilla and is therefore pressed upon.
4. Pressure on arteries can be used to stop haemorrhage in the area of its distribution. The common carotid artery can be compressed against the carotid tubercle (which is the anterior tubercle of transverse process of the sixth cervical vertebra). It should be remembered that pressure on the carotid sinus causes slowing of heart rate and fall of blood pressure. Also note that when the neck is extended the carotid sheath is retracted. It is because of this fact that in suicidal attempts at slitting the neck the cut often fails to reach the carotid arteries.

   Bleeding caused by severe injuries in the proximal part of the upper extremity can be controlled by pressure over the subclavian artery. Pressure is directed downwards and backwards (and somewhat medially). The artery gets compressed against the first rib.
5. We have seen that injury to the middle meningeal artery is an important cause of an extradural haemorrhage. To reach a bleeding anterior branch of this artery the surgeon takes a point 4 cm above the middle of the zygomatic arch and bores a hole through the skull. The region corresponds to the pterion.

   Extradural haemorrhage from an injured posterior division of the middle meningeal artery is less common. The blood can press upon the superior temporal gyrus and lead to deafness in the ear of the opposite side. To approach this branch the surgeon makes a hole in the skull over a point 4 cm above and 4 cm behind the external acoustic meatus.

THE VEINS

Variability: As in other parts of the body the arrangement of veins, specially that of superficial veins, is highly variable. In particular note that the anterior jugular vein (which is normally paired) may be represented by a single median vein, or may be absent on one side.

Injury to veins: Superficial veins are liable to be involved in injuries to the neck. The external jugular vein is particularly vulnerable. Normally when a vein is cut its walls retract thus limiting the amount of bleeding. However, it will be recalled that near its lower end the external jugular vein pierces the deep fascia. Here the wall of the vein is adherent to fascia, and this prevents the wall from retracting if the vein is injured. Also remember that during inspiration pressure in the vein can be negative and air can be sucked into the vein. This can have very serious consequences if it leads to air embolism.

Dangerous area of face: Near the medial angle of the eye the supraorbital vein, which is a tributary of the facial vein, communicates with the superior ophthalmic vein (lying in the orbit). The superior ophthalmic vein drains into the cavernous sinus. In this way the facial vein is brought into communication with the cavernous sinus. The facial vein also communicates with the cavernous sinus through the deep facial vein and the pterygoid plexus. Because of these communications an infection in the face can spread to the cavernous sinus leading to cavernous sinus thrombosis (see below). It has been observed that such spread of infection is most likely to take place if the infection is over the upper lip or the lower part of the nose. That is why this region is called the dangerous area of the face.

Venous pressure: Clinicians examining the cardiovascular system use the level of blood in the external jugular vein as an indication of venous pressure. When the patient lies flat the vein is at the same level as the right atrium and the entire vein is full of blood. When the head rests on a pillow the level of blood in the vein lies at junction of the lower and middle thirds of the neck. When the patient sits up the vein becomes empty. Venous pressure can be raised if there is right heart failure, raised intrathoracic pressure from any cause, or obstruction to the superior vena cava.

Increased venous pressure leads to dilatation of veins in the neck. The internal jugular vein can be markedly dilated.

Involvement in malignancy: Lymph nodes from all parts of the head and neck ultimately drain into the deep cervical lymph nodes which are therefore frequently involved in malignancy and in infections such as tuberculosis. In the treatment of malignancy the surgeon often has to remove these nodes. Enlarged nodes become adherent to the internal jugular vein and it is sometimes necessary for the surgeon to remove a segment of the vein along with the lymph nodes.

Intracranial Venous Sinuses

Intracranial venous sinuses are of importance because they receive blood from the brain. Infection in these sinuses can spread into brain tissue with serious consequences. Infections in the scalp can spread into the venous sinuses through emissary veins that pass through foramina in the skull. Recall that emissary veins traverse the layer of loose areolar tissue of the scalp which is therefore called the ***dangerous area of the scalp***. We have seen above that infection can reach the cavernous sinus from the face.

Thrombosis in the Cavernous Sinus

The cavernous sinus can be infected by spread of infection from the dangerous area of the face (see above). Infection can also reach it from the nose and paranasal sinuses.

Symptoms can be produced by (a) blockage to blood flow, (b) involvement of cranial nerves.

As veins of the orbit drain into the cavernous sinus they become congested. Accumulation of fluid in the orbit pushes the eyeball forwards (exophthalmos). The eyelids and the root of the nose show swelling.

Involvement of the ophthalmic nerve leads to severe pain in the region of distribution of the nerve (eye and over the forehead). Involvement of the oculomotor, trochlear and abducent nerves can lead to paralysis of extraocular muscles.

Thrombosis in the Superior Sagittal Sinus

Infection can spread to this sinus from the scalp or from the nasal cavities. It can also reach it from an infected sigmoid or transverse sinus.

The arachnoid granulations (made up of arachnoid villi) in the superior sagittal sinus are the main site at which CSF is absorbed into the blood stream. When the sinus is thrombosed this absorption is interfered with leading to increased pressure in the CSF. This leads to various signs of increased intracranial tension. In a child it can lead to hydrocephalus.

Venous blood from the cerebral hemisphere is drained predominantly by superior cerebral veins which open into the superior sagittal sinus. Infection from the sinus can extend along these veins to the cerebral hemisphere.

Thrombosis in the Sigmoid Sinus

The middle ear and the mastoid air cells are very frequent sites of infection. The close relationship of the sigmoid sinus to the middle ear (lying in the petrous temporal bone) and the mastoid process often leads to spread of infection to this sinus. Thrombosis in the sinus can extend downwards into the internal jugular vein. It can spread upwards along the transverse sinus into the superior sagittal sinus.

CLINICAL CORRELATIONS OF DEEP CERVICAL FASCIA

The arrangement of fascial layers in the neck determines the direction of spread of infections as follows.

a. In tuberculosis of the cervical vertebrae pus is formed and collects between the vertebral column and the prevertebral fascia. The pus can produce a swelling in the posterior wall of the pharynx, and such a swelling is in the midline. The swelling is referred to as a ***chronic retropharyngeal abscess*** (because of the chronic nature of tubercular infection).

   The pus from such an abscess can pass downwards (in front of the prevertebral muscles) and can appear under the skin of the posterior triangle of the neck. It can also descend into the axilla along the axillary sheath.

b. The retropharyngeal lymph nodes are located between the prevertebral fascia (behind) and the buccopharyngeal fascia (in front). In infection of these nodes an ***acute retropharyngeal abscess*** is formed. It is acute because of the nature of the infection. Unlike a chronic abscess which is situated in the midline, an acute abscess lies to one side of the midline. This is so because the prevertebral fascia and buccopharyngeal fascia are adherent to each other along the midline.

The pus can pass downwards behind the pharynx and oesophagus to reach the superior mediastinum, or even the posterior mediastinum .

c. An infection in the submandibular region is limited to a triangular area bounded by the two halves of the mandible and (posteriorly) by the hyoid bone. This is so because the investing layer of deep fascia is attached to these bones. Infection here produces a triangular swelling (***Ludwig's angina***). Collection of fluid can push the tongue upwards.

d. The deep cervical lymph nodes are often sites of tubercular infection. The pus formed may pierce through a small area of deep fascia and form a swelling under the skin. There is one collection of pus deep to the deep fascia, and another superficial to the fascia the two being in communication through the narrow opening (***collar stud abscess***).

The fascia covering the parotid gland (parotid fascia) is very strong. In infections of the parotid gland (e.g., mumps) the organ can, therefore, not expand. Nerves are pressed upon causing much pain.

THE SCALP

Wounds of the Scalp

The scalp is profusely supplied with blood, the arteries entering it from the sides, from the front and from the behind. Because of this wounds of the scalp bleed profusely. Bleeding can be difficult to stop because the walls of blood vessels are adherent to the dense subcutaneous fibrous tissue. Direct pressure over the wound is needed to stop bleeding.

The profuse blood supply also provides some advantages in dealing with scalp wounds. Portions of scalp that are torn off (evulsed) retain adequate blood supply (even through narrow areas of attachment), and heal well when stitched back into position. However, if a portion of scalp is completely detached the surgeon finds it difficult to fill the gap. Hence the surgeon makes it a point not to cut away parts of the scalp unless absolutely necessary.

In relation to wounds of the scalp it is necessary to remember that the skin and the epicranial aponeurosis are firmly united to each other by the layer of dense connective tissue. Also remember that the fibres of the aponeurosis run predominantly in an anteroposterior direction. A wound on the scalp does not gape (i.e., the edges do not separate) unless the epicranial aponeurosis is divided. Even if the aponeurosis is divided in an anteroposterior cut the wound will not gape because of the predominant direction of the fibres. It is only when the aponeurosis is cut transversely that the wound can gape widely.

Injuries on the head can lead to bleeding into various layers of the scalp. Bleeding into the superficial fascia is never extensive as the region is divided into small pockets by fibrous tissue. Bleeding into the layer of loose areolar tissue spreads widely reaching the orbital margin anteriorly, the nuchal lines posteriorly, and the temporal lines laterally. Bleeding deep to the pericranium (periosteum) does not extend beyond the margins of the bone as the pericranium is adherent to sutural ligaments which limit the spread of blood. The shape of the haematoma, therefore, corresponds to that of the underlying bone (***cephalhaematoma***).

Infections of the Scalp

An infection in the subcutaneous tissue is limited to a small area as the tissue is divided into small pockets by dense fibrous tissue. For the same reason pressure on nerves in the area becomes high and leads to severe pain.

An infection in the layer of loose areolar tissue can spread to the limits of the space (see above). This layer is traversed by emissary veins and infection can pass through these veins to intracranial venous sinuses. That is why the layer of loose areolar tissue is called the dangerous area of the scalp. Osteomyelitis of the skull bones can also be caused by spread of infection through emissary veins.

Swellings on the Scalp

Sebaceous cysts: Because of the presence of numerous hair follicles, and the sebaceous glands associated with them, the scalp is a common site for sebaceous systs. The cysts are often multiple.

A sebaceous cyst is caused by blockage to discharge of secretion of a sebaceous gland. The secretion accumulates and leads to formation of the cyst. The interior of the cyst is lined with epithelial cells.

Dermoid cysts. Dermoid cysts are formed by multiplication of epithelial cells that get burried under the skin surface. The cysts may be congenital, or may be caused by pricks. A dermoid cyst can lead to erosion of underlying bone.

Neoplasms. Various types types of tumours, benign and malignant, may occur in the scalp.

CRANIAL NERVES

The cranial nerves have been considered in detail in Chapter 9. Here we will consider how these nerves are tested during clinical examination, and some important features arising from damage to these nerves.

Olfactory Nerve

The olfactory nerve is tested by asking the patient to recognize various odours. The right and left nerves can be tested separately by closing one nostril and putting the substance near the open nostril.

OPTIC NERVE AND VISUAL PATHWAY

Testing the Optic Nerve

To test the optic nerve first ask the patient if his vision is normal. Acuity (sharpness) of vision can be tested by making the patient read letters of various sizes printed on a chart from a fixed distance. It must of course be remembered that loss of acuity of vision can be caused by errors of refraction, or by the presence of opacities in the cornea or the lens (cataract).

As part of a normal clinical examination the field of vision can be tested as follows. Ask the patient to sit opposite you (about half a meter away) and look straight forwards at you. As one eye to be tested at a time ask the patient to place a hand on one eye so that he can see only with the other eye. Stretch out one of your arms laterally so that your hand is about equal distance from your face and that of the patient. In this position you will probably not be able to see your hand. However, you may notice it if you move a finger. Keep moving your index finger and gradually bring the hand towards yourself until you can just see the movements of the finger. This gives you an idea of the extent of your own visual field in that direction. By asking the patient to tell you as soon as he can see the moving finger (making sure that he does not turn his head) you can get an idea of the patients field of vision in the direction of your hand. By repeating the test placing your hand in different directions a good idea of the field of vision of the patient can be obtained. If an abnormality is suspected detailed testing can be done using a procedure called ***perimetry***.

If there is any doubt about the integrity of optic nerve the retina is examined using an ***ophthalmoscope***. With this instrument we can see the interior of the eye through the pupil of the eye. The optic disc and blood vessels radiating from it can be seen

Effects of Injury to Visual Pathway

Injuries to different parts of the visual pathway can produce various kinds of defects. Loss of vision in one half (right or left) of the visual field is called ***hemianopia***. If the same half of the visual field is lost in both eyes the defect is said to be ***homonymous*** and if different halves are lost the defect is said to be ***heteronymous***. Note that the ***hemianopia is named in relation to the visual field*** and not to the retina.

Injury to the optic nerve will obviously produce total blindness in the eye concerned. Damage to the central part of the optic chiasma (e.g., by pressure from an enlarged hypophysis) interrupts the crossing fibres derived from the nasal halves of the two retinae resulting in ***bitemporal heteronymous hemianopia***. It has been claimed that macular fibres are more susceptible to damage by pressure than peripheral fibres and are affected first. When the lateral part of the chiasma is affected a nasal hemianopia results. This may be unilateral or bilateral. Complete destruction of the optic tract, the lateral geniculate body, the optic radiation or the visual cortex of one side, results in loss of the opposite half of the field of vision. A lesion on the right side leads to left homonymous hemianopia. Lesions anterior to the lateral geniculate body also interrupt fibres responsible for the ***pupillary light reflex*** (See below).

OCULOMOTOR, TROCHLEAR AND ABDUCENT NERVES

These three nerves are responsible for movements of the eyeball. In a routine clinical examination the movements are tested by asking the patient to keep his head fixed and to move his eyes in various directions i.e., upwards, downwards, inwards and outwards. An easy way is to ask the patient to keep his head fixed, and to follow the movements of your finger with his eyes. Such an examination can detect a gross abnormality in movement of the eyes.

Sometimes one of the ocular muscles may not be completely paralysed but may be weak. Two indications of such weakness are as follows.

Diplopia

This term means that objects are seen double. To understand this phenomenon remember that objects lying in different parts of the visual field produce images over different spots on the retina. The brain judges the position of an object by the position at which its image is formed on the retina. Normally the movements of the right and left eyes are in perfect alignment, and an object casts an image on corresponding spots on the two retinae so that only one image is perceived by the brain. When a muscle of the eyeball is weak, and a movement involving that muscle is performed, the movement of the defective eye is slightly less than that of the normal eye. As a result images of the object on the two retinae are not formed at corresponding points but over two points near each other. The brain therefore 'sees' two images, one from each retina.

To understand the causation of diplopia you can do a little experiment on yourself. Fix your gaze on any object. Place a finger below one eyeball and gently push it upwards. In addition to the normal bright image of the object you will see a second fainter image above the normal image. This illustrates that diplopia will be produced by any factor that distorts the normal alignment of the two eyes relative to each other.

Squint (or Strabismus)

This is a condition in which the two eyes do not look in the same direction. The squint becomes obvious when the eye movement involves a muscle that is paralysed or weak, because the weak muscle cannot keep up with the muscle of the normal side.

As explained above squint will be accompanied by diplopia. However, the patient compensates for lack of movement of the eyeball by turning the head in the direction of the object and on doing so the diplopia disappears.

If the normal eye is closed, the patient is unable to judge the position of objects in the field of vision correctly (because the image of the object does not fall on the part of the retina that corresponds to the true position of the object). All the features described above are those of ***paralytic squint***.

There is another type of squint called ***concomitant squint***. This condition is congenital, and manifests itself in early childhood. Squint is present in all positions of the eyeball. There is no muscular weakness and movements are normal in all directions. There is no diplopia.

Paralysis of Oculomotor Nerve

All movements of the eyeball are lost in the affected eye. When the patient is asked to look directly forwards the affected eye is directed laterally (by the lateral rectus) and downwards (by the superior oblique). There is lateral quint (external strabismus) and diplopia.

As the levator palpebrae superioris is paralysed there is drooping of the upper eyelid (***ptosis***). As parasympathetic fibres to the sphincter pupillae pass through the oculomotor nerve, the sphincter pupillae is paralysed. Unopposed action of sympathetic nerves produces a ***fixed and dilated pupil***.

Normally the pupil contracts when exposed to light (***light reflex***). It also contracts when the relaxed eye is made to concentrate on a near object (***accommodation reflex***). Both these reflexes are lost. The power of accommodation is lost because of paralysis of the ciliaris muscle.

Paralysis of Trochlear Nerve

The superior oblique muscle (supplied by the trochlear nerve) moves the eyeball downwards and laterally, and the inferior rectus (supplied by the oculomotor nerve) moves it downwards and medially. For direct downward movement synchronized action of both muscles is required. When the superior oblique muscle is paralysed the eyeball deviates medially on trying to look downwards.

Paralysis of Abducent Nerve

This nerve supplies the lateral rectus muscle which moves the eyeball laterally. In looking forwards the lateral pull of the lateral rectus is counteracted by the medial pull of the medial rectus and so the eye is maintained in the centre. When the lateral rectus is paralysed the affected eye deviates medially (***medial squint***, or ***internal strabismus***).

TRIGEMINAL NERVE

The trigeminal nerve has a wide sensory distribution. It also supplies the muscles of mastication.

The sensation of touch in the area of distribution of the nerve can be tested by touching different areas of skin with a wisp of cotton wool. The sensation of pain can be tested by gentle pressure with a pin.

Motor function is tested by asking the patient to clench his teeth firmly. Contraction of the masseter can be felt by palpation when the teeth are clenched.

Effects of Injury or Disease

Injury to the trigeminal nerve causes paralysis of the muscles supplied and loss of sensations in the area of supply. Some features of special importance are as follows:

1. Apart from their role in opening and closing the mouth, the muscles of mastication are responsible for side to side movements of the mandible. Contraction of these muscles on one side moves the chin to the opposite side. Normally the chin is maintained in the midline by the balanced tone of the muscles of the right and left sides. In paralysis of the pterygoid muscles of one side the chin is pushed to the ***paralysed side*** by muscles of the opposite side.
2. Loss of sensation in the ophthalmic division (specially the nasociliary nerve) is of great importance. Normally the eyelids close as soon as the cornea is touched (***corneal reflex***). Loss of sensation in the cornea abolishes this reflex leaving the cornea unprotected. This can lead to the formation of ulcers on the cornea which can in turn lead to blindness.
3. Pain arising in a structure supplied by one branch of the nerve may be felt in an area of skin supplied by another branch: this is called ***referred pain***. Some examples are as follows:
    a. Caries of a tooth in the lower jaw (supplied by the inferior alveolar nerve) may cause pain in the ear (auriculotemporal).
    b. If there is an ulcer or cancer on the tongue (lingual nerve) the pain may again be felt over the ear and temple (auriculotemporal).
    c. In frontal sinusitis (sinus supplied by a branch from the supraorbital nerve) the pain is referred to the forehead (skin supplied by supraorbital nerve). In fact headache is a common symptom when any structure supplied by the trigeminal nerve is involved (e.g., eyes, ears, teeth).
4. A source of irritation in the distribution of the nerve may cause severe persistent pain (***trigeminal neuralgia***). Removal of the cause can cure the pain. However, in some cases no cause can be found. In such cases pain can be relieved by injection of alcohol into the trigeminal ganglion, into one of the divisions of the nerve, or into its sensory root. In some cases it may be necessary to cut fibres of the sensory root. In this connection it is important to know that the fibres for the maxillary and mandibular divisions can be cut without destroying those for the ophthalmic division. This is possible as the fibres for the ophthalmic division lie separately in the upper medial part of the sensory root. Finally, it may be noted that trigeminal pain can also be relieved by cutting the spinal tract of the trigeminal nerve: this procedure is useful specially for relieving pain in the distribution of the ophthalmic division as pain can be abolished without loss of the sense of touch and, therefore, without the abolition of the corneal reflex.
5. ***Mandibular nerve block***: This is used for anaesthesia of the lower jaw (for extraction of teeth). Palpate the anterior margin of the ramus of the mandible. Just

medial to it you will feel the pterygomandibular raphe (ligament). The needle is inserted in the interval between the ramus and the raphe. The tip of the needle is now very near the inferior alveolar nerve, just before it enters the mandibular canal. Anaesthetic injected here blocks the nerve.

6. The lingual nerve lies very close to the medial side of the third molar tooth, just deep to the mucosa. The nerve can be injured in careless extraction of a third molar. In cases of cancer of the tongue, having intractable pain, the lingual can be cut at this site to relieve pain.

FACIAL NERVE

The facial nerve supplies the muscles of the face including the muscles that close the eyelids, and the mouth. The nerve is tested as follows.

1. Ask the patient to close his eyes firmly. In complete paralysis of the facial nerve the patient will not be able to close the eye on the affected side. In partial paralysis the closure is weak and the examiner can easily open the closed eye with his fingers (which is very difficult in a normal person).
2. Ask the person to smile. In smiling the normal mouth is more or less symmetrical, the two angles moving upwards and outwards. In facial paralysis the angle fails to move on the paralysed side.
3. Ask the patient to fill his mouth with air. Press the cheek with your finger and compare the resistance (by the buccinator muscle) on the two sides. The resistance is less on the paralysed side. On pressing the cheek air may leak out of the mouth because the muscles closing the mouth are weak.
4. The sensation of taste should be tested on the anterior two thirds of the tongue (as described under glossopharyngeal nerve).

Paralysis of Facial Nerve

Paralysis of the facial nerve is fairly common. It can occur due to injury or disease of the facial nucleus (***nuclear paralysis***) or of the nerve any where along its course (***infranuclear paralysis***). In the most common type of infranuclear paralysis called Bell's palsy the nerve is affected near the stylomastoid foramen. Facial muscles can also be paralysed by interruption of corticonuclear fibres running from the motor cortex to the facial nucleus: this is referred to as ***supranuclear paralysis***.

The effects of paralysis are due to the failure of the muscles concerned to perform their normal actions. Some effects are as follows:

1. The normal face is more or less symmetrical. When the facial nerve is paralysed on one side the most noticeable feature is the loss of symmetry. (Also see para 4 in this regard).
2. Normal furrows on the forehead are lost because of paralysis of the occipitofrontalis.
3. There is drooping of the eyelid and the palpebral fissure is wider on the paralysed side because of paralysis of the orbicularis oculi. The conjunctival reflex is lost for the same reason.
4. There is marked asymmetry of the mouth because of paralysis of the orbicularis oris and of muscles inserted into the angle of the mouth. This is most obvious when a smile is attempted. As a result of asymmetry the protruded tongue appears to deviate to one side, but is in fact in the midline.
5. During mastication food tends to accumulate between the cheek and the teeth. (This is normally prevented by the buccinator).

Additional effects are observed in injuries to the facial nerve at levels higher than the stylomastoid foramen, as follows:

a. If the injury is proximal to the origin of the chorda tympani there is loss of the sensation of taste on the anterior two thirds of the tongue.
b. The transmission of loud sounds to the internal ear is normally dampened by the stapedius muscle. When the lesion is proximal to the origin of the branch to the stapedius this muscle is paralysed. As a result even normal sounds appear too loud (***hyperacusis***).
c. In fractures of the temporal bone, or in lesions near the exit of the nerve from the brain the vestibulocochlear nerve may also be affected (leading to deafness).
d. In nuclear lesions (within the brainstem) other neighbouring nuclei may be affected leading to lesions of the abducent or trigeminal nerves.
e. Supranuclear lesions can be distinguished from nuclear or infranuclear lesions because these are usually accompanied by hemiplegia. Movements of the lower part of the face are more affected than those of the upper part: the explanation for this is that the corticonuclear fibres concerned with movements of the upper part of the face are bilateral, whereas those for movements of the lower part of the face are unilateral. Another difference is that while voluntary movements are affected, emotional expressions appear to be normal. It has been suggested that there are separate pathways from the cerebral cortex to the facial nucleus for voluntary and emotional movements; and that usually only the former are involved.

VESTIBULOCOCHLEAR NERVE

This nerve is responsible for hearing (cochlear part) and for equilibrium (vestibular part). Normally we test only the cochlear part.

1. The hearing of the patient can be tested by using a watch. First place the watch near one ear so that the patient knows what he is expected to hear. Next ask him to close his eyes and say so when he hears the ticking of the watch. The watch should be held away from the ear and then gradually brought towards it. The distance at which the sounds are first heard should be compared with the other ear.

In doing this test it must be remembered that loss of hearing can occur from various causes such as the presence of wax in the ear, or middle ear disease.

Nerve deafness can be distinguished from deafness due to a conduction defect (as in middle ear disease) by noting the following.

1. Sounds can be transmitted to the internal ear through air (normal way), and can also be transmitted through bone. Normally conduction through air is better than that through bone, but in defects of conduction the sound is better heard through bone.
2. Air conduction and bone conduction can be compared by using a tuning fork. Strike the tuning fork against an object so that it begins to vibrate producing sound. Place the tuning fork near the patients ear and then immediately put the base of the tuning fork on the mastoid process. Ask the patient where he hears the sound better. (This is called Rinne's test). In another test the base of a vibrating tuning fork is placed on the forehead. The sound is heard in both ears but is more clear in the ear with a conduction defect (This is Weber's test).

Defects in the vestibular apparatus or in the vestibular nerve are difficult to test and such cases need to be examined by a specialist.

GLOSSOPHARYNGEAL NERVE

Testing of this nerve is based on the fact that (a) the nerve carries fibres of taste from the posterior one third of the tongue; and (b) that it provides sensory innervation to the pharynx.

1. Sensations of taste can be tested by applying substances that are salty (salt), sweet (sugar), sour (lemon), or bitter (quinine) to the posterior one third of the tongue. The mouth should be rinsed and the tongue dried before the substance is applied.
2. Touching the pharyngeal mucosa causes reflex constriction of pharyngeal muscles. The glossopharyngeal nerve provides the afferent part of the pathway for this reflex.

VAGUS NERVE (AND CRANIAL PART OF ACCESSORY)

This nerve has an extensive distribution but testing is based on its motor supply to the soft palate and to the larynx.

1. Ask the patient to open the mouth wide and say 'aah'. Observe the movement of the soft palate. In a normal person the soft palate is elevated. When one vagus nerve is paralysed the palate is pulled towards the normal side. When the nerve is paralysed on both sides the soft palate does not move at all.
2. In injury to the ***superior laryngeal nerve*** the voice is weak due to paralysis of the cricothyroid muscle. At first there is hoarseness but after some time the opposite cricothyroid compensates for the deficit and hoarseness disappears.
3. Injury to the ***recurrent laryngeal nerve*** also leads to hoarseness, but this hoarseness is permanent. On examining the larynx through a laryngoscope it is seen that on the affected side the vocal fold does not move. It is fixed in a position midway between adduction and abduction. In cases where the recurrent laryngeal nerve is pressed upon by a tumour it is observed that nerve fibres that supply abductors are lost first.
4. In paralysis of both recurrent laryngeal nerves voice is lost as both vocal folds are immobile.
5. It may be remembered that the left recurrent laryngeal nerve runs part of its course in the thorax. It can be involved in bronchial or oesophageal carcinoma, or by secondary growths in mediastinal lymph nodes.

ACCESSORY NERVE (SPINAL PART)

This nerve is tested as follows.

1. Put your hands on the right and left shoulders of the patient and ask him to elevate (shrug) his shoulders. In paralysis the movement will be weak on one side (due to paralysis of the trapezius).
2. Ask the patient to turn his face to the opposite side (against resistance offered by your hand). In paralysis the movement is weak on the affected side (due to paralysis of the sternocleidomastoid muscle).

HYPOGLOSSAL NERVE

This nerve supplies muscles of the tongue. To test the nerve ask the patient to protrude the tongue. In a normal person the protruded tongue lies in the midline.

If the nerve is paralysed the tongue deviates to the ***paralysed side***. The explanation for this is as follows.

Protrusion of the tongue is produced by the pull of the right and left genioglossus muscles. The origin of the right and left genioglossus muscles lies anteriorly (on the hyoid bone), and the insertion lies posteriorly (on to the posterior part of the tongue). Each muscle draws the posterior part of the tongue forwards ***and medially***. Normally, the medial pull of the two muscles cancels out, but when one muscle is paralysed it is this medial pull of the intact muscle that causes the tongue to deviate to the opposite side.

Deviation of the tongue should be assessed with reference to the incisor teeth, and not to the lips. Remember that in facial paralysis the tongue may protrude normally, but may appear to deviate to one side because of asymmetry of the mouth.

SYMPATHETIC NERVES OF HEAD AND NECK

Interruption of sympathetic supply to the head and neck results in ***Horner's syndrome***. The features of this syndrome are as follows.

1. There is ***constriction of the pupil*** because of paralysis of the dilator pupillae. Unopposed action of the sphincter pupillae leads to constriction.
2. There is drooping of the upper eyelid (***ptosis***) because of paralysis of smooth muscle fibres present in the levator palpebrae superioris.
3. The eyeball is less prominent than normal (***enophthalmos***).
4. There is absence of sweating on the affected side of the face. (Remember that secretomotor supply to sweat glands is through sympathetic nerves).

HYPOPHYSIS CEREBRI

The hypophysis cerebri and its hormones have been described on page 373. Various types of tumours may arise in this organ. The effects of the tumour (adenoma) may be caused by pressure on surrounding structures, or by increased or decreased production of hormones.

An adenoma arising from chromophobe cells can become quite large and can produce pressure effects as follows.

a. Pressure on the walls of the hypophyseal fossa (sella turcica) leads to its enlargement, and this enlargement can be seen in a skiagram.
b. The enlarging tumour presses on and destroys other cells (acidophils, basophils) of the pars anterior, and gives rise to deficiency of the hormones produced by them. Pressure on the pars posterior can lead to diabetes insipidus (see below).
c. Pressure on the optic chiasma can lead to loss of vision in the temporal halves of vision in both eyes (***bitemporal hemianopia***). Stretching of the optic nerves can lead to optic atrophy.
d. Pressure on the hypothalamus can interfere with various visceral functions. It can lead to ***Frohlich's syndrome*** which is characterized by obesity, poor development of sex organs including the gonads, and altered secondary sex characters.
e. Pressure on the third ventricle, can result in obstruction to flow of CSF, and raised intracranial tension.

An adenoma can be removed surgically. The approach can be through the roof of the pharynx, through the sphenoidal sinuses. In extensive tumours the cranial cavity has to be opened so that the tumour can be seen directly.

In an ***eosinophil adenoma*** pressure effects are negligible. The main effects arise from excessive production of growth hormone. In a young individual (before the epiphyses have fused) the condition results in excessive growth (***gigantism***). If the adenoma is formed after the epiphyses have fused overgrowth mainly affects the head, the hands and the feet (***acromegaly***). The scalp, lips, tongue and face become thick because of increased amount of subcutaneous tissue, and the same happens to the hands and feet. The paranasal sinuses enlarge making the facial region prominent. There is overgrowth of hair, and the man's appearance tends to resemble that of an ape.

In a ***basophil adenoma*** there is excessive secretion of adrenotropic hormones. It leads to ***Cushings's syndrome*** which we have seen can also be caused by a tumour of the adrenal cortex. The syndrome is seen mostly in females. Abnormal deposition of fat takes place over the face, neck and trunk. The limbs remain thin and weak.

The posterior lobe of the hypophysis cerebri produces antidiuretic hormone (ADH) which is responsible for reabsorption of water from renal tubules. Destruction of the posterior lobe (e.g., by pressure from an adenoma), can result in ***diabetes insipidus***. In this condition large amounts of urine are passed (***polyuria***). The urine is of very low specific gravity and contains no sugar or albumin. The resultant dehydration leads to excessive thirst (***polydipsia***) and to dryness of skin.

Apart from pressure by a tumour diabetes insipidus can be caused by trauma to the region. In many cases there is no obvious cause.

PINEAL BODY

Tumours of the pineal gland can press on the tectum of the midbrain. This can damage the oculomotor nucleus and can thus lead to paralysis of the oculomotor nerve. Pressure of the tumour may obstruct the aqueduct and cause hydrocephalus.

THYROID GLAND

Congenital Anomalies

1. Parts of the thyroid (isthmus, or one lobe) may be absent. A ***pyrimidal lobe*** may pass upwards from the isthmus or from one of the lobes. It may be just a short stump or may reach right up to the hyoid bone.
2. Thyroid tissue is derived from a median diverticulum arising from the floor of the primitive pharynx. In later life the site of origin of the diverticulum lies over the posterior part of the tongue (foramen caecum). As the diverticulum elongates it grows downwards as the ***thyroglossal duct***. This duct lies in the midline of the neck. The tip of the diverticulum divides into two parts each of which forms one lobe of the thyroid gland.

   Abnormal thyroid tissue may develop anywhere along the course of the thyroglossal duct. Thyroid tissue present under the mucosa of the dorsum of the tongue is called a ***lingual thyroid***. Thyroid tissue may be embedded within the lingual musculature, may lie in the midline of the neck above or below the hyoid bone, or may even be found in the thorax. A fact of considerable surgical importance is that before removing an abnormally situated mass of thyroid tissue the surgeon must make sure that a thyroid gland is present at the normal site. Sometimes it may not be present.

3. Apart from these masses of thyroid tissue present along the path of the thyroglossal duct ***ectopic thyroid tissue*** may be present in other locations. These include the larynx, the trachea, the oesophagus, the pleura or pericardium, and the ovaries.
4. Remnants of the thyroglossal duct may persist and may form a thyroglossal cyst that may be seen any where along the course of the duct. When a cyst opens on to the surface of the neck a fistula is created. In treating these conditions the surgeon has to remove the entire track of the thyroglossal duct. The duct forms a loop deep to the hyoid bone, and part of this bone may have to be excised for complete removal of the duct. Finally note that remnants of the thyroglossal duct may give rise to a carcinoma.

Other Correlations

1. In examining a patient in which an enlargement of the thyroid is suspected, it is useful to remember that the thyroid moves up and down during swallowing.
2. Deficient intake of iodine (common in areas where drinking water does not contain iodine) can lead to benign enlargement of the thyroid gland. The enlarged thyroid is referred to as ***goitre***. The symptoms are those of hypothyroidism.
3. Hypothyroidism in infants leads to ***cretinism***. A child with cretinism has a puffed face with a protruding tongue, a bulky belly, and sometimes an umbilical hernia. Hypothyroidism in adults is manifested by symptoms including a slow pulse, cold intolerance, mental and physical lethargy, and a hoarse voice. In advanced cases the condition is called ***myxoedema***. There is deposition of mucopolysaccharides in subcutaneous tissue at various sites resulting in a non-pitting oedema. The face is bloated, the lips are thick and protuberant and the expression is dull.
   Hypothyroidism can be caused by underdevelopment of the thyroid gland and this can be caused by maternal and fetal iodine deficiency. It can also take place as a result of destruction of thyroid tissue because of carcinoma, thyroiditis, surgical removal of the thyroid gland, or prolonged use of antithyroid drugs.
4. Hyperthyroidism is also referred to as ***thyrotoxicosis***, or ***toxic goitre***. The condition is much more common in women than in men. The condition is marked by nervousness, loss of weight, tachycardia and palpitation, excitability, tremors of the outstretched hands, and exophthalmos. The most important causes are ***Grave's disease*** (or diffuse toxic goitre, in which no nodules are felt on palpation of the thyroid); multinodular goitre, and a toxic adenoma.
5. Tumours of the thyroid may be benign or malignant. A tumour can press upon or involve the trachea, or carotid sheath. Involvement of the recurrent laryngeal nerve may occur.
   Upward expansion of a tumour of the thyroid is limited by the fact that the sternothyroid muscles, which cover the thyroid gland in front, are attached above to the thyroid cartilage. The tumours therefore tend to grow downwards and can even enter the thorax (***retrosternal goitre***).
6. An operation for removal of the thyroid gland is called ***thyroidectomy***. This may be required in some cases of hyperthyroidism. Normally, the posterior part of the gland (and the parathyroids) are left behind. It is of interest to note that the part left behind receives an adequate blood supply through branches from the tracheal and oesophageal arteries (even after the main thyroid arteries have been ligated).
   In thyroidectomy the main arteries have to be cut and tied. The superior thyroid artery is intimately related to the external laryngeal artery at a high level, but they separate near the upper pole of the gland. The surgeon, therefore, always cuts this artery as near the gland as possible so that the nerve is not cut.

In contrast the inferior thyroid artery is closely related to the recurrent laryngeal nerve near the gland and has to be ligated as far away as possible from the gland.

7. Inflammation of the thyroid gland is called ***thyroiditis***. It can be caused by infection or by various other causes. The most important form of thyroiditis is caused by an ***autoimmune process*** (***autoimmune or lymphatic thyroiditis***). It is also called ***Hashimoto's disease***. The thyroid gland is enlarged and is infiltrated with lymphocytes.

PARATHYROID GLANDS

The parathyroid glands have been described on page 923 and variability in their position described. These variations are of considerable importance to a surgeon trying to locate the which outlines both thyroid and parathyroids. The areas where radioactive materials are located can be recorded on a gamma camera. Computer separation of the two images reveals the location of the parathyroids.

Hyperparathyroidism

Excessive amounts of circulating parathormone can be present in tumours of the parathyroid gland (parathyroid adenoma). As a result calcium is depleted from bones which become weak (and can fracture). Increased urinary excretion of calcium may lead to formation of urinary calculi.

Hypoparathyroidism

Calcium levels in blood fall leading to muscular irritability and convulsions. The condition may be spontaneous or may occur following accidental removal of parathyroid glands during thyroidectomy.

THE MOUTH, TEETH AND GUMS

The mouth is always examined as part of a general physical examination. Hence a doctor must be aware of common conditions affecting the region.

The lips are blue in cyanosis. Inflammation at the angles of the mouth (***angular stomatitis***) occurs in vitamin deficiencies. The number of teeth present should be compared with the age of the patient. The ages at which various teeth erupt have been described on page 877. Delayed eruption may be a sign of malnutrition or some other growth disorder. In older people who have lost some teeth the absence of sufficient teeth for mastication may result in digestive disorders. Peg shaped upper central incisors (***Hutchinson's teeth***) may be an indication of syphilis. In this condition the teeth may show notches. Notching may also be present in rickets. In acromegaly the lower jaw becomes relatively larger than the upper jaw so that the teeth go out of alignment.

Gums are often the site of chronic inflammation specially in persons with poor oral hygiene. Inflammation of gums is called ***gingivitis***. The gums may be inflamed and bleed easily. Pockets may form and pus may be present in them (***pyorrhea***). Infection in the gums can lead to digestive and respiratory problems. A blue line running along the edge of the gum may be a sign of lead poisoning. The gums are swollen and spongy and bleed easily in scurvy which is caused by a deficiency of vitamin C.

Dental caries is a very common disease of the teeth. Microorganisms produce small cavities that gradually enlarge. The patient is usually unaware of them until the cavity invades the dentine when the teeth become sensitive to hot and cold, or to sugar. If untreated the cavity ultimately reaches the pulp of the tooth resulting in severe pain. Dental caries can be prevented by teaching children to brush their teeth after meals. Prevention can also be ensured by regular check up by a dentist. If cavities are discovered early they can be filled up and the tooth can be saved.

Caries is common in milk teeth and is ignored on the assumption that these teeth are going to be replaced. However, caries can result in too early loss of milk teeth and this can result in abnormal eruption of permanent teeth.

Medicolegal Importance of Teeth

Being very hard, teeth are preserved for a very long time after death. They can be very useful in identifying a dead person specially if a dentists record of the state of the teeth is available.

For development of teeth and for various congenital malformations that may be seen consult the author's HUMAN EMBRYOLOGY.

HARELIP AND CLEFT PALATE

Embryologically, both the upper lip and the palate are derived from three elements. These are the right and left maxillary processes, and the frontonasal process which is a median structure.

Harelip

The frontonasal process forms the median part of the upper lip. This part is called the philtrum. On each side the frontonasal process fuses with the corresponding maxillary process. Abnormalities in fusion of these processes lead to clefts in the upper lip (called ***harelip*** because the hare normally has an upper lip with a cleft). The defect may be unilateral or bilateral. When defect in fusion is minimal only a small indentation may be seen in the margin of the lip. When non-union is complete the defect extends into the nostril, and is continuous with a defect in the palate as described below.

Cleft Palate

As stated above the palate is derived from the frontonasal process and the right and left maxillary processes. The frontonasal process forms the part of the palate that bears the incisor teeth. This part of the palate is also called the ***premaxilla***. It is triangular in shape, the apex of the triangle pointing backwards, and lying in the midline. The rest of the palate is formed by shelf like projections of the right and left maxillary process. These processes grow towards the midline. Anteriorly, each maxillary process fuses with the corresponding edge of the premaxilla. Behind the level of the premaxilla the two maxillary processes fuse with each other. From the manner of fusion it will be clear that the line of union of the three elements forming the palate is Y shaped

Defects in the process of union lead to the formation of different varieties of cleft palate as follows. Remember that fusion of components of the palate starts anteriorly and proceeds posteriorly.

a. Complete non-union gives rise to a Y-shaped cleft. Anteriorly the limbs of the 'Y' become continuous with a cleft in the upper lip. There will also be bilateral harelip.

b. The premaxilla may fuse with the maxillary process on one side, but not on the other side. At the same time the two maxillary processes do not fuse with each other. This results in a defect that is oblique anteriorly and median posteriorly. It will be associated with a unilateral hare lip.
c. Both the maxillary processes fuse with the premaxilla but their fusion to each other is deficient. This can give rise to median defects of varying extent. The cleft may involve both the hard palate and the soft palate, may be confined to the soft palate, or may be represented only by a cleft in the uvula.

It has been said above that fusion of the elements forming the palate begins anteriorly and progresses backwards. This statement does not apply to the upper lip. A harelip can exist without there being any cleft in the palate.

THE TONGUE

Congenital Malformations

The tongue may be too large (***macroglossia***), or too small (***microglossia***). Very rarely the tongue may be absent (***aglossia***). The tongue may be bifid.

The apical part of the tongue may be anchored to the floor of the mouth by a very short frenulum. The condition, which is called ***ankyloglossia*** or ***tongue tie***, interferes with speech.

Other rare anomalies include the presence of fissures on the tongue, the presence of a lingual thyroid, or the presence of remnants of the thyroglossal duct in the form of cysts.

Laceration of the Tongue

Laceration of the tongue can occur if the tongue gets caught between the teeth. This is likely to occur while eating, during epileptic attacks, and in injuries leading to fractures of the jaw.

Because of the vascularity of the tongue lacerations can cause serious bleeding. To stop bleeding pressure is applied posterior to the area of laceration (as the lingual artery runs forwards). Pressure is applied either by holding the tongue between the thumb and index finger; or by placing the thumb on the tongue and the index finger in the submental region.

Other Correlations

1. Muscles of the tongue are paralysed in lesions of the hypoglossal nerve.
2. Sensations of taste are lost from the anterior two thirds of the tongue in facial nerve paralysis; and from the posterior one third in lesions of the glossopharyngeal nerve. In some cases taste sensations over the anterior two thirds of the tongue may be affected in lesions of the trigeminal nerve.
3. The mucosa below the anterior part of the tongue is highly vascular. A drug placed here enters the blood stream faster than it does after an intramuscular injection. (Patients suffering from angina commonly find relief by placing a suitable tablet here).
4. In an unconscious patient care has to be taken that the tongue does not fall backwards towards the pharynx as this would obstruct respiration. The head is placed on one side and made to hang down.
5. Carcinoma of the tongue (and other parts of the mouth) is common in India because of tobacco chewing. To understand the various routes by which

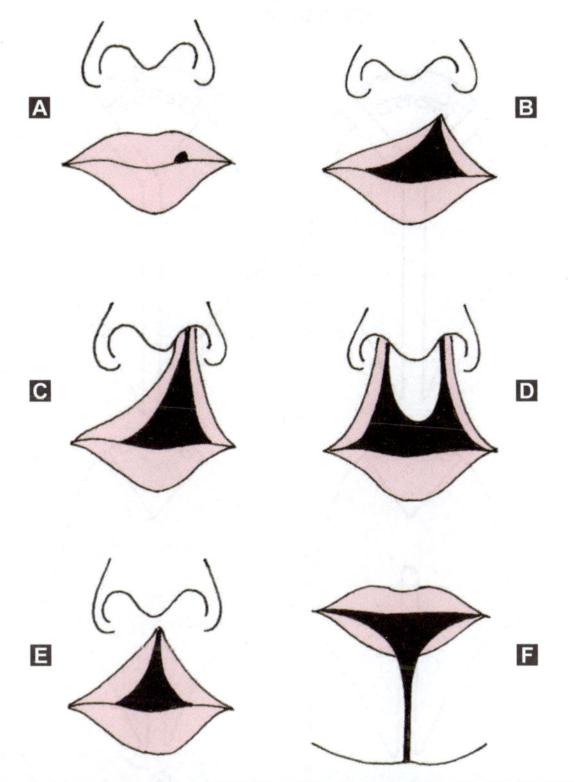

Fig. 15.1 Varieties of harelip. A to C. Different degrees of unilateral harelip. D. Bilateral harelip. E. Median harelip. F. Median cleft in lower lip.

carcinoma can spread see page 393 where the lymphatic drainage of the tongue is described.

SALIVARY GLANDS

1. The salivary glands are commonly infected with a virus that causes ***mumps***. It causes swelling and pain in the gland affected. It can involve more than one gland. The parotid is the most commonly infected salivary gland.
2. The salivary glands can also be infected by spread of infection from the mouth. An abscess may form in the gland.
3. The parotid fascia is very dense and allows very little expansion of the gland. Swellings of the parotid are therefore very painful.
4. Tumours may form in a salivary gland. They may be benign or malignant. Facial paralysis can occur by involvement in a malignant growth of the parotid gland, or by injury during removal of the gland. The surgeon tries to protect the nerve by removing the superficial and deep parts separately.

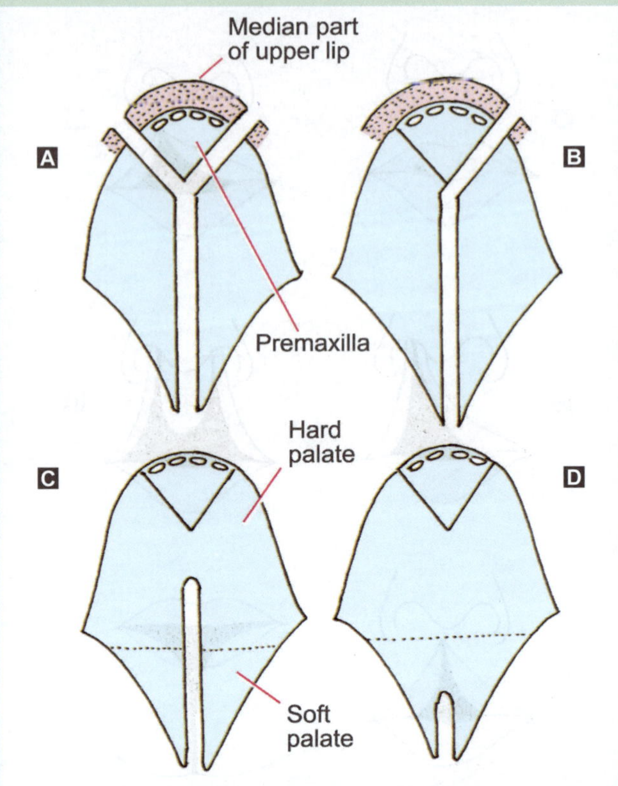

Fig. 15.2 Varieties of cleft palate. A. Complete non-fusion leading to a Y-shaped cleft accompanied by bilateral harelip. B. The left maxillary process has fused with the premaxilla, but not with the right maxillary process. The cleft is accompanied by unilateral harelip. C. Midline cleft involving both hard and soft palate. D. Cleft involving soft palate only.

5. A calculus may form in the submandibular gland. In operations on the submandibular gland the close relation of the facial artery to it has to be remembered.

TONSILS

PALATINE TONSILS

When we talk of tonsils we are really referring to palatine tonsils. Infections of the tonsils is common and is referred to as ***tonsillitis***. Infection can spread from them to peritonsillar tissues leading to a peritonsillar abscess (also called ***quinsy***). Infected tonsils can be responsible for spread of infection to the nasal cavities, the ears, and the respiratory passages.

An operation for surgical removal of the tonsils is called ***tonsillectomy***. The main danger during the operation is bleeding from the external palatine (peritonsillar) vein. The ascending branch of the facial artery (and sometimes the facial artery itself) are separated from the tonsil only by the superior constrictor muscle, and can in injured in a crudely performed tonsillectomy.

Palatine tonsils are best developed in children. Like other lymphoid tissue they undergo retrogression after puberty.

THE PHARYNGEAL TONSIL

This is a collection of lymphoid tissue present in relation to the roof of the nasopharynx. Hence it is also called the nasopharyngeal tonsil. When enlarged (because of chronic infection) the pharyngeal tonsils are referred to as adenoids. Adenoids lead to obstruction in the nasopharynx forcing the child to breathe through the mouth. A constantly open mouth can lead to deformities of the teeth and palate (as normal pressure of the tongue on the palate is not present). Infection frequently spreads to the middle ear (through the auditory tube). Removal of adenoids is called adenoidectomy.

PHARYNX

The inferior constrictor of the pharynx has been described on page 351. Its division into a cricopharyngeal part and a thyropharyngeal part has been noted. The cricopharyngeus is believed to act as a sphincter at the junction of the pharynx and oesophagus, and to prevent passage of air into the latter. The thyropharyngeus (along with other constrictors) helps to push the bolus of food down the pharynx. The posterior wall of the pharynx is weakest just above the cricopharyngeus. There may be a gap here between the thyropharyngeal and cricopharyngeal fibres. This gap is referred to as ***Killian's dehiscence***. Pressure of food over this area can lead to the formation of a pouch (diverticulum). This is more likely to occur if there is incoordination of muscles (the crico-pharyngeus failing to relax when the thyropharyngeus is contracting. The pharyngeal pouch thus formed cannot expand posteriorly (because of the presence of the vertebral column). It, therefore, grows downwards and can press on the oesophagus resulting in dysphagia (difficulty in swallowing).

NASAL CAVITY

Infection of the nasal cavity is called ***rhinitis***. (This term is derived from rhis which is the Greek word for nose). Infection from the nasal cavity can spread to paranasal sinuses, to the middle ear, to the pharynx and larynx, and even to the anterior cranial fossa (through the roof of the cavity). Rhinitis may be caused by viruses (as in common cold), by bacteria, and by allergy (allergic rhinitis). In allergic rhinitis the nasal mucosa can undergo hypertrophy resulting in chronic blockage.

Children often insert foreign bodies into the nose and they can get impacted there.

Bleeding from the nose is called ***epistaxis***. In most cases it is caused by rupture of blood vessels on the anterior inferior part of the nasal septum (***Little's area***).

The nasal septum is commonly deflected (i.e., it comes to lie to one side of the middle line). This can cause blocking of the nasal cavity on one side and may require surgical correction.

In cleft palate the nasal cavity is in communication with the mouth. Because of leakage of air into the nose during speech the person has a nasal twang.

PARANASAL SINUSES

Sinusitis

Paranasal sinuses are frequently sites of infection (sinusitis). The infection usually reaches them from the nasal cavity. As the sinuses open into the nasal cavity through narrow openings, slight swelling of the mucosa, or presence of thick secretions at the orifice, can block outflow of secretions that accumulate within the sinus. This is one reason why sinusitis so often becomes chronic.

This is specially true in the case of the ***maxillary sinus*** because the level of the opening of the maxillary air sinus into the nose is placed at a higher level than the floor of the sinus, so that natural drainage is difficult. To facilitate drainage it is sometimes necessary to make an artificial opening into the sinus through the inferior meatus of the nose. The sinus can also be drained through the vestibule of the mouth near the canine tooth.

A study of the anatomy of the lateral wall of the nose shows that secretions draining out of the frontal air sinus flow towards the opening into the maxillary sinus. For this reason frontal sinusitis often leads to maxillary sinusitis.

Infection in the maxillary sinus can spread to the orbit. [Remember that the plate of bone that forms the roof of the maxillary sinus also forms the floor of the orbit].

Diagnosis of Sinusitis

Infection in paranasal sinus leads to headache. In addition tenderness can often be elicited by pressure over the sinus. In frontal sinusitis tenderness is felt by upward pressure over the medial part of the superior orbital margin. In maxillary sinusitis there may be tenderness over the cheek below the inferior orbital margin. In ethmoidal sinusitis there can be tenderness over the medial wall of the orbit.

Pain originating in the paranasal sinuses may be referred to other sites. The frontal sinus is supplied by the supraorbital nerve which also supplies the skin of the forehead and anterior part of the scalp. Therefore frontal headache is almost always present in frontal sinusitis. In maxillary sinusitis pain may be felt in the upper jaw and teeth.

Diagnosis of maxillary sinusitis can be confirmed by transillumination. In a darkened room light (from a torch) is directed towards the wall of the sinus through the mouth or through the cheek. The presence of fluid, rather than air, reduces transmission of light. Radiography is also useful in confirming presence of sinusitis.

THE LARYNX AND TRACHEA

LARYNX

1. Entry of any foreign matter (including water or food) into the larynx can result in suffocation and death. The intense cough which is set up on the entry of even a small particle is a protective mechanism against suffocation.
2. Inflammation of the mucous membrane of the larynx (***laryngitis***) can cause hoarseness of voice, or even complete loss of voice, because of oedema above

the level of the vocal folds. [Note that laryngeal mucous membrane is firmly adherent to the vocal folds and that is why fluid accumulates above this level]. In the presence of severe inflammation or irritation the oedema may be of such a degree as to lead to suffocation. In such cases it may become necessary to create an artificial opening in the trachea (tracheostomy) to save the life of the person.

3. Paralysis of one or more muscles of the larynx also leads to hoarseness of voice. The hoarseness is temporary in case of injury to the external laryngeal nerve (as the function of the paralysed cricothyroid is gradually taken up by the muscle of the normal side). When the recurrent laryngeal nerve is injured hoarseness is permanent. In this connection it may be noted that in some cases only some groups of muscles may be affected. When all intrinsic laryngeal muscles are paralysed the vocal folds are immobile and lie midway between abduction and adduction. This is the position occupied by the vocal folds after death. Paralysis of abductors alone leads to adduction of the vocal folds (by unopposed action of the adductors): this leads to closure of the glottis with consequent suffocation. Hence paralysis of abductors alone is much more dangerous that paralysis of both abductors and adductors of the vocal folds.
   The interior of the larynx can be examined in a living person using an instrument called a laryngoscope. The procedure is called laryngoscopy.

THE FACE

In the preceding sections numerous references have been made to clinical correlations of the face. Some of these are as follows.

1. Horner's syndrome: see page 423.
2. Face in cretinism and myxoedema: see page 425.
3. Lips in cyanosis: page 426.
4. Hare lip : page 427.
5. Salivary glands: page 429.
6. Mouth in adenoids: 431.
7. Mandibulofacial dysostosis: page 407.
8. Injuries on the face: page 408.
9. Arteries: page 411.
10. Dangerous area of face: page 413.
11. Parotid fasçia: page 415.
12. Trigeminal nerve: page 419.
13. Facial paralysis: page 420.

NECK

In the preceding sections numerous references have been made to clinical correlations of the neck. Some of these are as follows.

1. Fracture of hyoid bone: page 409.
2. Torticolis: page 410.
3. Cervical spondylosis and other conditions affecting cervical vertebrae: page 410.
4. Large arteries of neck: page 411

5. Dysphagia lusoria: page 411.
6. Carotid angiography: page 412.
7. Cervical rib: page 412.
8. External jugular vein: page 413.
9. Venous pressure: page 413.
10. Deep cervical fascia: page 414.
11. Retropharyngeal abscesses: page 414.
12. Ludwig's angina: page 415.
13. Glossopharyngeal, and vagus nerves: page 422.
14. Superior laryngeal nerve: page 422.
15. Recurrent laryngeal nerve: page 422.
16. Spinal accessory nerve: page 422.
17. Thyroid gland: page 424.
18. Parathyroid glands: page 426.
19. Pharynx: page 431.
20. Larynx and trachea: page 432.
21. Tracheostomy: page 433.

Some additional facts of interest are as follows.

SWELLINGS IN THE NECK

Enlarged Lymph Nodes

Lymph nodes in the head and neck may be enlarged in various diseases. The most important of these are tuberculosis and malignancy. Physical examination of the neck involves systematic palpation of the nodes. The surgeon stands behind the patient whose neck is slightly flexed (to relax the muscles). Beginning with the suboccipital region the surgeon palpates the occipital nodes, the retroauricular or mastoid nodes, the parotid nodes, the submandibular and submental nodes, the anterior cervical nodes and the deep cervical nodes, the suprasternal nodes and the supraclavicular nodes..

In block dissection of the neck for removal of enlarged lymph nodes (in tuberculosis or malignancy), the submandibular gland is also removed. It has been noted that a segment of the internal jugular vein may also have to be removed. Removal of the vein on one side is compensated by drainage through the vein of the other side. However, if bilateral removal is required, an interval of a few weeks is given between operations on the two sides to allow collateral venous channels to open up. In block dissection special care is taken not to injure the carotid arteries, the vagus nerve, the spinal accessory nerve, the mandibular branch of the facial nerve and the hypoglosssal nerve. However, sometimes the vagus and hypoglossal nerves may have to be removed. Nerves lying deep to the prevertebral fascia (cervical and brachial plexus and their branches) remain intact. If necessary the sternocleidomastoid muscle is divided for better access.

Tumours of the Neck

We have seen above that lymph nodes in the neck may be involved in carcinoma at various sites. The primary growth may lie in the thyroid, the larynx, the base of the tongue, the laryngopharynx, and even the paranasal sinuses. Rarely secondaries from carcinoma of the breast, the bronchi the stomach or testis can reach these nodes.

Various other tumours may be seen in the neck. In infancy a swelling of the sternomastoid may be seen and later leads to torticolis. Tumours may form in remnants of the thyroglossal duct, or in the carotid body.

Midline Swellings

Common causes of swellings to be seen in the midline on the front of the neck include enlarged submental lymph nodes, cysts arising from remnants of the thyroglossal duct (thyroglossal cyst), enlargements of the thyroid gland, carcinoma of the larynx, and enlarged suprasternal lymph nodes.

Branchial Cysts and Fistulae

A series of branchial arches develop in the embryo in the region of the neck. The arches are separated (superficially) by ectodermal clefts. The first ectodermal cleft takes part in forming the external acoustic meatus. The second cleft is normally obliterated but sometimes remnants of it may form ***branchial cysts***. Such a cyst forms a swelling near the anterior border of the sternocleidomastoid muscle. If the cyst ruptures on to the surface it results in a ***branchial fistula***. For treatment it is necessary to excise the tract of the fistula.

Some other Infections of the Neck

While discussing the importance of the deep cervical fascia mention has been made of thc directions in which pus may pass from a retropharyngeal plexus.

The pharyngomaxillary space is a triangular interval into which infection can spread from the palatine tonsil or from a peritonsillar abscess. The base of the triangular space lies superiorly and is formed by the base of the skull. Medially there is the superior constrictor of the pharynx, and laterally the space is bounded by fascia covering the medial pterygoid muscle and the submandibular gland.

MENINGES AND CEREBROSPINAL FLUID

1. Inflammation of pia and arachnoid is called meningitis. The condition is characterized by fever and severe headache. Spasm of extensor muscles leads to rigidity of the neck. The spasm is a result of irritation of cervical nerve roots as they pass through the subarachnoid space. CSF pressure and chemical composition show alterations.
2. Samples of CSF may be obtained for examination by lumbar puncture. In some cases lumbar puncture may fail to yield CSF. In such cases CSF may be obtained by ***cisternal puncture***. A needle is introduced from behind, through the interval between the atlas and axis vertebrae. The needle is kept parallel to a plane joining the external acoustic meatus to the nasion. [The nasion is the point where the internasal suture meets the frontonasal suture]. The needle passes through the posterior atlanto-occipital membrane and enters the cisterna magna.
3. See hydrocephalus (page 407), extradural and subdural haemorrhage (page 409), and intracranial venous sinuses (page 413).

SPINAL CORD

Injuries to the spinal cord are very serious as they result in paralysis. Injury near the upper end of the cord can result in death by paralysis of respiratory muscles.

Injury in the cervical region can result in paralysis of all four limbs (***quadriplegia***), while injuries in the thoracic region can result in paralysis of both lower extremities (***paraplegia***).

The spinal cord can be injured or compressed in fractures and dislocations of the vertebral column. It can also be compressed by tumours. Compression by a tumour can also result in obstruction to the flow of CSF. This can be diagnosed by ***myelography***.

For effects of spinal cord injury on functioning of the urinary bladder see page 699.

In examining a patient having injury or disease of the spinal cord the physician has to determine the level of injury. In this connection it has to be remembered that the levels of spinal segments do not correspond to vertebral levels (page 119). The level of injury is determined by noting which muscles are paralysed and which areas of skin show anaesthesia. The status of reflexes also helps to localize the level of lesion.

EYES AND RELATED STRUCTURES

1. Infections are common in the eyelids (***blepharitis***). A pus filled swelling near the edge of the eyelid is a stye. It is caused by infection in large sebaceous glands present here. Inflammation of a tarsal gland results in a localized swelling called ***chalazion***. Inflammation of the conjunctiva is called ***conjunctivitis***. Other structures in the eye that may be infected are the iris (***iritis***), the ciliary body (***cyclitis***), and a combination of both these (***iridocyclitis***).

   Infection in the cornea is called ***keratitis***. It can lead to formation of a ***corneal ulcer***. Corneal ulcers can also be caused by injury or by foreign bodies that enter the eye.

   A superficial infection of the sclera is ***episcleritis***, and a deeper infection is ***scleritis***. Inflammation of the retina is ***retinitis***, and that of the optic nerve is ***optic neuritis***.
2. Injuries to the cornea can result in ***corneal opacities*** which can lead to blindness. Such blindness can be cured by corneal grafting. [The so called eye transplantations that are advertised so much in the lay press are really corneal transplants. A whole eye cannot be transplanted]. Alterations in the curvature of the cornea can lead to an error of refraction called astigmatism (see below).
3. An opacity in the lens of the eyeball is called ***cataract***. It occurs in many old persons and is a common cause of blindness. Vision can be restored by removing the lens, and this is one the most common operations done on the eyeball. Focussing power is restored by use of appropriate spectacles, or by implanting an artificial lens into the eye (***intraocular lens transplantation***).
4. Defects in the shape of the eyeball, or in refractive media, lead to errors of refraction in which images are not focussed on the retina. Common errors are as follows.

   In ***myopia*** (near sightedness) the image comes into focus in front of the plane of the retina. Objects can be seen clearly only when placed close to the eyes. Myopia is corrected with convex (plus) lenses.

   Hypermetropia is a condition in which the image comes to a focus behind the plane of the retina. Only distant objects can be seen. It is corrected with concave (minus) lenses.

Presbyopia is a condition caused by decreased elasticity of the lens in persons over 40 years old. It can be corrected by convex lenses.

In ***astigmatism*** the image is correctly focussed in some planes but not in others. This is due to abnormalities in curvature of the cornea or of the lens. Correction requires the use of cylindrical lenses.

The degree of refractive error is determined by a procedure called ***retinoscopy***.

5. Tumours may occur in the eye. A melanoma may arise from the iris or the choroid. Another tumour is a retinoblastoma.
6. The retina can be examined through an ophthalmoscope. The procedure is commonly referred to as ***fundus examination***. Apart from diagnosis diseases of the retina itself such examination also helps in assessing the status of patients in diseases like hypertension and diabetes.
7. The retina consists of a nervous layer (the retina proper) and an outer layer of pigment cells. In the embryo the two layers are separated by a cavity. Sometimes the nervous layer gets detached from the pigment layer (detachment of the retina). It causes serious impairment of vision.
8. See optic nerve (page 416), visual pathway (Chapter 23), squint (page 418), and corneal reflex (Chapter 26).

THE EAR

The anatomy of the external acoustic meatus, of the middle ear, and of the mastoid antrum are of great clinical importance as they are frequent sites of infection.

Middle ear infection is referred to as ***otitis media***. It is usually caused by extension of infection from the pharynx through the auditory tube. Such infections are more frequent in children as the tube is relatively wide in them. Infection in the middle ear can spread to the mastoid antrum and the mastoid air cells. This makes eradication of the infection much more difficult. Middle ear infection can also lead to perforation of the tympanic membrane. The pus then flows out of the external acoustic meatus. As the middle ear is closely related to the sigmoid sinus and the bulb of the internal jugular vein infection can spread to them. Through the sigmoid sinus infection can reach the temporal lobe of the brain.

Disease of the middle ear, of the ossicles, of the internal ear, and of the vestibulocochlear nerve can lead to deafness.

IMAGING OF THE HEAD AND NECK

As in other parts of the body, structures in the head and neck can be visualised in the living by plain radiography (Figs. 1.22, 1.23. 1.24A), and by injection of contrast media into blood vessels (Fig. 16.13) or into ducts (Fig. 1.24B)., Excellent visualisation of the brain can be obtained by use of computed tomography (CT) (Fig. 16.6) and by magnetic resonance imaging (MRI) (Figs. 16.14, 16.15). Some details of these procedures are given in the legends to the figures cited, and in Chapter 26.

PART TWO

Central Nervous System

CHAPTER

16

Colour Atlas of the Central Nervous System

This chapter presents a colour atlas of the central nervous system. The atlas should be used while reading the text from Chapter 17 onwards.

The pages at which illustrations of some important structures are to be found are given below. The last four plates are devoted to imaging methods.

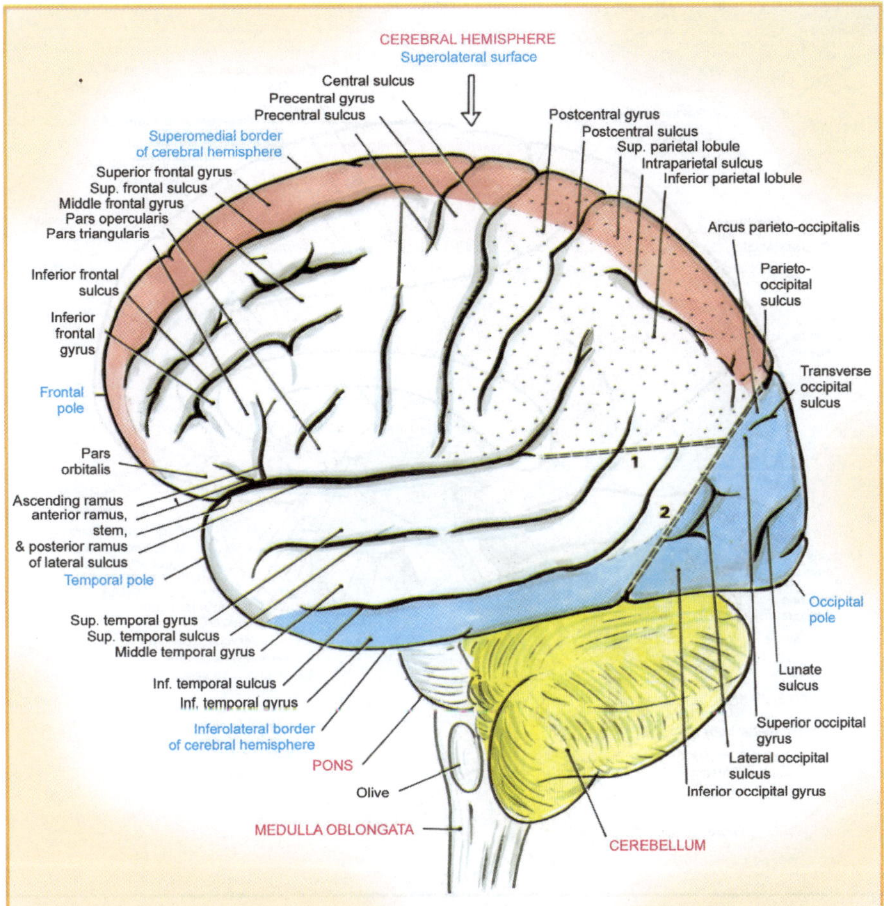

Fig. 16.1 Brain viewed from the lateral side (simplified). The interrupted double lines are imaginary: they are used to demarcate lobes. The area shaded in dots is the parietal lobe. The areas in front of it (above the posterior ramus of the lateral sulcus) is the frontal lobe. The temporal lobe is the area below the posterior ramus of the lateralsulcus and the imaginary line (1) that continues backwards in the line of the main part of the sulcus. The occipital lobe lies behind the parietal and temporal lobes being separated from them by the obliquely drawn imaginary line (2).The area of the cerebral cortex shaded pink is supplied by the anterior cerebral artery, and that shaded blue is supplied by the posterior cerebral artery. The uncoloured area is supplied by the middle cerebral artery.

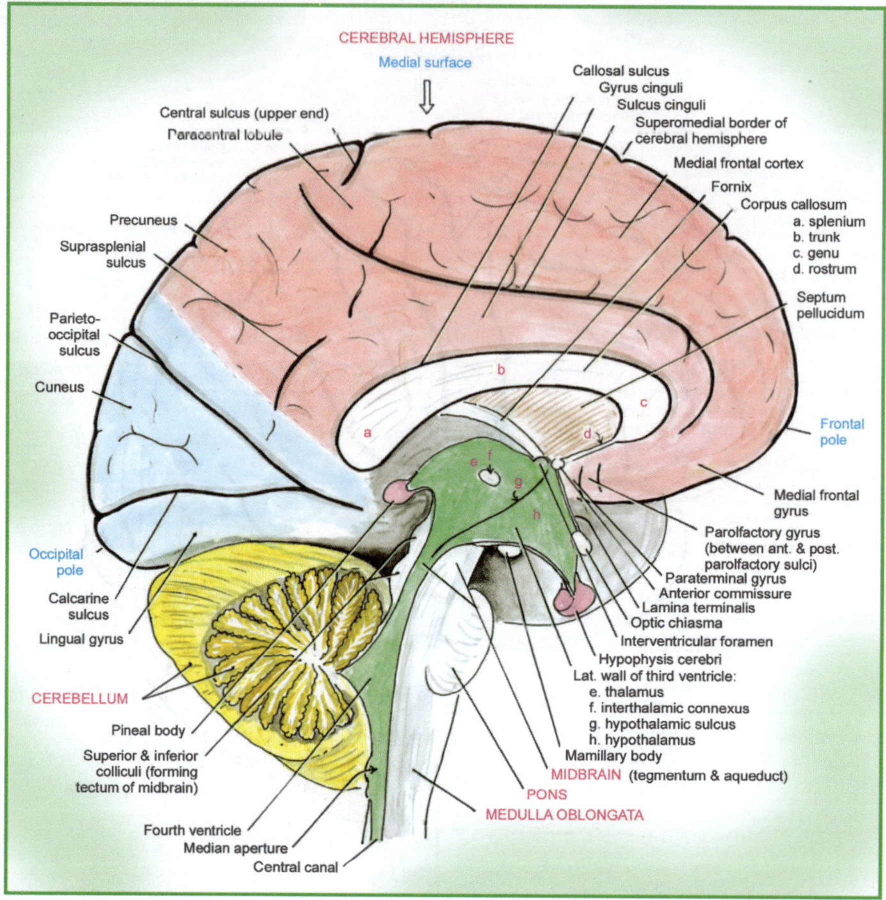

Fig. 16.2 Brain viewed from the medial side, after cutting it through the middle line (simplified). The area shaded in pink is supplied by the anterior cerebral artery, and that shaded blue is supplied by the posterior cerebral artery.

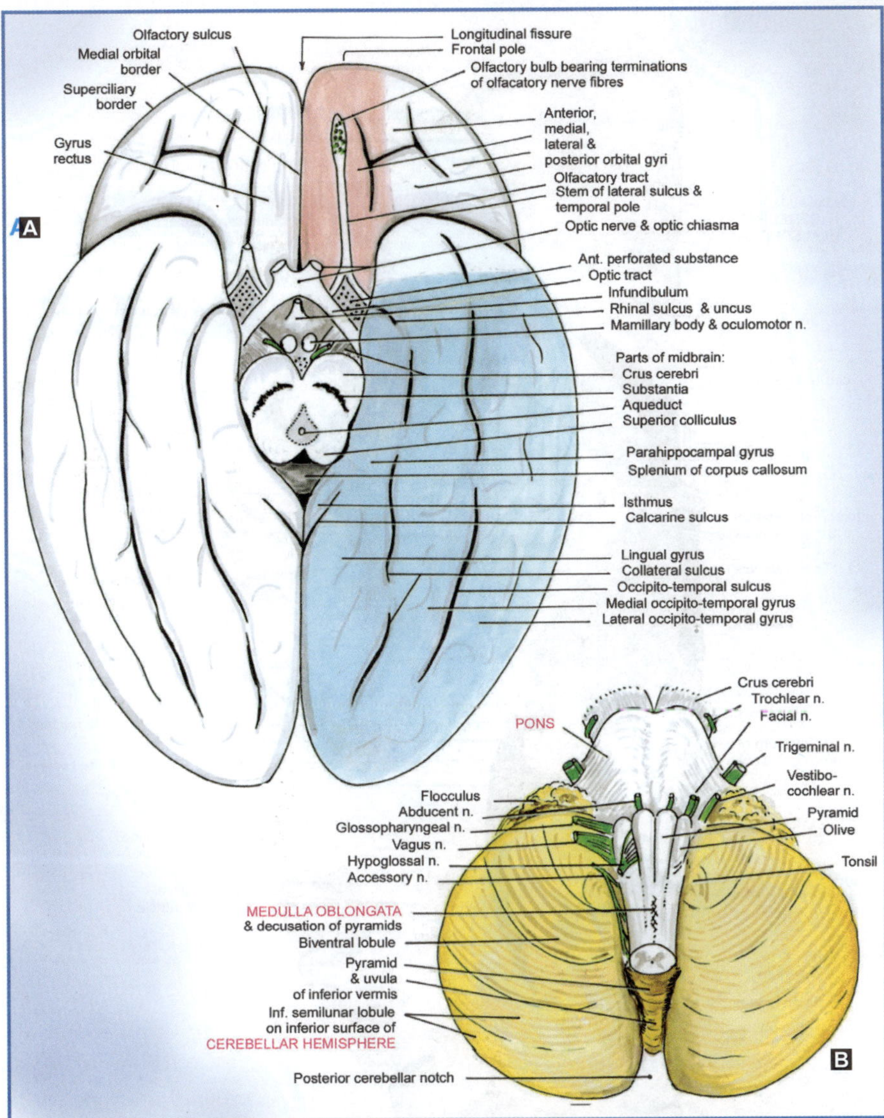

Figs 16.3A and B (A) Cerebrum seen from below. For significance of colours in the right half of the drawing see legend to Fig. 16.1. (B) Cerebellum and brainstem seen from below and in front.

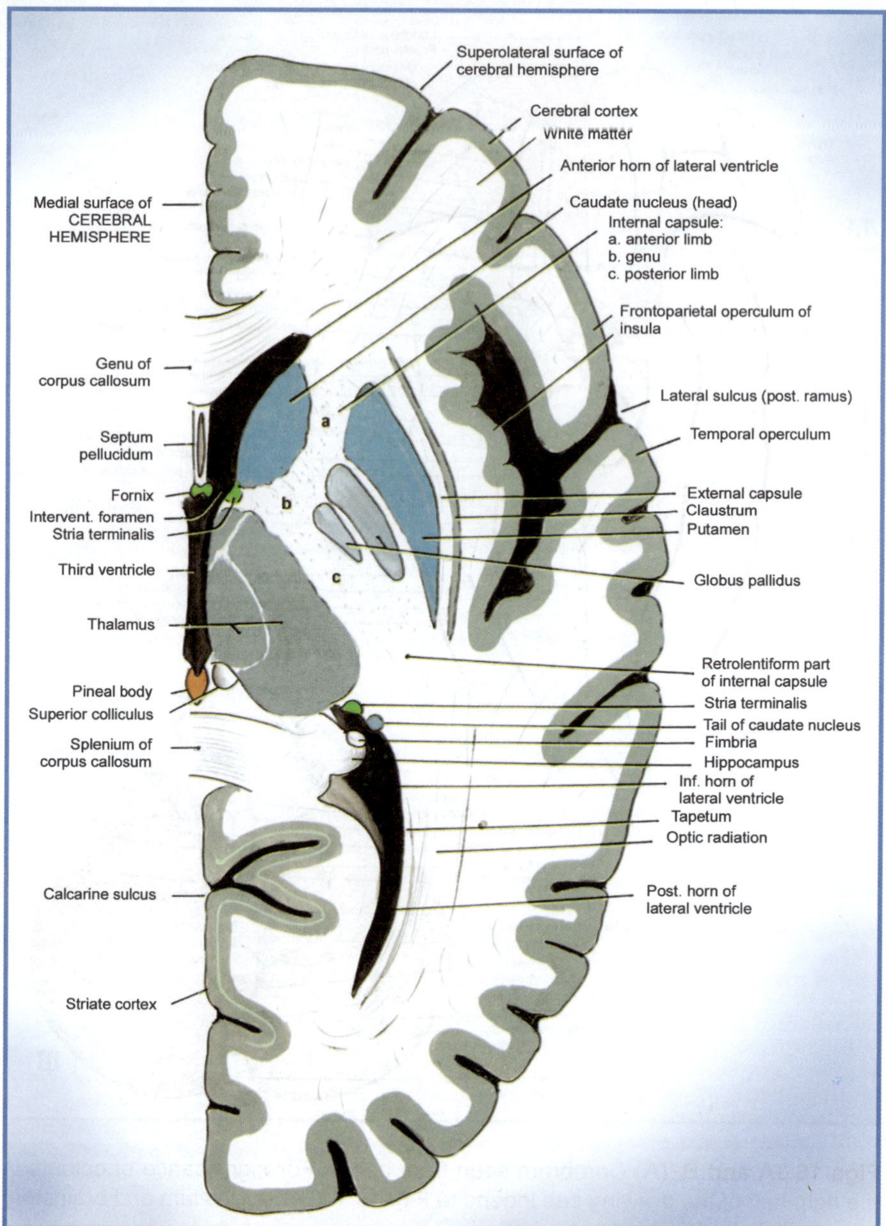

Fig. 16.4 Horizontal section through cerebral hemisphere to show the main features within it.

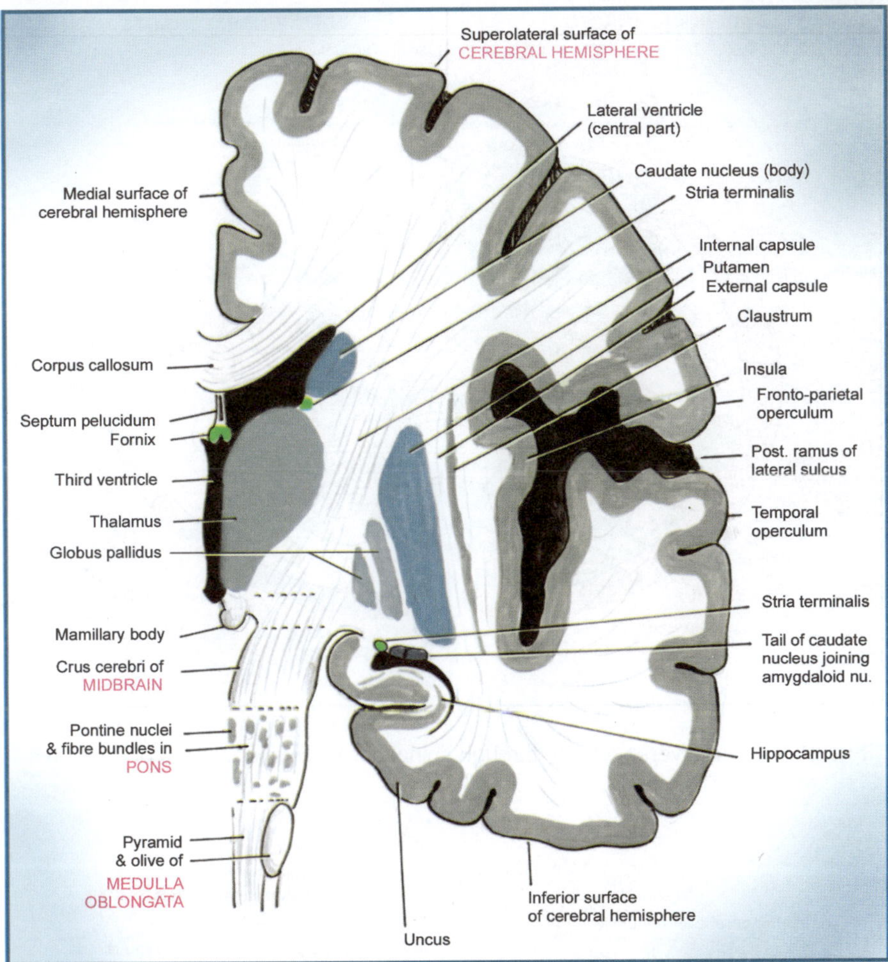

Fig. 16.5 Coronal section through cerebral hemisphere and brainstem (schematic). Note the continuity of fibres of the internal capsule with those of the crus cerebri.

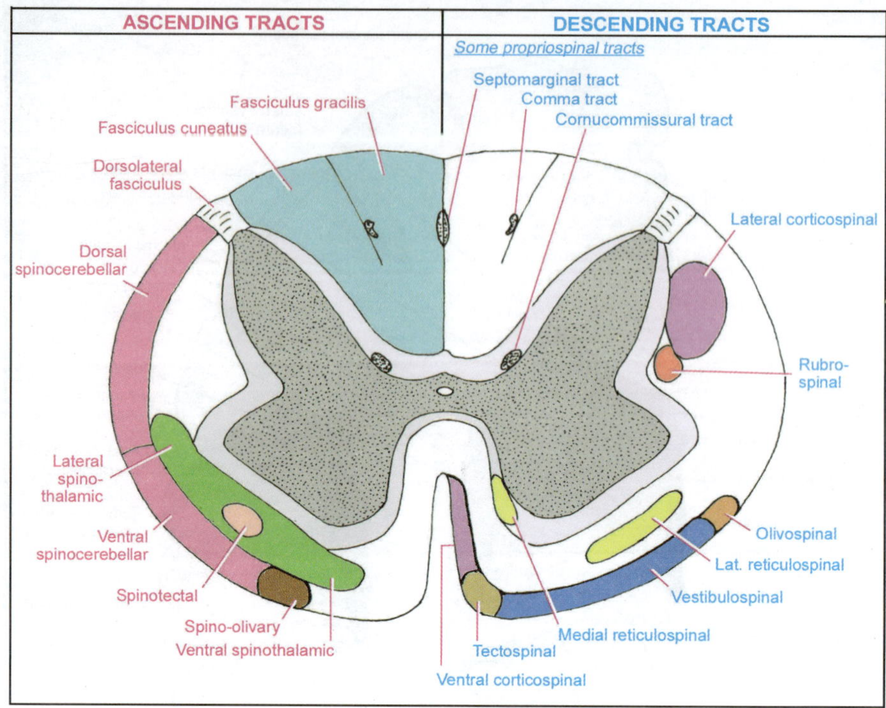

Fig. 16.6 A Transverse section through spinal cord showing position of tracts in it.

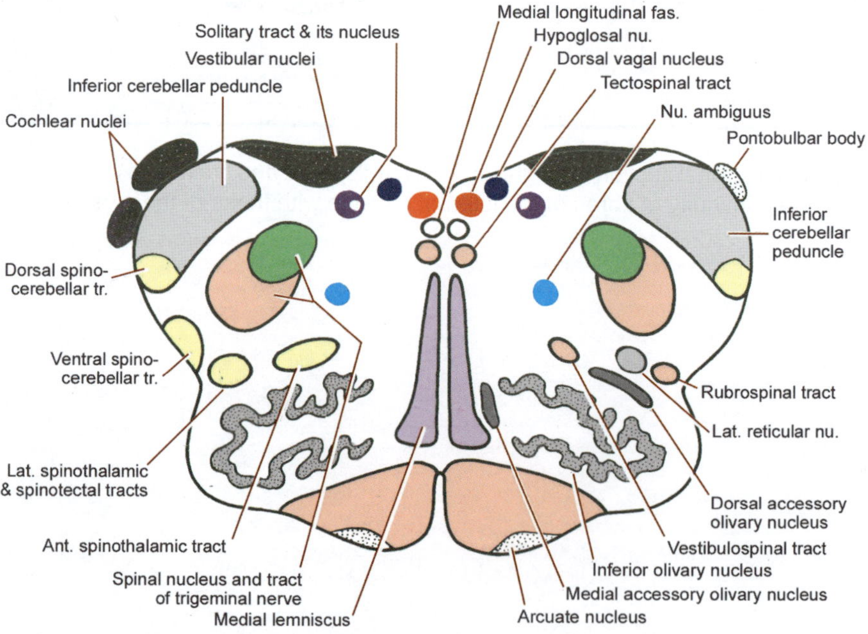

Fig. 16.6 B Transverse section through the medulla at the level of the olive.

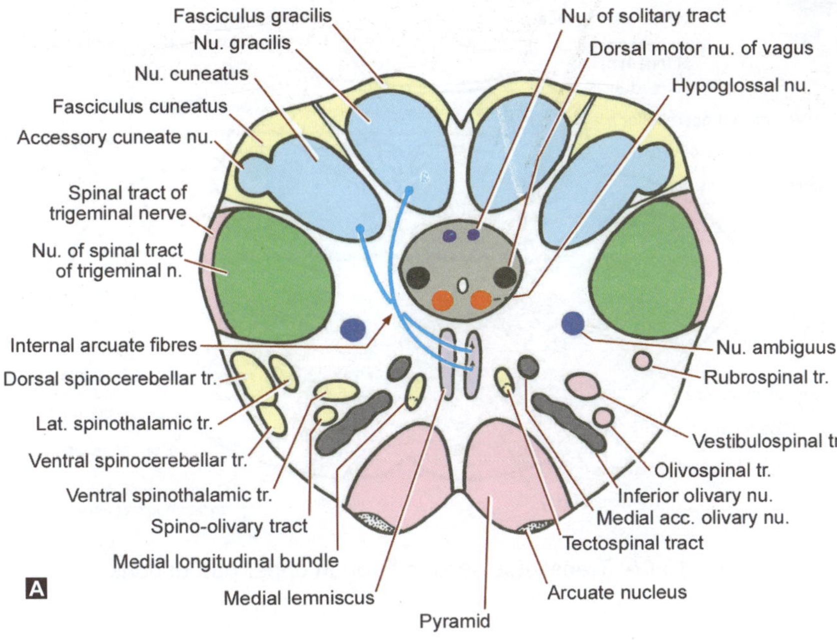

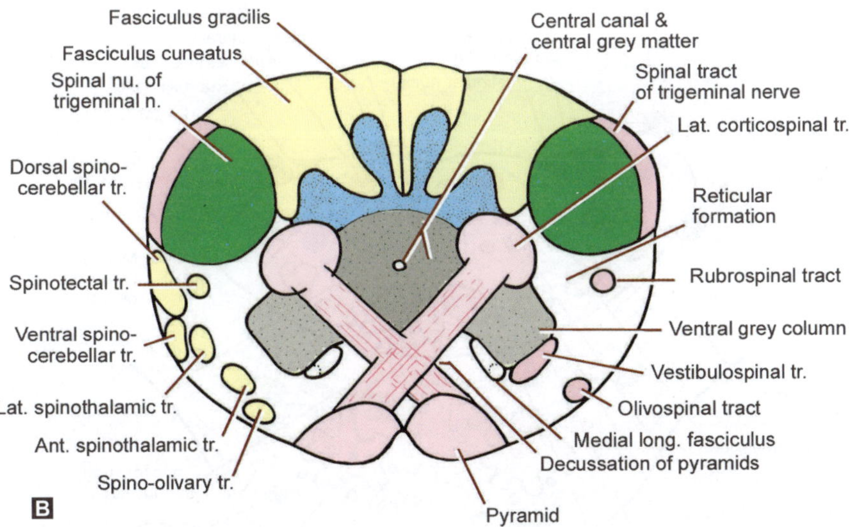

Fig. 16.7 Transverse sections through the medulla. A. At level of sensory decussation. B. At level of pyramidal decussation.

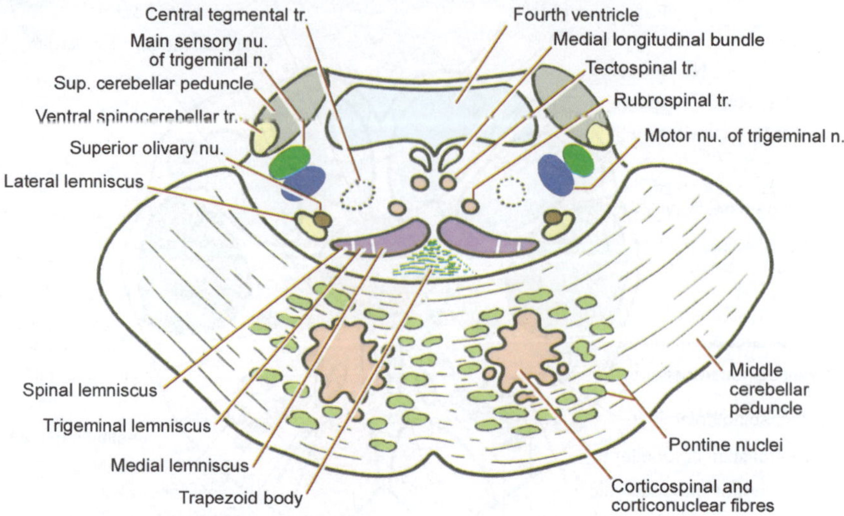

Fig. 16.8A Transverse section through upper part of pons.

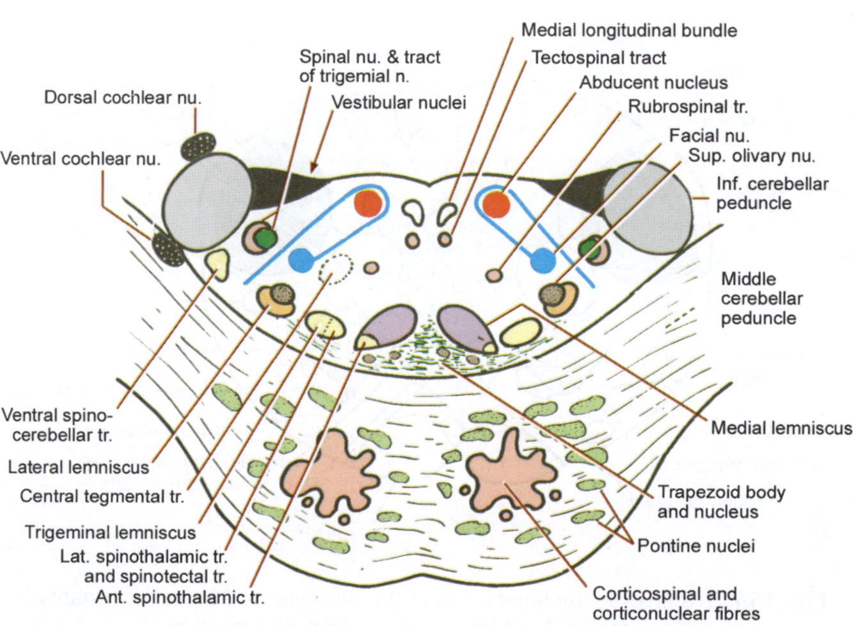

Fig. 16.8B Transverse section through lower part of pons.

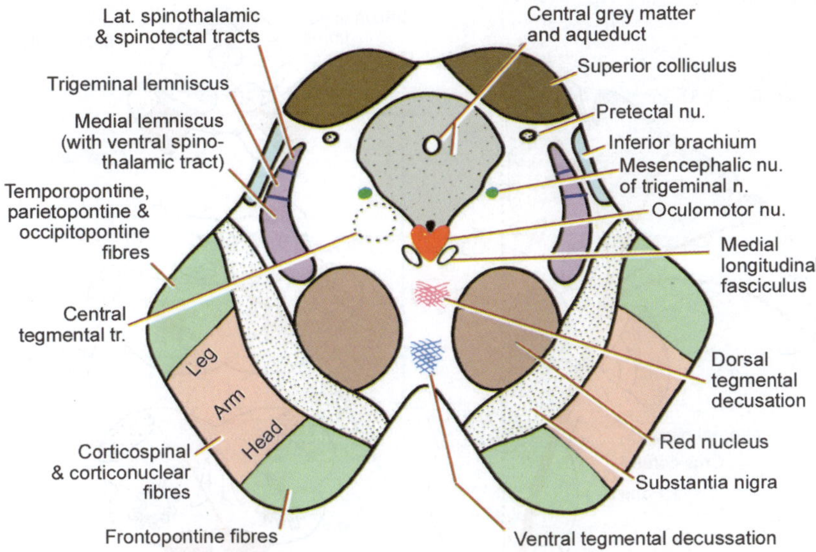

Fig. 16.9A Transverse section through upper part of midbrain.

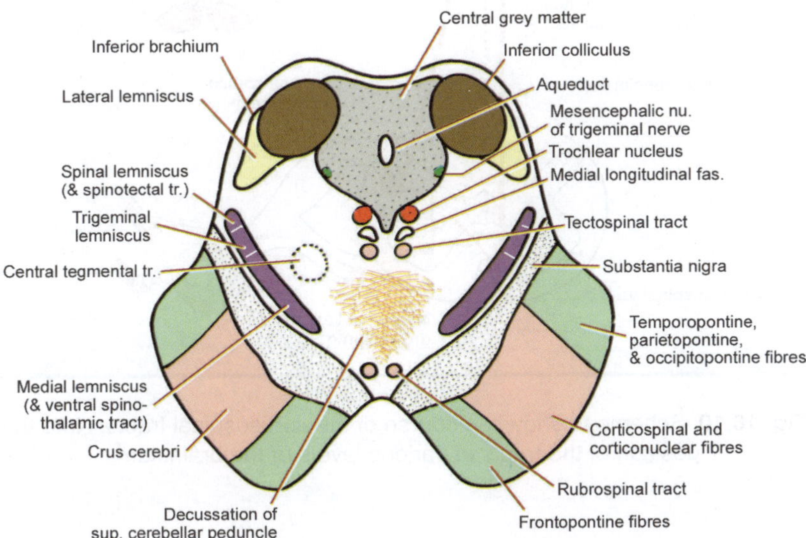

Fig. 16.9B Transverse section through lower part of midbrain.

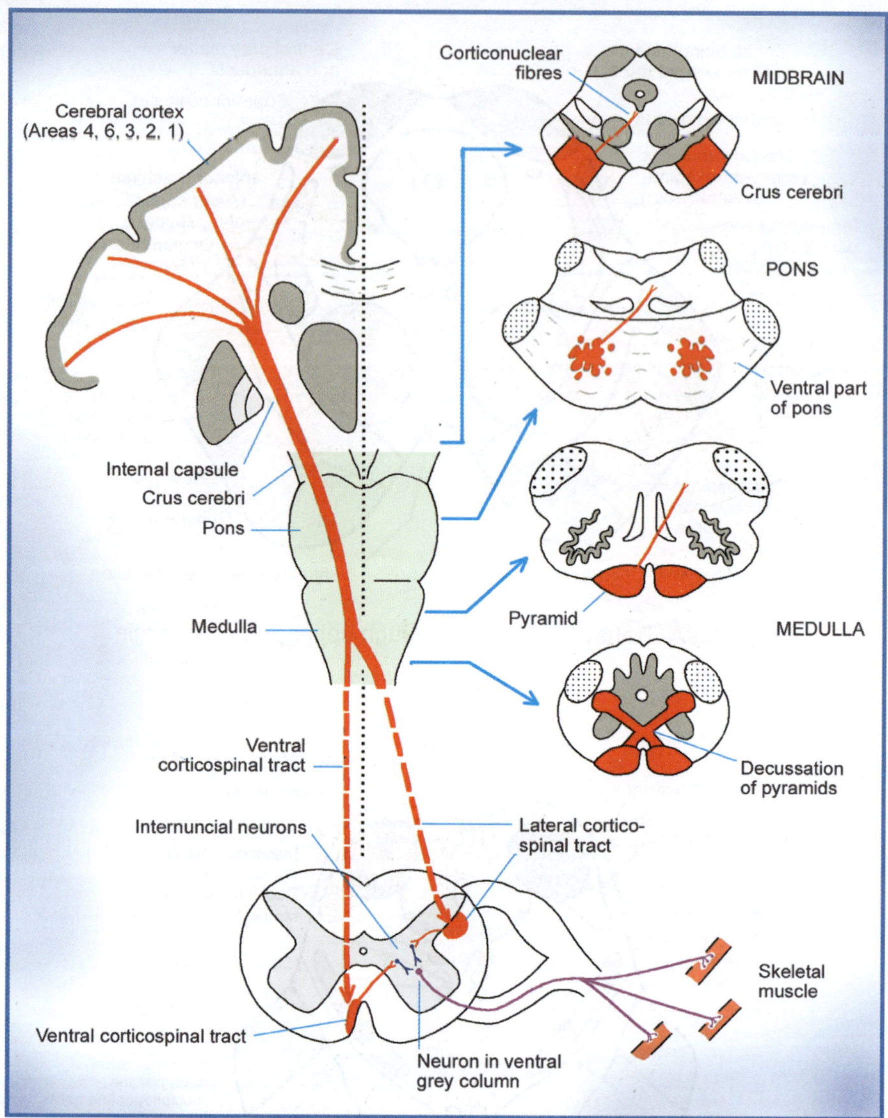

Fig. 16.10 Scheme to show the course of the corticospinal tracts. Note the position of the tracts at various levels of the brainstem.

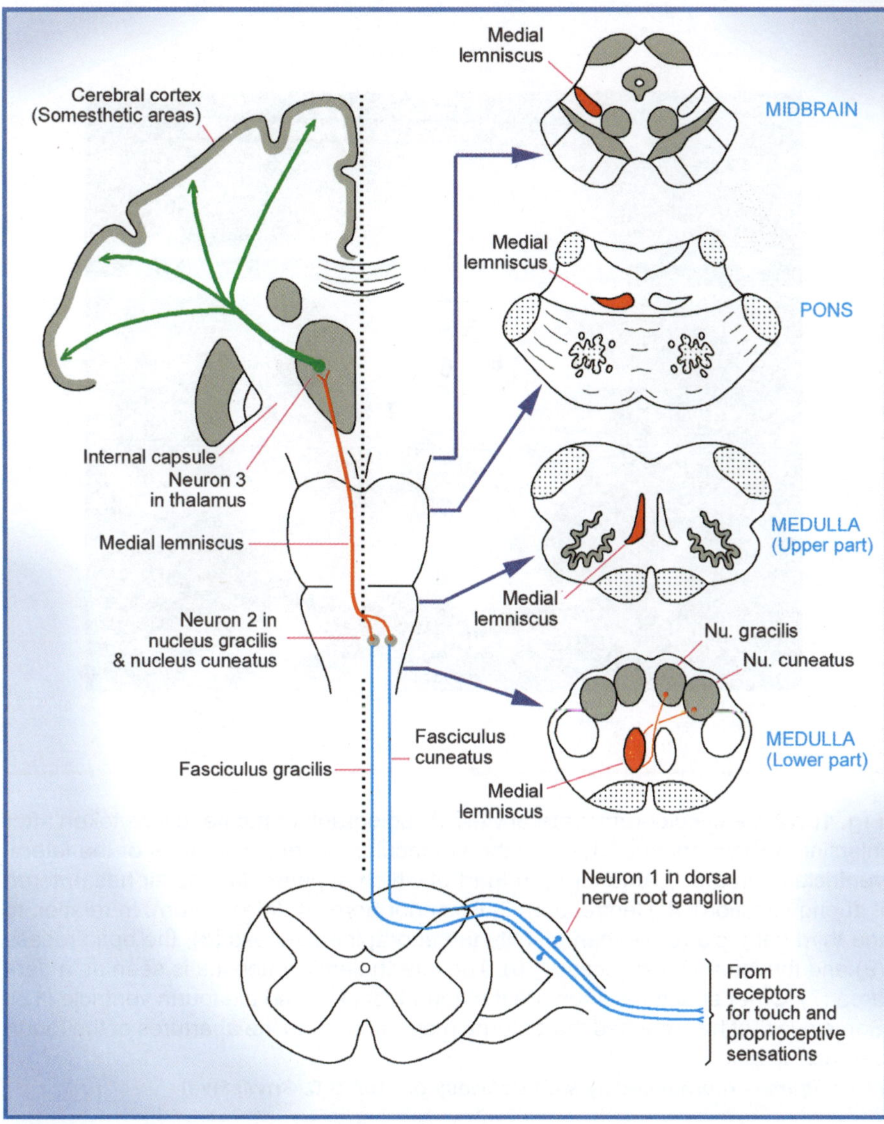

Fig. 16.11 Scheme to show the main features of the posterior column - medial lemniscus pathway. Note the position of the medial lemniscus at various levels of the brainstem.

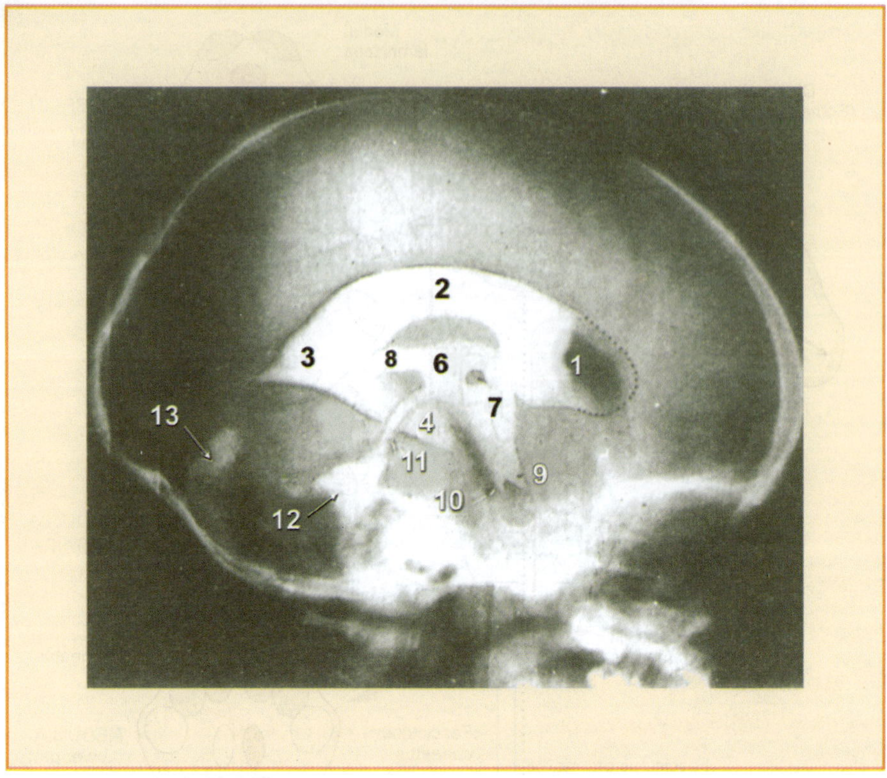

Fig. 16.12 Ventriculogram. Lateral view. A radiograph of the head was taken after injecting a radio-opaque dye into the ventricular system. The parts of the lateral ventricle seen are:1. Anterior horn (part of which appears dark as air has entered it during injection). 2. Central part. 3. Posterior horn. 4. Inferior horn. In relation to the third ventricle (6) we can identify the suprapineal recess (8), the optic recess (9) and the infundibular recess (10). The interthalamicconnexus is seen as a dark area (7). Other structures seen are the aqueduct (11), and the fourth ventricle (12). Some dye that has reached the cisterna magna (through the apertures of the fourth ventricle is also seen (13).

(This figure is reproduced by kind Courtesy of Prof. S.C. Srivastava)

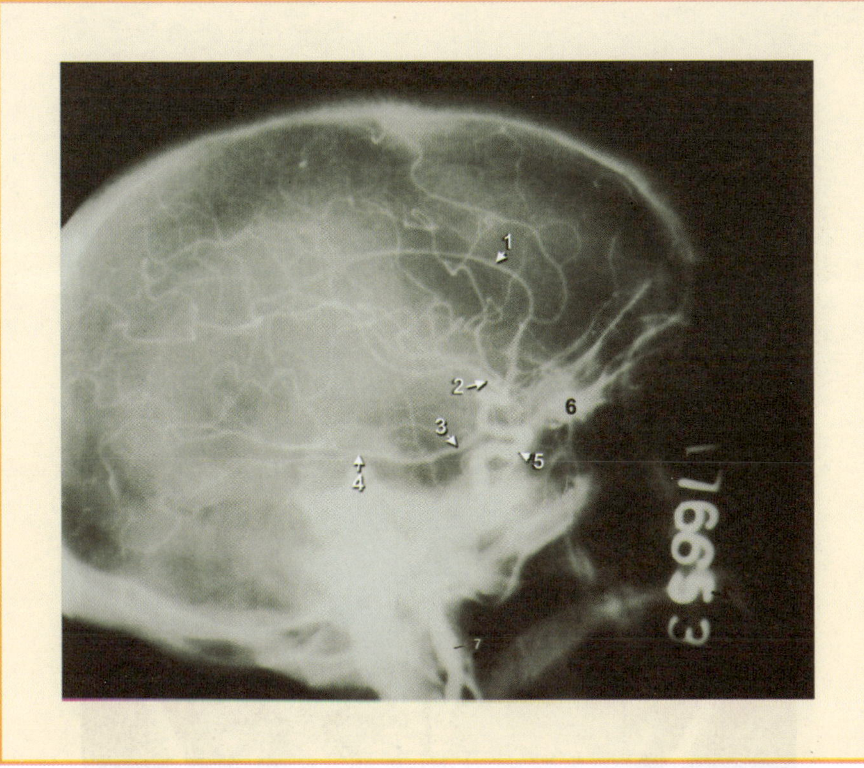

Fig. 16.13 Arteries of the brain visualised in a living person by the technique of carotid angiography. Lateral view. 1. Anterior cerebral artery. 2. Middle cerebral artery. 3. Posterior communicating artery. In this patient this artery appears to continue into the posterior cerebral artery (4). This is unusual. 5. Internal carotid artery in the cavernous sinus. 6. Branches of ophthalmic artery. 7. Internal carotid artery in the neck.

(This figure is reproduced by Courtesy of Dr. R.K. Yadav).

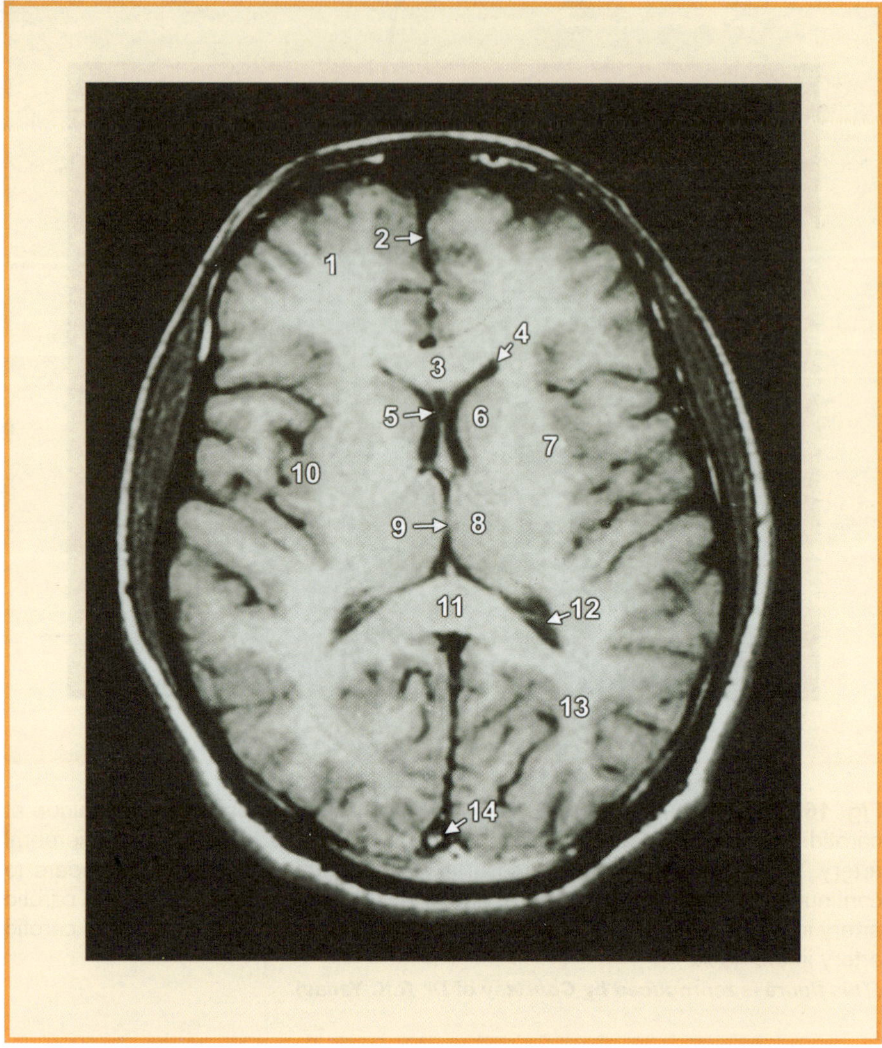

Fig. 16.14 Sectional view of cerebral hemisphere obtained in a living person by the technique of magnetic resonance imaging (MRI). 1. Frontal lobe. 2. Median longitudinal fissure. 3. Genu of corpus callosum. 4. Anterior horn of lateral ventricle. 5. Septum pellucidum (double layered). 6. Caudate nucleus. 7. Lentiform nucleus. 8. Thalamus. 9. Third ventricle. 10. Insula. 11. Splenium of corpus callosum. 12. Posterior horn of lateral ventricle. 13. Occipital lobe. 14. Superior sagittal sinus. ***(This figure is reproduced by Courtesy of Dr. R.K. Yadav).***

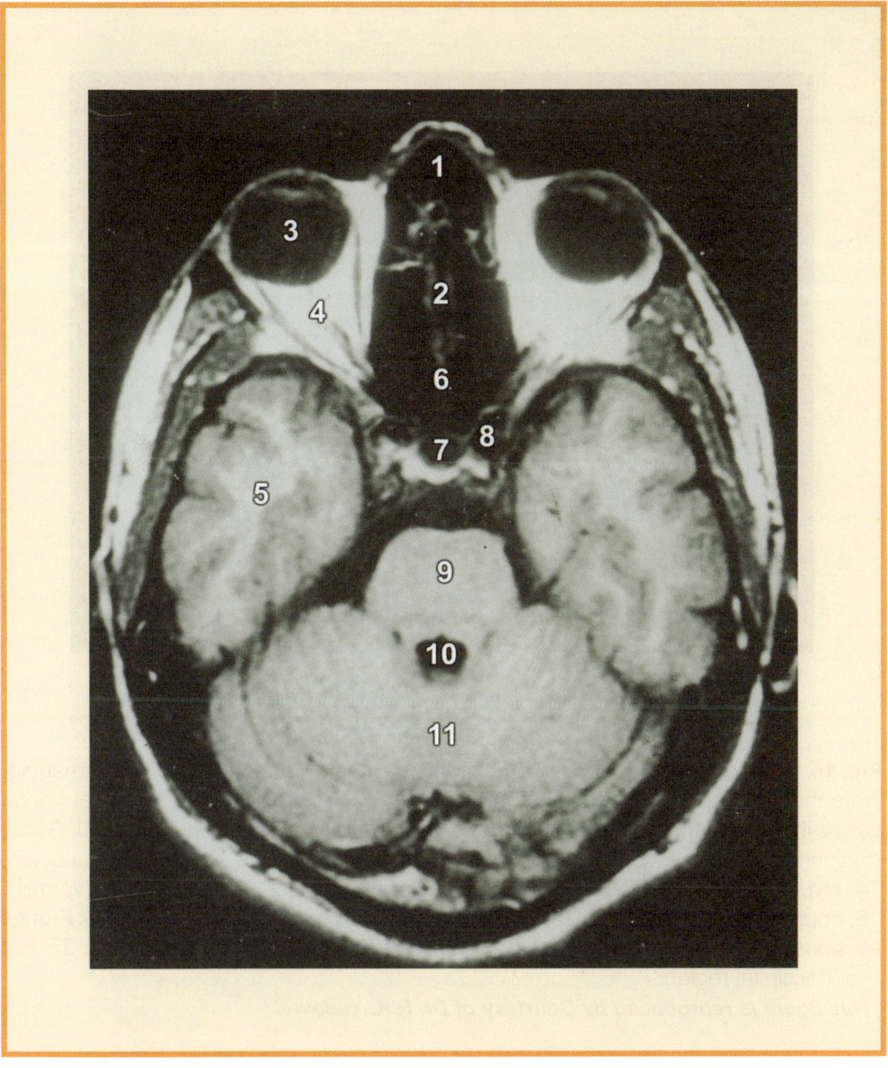

Fig. 16.15 Magnetic resonance imaging. Transverse sectional view of head passing through the orbit, and the middle and posterior cranial fossae. 1. Nasal cavity. 2. Nasal septum. 3. Eyeball. 4. Retroocular part of orbit. 5. Temporal lobe of cerebral hemisphere. 6. Nasopharynx. 7. Hypophyseal fossa. 8. Sphenoidal sinus. 9. Pons. 10. Fourth ventricle. 11. Cerebellum.

(This figure is reproduced by Courtesy of Dr. R.K. Yadav).

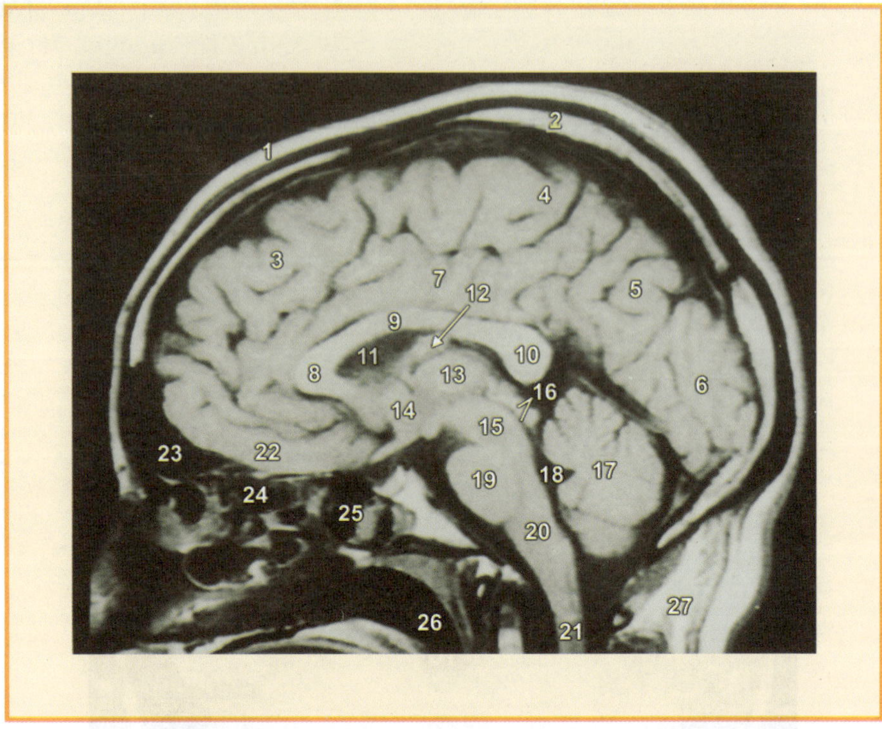

Fig. 16.16 Sagittal sectional view of the brain obtained by magnetic resonance imaging. Note the vast amount of detail that can be seen. 1. Scalp. 2. Skull. 3. Medial frontal gyrus. 4. Paracentral lobule. 5. Precuneus. 6. Cuneus. 7. Gyrus cinguli. 8. 9. 10. Genu, trunk and splenium of corpus callosum. 11. Lateral ventricle. 12. Fornix. 13. Thalamus. 14. Hypothalamus. 15. Midbrain. 16. Colliculi and aqueduct. 17. Cerebellum (vermis). 18. Fourth ventricle. 19. Pons. 20. Medulla. 21. Spinal cord. 22. Gyrus rectus. 23. Frontal air sinus. 24. Ethmoidal air sinuses. 25. Sphenoidal sinus. 26. Nasopharynx. 27. Fat in suboccipital region.

(This figure is reproduced by Courtesy of Dr. R.K. Yadav)○.

CHAPTER

17

Introduction to the Central Nervous System Internal Structure of Spinal Cord

INTRODUCTION TO THE CENTRAL NERVOUS SYSTEM

The ***central nervous system*** is made up of the brain and spinal cord; and that the ***peripheral nervous system*** consists of the cranial nerves and the spinal nerves. The brain consists of the cerebrum, made up of two large cerebral hemispheres; the cerebellum; and the brainstem consisting of the midbrain, the pons and the medulla oblongata. The medulla oblongata is continuous with the spinal cord.

The nerves that make up the peripheral nervous system have been considered in the appropriate sections. In this section we will consider the main features of the central nervous system. The account given here should meet the requirements of most undergraduate students. Those desiring a more detailed account should consult the author's HUMAN NEUROANATOMY.

Some Elementary Facts about Neurons

The nervous system is made up, predominantly, of tissue that has the special property of being able to conduct impulses rapidly from one part of the body to another. The specialised cells that constitute the functional units of the nervous system are called ***neurons***. Within the brain and spinal cord neurons are supported by a special kind of connective tissue that is called ***neuroglia.*** Nervous tissue, composed of neurons and neuroglia, is richly supplied with blood, but lymph vessels are not present.

A neuron consists of a ***cell body*** which gives off a variable number of ***processes***. The cell body is also called the ***soma*** or ***perikaryon***. The processes arising from the cell body of a neuron are called ***neurites.*** These are of two kinds. Most neurons give off a number of short branching processes called ***dendrites*** and one longer process called an ***axon.*** There are various structural differences between dendrites and axons. However, the most important difference is functional. In a dendrite, the nerve impulse travels ***towards the cell body*** whereas in an axon the impulse travels ***away***

from the cell body. Peripheral nerves are made up of aggregations of axons (and in some cases of dendrites).

During its formation each axon (and some dendrites) comes to be associated with certain cells that provide a sheath for it. The cells providing this sheath for axons lying outside the central nervous system are called ***Schwann cells***. Axons lying within the central nervous system are provided a similar covering by a kind of neuroglial cell called an ***oligodendrocyte***.

All nerve fibres in peripheral nerves have an outer sheath called the ***neurilemma***. This forms the outer covering of the nerve fibre. Deep to the neurilemma most nerve fibres also have a second sheath that is rich in lipids. This is the ***myelin sheath***.

Axons having a myelin sheath are called ***myelinated axons***. Those without this sheath are ***unmyelinated axons***.

An axon (or its branches) can terminate in two ways. Within the central nervous system, it always terminates by coming in intimate relationship with another neuron, the junction between the two neurons being called a ***synapse***. Outside the central nervous system, the axon may end in relation to an effector organ (e.g., muscle or gland), or may end by synapsing with neurons in a peripheral ganglion.

Neurons vary considerably in the size and shape of their cell bodies (somata) and in the length and manner of branching of their processes. The shape of the cell body is dependent on the number of processes arising from it. The most common type of neuron gives off several processes and the cell body is, therefore, ***multipolar***. Some neurons have only one axon and one dendrite and are ***bipolar.*** Another type of neuron has a single process and is therefore described as ***unipolar***. However, this process almost immediately divides into two. One of the divisions represents the axon; the other is functionally a dendrite, but its structure is indistinguishable from that of an axon. Depending on the shapes of their cell bodies some neurons are referred to as ***stellate*** (star shaped) or ***pyramidal.***

The above account of the structure of neurons is confined to the barest facts. For detailed descriptions of neuron structure consult the author's HUMAN NEUROANATOMY.

Apart from structural differences neurons can also be classified on the basis of their functions. A classification of types of nerve fibres to be seen in peripheral nerves; and the arrangement of neurons giving origin to various functional types of nerve fibres has been discussed in Chapter 9. These descriptions will be essential to understanding of some aspects of the structure of the brain.

Grey and White Matter

Sections through the spinal cord or through any part of the brain show certain regions that appear whitish, and others that have a darker greyish colour. These constitute the ***white*** and ***grey matter*** respectively. Microscopic examination shows that the cell bodies of neurons are located only in grey matter which also contains dendrites and axons starting from or ending on the cell bodies. Most of the fibres within the grey matter are unmyelinated. On the other hand the white matter consists predominantly of myelinated fibres. It is the reflection of light by myelin that gives this region its whitish appearance. Neuroglia and blood vessels are present in both grey and white matter.

The arrangement of the grey and white matter differs at different situations in the brain and spinal cord. In the spinal cord and brainstem the white matter is on the outside whereas the grey matter forms one or more masses embedded within the white matter. In the cerebrum and cerebellum there is an extensive, but thin, layer of grey matter on the surface. This layer is called the ***cortex*** (Fig. 16.4). Deep to the cortex there is white matter, but within the latter several isolated masses of grey matter are present. Such isolated masses of grey matter, present anywhere in the central nervous system, are referred to as ***nuclei.*** As grey matter is made of cell bodies of neurons (and the processes arising from or terminating on them) nuclei can be defined as groups of cell bodies of neurons. Aggregations of the cell bodies of neurons may also be found outside the central nervous system. Such aggregations are referred to as ***ganglia.***

Ganglia are of two distinct functional types. ***Sensory ganglia*** contain neurons which give off processes that form the afferent fibres of peripheral nerves. Examples of sensory ganglia are the dorsal nerve root ganglia of spinal nerves, and the trigeminal ganglion. ***Autonomic ganglia*** include ***sympathetic ganglia*** located on the sympathetic chain, and ***parasympathetic ganglia***. Examples of the latter are the ciliary ganglion and the submandibular ganglion. Some autonomic neurons are located in ***nerve plexuses*** (often called ganglia) present in close relationship to some viscera.

The axons arising in one mass of grey matter terminate very frequently by synapsing with neurons in other masses of grey matter. The axons connecting two (or more) masses of grey matter are frequently numerous enough to form recognisable bundles. Such aggregations of fibres are called ***tracts***. Larger collections of fibres are also referred to as ***funiculi, fasciculi*** or ***lemnisci***. Large bundles of fibres connecting the cerebral or cerebellar hemispheres to the brainstem are called ***peduncles.***

Arrangement of Neurons within the Central Nervous System

The various functional categories of nerve fibres present in peripheral nerves, and the arrangement of neurons associated with these fibres, has been described in Chapter 9. We have seen that neurons giving rise to fibres of peripheral nerves are basically of two types as follows.

a. Neurons having cell bodies that lie within the brain and spinal cord, send out efferent processes that leave the CNS to form the motor fibres of peripheral nerves.
b. Neurons having cell bodies located in ganglia outside the CNS, give origin to peripheral processes that form afferent nerve fibres of peripheral nerves. Their central processes form the sensory roots of the nerves in question. They enter the brain or spinal cord and synapse with neurons within them.

The bulk of the CNS is, however, made up of neurons that lie entirely within it. As explained earlier, the cell bodies of these neurons are invariably located in masses of grey matter. The axons may be short, ending in close relation to the

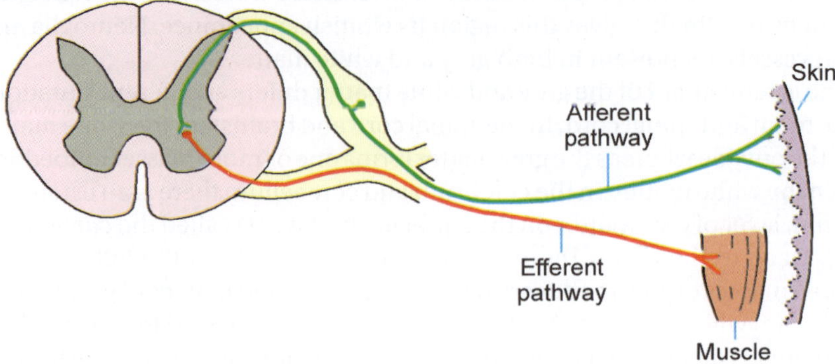

Fig. 17.1 A spinal reflex arc composed of two neurons.

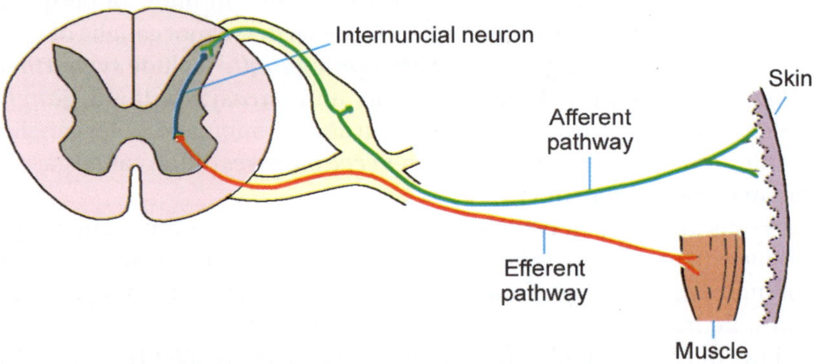

Fig. 17.2 A spinal reflex arc composed of three neurons.

cell body, or may be long and may travel to other masses of grey matter lying at considerable distances from the grey matter of origin. The neurons within the CNS are interconnected in an extremely intricate manner. The description that follows illustrates some of the basic arrangements encountered.

The simplest pathways are those concerned with reflex activities, such as the contraction of a muscle in response to an external stimulus. For example, if the skin of the sole of a sleeping person is scratched, the leg is reflexly drawn up. Let us see how this happens. The simplest possible arrangement is shown in Fig. 17.1. The stimulus applied to skin gives rise to a nerve impulse which is carried by the peripheral process of a unipolar neuron to the dorsal nerve root ganglion. From here the impulse passes into the central process which terminates by directly synapsing with an anterior grey column cell supplying the muscle which draws the leg up. The complete pathway constitutes a ***reflex arc*** and in the above example it consists of two neurons — one afferent and the other efferent. In actual practice, however, the reflex arc is generally made up of three neurons as shown in Fig. 17.2. The central process of the dorsal nerve root ganglion cell ends by synapsing with a neuron lying in the posterior grey column. This neuron has a short axon that ends by synapsing with a neuron in the anterior grey column, thus completing the reflex arc. The third neuron interposed between the afferent and efferent neurons is called an ***internuncial neuron,*** or simply an ***interneuron.***

The purpose served by an interneuron may be basically of three types. Firstly, the axon arising from an interneuron may divide into a number of branches and may synapse with a number of different efferent neurons. As a result an impulse coming along a single afferent neuron may result in an effector response by a large number of efferent neurons. Secondly, afferent impulses brought by a number of afferent neurons may converge on a single efferent neuron through the agency of interneurons. Some of these impulses tend to induce activity in the efferent neuron (i.e., they are ***facilitatory)*** while others tend to suppress activity (i.e., they are ***inhibitory).*** Thirdly, through interneurons an afferent neuron may establish contact with efferent neurons in the opposite half of the spinal cord, or in a higher or lower segment of the cord.

Every time a stimulus reaches a neuron it does not mean that it must become active and must produce an impulse. A neuron receives inputs from many neurons (in some cases from hundreds of them). Some of these inputs are facilitatory and others are inhibitory. Activity in the neuron (in the form of initiation of an impulse) depends on the sum total of these inputs. Thus, each neuron may be regarded as a decision making centre. The greater the number of neurons involved in any pathway, the greater the possibility of such interactions. Viewed in this light it will become clear that interneurons interposed in a pathway increase the number of levels at which 'decisions' can be taken. It will also be appreciated that most of the neurons within the nervous system are, in this sense, interneurons which are involved in numerous highly complex interactions on which the working of the nervous system depends.

From what has been said above it will be seen that some activities occur due to reflex action, and may involve only neurons within the spinal cord. However, most activities of the spinal cord are subjected to influence from higher centres. In the more complicated types of activity several higher centres may be involved and the pathways may be extremely complicated. Afferent impulses reaching these higher centres (e.g., the cerebral cortex) would appear to be somehow stored and this stored information (of which we may or may not be conscious) is used to guide responses to similar stimuli received in future. This accounts for memory and for learning processes.

From the above it will be appreciated that in a study of the nervous system we must first of all have some knowledge of the various masses of grey matter in the CNS and of their interconnections. To this end we will begin by studying the internal structure of the spinal cord below.

Projection, Association and Commissural Fibres

When a considerable number of fibres pass from a mass of grey matter in one part of the brain to another mass of grey matter in another part of the brain or spinal cord these are referred to as ***projection fibres.*** Fibres interconnecting different areas of the cerebral cortex or of the cerebellar cortex are called ***association fibres***, while fibres connecting identical areas of the two halves of the brain are called ***commissural fibres.*** All fibres crossing from one side of the brain or spinal cord to the opposite side are not commissural. When fibres originating in a mass of grey matter in one half of the CNS end in some other mass of grey matter in the opposite half they are referred to as ***decussating fibres,*** and the sites where such crossings take place are referred to as ***decussations.***

INTERNAL STRUCTURE OF SPINAL CORD

The gross anatomy of the spinal cord, and some elementary facts about its internal structure have been described in Chapter 56. The concept of spinal segments, and the relationship of the spinal cord to spinal nerves has also been examined therein.

We have seen that the grey matter of the spinal cord is divided into ventral, dorsal and lateral columns, and that the white matter is divided into anterior, posterior, and lateral funiculi.

The relative amount of grey and white matter, and the shape and size of the grey columns, vary at different levels of the spinal cord (Fig. 17.3). The amount of grey matter to be seen at a particular level can be correlated with the mass of tissue to be supplied. It is, therefore, greatest in the region of the cervical and lumbar enlargements which supply the limbs. The amount of white matter undergoes progressive increase as we proceed up the spinal cord. This is a result of the fact that (a) progressively more and more ascending fibres are added as we pass up the cord, and (b) the number of descending fibres decreases as we go down the cord as some of them terminate in each segment.

Subdivisions of Grey Matter

The grey matter of the spinal cord may be subdivided in more than one manner.

1. Traditionally, the ventral grey column has been divided into a ventral part, the ***head***, and a dorsal part, the ***base.*** Similarly, the dorsal grey column has been subdivided (from anterior to posterior side) into a ***base,*** a ***neck***, and a ***head***. These subdivisions have, however, been found to have little importance.
2. An attempt has been made to recognise discrete collections of neurons (or nuclei) in various regions of the spinal grey matter. These are illustrated in the left half of Fig. 17.4.

The ***ventral column neurons*** are arranged in the form of several discrete and elongated groups. We can recognise (a) a ***medial group*** which may be subdivided into ***dorsomedial*** and ***ventromedial*** parts; (b) a ***lateral group*** consisting of ***dorsolateral, ventrolateral*** and ***retrodorsolateral*** parts; and a ***central group*** represented by the ***phrenic*** and ***accessory*** nuclei (in the cervical region) and by the ***lumbosacral nucleus*** (in the lumbosacral region). Some large cells present along the anterior margin of the ventral grey column are called ***spinal border cells.***

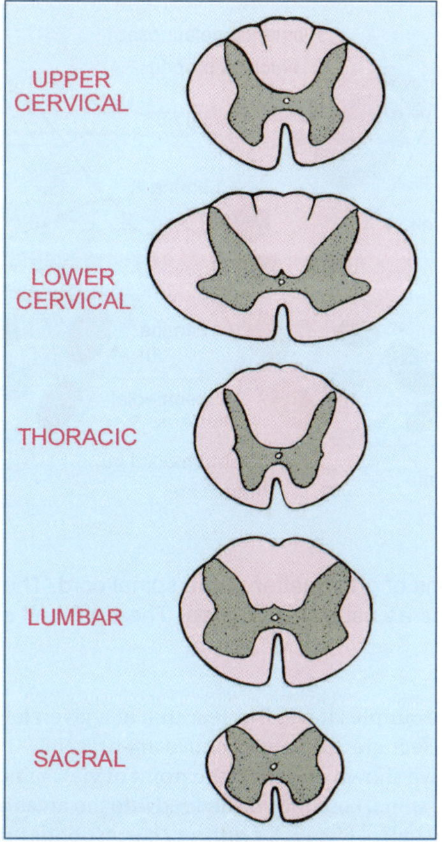

Fig. 17.3 Diagrams to show differences in appearance of transverse sections through various levels of the spinal cord.

Within the ***dorsal grey column*** the following relatively discrete areas may be recognised.

a. ***Substantia gelatinosa*** near the apex.
b. ***Nucleus proprius*** (or dorsal funicular group).
c. ***Dorsal nucleus*** (also called the thoracic nucleus or Clark's column) lying on the medial side of the base.
d. A thin layer of cells lying superficial to the substantia gelatinosa and constituting the ***posteromarginal nucleus***, also called the marginal zone.

Between the ventral and dorsal grey columns an intermediate zone is sometimes described. This contains the ***intermedio-lateral*** and ***intermedio-medial*** nuclei.

In Fig. 17.4. the ventral grey column is shown to be subdivided by a line passing forwards and medially. The part of the column lateral to this line (containing the greater part of the lateral group of nuclei) is present only in the region of the cervical and lumbar enlargements of the spinal cord. From this it can be inferred that the lateral group of nuclei innervate the musculature of the limbs. The dorsal nucleus is present only in the thoracic and upper lumbar segments. The intermediolateral group of neurons is present (a) from segments T1 to L2, and (b) in segments S2, S3

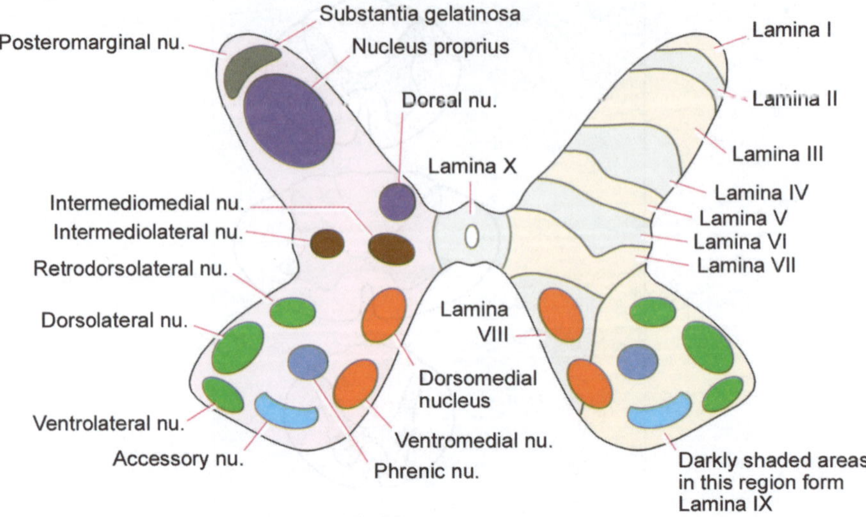

Fig. 17.4 Subdivisions of grey matter of the spinal cord. The left half of the figure shows the cell groups as usually described. The right half shows the concept of laminae.

and S4. From these examples it will be clear that at a given level of the spinal cord only some of the nuclear groups named above are present.

Recent studies have shown that from the point of view of neuronal connections the grey matter of the spinal cord may be divided into ten areas or laminae. These are illustrated in the right half of Fig. 17.4. ***Lamina I*** corresponds to the posteromarginal nucleus (lamina marginalis), ***lamina II*** to the substantia gelatinosa, and ***laminae III and IV*** to the nucleus proprius. ***Lamina V*** and ***lamina VI*** correspond to the base of the dorsal grey column. The lateral part of lamina V corresponds to the formatio reticularis. ***Lamina VII*** corresponds to the intermediate grey matter and includes the intermedio-medial, intermedio-lateral, and dorsal nuclei. It is believed to be made up predominantly of interneurons. At the level of the cervical and lumbar enlargements this lamina extends into the lateral part of the ventral horn. ***Lamina VIII*** occupies most of the ventral horn in the thoracic segments, but at the level of the limb enlargements it is confined to the medial part of the ventral horn. ***Lamina IX*** is made up of the various discrete groups of ventral column neurons already described. ***Lamina X*** forms the grey matter around the central canal.

Significance of Neurons in Grey Matter of Spinal Cord

The ***ventral column neurons*** of the spinal cord may be functionally divided into three major categories as follows.

a. The most prominent neurons with large cell bodies and prominent Nissl substance are designated ***alpha neurons***. These are somatic efferent neurons. Their axons (***alpha efferents)*** leave the spinal cord through the ventral nerve roots of spinal nerves and innervate striated muscle.
b. Some smaller neurons designated as ***gamma neurons*** are also located in lamina IX. They supply intrafusal fibres of muscle spindles.

c. A considerable number of smaller neurons in the ventral grey column are internuncial neurons.

We may now note certain additional facts about the ventral column neurons.

1. Alpha neurons occupy lamina IX of the ventral grey column.
2. Sensory impulses arising in muscle spindles travel to the spinal cord and reach the alpha neurons. The gamma neurons thus influence the activity of alpha neurons indirectly through muscle spindles.
3. Internuncial neurons are most abundant in Lamina VII. Some ramifications of the central processes of cells in the dorsal nerve root ganglia (bringing afferent impulses from the periphery), and axons descending from higher centres, terminate in relation to these internuncial neurons. The axons of internuncial neurons convey these impulses to alpha and gamma neurons.
4. Another variety of neuron that is believed (on physiological grounds) to exist in the ventral grey column is the so called ***Renshaw cell***. These cells receive the terminations of collaterals arising from the axons of alpha neurons. The axons of Renshaw cells carry the impulses back to the cell bodies of the same alpha neurons, and thus help to regulate their activity.

The ***neurons of the dorsal grey column*** may be subdivided as follows.

a. Some of these are internuncial neurons similar to those in the ventral grey column.
b. Many dorsal column neurons receive afferent impulses through the central processes of neurons in dorsal nerve root ganglia. These dorsal column neurons give off axons that enter the white matter of the spinal cord either on the same or opposite side. These axons may behave in one of the following ways.
   1. They may ascend or descend for some segments before terminating in relation to neurons at other levels of the spinal cord. Such axons constitute ***intersegmental tracts.***
   2. A considerable number of axons arising from dorsal column neurons run upwards in the spinal cord and constitute ***ascending tracts*** which terminate in various masses of grey matter in the brain. These tracts form a considerable part of the white matter of the spinal cord.

The ***neurons of the intermediolateral group*** (lateral grey column) are visceral efferent neurons. They are present at two levels of the spinal cord.

a. One group is present in the thoracic and upper two or three lumbar segments. These are preganglionic neurons of the sympathetic nervous system. Their axons terminate in relation to postganglionic neurons in sympathetic ganglia (and occasionally in some other situations). Axons of these postganglionic neurons are distributed to various organs, and to blood vessels.
b. The second group of visceral efferent neurons is found in the second, third and fourth sacral segments of the spinal cord. These are preganglionic neurons of the parasympathetic nervous system. Their axons leave the spinal cord through the ventral nerve roots to reach spinal nerves. They leave the spinal nerves as the ***pelvic splanchnic nerves*** which are distributed to some viscera in the pelvis and abdomen. They end by synapsing with

ganglion cells located in intimate relationship to the viscera concerned. The postganglionic fibres arising in these ganglia are short and supply smooth muscle and glands in these viscera.

WHITE MATTER OF THE SPINAL CORD

The anterior, lateral and posterior funiculi of the spinal cord are made up of nerve fibres running up or down the cord. These constitute the ascending and descending tracts which are described in Chapter 19.

CHAPTER

18

Gross Anatomy of the Brain

GROSS ANATOMY OF THE BRAINSTEM

The brainstem consists (from above downwards) of the midbrain, the pons and the medulla (Fig. 18.1, 18.2). The midbrain is continuous, above, with the cerebral hemispheres. The medulla is continuous, below, with the spinal cord. Posteriorly, the pons and medulla are separated from the cerebellum by the fourth ventricle (Fig. 18.3). The ventricle is continuous, below, with the central canal, which traverses the lower part of the medulla, and becomes continuous with the central canal of the spinal cord. Cranially, the fourth ventricle is continuous with the aqueduct, which passes through the midbrain. The midbrain, pons and medulla are connected to the cerebellum by the superior, middle and inferior cerebellar peduncles, respectively.

A number of cranial nerves are attached to the brainstem. The third and fourth nerves emerge from the surface of the midbrain; and the fifth from the pons. The sixth, seventh and eighth nerves emerge at the junction of the pons and medulla. The ninth, tenth, eleventh and twelfth cranial nerves emerge from the surface of the medulla.

Gross Anatomy of the Medulla

The medulla is broad above, where it joins the pons; and narrows down below, where it becomes continuous with the spinal cord. The junction of the medulla and cord is usually described as lying at the level of the upper border of the atlas vertebra. The transition is, in fact, not abrupt but occurs over a certain distance. The medulla is divided into a lower ***closed part***, which surrounds the central canal; and an upper ***open part***, which is related to the lower part of the fourth ventricle. The surface of the medulla is marked by a series of fissures or sulci that divide it into a number of regions. The ***anterior median fissure*** and the ***posterior median sulcus*** are upward continuations of the corresponding features seen on the spinal cord. On each side the ***anterolateral sulcus*** lies in line with the ventral roots of spinal nerves. The rootlets of the hypoglossal

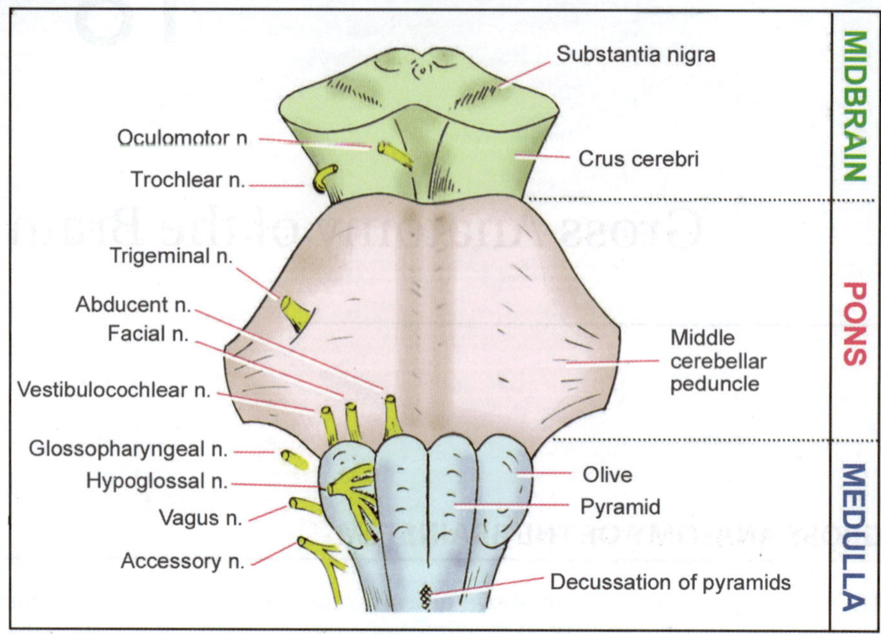

Fig. 18.1 Ventral aspect of the brainstem.

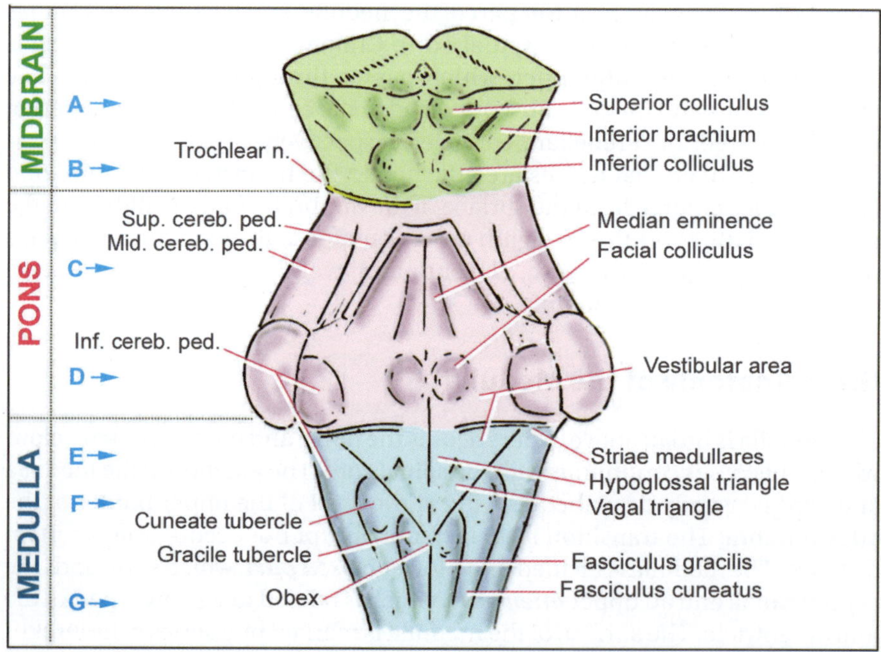

Fig. 18.2 Dorsal aspect of the brainstem. Letters G to A represent levels at which transverse sections are shown in Figs. 18.4 to 18.10. More detailed transverse sections are given in Figs. 16.6 to 16.9.

nerve emerge from this sulcus. The ***posterolateral sulcus*** lies in line with the dorsal nerve roots of spinal nerves, and gives attachment to rootlets of the glossopharyngeal, vagus and accessory nerves. The region between the anterior median sulcus and the anterolateral sulcus is occupied (on either side of the midline) by an elevation called the ***pyramid.*** The elevation is caused by a large bundle of fibres that descend from the cerebral cortex to the spinal cord. Some of these fibres cross from one side to the other in the lower part of the medulla, obliterating the anterior median fissure. These crossing fibres constitute the ***decussation of the pyramids***. Some other fibres emerge from the anterior median fissure, above the decussation, and wind laterally over the surface of the medulla. These are the ***anterior external arcuate fibres.*** In the upper part of the medulla, the region between the anterolateral and posterolateral sulci shows a prominent, elongated, oval swelling named the ***olive.*** It is produced by a large mass of grey matter called the ***inferior olivary nucleus.*** The posterior part of the medulla, between the posterior median sulcus and the posterolateral sulcus, contains tracts that enter the medulla from the posterior funiculus of the spinal cord. These are the ***fasciculus gracilis*** lying medially, next to the middle line, and the ***fasciculus cuneatus*** lying laterally. These fasciculi end in rounded elevations called the ***gracile*** and ***cuneate tubercles.*** These tubercles are produced by masses of grey matter called the ***nucleus gracilis*** and the ***nucleus cuneatus*** respectively.

Just above these tubercles the posterior aspect of the medulla is occupied by a triangular fossa which forms the lower part of the floor of the fourth ventricle. This fossa is bounded on either side by the inferior cerebellar peduncle. The lower part of the medulla, immediately lateral to the fasciculus cuneatus, is marked by another longitudinal elevation called the ***tuberculum cinereum.*** This elevation is produced by an underlying collection of grey matter called the ***spinal nucleus of the trigeminal nerve.*** The grey matter of this nucleus is covered by a layer of nerve fibres that form the ***spinal tract of the trigeminal nerve.***

Gross Anatomy of the Pons

The pons shows a convex ***anterior surface***, marked by prominent transversely running fibres. Laterally, these fibres collect to form a bundle, the ***middle cerebellar peduncle***. The trigeminal nerve emerges from the anterior surface, and the point of its emergence is taken as a landmark to define the plane of junction between the pons and the middle cerebellar peduncle. The anterior surface of the pons is marked, in the midline, by a shallow groove, the ***sulcus basilaris,*** which lodges the basilar artery. The line of junction between the pons and the medulla is marked by a groove through which a number of cranial nerves emerge. The abducent nerve emerges just above the pyramid and runs upwards in close relation to the anterior surface of the pons. The facial and vestibulo-cochlear nerves emerge in the interval between the olive and the pons. The posterior aspect of the pons forms the upper part of the floor of the fourth ventricle.

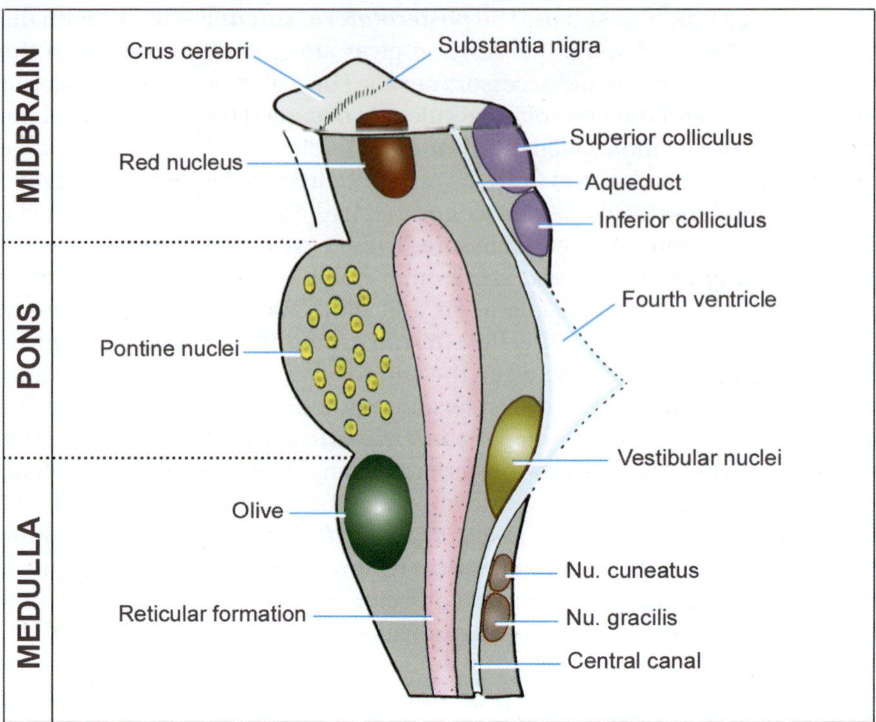

Fig. 18.3 Median section through the brainstem. Some important masses of grey matter are shown projected on to the median plane.

Gross Anatomy of the Midbrain

When the midbrain is viewed from the anterior aspect, we see two large bundles of fibres, one on each side of the middle line. These are the ***crura*** of the midbrain. The crura are separated by a deep fissure. Near the pons the fissure is narrow, but broadens as the crura diverge to enter the corresponding cerebral hemispheres. The parts of the crura just below the cerebrum form the posterior boundary of a space called the ***interpeduncular fossa*** (Fig. 18.21). The oculomotor nerve emerges from the medial aspect of the crus (singular of crura) of the same side.

The posterior aspect of the midbrain is marked by four rounded swellings. These are the ***colliculi,*** one ***superior*** and one ***inferior*** on each side. Each colliculus is related laterally to a ridge called the ***brachium.*** The ***superior brachium*** connects the superior colliculus to the lateral geniculate body, while the ***inferior brachium*** connects the inferior colliculus to the medial geniculate body. Just below the colliculi, there is the uppermost part of a membrane, the ***superior medullary velum,*** which stretches between the two superior cerebellar peduncles, and helps to form the roof of the fourth ventricle. The trochlear nerve emerges from the velum, and then winds round the side of the midbrain to reach its ventral aspect.

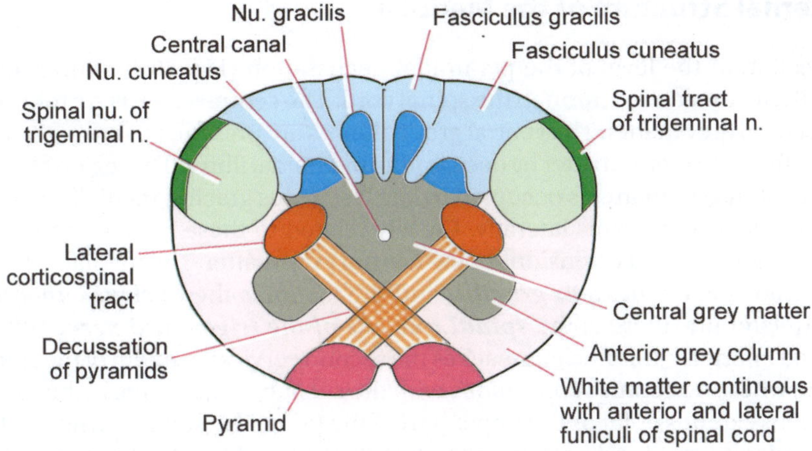

Fig. 18.4 Main features to be seen in a transverse section through the medulla at the level of the pyramidal decussation.

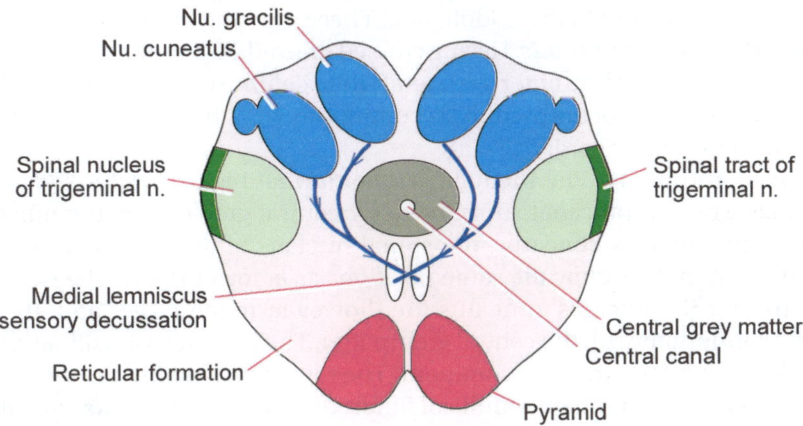

Fig. 18.5 Transverse section through the medulla to show the main features seen at the level of the sensory decussation.

PRELIMINARY REVIEW OF THE INTERNAL STRUCTURE OF THE BRAINSTEM

The following description is confined to those features of internal structure that can be seen with the naked eye. A detailed consideration of the internal structure of the brainstem will be taken up in Chapter 20.

The main features of the internal structure of the brainstem are most easily reviewed by examining transverse sections at various levels. These are illustrated in Figs. 18.4 to 18.8. The levels represented in these figures are indicated in Fig. 18.2.

Internal Structure of the Medulla

A section at the level of the pyramidal decussation (Fig. 18.4) shows some similarity to sections through the spinal cord. The central canal is surrounded by central grey matter. The ventral grey columns are present, but are separated from the central grey matter by decussating pyramidal fibres. The region behind the central grey matter is occupied by the fasciculus gracilis, medially; and by the fasciculus cuneatus laterally. Closely related to these fasciculi there are two tongue-shaped extensions of the central grey matter. The medial of these extensions is the ***nucleus gracilis***, and the lateral is the ***nucleus cuneatus***. More laterally, there is the ***spinal nucleus of the trigeminal nerve***. When traced inferiorly, this nucleus reaches the second cervical segment of the spinal cord, where it becomes continuous with the substantia gelatinosa. Above, the nucleus extends as far as the upper part of the pons. The spinal nucleus of the trigeminal nerve is related superficially to the ***spinal tract*** of the nerve. The ventral part of the medulla is occupied, on either side of the middle line, by a prominent bundle of fibres: these fibres form the ***pyramid***. The fibres of the pyramids are ***corticospinal fibres*** on their way from the cerebral cortex to the spinal cord. At this level in the medulla many of these fibres run backwards and medially to cross in the middle line. These crossing fibres constitute the ***decussation of the pyramids***. Having crossed the middle line, the corticospinal fibres turn downwards to enter the lateral white column of the spinal cord. The anterolateral region of the medulla is continuous with the anterior and lateral funiculi of the spinal cord.

A section thorough the medulla at a somewhat higher level is shown in Fig. 18.5. The central canal surrounded by central grey matter, the nucleus gracilis, the nucleus cuneatus, the spinal nucleus of the trigeminal nerve, and the pyramids occupy the same positions as at lower levels. The nucleus gracilis and the nucleus cuneatus are, however, much larger and are no longer continuous with the central grey matter. The fasciculus gracilis and the fasciculus cuneatus are less prominent. The region just behind the pyramids is occupied by a prominent bundle of fibres, the ***medial lemniscus,*** on either side of the middle line. The medial lemniscus is formed by fibres arising in the nucleus gracilis and the nucleus cuneatus. These fibres cross the middle line and turn upwards in the lemniscus of the opposite side. Crossing fibres of the two sides constitute the ***sensory decussation.*** The region lateral to the medial lemniscus contains scattered neurons mixed with nerve fibres. This region is the ***reticular formation***. More laterally there is a mass of white matter containing various tracts.

A section through the medulla at the level of the olive is shown in Fig. 18.6. The pyramids, the medial lemniscus, the spinal nucleus and tract of the trigeminal nerve, and the reticular formation are present in the same relative position as at lower levels. The medial lemniscus is, however, much more prominent and is somewhat expanded anteriorly. Lateral to the spinal nucleus (and tract) of the trigeminal nerve we see a large compact bundle of fibres. This is the ***inferior cerebellar peduncle*** which connects the medulla to the

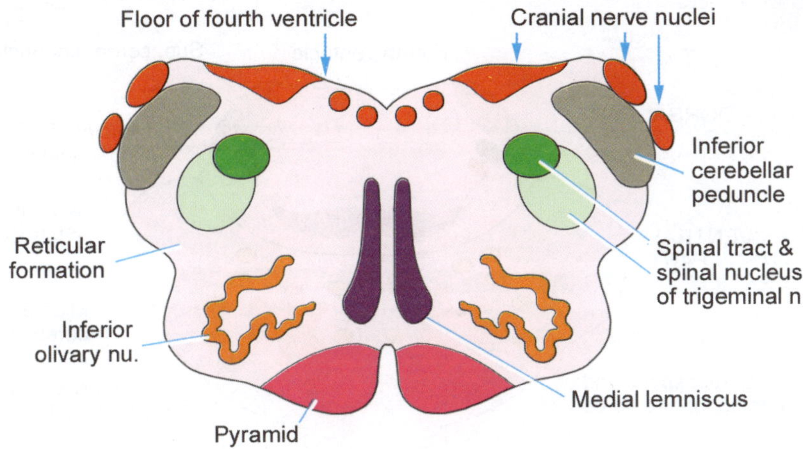

Fig. 18.6 Main features to be seen in a transverse section through the medulla at the level of the olive.

cerebellum. Posteriorly, the medulla forms the floor of the fourth ventricle. Here it is lined by a layer of grey matter in which are located several important cranial nerve nuclei. The ***inferior olivary nucleus*** forms a prominent feature in the anterolateral part of the medulla at this level. It is made up of a thin lamina of grey matter that is folded on itself like a crumpled purse. The nucleus has a hilum that is directed medially.

Internal Structure of the Pons

The pons is divisible into a ventral part and a dorsal part (Fig. 18.7).

The ***ventral (or basilar) part*** consists of transverse and vertical fibres. Amongst the fibres are groups of cells that constitute the ***pontine nuclei***. When traced laterally the transverse fibres form the ***middle cerebellar peduncle***. The vertical fibres are of two types. Some of them descend from the cerebral cortex to end in the pontine nuclei. Others are corticospinal fibres that descend through the pons into the medulla where they form the pyramids.

The ***dorsal part (or tegmentum)*** of the pons may be regarded as an upward continuation of the part of the medulla behind the pyramids. Superiorly, it is continuous with the tegmentum of the midbrain. It is bounded posteriorly by the fourth ventricle. Laterally, it is related to the ***superior cerebellar peduncles*** in its upper part (Fig. 18.7); and to the inferior cerebellar peduncles in its lower part (Fig. 18.8). The spinal nucleus and tract of the trigeminal nerve lie just medial to these peduncles. The medial lemniscus forms a transversely elongated band of fibres just behind the ventral part of the pons.

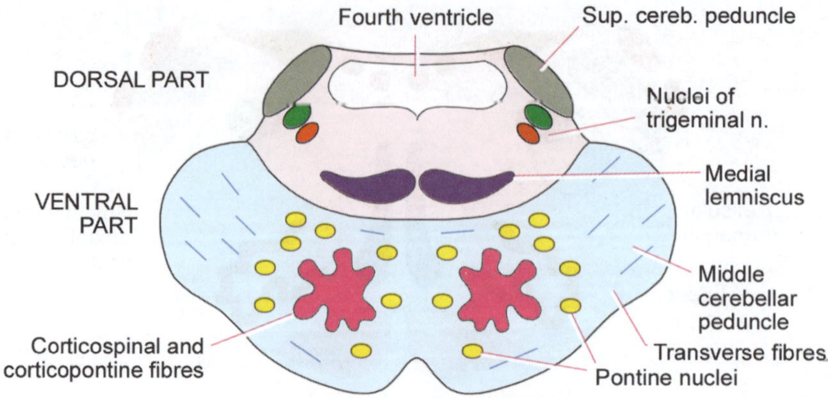

Fig. 18.7 Main features to be seen in a transverse section through the upper part of the pons.

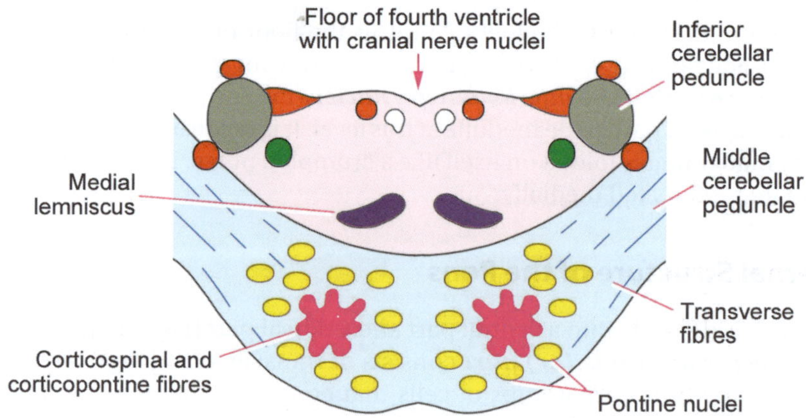

Fig. 18.8 Main features to be seen in a transverse section through the lower part of the pons.

Internal Structure of the Midbrain

For convenience of description, the midbrain may be divided as follows (Fig. 18.9).

(i) The part lying behind a transverse line drawn through the cerebral aqueduct is called the ***tectum.*** It consists of the superior and inferior colliculi of the two sides.

(ii) The part lying in front of the transverse line is made up of right and left halves called the ***cerebral peduncles.*** Each peduncle consists of three parts. From anterior to posterior side these are the ***crus cerebri*** (or ***basis pedunculi),*** the ***substantia nigra*** and the ***tegmentum.***

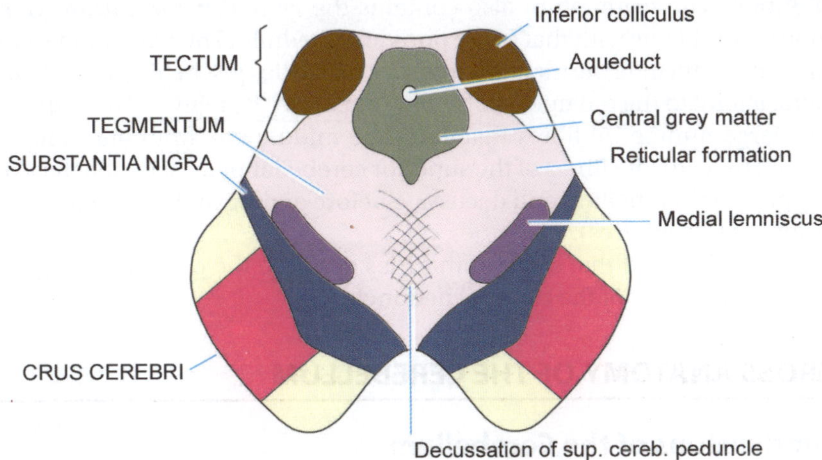

Fig. 18.9 Main features to be seen in a transverse section through the lower part of the midbrain.

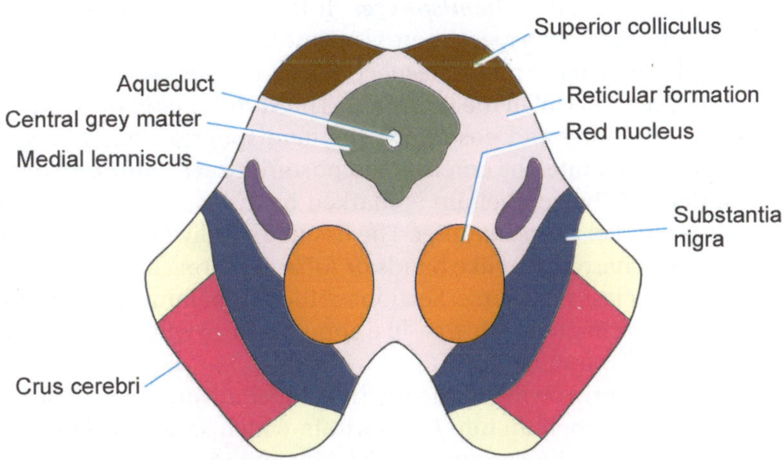

Fig. 18.10 Main features to be seen in a transverse section through the upper part of the midbrain.

The ***crus cerebri*** consists of a large mass of vertically running fibres. These fibres descend from the cerebral cortex. Some of these pass through the midbrain to reach the pons, while others reach the spinal cord. The two crura are separated by a notch seen on the anterior aspect of the midbrain.

The ***substantia nigra*** is made up of pigmented grey matter and, therefore, appears dark in colour.

The ***tegmentum*** of the two sides is continuous across the middle line. It contains important masses of grey matter as well as fibre bundles. The largest of the nuclei is the ***red nucleus*** (Fig. 18.10) present in the upper half of the midbrain. The tegmentum also contains the ***reticular formation*** which is continuous below with that of the pons and medulla. The fibre bundles of the tegmentum include the medial lemniscus which lies just behind the substantia nigra, lateral to the red nucleus. The lower part of the tegmentum is traversed by a large number of fibres that cross the middle line from one side to the other. These are the fibres of the superior cerebellar peduncles that have their origin in the cerebellum and decussate before ending in the red nucleus (and in some other centres).

It may be noted that some authorities describe the corresponding half of the tectum as part of the cerebral peduncle.

GROSS ANATOMY OF THE CEREBELLUM

Subdivisions of the Cerebellum

The cerebellum lies in the posterior cranial fossa, behind the pons and the medulla. It is separated from the cerebrum by a fold of dura mater called the ***tentorium cerebell***.

The cerebellum consists of a part lying near the middle line called the ***vermis,*** and of two lateral ***hemispheres.*** It has two surfaces, ***superior*** and ***inferior.*** On the superior aspect, there is no line of distinction between vermis and hemispheres. On the inferior aspect, the two hemispheres are separated by a deep depression called the ***vallecula.*** The vermis lies in the depth of this depression. Anteriorly and posteriorly the hemispheres extend beyond the vermis and are separated by anterior and posterior ***cerebellar notches.***

The surface of the cerebellum is marked by a series of fissures that run more or less parallel to one another. The fissures subdivide the surface of the cerebellum into narrow leaf like bands or ***folia***. The long axis of the majority of folia is more or less transverse. Sections of the cerebellum cut at right angles to this axis have a characteristic tree-like appearance to which the term ***arbor-vitae*** (tree of life) is applied.

Some of the fissures on the surface of the cerebellum are deeper than others. They divide the cerebellum into ***lobes*** within which smaller ***lobules*** may be recognised. To show the various subdivisions of the cerebellum in a single illustration it is usual to represent the organ as if it has been 'opened out' so that the superior and inferior aspects can both be seen. Such an illustration is shown in Fig. 18.11. This should be compared with Figs. 18.12 A, B which are more realistic drawings of the superior and inferior surfaces, and with Fig. 18.13 which is a middle line section showing the subdivisions of the vermis.

The deepest fissures in the cerebellum are (i) the ***primary fissure*** seen on the superior surface, and (ii) the ***posterolateral fissure*** seen on the inferior aspect. These fissures divide the cerebellum into three lobes. The part anterior to the primary fissure is the ***anterior lobe.*** The part between the two fissures is the ***middle lobe*** (sometimes called the ***posterior lobe***). The remaining part is the ***flocculonodular lobe.*** The anterior and middle lobes together form the ***corpus cerebelli.***

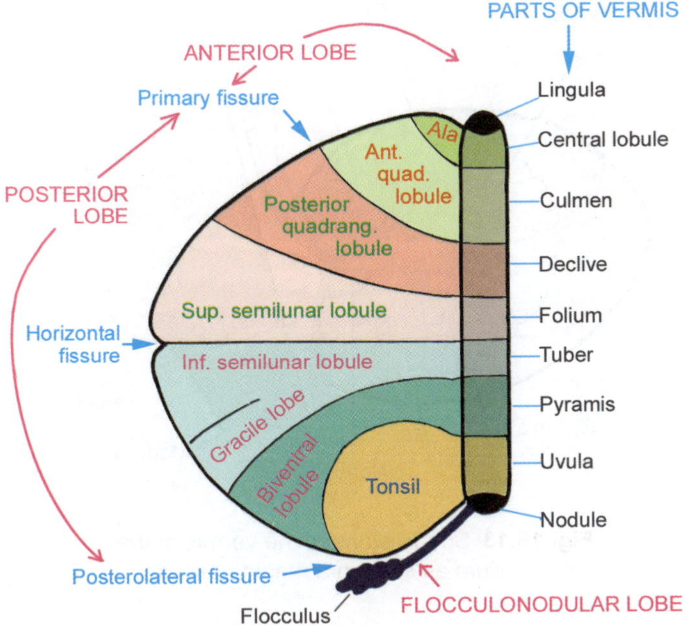

Fig. 18.11 Scheme to show the subdivisions of the cerebellum.

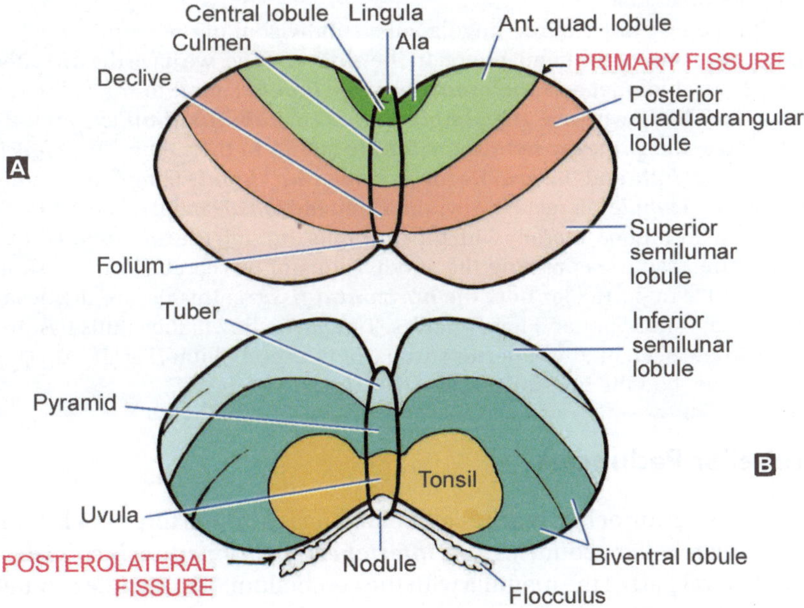

Fig. 18.12 Subdivisions of the cerebellum. A. As seen on the superior aspect. B. As seen on the inferior aspect.

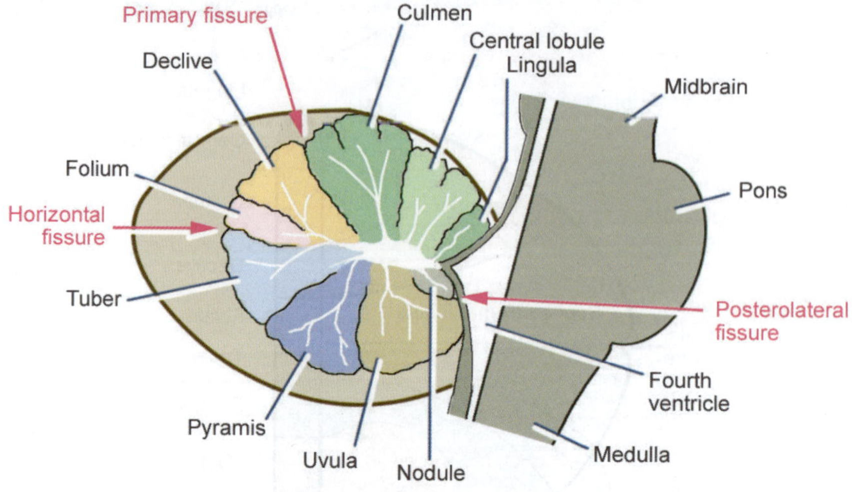

Fig. 18.13 Subdivisions of the vermis of the cerebellum as seen in a median section.

The vermis is so called because it resembles a worm. Proceeding from above downwards in Fig. 18.11 it is seen to consist of the ***lingula, central lobule*** and ***culmen*** (in the anterior lobe); the ***declive, folium*** (or ***folium vermis***), ***tuber*** (or ***tuber vermis), pyramid*** and ***uvula*** (in the middle lobe); and the ***nodule*** (in the flocculonodular lobe).

With the exception of the lingula each subdivision of the vermis is related laterally to a part of the hemisphere. In the anterior lobe, we have the ***ala*** lateral to the central lobule; and the ***quadrangular lobule*** lateral to the culmen. In the middle lobe, we have the ***simple lobule*** (or ***lobulus simplex)*** lateral to the declive; the ***superior semilunar lobule*** lateral to the folium; the ***inferior semilunar lobule*** and the ***gracile*** (or ***paramedian) lobule*** lateral to the tuber; the ***biventral lobule*** lateral to the pyramid; and the ***tonsil*** lateral to the uvula. The nodule is continuous laterally with the flocculus through the inferior medullary velum. The fissures separating the subdivisions of the cerebellum are shown in Fig. 18.11. In particular note the ***horizontal fissure***: this fissure divides the cerebellum into upper and lower halves. The parts shown above this fissure in Fig. 18.11 are seen on the superior surface of the cerebellum (Fig. 18.12A), and those below it on the inferior surface (Fig. 18.12B).

Cerebellar Peduncles

The fibres entering or leaving the cerebellum pass through three thick bundles called the cerebellar peduncles. The ***inferior cerebellar peduncle*** connects the posterolateral part of the medulla with the cerebellum. The ***middle cerebellar peduncle*** looks like a lateral continuation of the ventral part of the pons. It connects the pons to the cerebellum. The ***superior cerebellar peduncle*** is

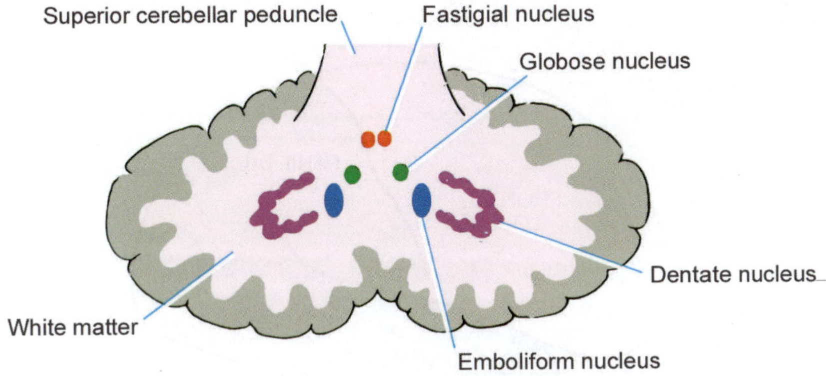

Fig. 18.14 Scheme to show the cerebellar nuclei.

the main connection between the midbrain and the cerebellum. The fibres passing through each peduncle are enumerated in Chapter 19.

White Matter of the Cerebellum

The central core of each cerebellar hemisphere is formed by white matter. The peduncles are continued into this white matter. The white matter of the two sides is connected by a thin lamina of fibres that are closely related to the fourth ventricle. The upper part of this lamina forms the superior medullary velum, and its inferior part forms the inferior medullary velum. Both these take part in forming the roof of the fourth ventricle.

Grey Matter of the Cerebellum

Most of the grey matter of the cerebellum is arranged as a thin layer covering the central core of white matter. This layer is the ***cerebellar cortex***. The subdivisions of the cerebellar cortex correspond to the subdivisions of the cerebellum described above. Embedded within the central core of white matter there are masses of grey matter which constitute the ***cerebellar nuclei.*** These are as follows (Fig. 18.14).

1. The ***dentate nucleus*** lies in the centre of each cerebellar hemisphere. Cross sections through the nucleus have a striking resemblance to those through the inferior olivary nucleus. Like the latter it is made up of a thin lamina of grey matter that is folded upon itself so that it resembles a crumpled purse. Both the nuclei have a hilum directed medially.
2. The ***emboliform nucleus*** lies on the medial side of the dentate nucleus.
3. The ***globose nucleus*** lies medial to the emboliform nucleus.
4. The ***fastigial nucleus*** lies close to the middle line in the anterior part of the superior vermis.

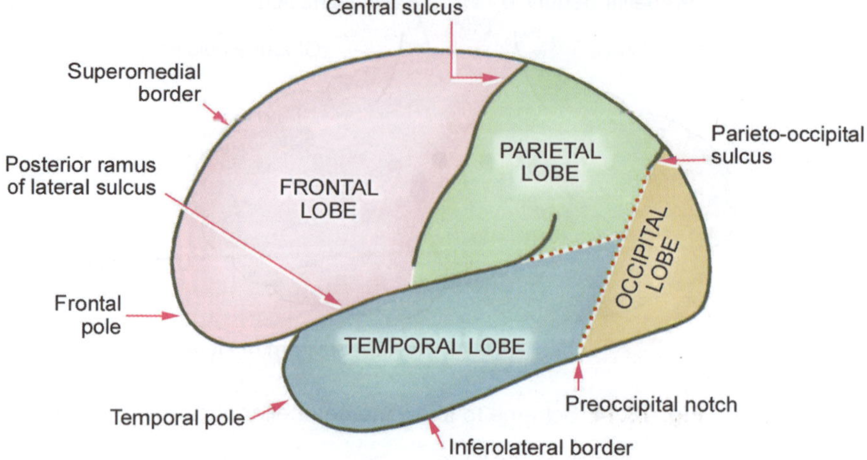

Fig. 18.15 Lateral aspect of the cerebral hemisphere to show borders, poles and lobes.

GROSS ANATOMY OF THE CEREBRAL HEMISPHERES

EXTERIOR OF THE CEREBRAL HEMISPHERES

Poles, Surfaces, and Borders

The cerebrum consists of two cerebral hemispheres that are partially connected with each other. When viewed from the lateral aspect each cerebral hemisphere has the appearance shown in Fig. 18.15. Three somewhat pointed ends or ***poles*** can be recognised. These are the ***frontal pole*** anteriorly, the ***occipital pole*** posteriorly, and the ***temporal pole*** that lies between the frontal and occipital poles, and points forwards and somewhat downwards. A coronal section through the cerebral hemispheres (Fig. 18.16) shows that each hemisphere has three borders, ***superomedial, inferolateral*** and ***inferomedial.*** These borders divide the surface of the hemisphere into three large surfaces, ***superolateral, medial*** and ***inferior.*** The inferior surface is further subdivided into an anterior ***orbital*** part and a posterior ***tentorial*** part (Fig. 18.16). Corresponding to these subdivisions, the inferomedial border is divided into an anterior part called the ***medial orbital border*** and a posterior part called the ***medial occipital border.*** The orbital part of the inferolateral border is called the ***superciliary border*** (as it lies just above the level of the eyebrows). The surfaces of the cerebral hemisphere are not smooth. They show a series of grooves or ***sulci*** which are separated by intervening areas that are called ***gyri.***

Lobes

For convenience of description each cerebral hemisphere is divided into four major subdivisions or ***lobes.*** To consider the boundaries of these lobes

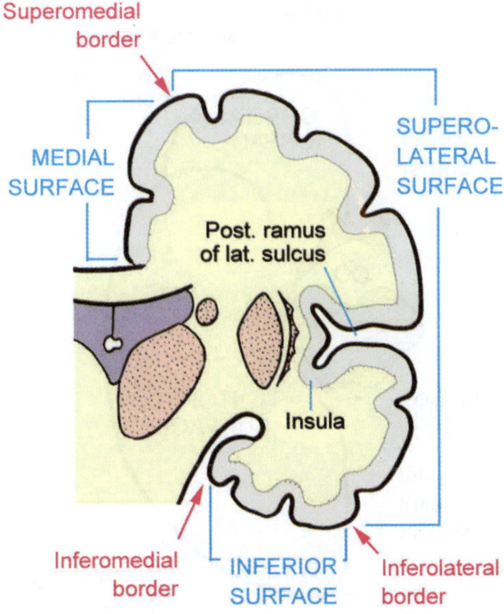

Fig. 18.16 Coronal section through a cerebral hemisphere to show its borders and surfaces.

reference has to be made to some sulci and other features to be seen on each hemisphere (Fig. 18.15).

1. On the superolateral surface of the hemisphere there are two prominent sulci. One of these is the ***posterior ramus of the lateral sulcus*** which begins near the temporal pole and runs backwards and slightly upwards. Its posteriormost part curves sharply upwards. The second sulcus that is used to delimit the lobes is the ***central sulcus.*** It begins on the superomedial margin a little behind the midpoint between the frontal and occipital poles, and runs downwards and forwards to end a little above the posterior ramus of the lateral sulcus.
2. On the medial surface of the hemisphere, near the occipital pole, there is a sulcus called the ***parieto-occipital sulcus*** (Fig. 18.19). The upper end of this sulcus reaches the superomedial border and a small part of it can be seen on the superolateral surface (Fig. 18.15).
3. A little anterior to the occipital pole the inferolateral border shows a slight indentation called the ***preoccipital notch*** (or ***preoccipital incisure***).

   To complete the subdivision of the hemisphere into lobes we now have to draw two imaginary lines. The first imaginary line connects the upper end of the parieto-occipital sulcus to the preoccipital notch. The second imaginary line is a backward continuation of the posterior ramus of the lateral sulcus (excluding the posterior upturned part) to meet the first line. We are now in a position to define the limits of the various lobes as follows.

   a. The ***frontal lobe*** lies anterior to the central sulcus, and above the posterior ramus of the lateral sulcus.

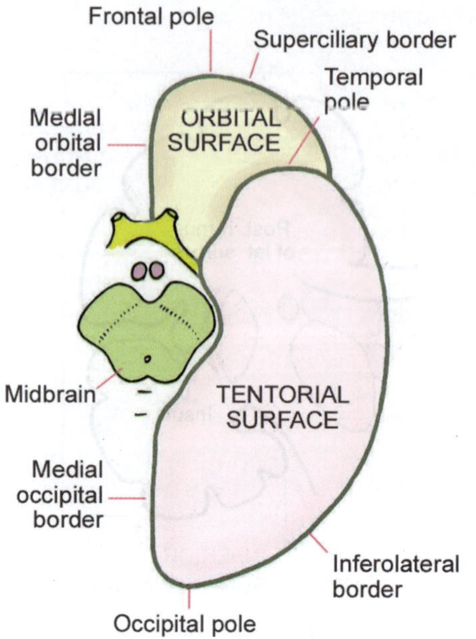

Fig. 18.17 Inferior aspect of a cerebral hemisphere to show its borders, poles and surfaces.

b. The ***parietal lobe*** lies behind the central sulcus. It is bounded below by the posterior ramus of the lateral sulcus and by the second imaginary line; and behind by the upper part of the first imaginary line.

c. The ***occipital lobe*** is the area lying behind the first imaginary line.

d. The ***temporal lobe*** lies below the posterior ramus of the lateral sulcus and the second imaginary line. It is separated from the occipital lobe by the lower part of the first imaginary line.

Before going on to consider further subdivisions of each of the lobes named above, attention has to be directed to details of some structures already mentioned.

a. The upper end of the central sulcus winds round the superomedial border to reach the medial surface. Here its end is surrounded by a gyrus called the ***paracentral lobule*** (Fig. 18.19). The lower end of the central sulcus is always separated by a small interval from the posterior ramus of the lateral sulcus (Fig. 18.15).

b. The lateral sulcus begins on the inferior aspect of the cerebral hemisphere where it lies between the orbital surface and the anterior part of the temporal lobe (Fig. 18.21). It runs laterally to reach the superolateral surface. On reaching this surface it divides into three rami (branches). These rami are ***anterior*** (or ***anterior horizontal***), ***ascending*** (or ***anterior ascending***) and ***posterior*** (Fig. 18.18). The anterior and ascending rami are short and run into the frontal lobe in the directions indicated by their names. The posterior ramus has already been considered. Unlike most

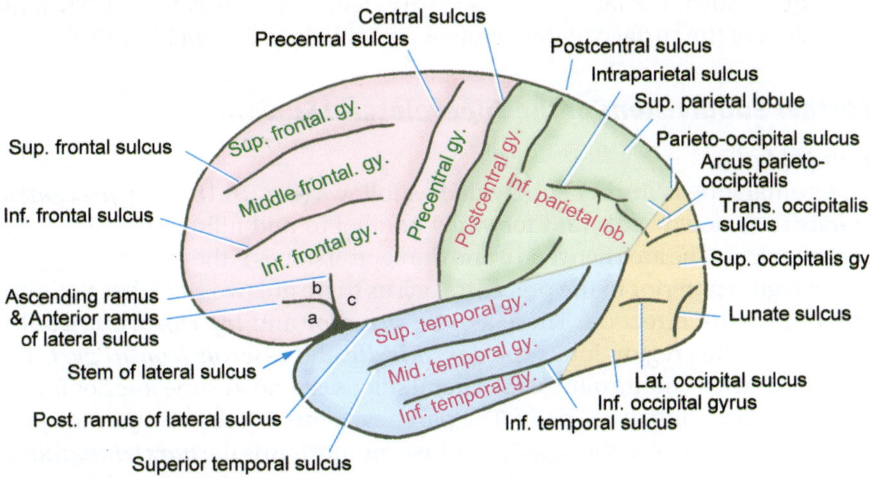

Fig. 18.18 Simplified presentation of sulci and gyri on the superolateral surface of the cerebral hemisphere. a = pars orbitalis. b = pars triangularis. c = pars opercularis. Also see Fig. 16.1.

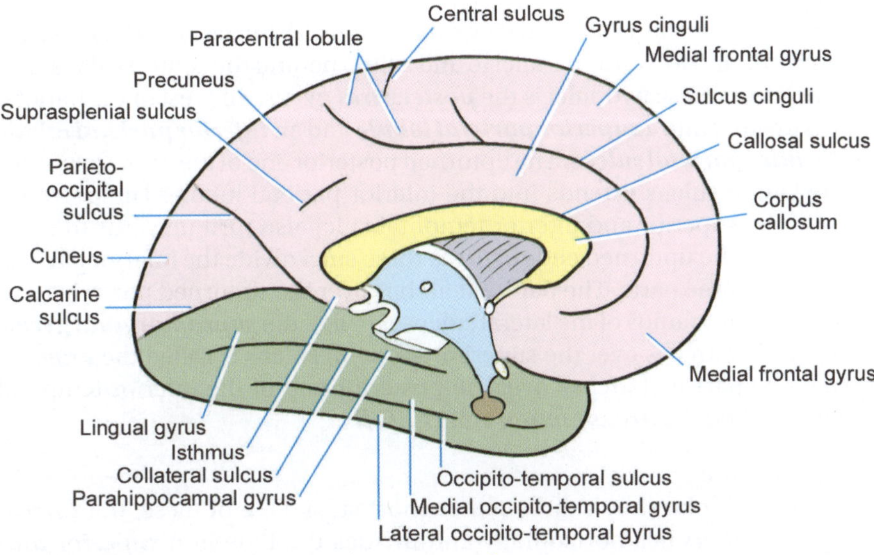

Fig. 18.19 Simplified presentation of sulci and gyri on the cerebral hemisphere as seen from the medial aspect. The medial surface and the tentorial surface (shaded in dots) are seen. The corpus callosum and some other median structures have been cut across.

other sulci, the lateral sulcus is very deep. Its walls cover a fairly large area of the surface of the hemisphere called the ***insula*** (Fig. 18.17).

Further Subdivisions of the Superolateral Surface

Frontal Lobe

The frontal lobe is further subdivided as follows (Fig. 18.18). The ***precentral sulcus*** runs downwards and forwards parallel to and a little anterior to the central sulcus. The area between it and the central sulcus is the ***precentral gyrus.*** In the region anterior to the precentral gyrus there are two sulci that run in an anteroposterior direction. These are the ***superior*** and ***inferior frontal sulci.*** They divide this region into ***superior, middle*** and ***inferior frontal gyri.*** The anterior and ascending rami of the lateral sulcus extend into the inferior frontal gyrus dividing it into three parts. The part below the anterior ramus is the ***pars orbitalis***; that between the anterior and ascending rami is the ***pars triangularis***; and the part posterior to the ascending ramus is the ***pars opercularis.***

Temporal Lobe

The temporal lobe has two sulci that run parallel to the posterior ramus of the lateral sulcus. They are termed the ***superior and inferior temporal sulci.*** They divide the superolateral surface of this lobe into ***superior, middle and inferior temporal gyri.***

Parietal Lobe

The parietal lobe shows the following subdivisions. The ***postcentral sulcus*** runs downwards and forwards parallel to and a little behind the central sulcus. The area between these two sulci is the ***postcentral gyrus.*** The rest of the parietal lobe is divided into a ***superior parietal lobule*** and an ***inferior parietal lobule*** by the ***intraparietal sulcus.*** The upturned posterior end of the posterior ramus of the lateral sulcus extends into the inferior parietal lobule. The posterior ends of the superior and inferior temporal sulci also turn upwards to enter this lobule. The upturned ends of these three sulci divide the inferior parietal lobule into three parts. The part that arches over the upturned posterior end of the posterior ramus of the lateral sulcus is called the ***supramarginal gyrus.*** The part that arches over the superior temporal sulcus is called the ***angular gyrus.*** The part that arches over the posterior end of the inferior temporal sulcus is called the ***arcus temporo-occipitalis.***

Occipital Lobe

The occipital lobe shows three rather short sulci. One of these, the ***lateral occipital sulcus*** lies horizontally and divides the lobe into ***superior and inferior occipital gyri.*** The ***lunate sulcus*** runs downwards and slightly forwards just in front of the occipital pole. The vertical strip just in front of it is the ***gyrus descendens.*** The ***transverse occipital sulcus*** is located in the uppermost part of the occipital lobe. The upper end of the parieto-occipital sulcus (which just reaches the superolateral surface from the medial surface) is surrounded by the ***arcus parieto-occipitalis.*** As its name suggests, it belongs partly to the parietal lobe and partly to the occipital lobe.

Insula

In the depth of the stem and posterior ramus of the lateral sulcus there is a part of the cerebral hemisphere called the insula (insula = insulated or hidden). It is surrounded by a ***circular sulcus.*** During development of the cerebral hemisphere this area grows less than surrounding areas which, therefore, come to overlap it and occlude it from surface view. These surrounding areas are called ***opercula*** (= lids). The ***frontal operculum*** lies between the anterior and ascending rami of the lateral sulcus. The ***frontoparietal operculum*** lies above the posterior ramus of the lateral sulcus. The ***temporal operculum*** lies below this sulcus. The temporal operculum has a superior surface hidden in the depth of the lateral sulcus (Figs. 18.17, 18.26B). On this surface we see two gyri called the ***anterior and posterior transverse temporal gyri.***

Medial Surface of Cerebral Hemisphere

When the two cerebral hemispheres are separated from each other by a cut in the middle line the appearances seen are shown in Figs. 18.19 and 18.20. The structures seen are as follows.

The ***corpus callosum*** is a prominent arched structure consisting of commissural fibres passing from one hemisphere to the other (Fig. 18.20). It consists of a central part called the ***trunk,*** a posterior end or ***splenium,*** and an anterior end or ***genu.*** A little below the corpus callosum we see the third ventricle of the brain. A number of structures can be identified in relation to this ventricle. The ***interventricular foramen*** through which the third ventricle communicates with the lateral ventricle can be seen in the upper and anterior part. Posteroinferiorly, the ventricle is continuous with the ***cerebral aqueduct.*** The lateral wall of the ventricle is formed in greater part by a large mass of grey matter called the ***thalamus.*** The right and left thalami are usually interconnected (across the middle line) by a strip of grey matter called the ***interthalamic connexus.*** The anteroinferior part of the lateral wall of the third ventricle is formed by a collection of grey matter that constitutes the ***hypothalamus.***

Above the thalamus there is a bundle of fibres called the ***fornix.*** Posteriorly, the fornix is attached to the undersurface of the corpus callosum, but anteriorly it disappears from view just in front of the interventricular foramen. Extending between the fornix and the corpus callosum there is a thin lamina called the ***septum pellucidum*** (or ***septum lucidum***), which separates the right and left lateral ventricles from each other. Removal of the septum pellucidum brings the interior of the lateral ventricle into view.

In the anterior wall of the third ventricle there are the ***anterior commissure*** and the ***lamina terminalis.*** The anterior commissure is attached to the genu of the corpus callosum through a thin lamina of fibres that constitutes the ***rostrum*** of the corpus callosum. Below, the anterior commissure is continuous with the lamina terminalis which is a thin lamina of nervous tissue. The lower end of the lamina terminalis is attached to the optic chiasma. Posteriorly, the third ventricle is related to the ***pineal gland*** and inferiorly to the ***hypophysis cerebri.***

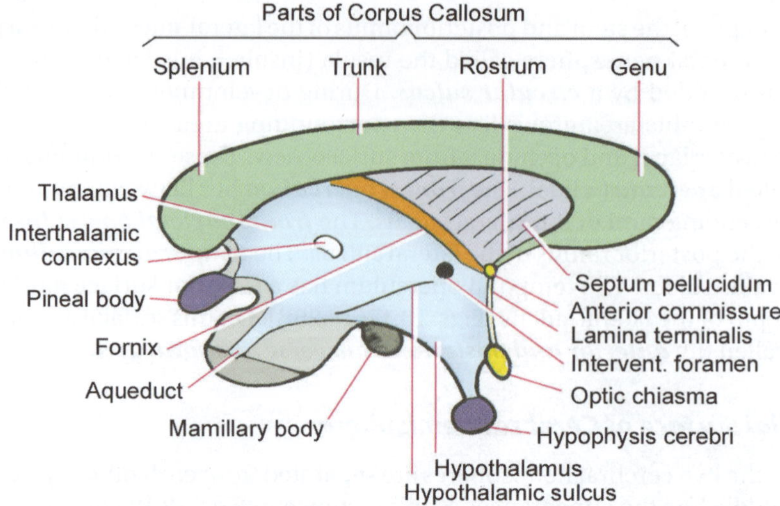

Fig. 18.20 Enlarged view of part of Fig. 18.19 to show some structures to be seen on the medial aspect of the cerebral hemisphere.

Above the corpus callosum (and also in front of and behind it) we see the sulci and gyri of the medial surface of the hemisphere (Fig. 18.19). The most prominent of the sulci is the ***cingulate sulcus*** which follows a curved course parallel to the upper convex margin of the corpus callosum. Anteriorly, it ends below the rostrum of the corpus callosum. Posteriorly, it turns upwards to reach the superomedial border a little behind the upper end of the central sulcus. The area between the cingulate sulcus and the corpus callosum is called the ***gyrus cinguli.*** It is separated from the corpus callosum by the ***callosal sulcus.*** The part of the medial surface of the hemisphere between the cingulate sulcus and the superomedial border consists of two parts. The smaller posterior part which is wound around the end of the central sulcus is called the ***paracentral lobule***. The large anterior part is called the ***medial frontal gyrus.*** These two parts are separated by a short sulcus continuous with the cingulate sulcus.

The part of the medial surface behind the paracentral lobule and the gyrus cinguli shows two major sulci that cut off a triangular area called the ***cuneus.*** The triangle is bounded anteriorly and above by the ***parieto-occipital sulcus***; inferiorly by the ***calcarine sulcus***; and posteriorly by the superomedial border of the hemisphere. The calcarine sulcus extends forwards beyond its junction with the parieto-occipital sulcus and ends a little below the splenium of the corpus callosum. The small area separating the splenium from the calcarine sulcus is called the ***isthmus.*** Between the parieto-occipital sulcus and the paracentral lobule there is a quadrilateral area called the ***precuneus.*** Anteroinferiorly the precuneus is separated from the posterior part of the gyrus cinguli by the ***suprasplenial (or subparietal) sulcus.***

The precuneus and the posterior part of the paracentral lobule form the medial surface of the parietal lobe.

Although the parieto-occipital and calcarine sulci appear to be continuous with each other on surface view, they are separated by the cuneate gyrus which lies in the depth of the area where the two sulci meet. The parts of the calcarine sulcus anterior and posterior to the junction with the parieto-occipital sulcus are separated by a deeply situated anterior cuneolingual gyrus.

A small area anterior to the lamina terminalis shows certain small sulci and gyri that are consideredin Chapter 21.

Inferior Surface of Cerebrum

When the cerebrum is separated from the hindbrain by cutting across the midbrain, and is viewed from below, the appearances seen are shown in Fig. 18.21. Posterior to the midbrain we see the undersurface of the splenium of the corpus callosum. Anterior to the midbrain there is a depressed area called the ***interpeduncular fossa***. The fossa is bounded in front by the ***optic chiasma*** and on the sides by the right and left ***optic tracts***. The optic tracts wind round the sides of the midbrain to terminate on its posterolateral aspect. In this region two swellings, the ***medial and lateral geniculate bodies***, can be seen.

Certain structures are seen within the interpeduncular fossa. These are closely related to the floor of the third ventricle (see also Fig. 18.20). Anterior and medial to the crura of the midbrain there are two rounded swellings called the ***mamillary bodies.*** Anterior to these bodies there is a median elevation called the ***tuber cinereum,*** to which the infundibulum of the hypophysis cerebri is attached. The triangular interval between the mamillary bodies and the midbrain is pierced by numerous small blood vessels and is called the ***posterior perforated substance.*** A similar area lying on each side of the optic chiasma is called the ***anterior perforated substance***. The anterior perforated substance is bounded anterolaterally by the lateral olfactory stria and posterolaterally by the uncus (see below). The anterior perforated substance is connected to the insula by a band of grey matter called the ***limen insulae*** which lies in the depth of the stem of the lateral sulcus.

In addition to these structures we see the sulci and gyri on the orbital and tentorial parts of the inferior surface of the each cerebral hemisphere (described below). The orbital and tentorial parts of the inferior surface are separated from each other by the stem of the lateral sulcus.

Orbital Surface

Close to the medial border of the orbital surface there is an anteroposterior sulcus: it is called the ***olfactory sulcus*** because the olfactory bulb and tract lie superficial to it. The area medial to this sulcus is called the ***gyrus rectus***. The rest of the orbital surface is divided by an H-shaped ***orbital sulcus*** into ***anterior***, ***posterior***, ***medial*** and ***lateral orbital gyri.***

Tentorial Surface

The tentorial surface is marked by two major sulci that run in an anteroposterior direction. These are the ***collateral sulcus*** medially, and the ***occipito-temporal sulcus*** laterally. The posterior part of the collateral sulcus runs parallel to the calcarine sulcus: the area between them is the ***lingual gyrus.*** Anteriorly,

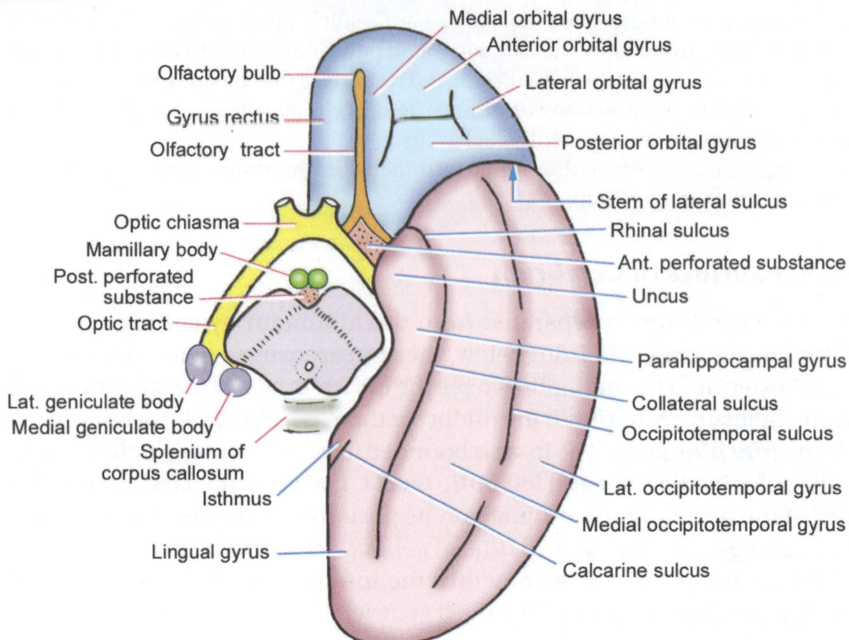

Fig. 18.21 Structures to be seen on the inferior aspect of the cerebral hemisphere. Also see Fig. 16.3.

the lingual gyrus becomes continuous with the ***parahippocampal gyrus*** which is related medially to the midbrain and to the interpeduncular fossa. The anterior end of the parahippo-campal gyrus is cut off from the curved temporal pole of the hemisphere by a curved ***rhinal sulcus.*** This part of the parahippocampal gyrus forms a hook-like structure called the ***uncus.*** Posteriorly, the parahippocampal gyrus becomes continuous with the gyrus cinguli through the isthmus (Fig. 18.19). The area between the collateral sulcus and the rhinal sulcus medially, and the occipitotemporal sulcus laterally, is the ***medial occipitotemporal gyrus.*** The area lateral to the occipitotemporal sulcus is called the ***lateral occipitotemporal gyrus.*** This gyrus is continuous (around the inferolateral margin of the cerebral hemisphere) with the inferior temporal gyrus.

The inferior surface of the cerebral hemisphere presents several additional features of interest. These are considered in Chapter 21 while describing the olfactory region.

AN INTRODUCTION TO SOME STRUCTURES WITHIN THE CEREBRAL HEMISPHERES

For a proper understanding of the structure of the cerebrum, brief reference to the development of the brain is necessary. At an early stage of development

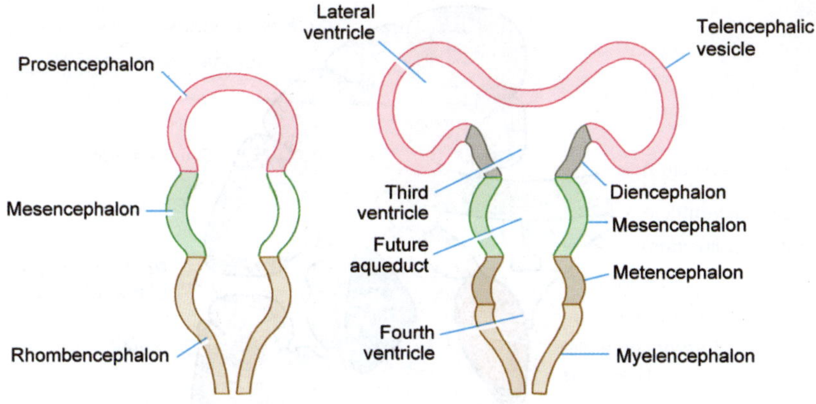

Fig. 18.22 Two stages in the development of the brain.

the brain is made up of three hollow vesicles. These are the ***prosencephalon,*** the ***mesencephalon*** and the ***rhombencephalon*** (in craniocaudal sequence) (Fig. 18.22). The mesencephalon gives rise to the midbrain, while the rhombencephalon forms the hindbrain (i.e., the pons, the medulla, and the cerebellum). The cerebrum develops from the prosencephalon which soon shows a subdivision into a median part, the ***diencephalon,*** and two lateral evaginations (the ***telencephalic vesicles***) which together constitute the ***telencephalon.*** In subsequent development, the telencephalic vesicles grow much faster than the diencephalon. As they enlarge they eventually overlap the diencephalon and fuse with its lateral aspect. One telencephalic vesicle, along with the corresponding half of the diencephalon constitutes one cerebral hemisphere. From what has been said above it will be clear that the diencephalic part of the hemisphere lies medially and inferiorly relative to the part derived from the telencephalon.

The developing brain has a series of cavities within it. The cavity of each telencephalic vesicle becomes one ***lateral ventricle.*** The ***third ventricle*** may be regarded as the cavity of the diencephalon. The interventricular foramina connecting the lateral ventricles to the third ventricle represent the sites of the original telencephalic evaginations.

Keeping these facts in mind we may now examine the basic structure of the cerebral hemispheres as seen in a coronal section (Fig. 18.23).

The surface of the cerebral hemisphere is covered by a thin layer of grey matter called the ***cerebral cortex***. The cortex follows the irregular contour of the sulci and gyri of the hemisphere and extends into the depths of the sulci. As a result of this folding of the cerebral surface, the cerebral cortex acquires a much larger surface area than the size of the hemispheres would otherwise allow.

The greater part of the cerebral hemisphere deep to the cortex is occupied by white matter within which are embedded certain important masses of grey matter. Immediately lateral to the third ventricle there are the ***thalamus*** and ***hypothalamus*** (and certain smaller masses) derived from the diencephalon.

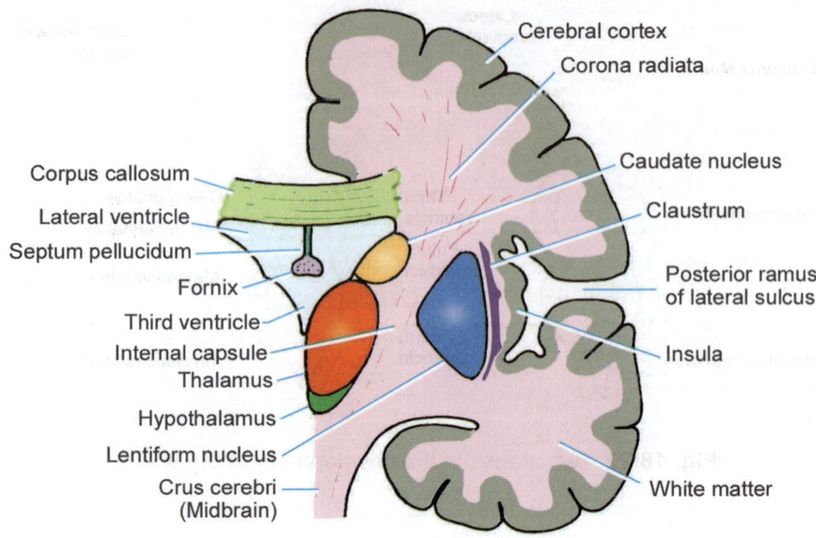

Fig. 18.23 Coronal section through a cerebral hemisphere to show some important masses of grey matter, and sorne other structures within it. Also see Fig. 16.5.

More laterally there is the ***corpus striatum*** which is derived from the telecephalon. It consists of two masses of grey matter, the ***caudate nucleus*** and the ***lentiform nucleus***. A little lateral to the lentiform nucleus we see the cerebral cortex in the region of the insula. Between the lentiform nucleus and the insula there is a thin layer of grey matter called the ***claustrum.*** The caudate nucleus, the lentiform nucleus, the claustrum and some other masses of grey matter (all of telencephalic origin) are referred to as ***basal ganglia.***

The white matter that occupies the interval between the thalamus and caudate nucleus medially, and the lentiform nucleus laterally, is called the ***internal capsule.*** It is a region of considerable importance as major ascending and descending tracts pass through it. The white matter that radiates from the upper end of the internal capsule to the cortex is called the ***corona radiata.***

The two cerebral hemispheres are interconnected by fibres passing from one to the other. These fibres constitute the ***commissures*** of the cerebrum. The largest of these is the ***corpus callosum*** which is seen just above the lateral ventricles in Fig. 18.23.

IMPORTANT FUNCTIONAL AREAS OF THE CEREBRAL CORTEX

Some areas of the cerebral cortex can be assigned specific functions. These areas can be defined in terms of sulci and gyri described in preceding pages. However, some areas are commonly referred to by numbers and it is necessary to know what these numbers mean. Various workers who have studied the microscopic structure of the cerebral cortex have found that there

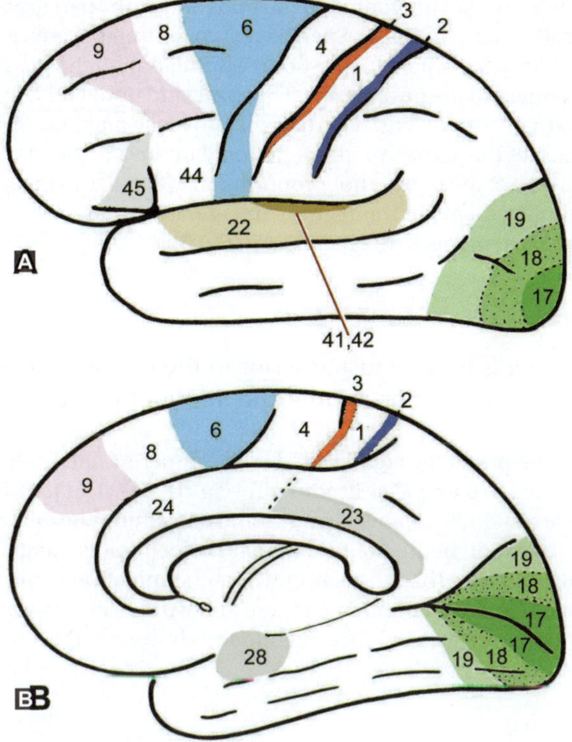

Fig. 18.24 Location of some of the areas of Brodmann on the superolateral aspect (A) and on the medial aspect (B) of the cerebral hemisphere.

is considerable variation from region to region. They have also found that these variations do not necessarily follow the boundaries of sulci and gyri, but often cut across them. Various authors have worked out 'maps' of the cerebral cortex indicating areas of differing structure. The best known scheme is that of Brodmann who represented different areas by numbers. Although the functional significance of the areas is open to question, areas of the cortex are very frequently referred to by Brodmann's numbers. It is, therefore, necessary to be familiar with them. The numbers most commonly referred to are shown in Fig. 18.24 A, B.

The concepts regarding the different functional areas of the cerebral cortex have undergone considerable modification in recent years, but in clinical work reference continues to be made to classical subdivisions which are as follows. For more recent views see the author's HUMAN NEUROANATOMY.

Motor Area

The motor area of classical description is located in the precentral gyrus on the superolateral surface of the hemisphere (Fig. 18.25), and in the anterior part of the paracentral lobule on the medial surface.

It corresponds to area 4 of Brodmann (and possibly to the part of area 6 which lies in the precentral gyrus, Fig. 18.24). Specific regions within the area are responsible for movements in specific parts of the body. Stimulation of the paracentral lobule produces movement in the lower limbs. The trunk and upper limb are represented in the upper part of the precentral gyrus, while the face and head are represented in the lower part of the gyrus. Another feature of interest is that the area of cortex representing a part of the body is not proportional to the size of the part, but rather to intricacy of movements in the region. Thus relatively large areas of cortex are responsible for movements in the hands or in the lips.

Premotor Area

The premotor area is located just anterior to the motor area. It occupies the posterior parts of the superior, middle and inferior frontal gyri (Fig. 18.25).

The part of the premotor area located in the superior and middle frontal gyri corresponds to areas 6 and 8 of Brodmann (Fig. 18.24). The part in the inferior frontal gyrus corresponds to areas 44 and 45 and constitutes the ***motor speech area (of Broca).*** Stimulation of the premotor area results in movements, but these are somewhat more intricate than those produced by stimulation of the motor area.

Closely related to the premotor area there are two specific areas of importance. One is the motor speech area of Broca, mentioned above; and the other is the frontal eye field.

Motor Speech Area

The motor speech area of Broca lies in the inferior frontal gyrus (areas 44 and 45, Fig. 18.24A). Injury to this region results in inability to speak (***aphasia)*** even though the muscles concerned are not paralysed. These effects occur only if damage occurs in the left hemisphere in right handed persons; and in the right hemisphere in left handed persons. In other words motor control of speech is confined to one hemisphere: that which controls the dominant upper limb.

Frontal Eye Field

The frontal eye field lies in the middle frontal gyrus just anterior to the precentral gyrus. It includes parts of areas 6, 8, and 9. Stimulation of this area causes both eyes to move to the opposite side. These are called ***conjugate movements.*** Movements of the head and dilatation of the pupil may also occur. This area is connected to the cortex of the occipital lobe which is concerned with vision.

Sensory Area

The sensory area of classical description is located in the postcentral gyrus (Fig. 18.25). It corresponds to areas 1, 2, and 3 of Brodmann. It also extends on to the medial surface of the hemisphere where it lies in the posterior part of the paracentral lobule. Responses can be recorded from the sensory area when individual parts of the body are stimulated. A definite representation of various parts of the body can be mapped out in the sensory area. It corresponds to that in the motor area in that the body is represented upside down. The area of cortex that receives sensations from a particular part of the body is not proportional

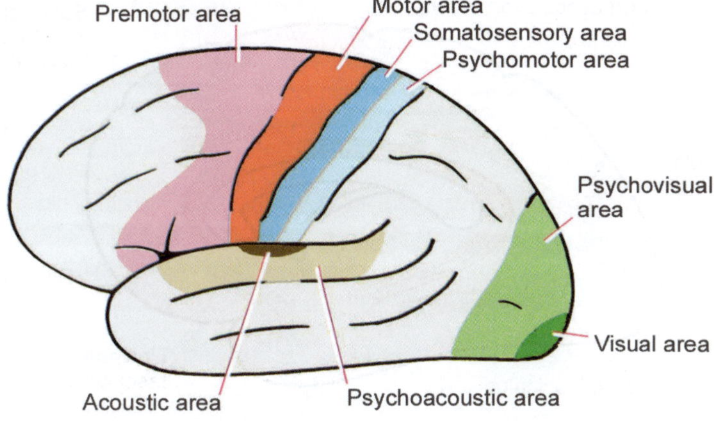

Fig. 18.25 Functional areas on the superolateral aspect of the cerebral hemisphere.

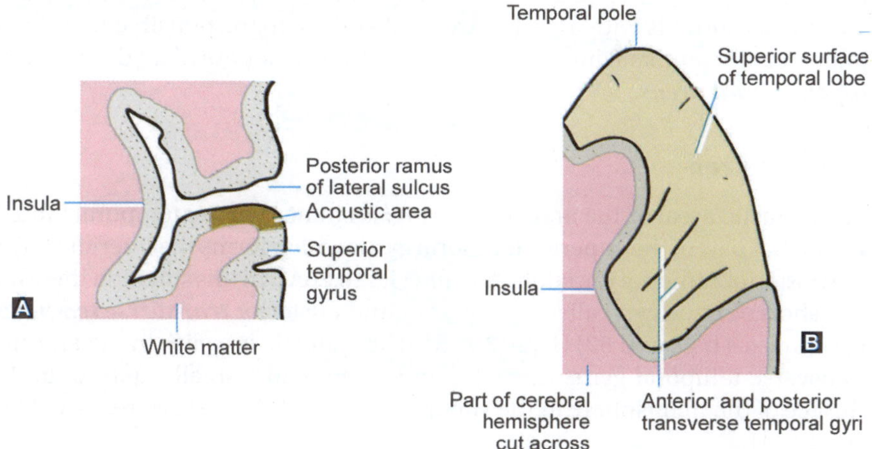

Fig. 18.26 (A) Location of the acoustic area in relation to the superior temporal gyrus. (B) Superior aspect of the superior temporal gyrus to show the transverse temporal gyri.

to the size of that part, but rather to the complexity of sensations received from it. Thus the digits, the lips and the tongue have a disproportionately large representation.

Visual Areas

The areas concerned with vision are located in the occipital lobe, mainly on the medial surface, both above and below the calcarine sulcus (area 17). Area 17 extends into the cuneus, and into the lingual gyrus (Fig. 18.24). Posteriorly,

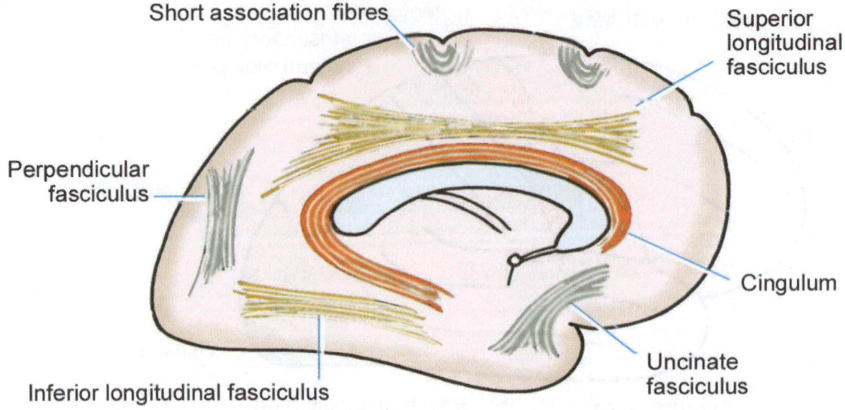

Fig. 18.27 Large bundles of association fibres present within the cerebral hemisphere.

it may extend onto the superolateral surface where it is limited (anteriorly) by the lunate sulcus. Area 17 is continuous, both above and below, with area 18 and beyond this with area 19. Areas 18 and 19 are responsible mainly for interpretation of visual impulses reaching area 17: they are often described as ***psychovisual areas***.

Acoustic Area

The acoustic area, or the area for hearing, is situated in the temporal lobe. It lies in that part of the superior temporal gyrus which forms the inferior wall of the posterior ramus of the lateral sulcus (Fig. 18.26A). In this situation there are two short oblique gyri called the anterior and posterior ***transverse temporal gyri*** (areas 41, 42 and 52) (Fig. 18.26B). The acoustic area lies in the anterior transverse temporal gyrus (area 41) and extends to a small extent onto the surface of the hemisphere in the superior temporal gyrus (See areas 41, 42 in Fig. 18.24).

WHITE MATTER OF CEREBRAL HEMISPHERES

Deep to the cerebral cortex the greater part of each cerebral hemisphere is occupied by nerve fibres that constitute the white matter. These fibres may be:

a. ***Association fibres*** that interconnect different regions of the cerebral cortex.
b. ***Projection fibres*** that connect the cerebral cortex with other masses of grey matter; and ***vice versa.***
c. ***Commissural fibres*** that interconnect identical areas in the two hemispheres.

Association Fibres

These may be short and may connect adjoining gyri. Alternatively, they may be long and may connect distant parts of the cerebral cortex. Many of

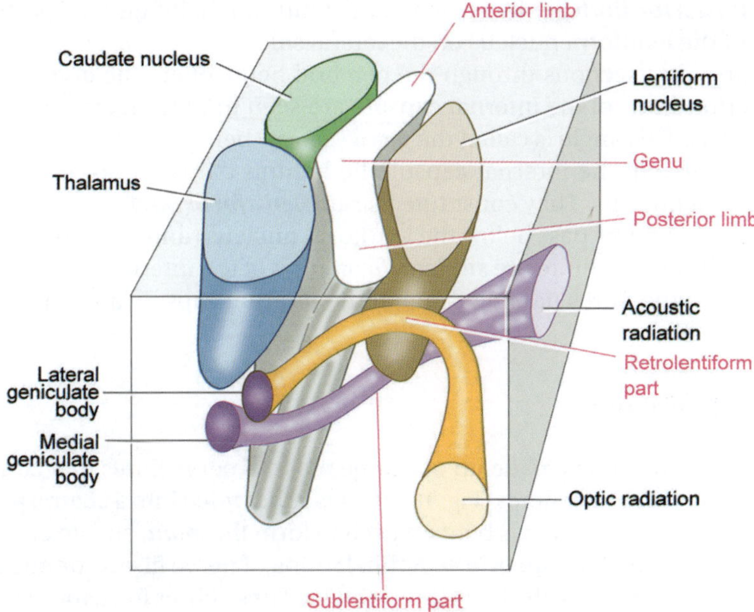

Fig. 18.28 Scheme to show the subdivisions of the internal capsule.

the association fibres form bundles that can be seen by gross dissection. Some of these are shown in Fig. 18.27. Some association fibres pass through commissures to connect ***dissimilar*** areas in the two cerebral hemispheres.

Projection Fibres

These fibres connect the cerebral cortex to centres in the brainstem and spinal cord, in both directions. Fibres to the cortex are often referred to as ***corticopetal fibres***, while those going away from the cortex are referred to as ***corticofugal fibres.*** Fibres connecting the cortex with the thalamus, the hypothalamus and the basal ganglia, are also projection fibres. Many of the major projection fibres pass through the internal capsule, which is considered below.

The Internal Capsule

We have seen that a large number of nerve fibres interconnect the cerebral cortex with centres in the brainstem and spinal cord, and with the thalamus. Most of these fibres pass through the interval between the thalamus and caudate nucleus medially, and the lentiform nucleus laterally. This region is called the ***internal capsule.*** Superiorly, the internal capsule is continuous with the corona radiata; and, below, with the crus cerebri (of the midbrain). The internal capsule may be divided into the following parts (Fig. 18.28).

a. The ***anterior limb*** lies between the caudate nucleus medially, and the anterior part of the lentiform nucleus laterally.

b. The ***posterior limb*** lies between the thalamus medially, and the posterior part of the lentiform nucleus on the lateral side.
c. In transverse sections through the cerebral hemisphere the anterior and posterior limbs of the internal capsule are seen to meet at an angle open outwards. This angle is called the ***genu*** (genu = bend).
d. Some fibres of the internal capsule lie behind the posterior end of the lentiform nucleus. They constitute its ***retrolentiform part.***
e. Some other fibres pass below the lentiform nucleus (and not medial to it). These fibres constitute the ***sublentiform part*** of the internal capsule.

Details of the fibres passing through the internal capsule are considered in Chapter 22.

Corpus Callosum

The corpus callosum is made up of a large mass of nerve fibres that connect the two cerebral hemispheres (Fig. 18.20). It is subdivided into a central part or ***trunk,*** an anterior end that is bent on itself to form the ***genu***, and an enlarged posterior end called the ***splenium.*** A thin lamina of nerve fibres connects the genu to the upper end of the lamina terminalis. These fibres form the ***rostrum*** of the corpus callosum. The corpus callosum is intimately related to the lateral ventricles. Its undersurface gives attachment to the septum pellucidum (Fig. 18.20).

The fibres of the corpus callosum interconnect the corresponding regions of almost all parts of the cerebral cortex of the two hemispheres. The fibres of the genu run forwards into the frontal lobes, the fibres of the two sides forming a fork-like structure called the ***forceps minor***. Many fibres of the splenium run backwards into the occipital lobe to form a similar structure called the ***forceps major.*** (Each half of the forceps major bulges into the posterior horn of the corresponding lateral ventricle, forming the ***bulb of the posterior horn***). The fibres of the trunk of the corpus callosum (and some from the splenium) run laterally and as they do so they intersect the fibres of the corona radiata. Some fibres of the trunk and of the splenium, of the corpus callosum form a flattened band called the ***tapetum***. The tapetum is closely related to the posterior and inferior horns of the lateral ventricle.

As mentioned above all fibres passing through the corpus callosum are not strictly commissural. Some fibres that interconnect dissimilar areas in the two hemispheres are really association fibres.

CHAPTER

19

Tracts of Spinal Cord and Brainstem Cerebellar Connections

TRACTS OF SPINAL CORD AND BRAINSTEM

We have seen that a collection of nerve fibres within the central nervous system, that connects two masses of grey matter, is called a tract. A tract may be defined as a collection of nerve fibres having the same origin, course, and termination. Tracts may be ascending or descending. They are usually named after the masses of grey matter connected by them. Thus a tract beginning in the cerebral cortex and descending to the spinal cord is called the corticospinal tract, while a tract ascending from the spinal cord to the thalamus is called the spinothalamic tract. We have noted that tracts are sometimes referred to as fasciculi or lemnisci. The major tracts passing through the spinal cord and brainstem are shown schematically in Fig. 19.1. The position of the tracts in a transverse section of the spinal cord is shown in Fig. 16.6A, and at ascending levels of the brainstem in Figs. 16.6B to 16.9. It will be a useful exercise for the student to follow the course of each tract described below by noting its position in each of these figures. In studying these figures it must be remembered that in actual fact the boundaries of areas occupied by the fibres of each tract are not clear cut.

There is considerable overlap of the territories of various tracts. The lines of demarcation are, therefore, approximate and artificial. It may also be remembered that the position of a particular tract varies at different levels of the spinal cord; and that some of the tracts shown in Fig. 16.6A are present only in the upper part of the cord.

DESCENDING TRACTS ENDING IN THE SPINAL CORD

Corticospinal Tract

The corticospinal tract is made up, predominantly, of axons of cells lying in the motor area of the cerebral cortex (area 4). Some fibres also arise from the

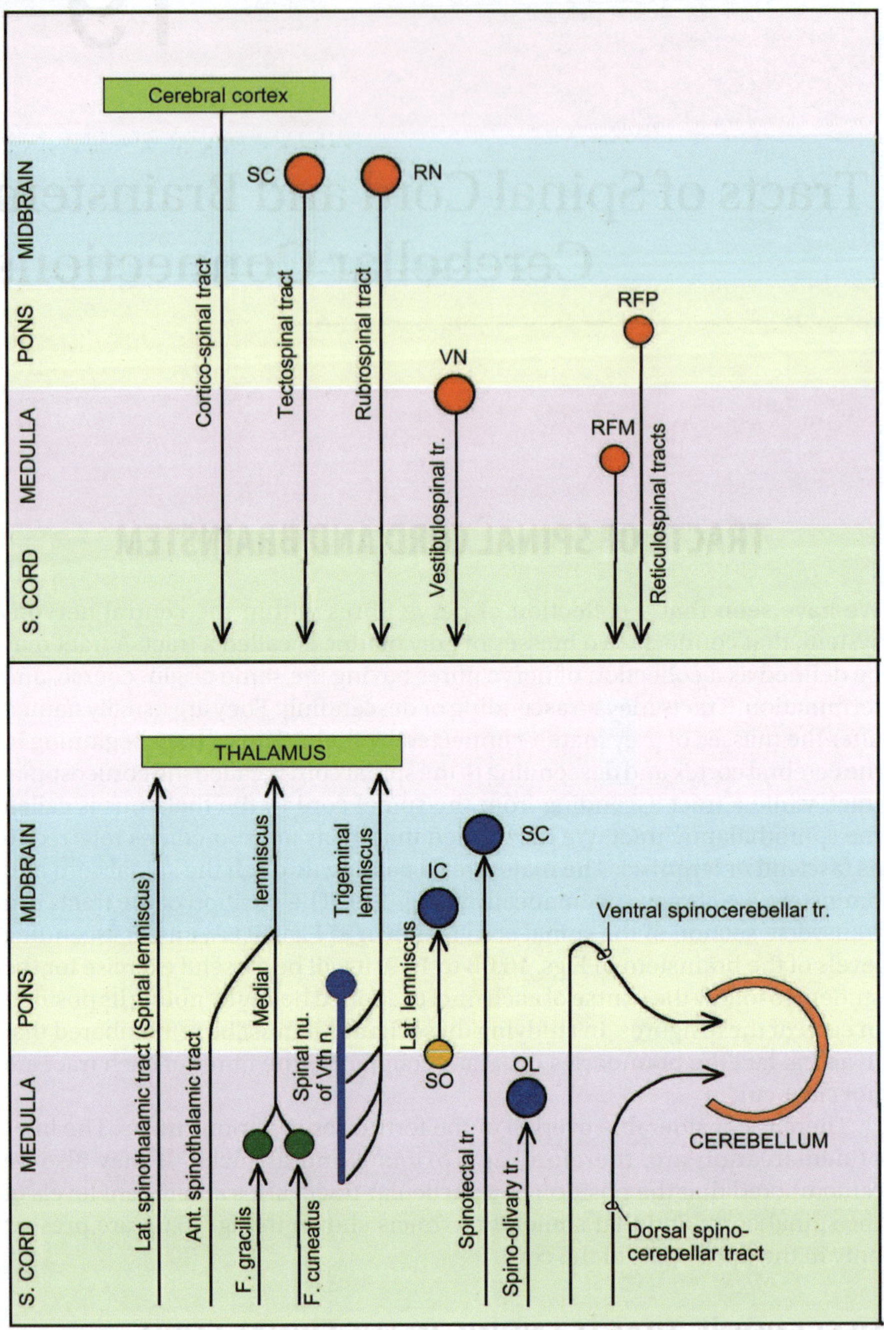

Fig. 19.1 Scheme to show the various tracts passing through the brainstem. SC = superior colliculus; RN = red nucleus; VN = vestibular nuclei; OL = inferior olivary nucleus. RFP = reticular formation of pons. RFM = reticular formation of medulla; IC = inferior collicus; SO = superior olivary nucleus.

premotor area (area 6) and some from the somatosensory area (areas 3, 2, 1) (Figs. 16.10, 18.24). From this origin fibres pass through the corona radiata to enter the internal capsule where they lie in the posterior limb (Figs. 16.10 and 22.2A). After passing through the internal capsule the fibres enter the crus cerebri (of the midbrain): they occupy the middle two-thirds of the crus. The fibres then descend through the ventral part of the pons to enter the pyramids in the upper part of the medulla. Near the lower end of the medulla about 80 percent of the fibres cross to the opposite side. (The crossing fibres of the two sides constitute the decussation of the pyramids.)

The fibres that have crossed in the medulla enter the lateral funiculus of the spinal cord and descend as the ***lateral corticospinal tract*** (Fig. 16.6). The fibres of this tract terminate in grey matter at various levels of the spinal cord. Most of them end by synapsing with internuncial neurons in the bases of the dorsal and ventral grey columns (laminae IV to VII). The internuncial neurons carry the impulses brought by fibres of the tract to ventral column neurons. A few fibres of the tract may terminate directly on ventral column neurons.

The corticospinal fibres that do not cross in the pyramidal decussation enter the anterior funiculus of the spinal cord to form the ***anterior corticospinal tract.*** On reaching the appropriate level of the spinal cord the fibres of this tract cross the middle line to reach grey matter on the opposite side of the cord. Their manner of termination is similar to that of fibres of the lateral corticospinal tract. In this way the corticospinal fibres of both the lateral and anterior tracts ultimately connect the cerebral cortex of one side with ventral column neurons in the opposite half of the spinal cord.

The cerebral cortex controls voluntary movement through this tract. Interruption of the tract anywhere in its course leads to paralysis of the muscles concerned. As the fibres are closely packed in their course through the internal capsule and brainstem small lesions here can cause widespread paralysis.

The neurons that give origin to the fibres of the corticospinal tracts are often referred to as ***upper motor neurons*** in distinction to the ventral column neurons and their processes which constitute the ***lower motor neurons.*** Interruption of either of these neurons leads to paralysis, but the nature of the paralysis is distinctive in each case.

Rubrospinal Tract

This tract is made up of axons of neurons lying in the red nucleus (which lies in the upper part of the midbrain). The fibres of the tract cross to the opposite side in the lower part of the tegmentum of the midbrain. The crossing fibres constitute the ***ventral tegmental decussation*** (Fig. 16.9A). The tract descends through the pons and medulla to enter the lateral funiculus of the spinal cord (Fig. 16.6). The fibres of the tract end by synapsing with ventral column neurons through internuncial neurons located in laminae V to VII of the spinal grey matter.

Tectospinal Tract

The fibres of this tract arise from neurons in the superior colliculus (midbrain). The fibres cross to the opposite side in the upper part of the tegmentum of the midbrain. The crossing fibres form the ***dorsal tegmental decussation*** (Fig. 16.9A). The tract descends through the pons and medulla into the anterior funiculus of the spinal cord. The fibres terminate by synapsing with ventral column neurons in cervical segments of the cord, through internuncial neurons located in laminae VI to VIII of the spinal grey matter.

Vestibulospinal Tract

The neurons of origin of the vestibulospinal tract lie in the lateral vestibular nucleus. This tract is uncrossed and lies in the anterior funiculus of the spinal cord (Fig. 16.6). Its fibres end in relation to neurons in the ventral grey column (laminae VII and VIII). This tract is an important efferent path for equilibrium.

Olivospinal Tract

This tract is generally described as arising from the inferior olivary nucleus (medulla) and terminating in relation to ventral column neurons of the spinal cord. Its exact connections are, however, unknown.

Reticulospinal Tracts

Fibres arising in the reticular formation of the brainstem descend to end in relation to internuncial neurons in laminae VII and VIII of the spinal cord. Reticulospinal fibres are widely scattered in the anterior and lateral funiculi. Usually, two tracts medial and lateral are recognised. The ***medial reticulospinal tract*** begins in the reticular formation of the pons. Most of its fibres are uncrossed. The ***lateral reticulospinal tract*** begins in the reticular formation of the medulla. It contains both crossed and uncrossed fibres.

The fibres of the reticulospinal tracts influence the alpha and gamma motor neurons.

Significance of Descending Tracts

The various descending tracts described above, that end in relation to ventral column neurons, influence their activity, and thereby have an effect on contraction and tone of skeletal muscle. Although a small number of the fibres of these tracts may synapse directly with ventral column neurons, most of them influence these cells through intervening internuncial neurons. This influence is exerted both on alpha neurons and gamma neurons. We have already seen that gamma neurons indirectly influence the activity of alpha neurons via muscle spindles. Hence all these influences ultimately reach the alpha neurons. Such influences may be either facilitatory or inhibitory.

The corticospinal and rubrospinal tracts are described as being facilitatory to flexors and inhibitory to extensors, while the vestibulospinal tract is said to have the opposite effect. The medial reticulospinal tract is generally regarded as facilitatory and the lateral tract as inhibitory.

The corticospinal tracts are often referred to as ***pyramidal tracts***. Traditionally all other descending tracts have been collectively referred to as ***extrapyramidal tracts***. It has often been presumed that the pyramidal and extrapyramidal tracts act in opposition to each other. It has also been said that the pyramidal fibres end in relation to alpha neurons, and

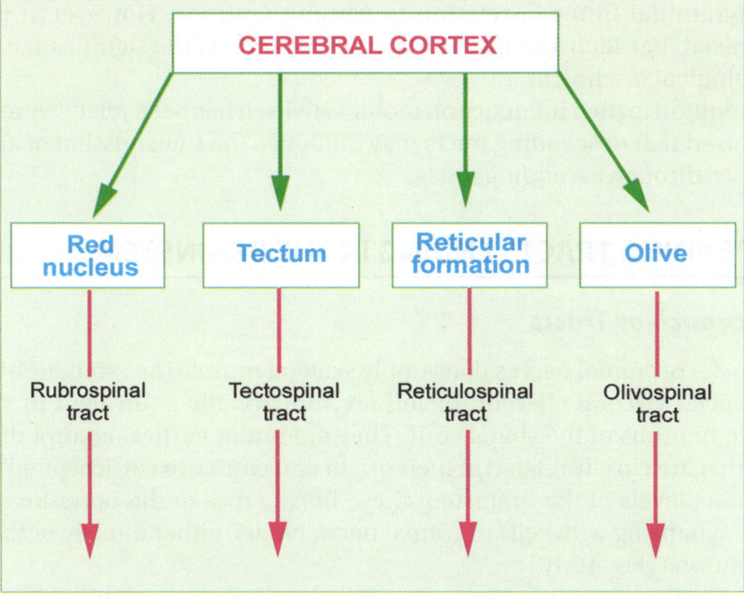

Fig. 19.2 Indirect pathways through which the cerebral cortex may influence the spinal cord. These are often described as extra-pyramidal tracts.

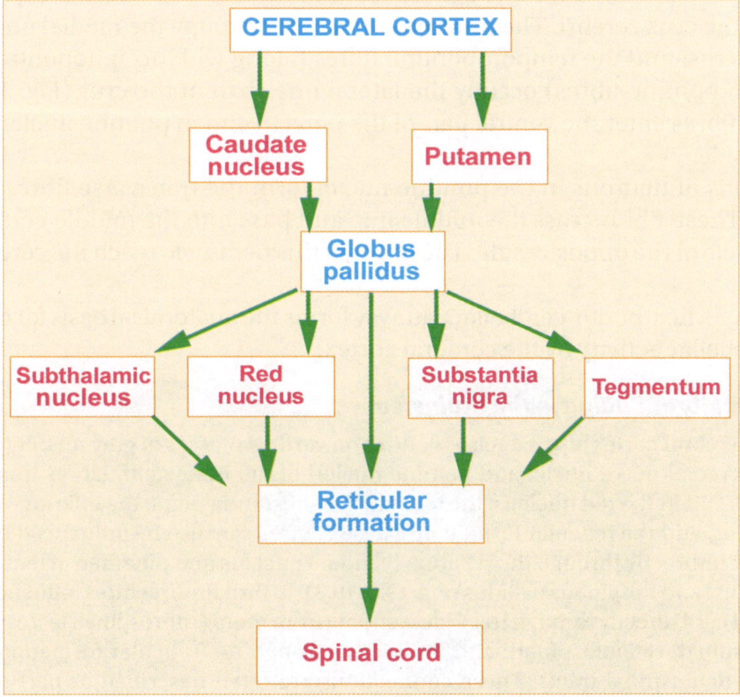

Fig. 19.3 Indirect pathways through which the corpus striatum may influence the spinal cord.

extrapyramidal fibres in relation to gamma neurons. However, it is now recognised that such a distinction is artificial and of little significance either physiological or clinical.

In addition to their influence on motor activity, it has been relatively recently recognised that descending tracts may influence the transmission of afferent impulses through ascending tracts.

DESCENDING TRACTS ENDING IN THE BRAINSTEM

Corticonuclear Tracts

The nuclei of cranial nerves that supply skeletal muscle (i.e., somatic efferent and special visceral efferent nuclei) are functionally equivalent to ventral column neurons of the spinal cord. They are under cortical control through fibres that are closely related in their origin and course to corticospinal fibres. At various levels of the brainstem these fibres cross to the opposite side to end by synapsing with cells in cranial nerve nuclei, either directly or through interneurons (Fig. 16.10) .

Cortico-ponto-cerebellar Pathway

Fibres arising in the cerebral cortex of the frontal, temporal, parietal and occipital lobes descend through the corona radiata and internal capsule to reach the crus cerebri. The frontopontine fibres occupy the medial one sixth of the crus; and the temporopontine fibres (along with occipitopontine and parieto-pontine fibres) occupy the lateral one sixth of the crus (Fig. 16.9B). These fibres enter the ventral part of the pons to end in pontine nuclei of the same side.

Axons of neurons in the pontine nuclei form the transverse fibres of the pons. These fibres cross the middle line and pass into the middle cerebellar peduncle of the opposite side. The fibres of this peduncle reach the cerebellar cortex.

The cortico-ponto-cerebellar pathway forms the anatomical basis for control of cerebellar activity by the cerebral cortex.

Other Fibres Ending in the Brainstem

The cerebral cortex also exercises control on various masses of grey matter (other than cranial nerve nuclei and pontine nuclei) of the brainstem. Fibres from the cortex end in the red nucleus, the tectum, the substantia nigra, the inferior olivary nucleus, and the reticular formation. These centres can also be influenced by the cortex indirectly through the striatum (caudate nucleus and putamen of lentiform nucleus) and the globus pallidus (Fig. 19.2, 19.3). In turn these centres influence the spinal cord directly through tracts descending from them (rubrospinal, tectospinal, olivospinal, reticulospinal); and indirectly through the reticular formation and the reticulospinal tracts. These connections are often described as part of the extrapyramidal pathways referred to above.

ASCENDING TRACTS

Introductory Remarks

The ascending tracts of the spinal cord and brainstem represent one stage of multineuron pathways by which afferent impulses arising in various parts of the body are conveyed to different parts of the brain. The ***first order neurons*** of these pathways are usually located in spinal (dorsal nerve root) ganglia (Fig. 9.17). We have seen that the neurons in these ganglia are unipolar (pseudounipolar). Each neuron gives off a peripheral process and a central process. The peripheral processes of the neurons form the afferent fibres of peripheral nerves. They end in relation to sensory end organs (receptors) situated in various tissues. The central processes of these neurons enter the spinal cord through the dorsal nerve roots. Having entered the cord the central processes, as a rule, terminate by synapsing with cells in spinal grey matter. Some of them may run upwards in the white matter of the cord to form ascending tracts (Fig. 16.11). The majority of ascending tracts are, however, formed by axons of cells in spinal grey matter. These are ***second order*** sensory neurons (Fig. 19.5). In the case of pathways that convey sensory information to the cerebral cortex the second order neurons end by synapsing with neurons in the thalamus. ***Third order*** sensory neurons located in the thalamus carry the sensations to the cerebral cortex.

The following additional points may now be noted.

1. The axons of the second orders neurons may enter white matter on the same side, forming an uncrossed tract; or on the opposite side, forming a crossed tract.
2. In the case of the head (and other parts supplied by cranial nerves) the first order neurons are located in sensory ganglia situated on the cranial nerves. (In some of these ganglia ***viz.,*** cochlear and vestibular, the neurons are bipolar, not unipolar as in most ganglia). The central processes of these neurons end in relation to afferent nuclei of cranial nerves. The neurons in these nuclei constitute second order neurons.
3. Only those afferent impulses which reach the cerebral cortex are consciously perceived. One exception to this may be perception of some degree of pain in the thalamus. Afferent impulses ending in the cerebellum or in the brainstem influence the activities of these centres.

ASCENDING PATHWAYS CONNECTING THE SPINAL CORD TO THE CEREBRAL CORTEX

The Posterior Column — Medial Lemniscus Pathway

Fasciculus Gracilis and Fasciculus Cuneatus:

These tracts occupy the posterior funiculus of the spinal cord and are, therefore, often referred to as the ***posterior column tracts*** (Fig. 16.6). They are unique in that they are formed predominantly by central processes of neurons located in dorsal nerve root ganglia i.e., by first order sensory neurons (Fig. 16.11). The fibres derived from the lowest ganglia are situated most medially; while those from the highest ganglia are most lateral. The fasciculus gracilis, which lies medially is, therefore, composed of fibres from the sacral, lumbar and lower thoracic ganglia; while the fasciculus cuneatus which lies laterally consists of fibres from upper thoracic and cervical ganglia. The fibres of these fasciculi extend upwards as far as the lower part of the medulla. Here the fibres of the gracile and cuneate fasciculi terminate by synapsing with neurons in the nucleus gracilis and nucleus cuneatus respectively.

Medial Lemniscus

The neurons of the gracile and cuneate nuclei are second order sensory neurons. Their axons run forwards and medially (as ***internal arcuate fibres***) to cross the middle line. The crossing fibres of the two sides constitute the ***sensory decussation.*** Having crossed the middle line, the fibres turn upwards to form a prominent bundle called the medial lemniscus (Fig. 16.11). The medial lemniscus runs upwards through the medulla, pons and midbrain to end in the thalamus (ventral posterolateral nucleus). Note the position of the medial lemniscus at different levels of the brainstem in Fig. 16.11.

The pathway described above carries:

1. Some components of the sense of touch. These include deep touch and pressure, the ability to localise exactly the part touched (tactile localisation), the ability to recognise as separate two points on the skin that are touched simultaneously (tactile discrimination), and the ability to recognise the shape of an object held in the hand (stereognosis).
2. Proprioceptive impulses that convey the sense of position and of movement of different parts of the body.
3. The sense of vibration.

Spinothalamic Pathway

a. The first order neurons of this pathway are located in spinal ganglia. The central processes of these neurons enter the spinal cord and terminate in relation to spinal grey matter. They may ascend in the dorsolateral tract (situated near the tip of the dorsal grey column, Fig. 16.6) for one or more segments before ending in grey matter.
b. The second order neurons of this pathway are located in the spinal grey matter,
c. Third order sensory neurons located in the thalamus give off axons that pass through the internal capsule and the corona radiata to reach the somatosensory areas of the cerebral cortex.

> Their exact location is uncertain. Most of them are probably located in laminae IV, V and VI.

The axons of these neurons constitute the anterior and lateral spinothalamic tracts. They cross to the opposite side of the spinal cord in the white

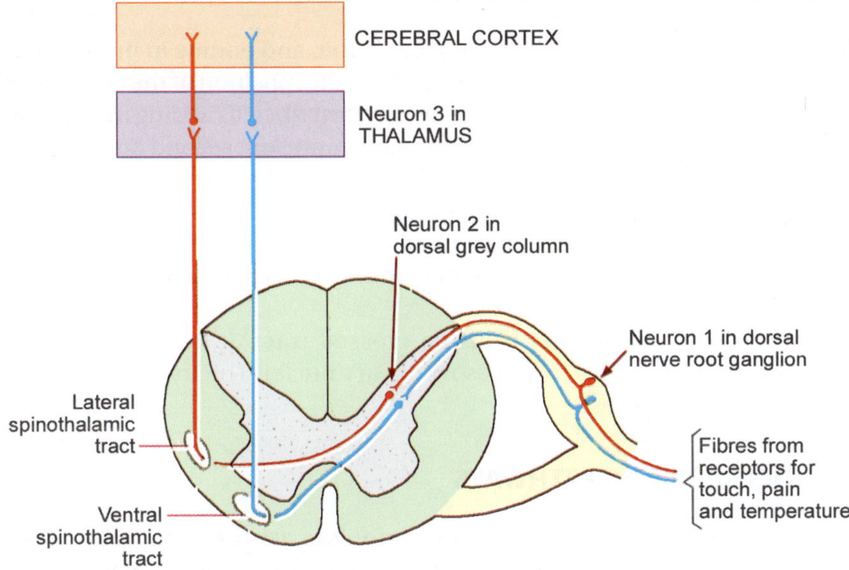

Fig. 19.4 Scheme to illustrate the main features of the spinothalamic tracts.

commissure. This crossing is oblique. The fibres for the lateral spinothalamic tract cross within the same segment of the cord, while those of the anterior spinothalamic tract may ascend for one or more segments before they cross to the opposite side.

The fibres for the anterior spinothalamic tract enter the anterior funiculus (Figs. 16.6, 19.4) and ascend to the medulla. The course of this tract through the brainstem is controversial. According to some authorities this tract merges with the medial lemniscus in the medulla and travels in the lemniscus to the thalamus. According to other authorities the tract runs upwards in the medulla and pons in a bundle common to it and the lateral spinothalamic tract and joins the medial lemniscus in the upper part of the pons (Fig. 19.1). The fibres ultimately end in the thalamus (ventral posterolateral nucleus).

The fibres for the lateral spinothalamic tract enter the lateral funiculus. They ascend through the medulla, pons and midbrain (where this tract is often referred to as the ***spinal lemniscus***) to end in the thalamus (ventral posterolateral nucleus).

Traditionally it has been said that the anterior spinothalamic tract carries sensations of crude touch and pressure, while the lateral tract has been said to carry sensations of pain and temperature. It is now realised that although different fibres within the spinothalamic tracts carry different types of sensations, the anterior and lateral spinothalamic tracts constitute a single functional unit.

ASCENDING PATHWAYS ENDING IN THE BRAINSTEM

A number of tracts arising in spinal grey matter, and ending in masses of grey matter in the brainstem, are described. The exact position of the cells of origin of the tracts is unknown. They are generally described as arising from neurons in the dorsal grey columns, and presumably represent second order neurons.

The ***spinotectal tract*** connects the spinal grey matter to the superior colliculus. It is a crossed tract. It carries impulses that regulate reflex movements of the head and eyes in response to stimulation of some parts of the body. According to some authorities the tract may also carry sensations of pain and temperature.

The ***spino-olivary tract*** is also a crossed tract. It is believed to carry proprioceptive impulses to accessory olivary nuclei. The tract may also carry exteroceptive impulses.

SPINOCEREBELLAR PATHWAYS

These pathways carry proprioceptive impulses arising in muscle spindles, Golgi tendon organs, and other receptors to the cerebellum. They constitute the afferent component of reflex arcs involving the cerebellum for control of posture. Recent investigations have shown that some exteroceptive sensations (e.g., touch) may reach the cerebellum through these pathways.

a. The first order neurons of these pathways are located in dorsal nerve root ganglia. Their peripheral processes end in relation to muscle spindles, Golgi tendon organs and other proprioceptive receptors. The central processes of the neurons concerned ascend in the posterior funiculi for varying distances before ending in spinal grey matter. Some of them ascend all the way to the medulla and end in the accessory cuneate nucleus.
b. The second order neurons of the pathway are arranged in a number of groups.
   i. Neurons located in the dorsal nucleus (situated on the medial side of the base of the dorsal grey column in segments C8 to L3 of the spinal cord: Fig. 17.4) give origin to fibres of the ***dorsal (posterior) spinocerebellar tract.*** This is an uncrossed tract lying in the lateral funiculus (Fig. 16.6). It ascends to the medulla where its fibres become incorporated in the inferior cerebellar peduncle and pass through it to reach the cerebellum (Fig. 19.5).
   ii. The location of neurons giving origin to the ***ventral (anterior) spinocerebellar tract*** is uncertain. They are probably located in the junctional area between the ventral and dorsal grey columns (laminae V, VI, VII) in the lumbar and sacral segments of the cord. Some of the neurons concerned may lie in the ventral grey column. The fibres of this tract are predominantly crossed. They ascend in the lateral funiculus, anterior to the fibres of the dorsal spinocerebellar tract (Fig. 16.6), and pass through the medulla and pons. At the upper end of the pons the fibres turn downwards to enter the superior cerebellar peduncle through which they reach the cerebellum (Fig. 19.5).

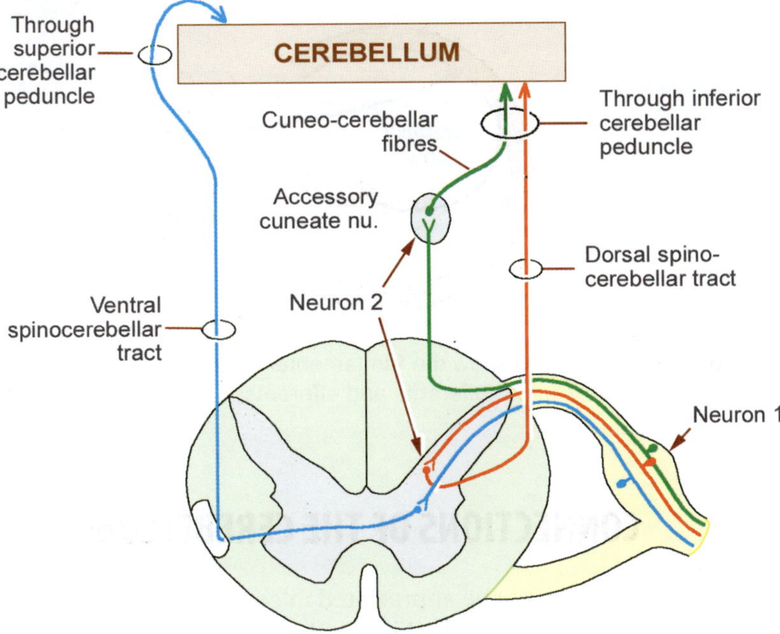

Fig. 19.5 Scheme to illustrate the main features of spinocerebellar pathways.

From a functional point of view both the ventral and dorsal spinocerebellar tracts are concerned mainly with the lower limbs. The dorsal tract is believed to carry impulses concerned with fine coordination of muscles controlling posture, and with movements of individual muscles. On the other hand the ventral tract is concerned with movements of the limb as a whole.

iii. We have seen that the central processes of some first order neurons (related to cervical segments) reach the accessory cuneate nucleus in the medulla. Second order neurons lying in this nucleus give origin to ***posterior external arcuate fibres*** which enter the inferior cerebellar peduncle to reach the cerebellum. This ***cuneocerebellar tract*** carries impulses from the upper limb. It may be regarded as the forelimb equivalent of the dorsal spinocerebellar tract.

iv. ***Rostral spinocerebellar pathway:*** This tract is believed to arise from spinal grey matter in cervical regions of the spinal cord. The locations of the neurons of origin is, however, unknown. Most fibres of the pathway are uncrossed. They reach the cerebellum through the inferior and superior cerebellar peduncles. This pathway is regarded, functionally, as the forelimb equivalent of the ventral spinocerebellar tract.

From the above account of spinocerebellar pathways it will be seen that these are two neuron pathways in contrast to three neuron pathways to the cerebral cortex.

v. Impulses from the spinal cord may reach the cerebellum indirectly by travelling through the spino-olivary tract, and through olivocerebellar fibres. Similarly, impulses may reach the cerebellum after travelling through spinoreticular and reticulocerebellar fibres.

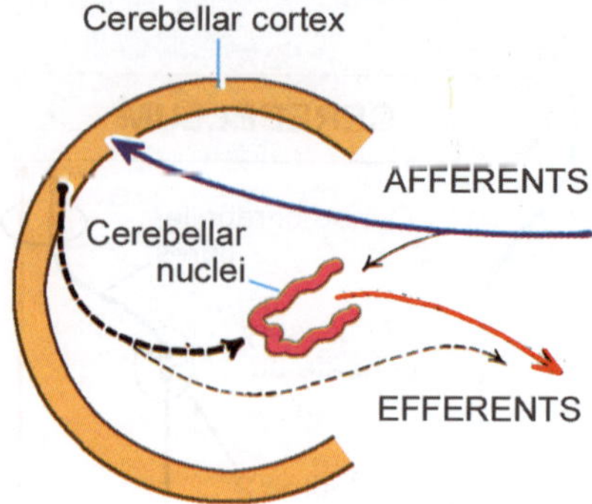

Fig. 19.6 Scheme to show the fundamental arrangement of cerebellar afferents and efferents.

CONNECTIONS OF THE CEREBELLUM

The fundamental points to be appreciated in considering the connections of the cerebellum are that, as a rule (Fig. 19.6):

a. afferent fibres terminate in the cortex;
b. efferent fibres arising in the cortex end in cerebellar nuclei; and
c. fibres arising in the nuclei project to centres outside the cerebellum.

There are, however, important exceptions to these rules. Some fibres (notably vestibular) project directly to the cerebellar nuclei. Some parts of the cortex give off efferents that bypass the nuclei to reach centres outside the cerebellum.

Afferent Fibres Entering the Cerebellum

The cerebellum receives direct afferents from the spinal cord and from various centres in the brainstem. The main afferents are (Fig. 19.7):

1. ***Spinocerebellar*** (through the various tracts described above). These terminate predominantly in the paleocerebellum.
2. ***Pontocerebellar***. These are part of the cortico-ponto-cerebellar pathway. They end predominantly in the neocerebellum.
3. ***Olivocerebellar***. These end mainly in the neocerebellum and partly in the paleo-cerebellum.
4. ***Vestibulocerebellar***, from the vestibular nuclei, and also direct fibres of the vestibular nerve.
5. ***Reticulocerebellar*** fibres from the reticular formation of the pons and of the medulla.

The cerebellum also receives fibres from the tectum, the arcuate nuclei, the accessory cuneate nucleus, and from the sensory nuclei of the trigeminal nerve.

Efferent Fibres Leaving the Cerebellum

The main efferents of the cerebellum are (Fig. 19.7):

1. ***Cerebello-rubral***, to the red nucleus of the opposite side.
2. ***Cerebello-thalamic***, to the thalamus of the opposite side.
3. ***Cerebello-vestibular***, to the vestibular nuclei.
4. ***Cerebello-reticular***, to the reticular formation.

Some fibres from the cerebellum are also believed to reach the inferior olivary nucleus, the nucleus of the oculomotor nerve, and the tectum.

CEREBELLAR PEDUNCLES

The various fibres entering or leaving the cerebellum pass through the superior, middle and inferior cerebellar peduncles. These connect the cerebellum to the midbrain, the pons and the medulla respectively. The main fibres composing each peduncle are enumerated below. (For additional details see the author's HUMAN NEUROANATOMY).

Superior Cerebellar Peduncle

A. Fibres entering the cerebellum

1. Ventral spinocerebellar tract.
2. Rostral (or superior) spino-cerebellar tract.

B. Fibres leaving the cerebellum

1. Cerebello-rubral fibres.
2. Cerebello-thalamic fibres.
3. Cerebello-reticular fibres (from dentate nucleus, some from the fastigial nucleus).

Middle Cerebellar Peduncle

This is made up of ponto-cerebellar fibres.

Inferior Cerebellar Peduncle

A. Fibres entering the cerebellum

1. Posterior spino-cerebellar tract.
2. Cuneo-cerebellar tract (posterior external arcuate fibres.
3. Olivo-cerebellar fibres from inferior olivary nucleus.
4. Reticulo-cerebellar fibres.
5. Vestibulo-cerebellar fibres.
6. Parolivo-cerebellar fibres from accessory olivary nuclei.
7. Anterior external arcuate fibres from arcuate nuclei.

B. Fibres leaving the cerebellum

1. Cerebello-olivary fibres
2. Cerebello-vestibular fibres.

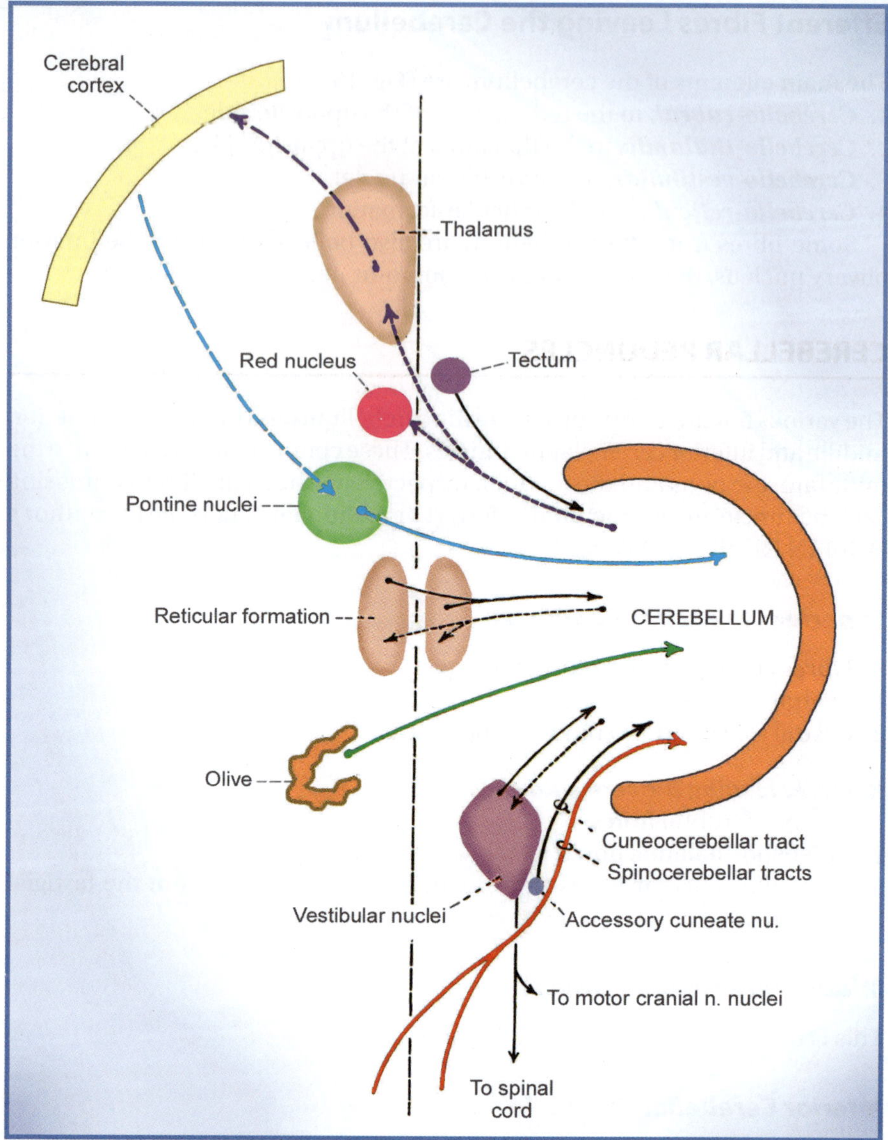

Fig. 19.7 Scheme to show the connections of the cerebellum as a whole.

3. Cerebello-reticular fibres (from fastigial nucleus).
4. Some cerebello-spinal and cerebello-nuclear fibres are also present.

FURTHER DETAILS OF CEREBELLAR CONNECTIONS

Vestibulo-Cerebellar Connections

The vestibular nerves carry impulses necessary for maintaining equilibrium (from semicircular ducts, utricle and saccule) to the cerebellum. The fibres of this nerve are constituted by central processes of bipolar neurons in the vestibular ganglion. They terminate in vestibular nuclei. New fibres arising in the nuclei carry these impulses to the cortex of the flocculonodular lobe (and some adjoining areas). Fibres arising in the flocculonodular lobe project to the fastigial nuclei. Finally, fibres arising in the fastigial nuclei project to the vestibular nuclei. The vestibular nuclei project to the spinal cord through the vestibulospinal tract. Through these connections the cerebellum is able to influence the musculature of the limbs in response to vestibular stimuli.

Olivo-Cerebellar Connections

The inferior olivary nucleus (and the accessory olivary nuclei) send numerous fibres to the opposite half of the cerebellum. Various parts of this nucleus exhibit a point to point relationship with the cerebellar hemisphere. The accessory olivary nuclei (lying most medially) project to the vermis; while medial, intermediate and lateral parts of the inferior olivary nucleus project to corresponding regions of the hemispheres.

Reticulo-Cerebellar Connections

The cerebellum receives fibres from and sends fibres to the reticular formation. Impulses passing from the cerebellum to the reticular formation are relayed to the spinal cord and to cranial nerve nuclei through reticulospinal and reticulonuclear pathways; and to the thalamus through reticulothalamic fibres.

Cerebello Rubral Connections

Fibres arising in the emboliform and globose nuclei (and some from the dentate nucleus) pass through the superior cerebellar peduncle to reach the red nucleus. These enable the cerebellum to influence the spinal cord through the rubrospinal tract. In this cerebello-rubro-spinal pathway, there is a double decussation. The cerebellorubral fibres cross in the decussation of the superior cerebellar peduncle while the rubrospinal fibres cross in the ventral tegmental decussation. As a result the cerebellum influences the same side of the spinal cord.

Cerebello-Thalamic Connections

Fibres arising in the dentate nucleus (and a few in the emboliform and globose nuclei) pass through the superior cerebellar peduncle, to reach the thalamus of the opposite side, either directly, or after relay in the red nucleus.

Connections of Cerebellar Nuclei

We have seen that the cerebellar nuclei receive afferents from the cerebellar cortex. As a broad generalisation it can be said that the fastigial nuclei receive fibres from the flocculonodular lobe and other parts of the vermis (archicerebellum); the emboliform and globose nuclei from the paravermal cortex (mainly paleocerebellum); and the dentate nuclei from the lateral part of the cerebellar hemispheres.

Efferent fibres from the dentate nucleus (accompanied by some fibres from the emboliform and globose nuclei) constitute the greater part of the superior cerebellar peduncle. On reaching the lower part of the midbrain most of these fibres cross the middle line (in the decussation of the superior cerebellar peduncle) and ascend to the red nucleus and to the thalamus. For details see Fig. 19.10.

Fibres arising in fastigial nuclei pass through the inferior cerebellar peduncle and reach the vestibular nuclei and the reticular formation.

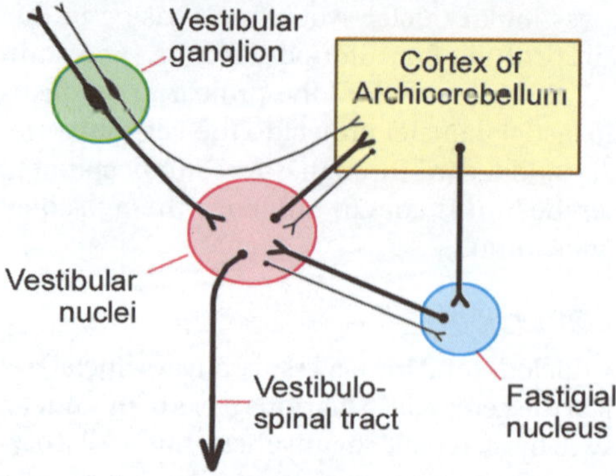

Fig. 19.8 Scheme to show the vestibulo-cerebellar connections.

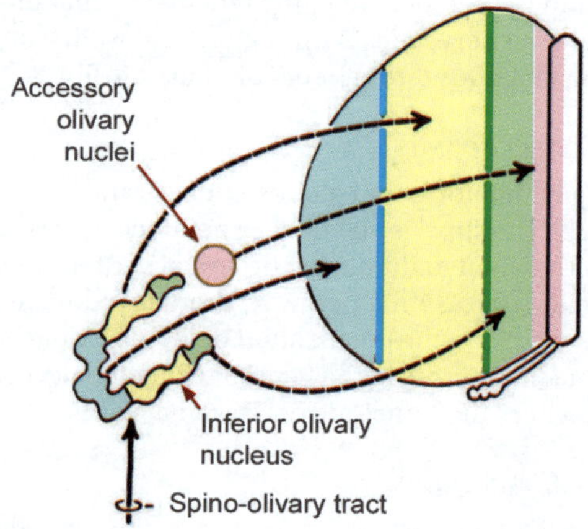

Fig. 19.9 Scheme to show the olivo-cerebellar connections.

Summary of Pathways Interconnecting the Cerebellum and Spinal Cord

Spinocerebellar pathways convey to the cerebellum proprioceptive information necessary for controlling muscle tone and for maintaining body posture. These pathways also carry exteroceptive impulses.

Direct Pathways from Spinal Cord to Cerebellum

These are the ventral spinocerebellar tract, and the dorsal spinocerebellar tract which convey information from the hindlimb. Information from the forelimb is probably conveyed by the rostral spinocerebellar tract and the cuneocerebellar

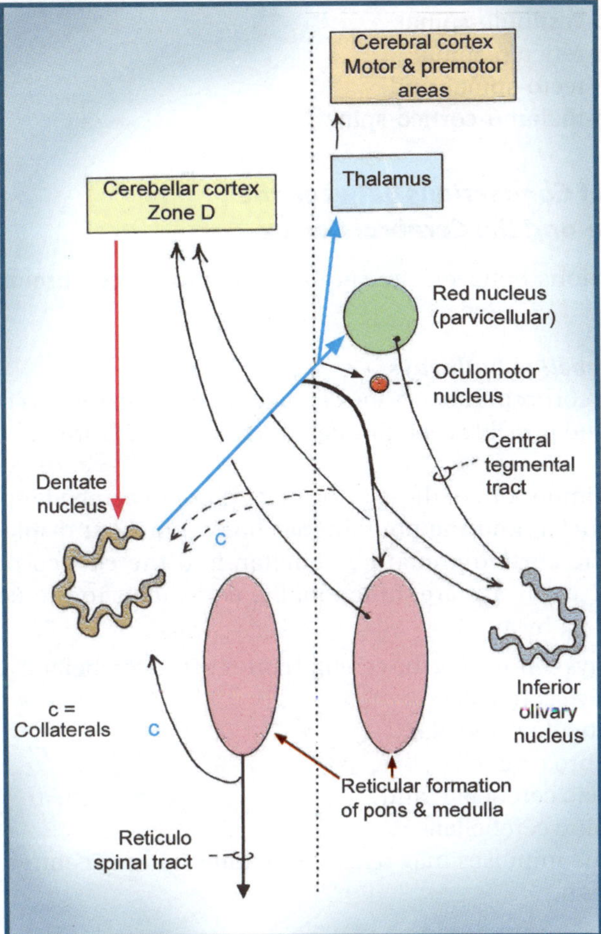

Fig. 19.10 Scheme to show the connections of the dentate nucleus.

tract. The cuneocerebellar tract begins in the medulla, but is included here as it is functionally equivalent to spinocerebellar tracts.

Indirect Pathways from Spinal Cord to Cerebellum

These are:
a. Spino-olivo-cerebellar;
b. Spino-reticulo-cerebellar;
c. Spino-vestibulo-cerebellar; and
d. Spino-tecto-cerebellar pathways.

Cerebello-Spinal Pathways

The cerebellum can influence the spinal cord through the following pathways:
a. Cerebello-rubro-spinal;

b. Cerebello-vestibulo-spinal;
c. Cerebello-reticulo-spinal;
d. Cerebello-tecto-spinal; and
e. Cerebello-thalamo-cortico-spinal.

Summary of Connections between the Cerebellum and the Cerebral Cortex

The connections between the cerebellum and the cerebral cortex are all indirect.

Cortico-Cerebellar Pathways

The cerebral cortex influences the cerebellum through various centres in the brainstem (and possibly even through the spinal cord) through the following pathways.

a. The most important of these is the cortico ponto cerebellar pathway. The arcuate nuclei and the pontobulbar body represent displaced pontine nuclei. The cortico arcuato cerebellar, and the cortico ponto bulbar cerebellar pathways are, functionally, equivalent to the cortico ponto cerebellar pathway.

Other pathways connecting the cerebral cortex to the cerebellum are as follows.

b. Cortico olivo cerebellar;
c. Cortico reticulo cerebellar;
d. Cortico rubro cerebellar;
e. Cortico tecto cerebellar; and
f. Cortico spino cerebellar.

Some of the impulses may reach these intermediary centres through the corpus striatum.

Cerebello-Cortical Pathways

We have seen that the cerebellum projects upon the cerebellar nuclei from where fresh fibres relay to the thalamus. Thalamocortical fibres carry these impulses to the cerebral cortex.

FUNCTIONS OF THE CEREBELLUM

The cerebellum plays an essential role in the control of movement. It is responsible for ensuring that movement takes place smoothly, in the right direction, and to the right extent. It is responsible for maintaining the equilibrium of the body.

These functions are possible because the cerebellum receives constant information regarding the state of contraction of muscles, and of the position of various joints. It also receives information from the eyes, the ears, the vestibular apparatus, the reticular formation and the cerebral cortex. All this information is integrated, and is used to influence movement through motor centres in the brainstem and spinal cord, and also through the cerebral cortex.

Some effects of ***cerebellar dysfunction*** are considered in Chapter 26.

CHAPTER

20

Internal Structure of Brainstem

A brief outline of the internal structure of the brainstem has been given in Chapter 8. (This chapter should be revised before proceeding further). We have also considered the cranial nerve nuclei and their connections, and the tracts passing through the brainstem (Chapter 19). With this background we will now consider the internal structure of the brainstem as seen in transverse sections at various levels. The illustrations are given in the atlas section (Figs. 16.6 to 16.9).

THE MEDULLA

(1) A section through the medulla ***at the level of the pyramidal decussation*** is shown in Fig. 16.7B. Some features to be seen at this level have been reviewed on page 474 (Fig. 18.4). The pyramids and their decussation, the nucleus gracilis, the nucleus cuneatus, the spinal nucleus of the trigeminal nerve, the central grey matter, the central canal, and the uppermost part of the ventral grey column have been identified.

The ventral grey column is separated from the central grey matter by decussating pyramidal fibres. The neurons in it give origin to the uppermost rootlets of the first cervical nerve, and to some fibres in the spinal root of the accessory nerve. The area between the ventral grey column and the spinal nucleus of the trigeminal nerve is occupied by the lower part of the reticular formation.

The main descending fibres to be seen at this level are the corticospinal fibres that form the pyramids. After crossing the midline these fibres turn downwards in the region lateral to the central grey matter to form the lateral corticospinal tract. We have already seen that those fibres of the pyramids that do not cross descend into the ventral funiculus of the spinal cord to form the ventral corticospinal tract. Other descending tracts to be seen at this level (in the anterolateral part of the medulla, Fig. 16.7B, right half) are the rubrospinal tract, the vestibulospinal tract, the olivospinal tract and the tectospinal tract. The tectospinal tract is incorporated within the medial longitudinal fasciculus. Among descending tracts we may also include the spinal tract of the trigeminal nerve, which forms a layer of fibres superficial to the spinal nucleus of this nerve.

The ascending tracts to be seen at this level include the fasciculus gracilis and fasciculus cuneatus which occupy the areas behind the corresponding nuclei; and the spinothalamic, spinocerebellar, spinotectal and spino-olivary tracts that occupy the anterolateral region.

(2) A section through the medulla ***at the level of the sensory decussation*** is shown in Fig. 16.7A. Some features of a section at this level have already been seen (page 473, Fig. 18.5). The central canal surrounded by central grey matter, the medial lemniscus, the pyramids, the nucleus gracilis, the nucleus cuneatus, the spinal nucleus of the trigeminal nerve, and the reticular formation have been identified.

The nucleus gracilis and the nucleus cuneatus are much larger than at lower levels. Internal arcuate fibres arising in these nuclei arch forwards and medially around the central grey matter to cross the middle line. Having crossed the middle line these fibres turn cranially to constitute the medial lemniscus. As the fibres from the nucleus gracilis and the nucleus cuneatus pass forwards they intercross so that the fibres from the nucleus gracilis come to lie ventral to those from the nucleus cuneatus. The most medial fibres (from the legs) come to lie most anteriorly in the medial lemniscus. These are followed by fibres from the trunk and from the upper limb in that order. Higher up in the brainstem the medial lemniscus changes its orientation, its long axis (as seen in cross section) becoming transverse (Fig. 16.8A). The most anterior fibres become lateral, and the posterior fibres become medial. In its course through the medulla the medial lemniscus is probably joined by the anterior spinothalamic tract.

A number of cranial nerve nuclei can be identified at this level. Several of these are present in relation to the central grey matter. The hypoglossal nucleus is located ventral to the central canal just lateral to the middle line. The dorsal vagal nucleus lies dorsolateral to the hypoglossal nucleus. The nucleus of the solitary tract is seen dorsal to the central canal near the middle line. The lower ends of these nuclei of the two sides become continuous with each other to form the ***commissural nucleus*** of the vagus. The nucleus ambiguus lies in the reticular formation medial to the spinal nucleus of the trigeminal nerve.

Other masses of grey matter that may be recognized at this level are:

a. the lowest part of the ***inferior olivary nucleus***;
b. the ***medial accessory olivary nucleus*** which lies dorsal to the medial part of the inferior olivary nucleus (see below);
c. the ***lateral reticular nucleus*** lying in the lateral part of the reticular formation ; and
d. ***arcuate nuclei*** lying on the anterior aspect of the pyramids.

The gracile and cuneate fasciculi are much smaller than at lower levels as the fibres of these tracts progressively terminate in the gracile and cuneate nuclei. Other ascending tracts to be seen at this level are the spinothalamic, spinocerebellar, spinotectal and spino-olivary tracts all of which lie in the anterolateral region (Fig. 16.7A, left half).

The descending tracts present are (Fig. 16.7A, right half) the pyramids, the rubro-spinal, vestibulospinal and olivospinal tracts, and the medial longitudinal fasciculus which includes the tectospinal tract.

(3) A section through the medulla ***at the level of the olive*** is shown in Fig. 16.6B. Some features of a transverse section at this level have been introduced on page 473 (Fig. 18.6). The floor of the fourth ventricle lined by grey matter, the reticular formation, the spinal nucleus and tract of the trigeminal nerve, the inferior cerebellar peduncle, the inferior olivary nucleus, the medial lemniscus and the pyramids have been briefly considered.

Several cranial nerve nuclei can be recognized in relation to the floor of the fourth ventricle. From medial to lateral side these are the hypoglossal nucleus, the dorsal vagal nucleus, and the vestibular nuclei. The solitary tract and its nucleus lie ventrolateral to the dorsal vagal nucleus. The nucleus ambiguus lies much more ventrally within the reticular formation.

The dorsal and ventral cochlear nuclei can be seen in relation to the inferior cerebellar peduncle. (They are shown schematically in Fig. 16.6B. They are actually seen at higher levels of the medulla, near its junction with the pons).

Other masses of grey matter present are the medial and dorsal accessory olivary nuclei (lying medial and dorsal, respectively, to the inferior olivary nucleus), and the lateral reticular nucleus and arcuate nuclei which occupy the same relative positions as at lower levels. The pontobulbar body lies on the dorsolateral aspect of the inferior cerebellar peduncle (Fig. 16.6B, right).

The descending tracts to be seen at this level (Fig. 16.6B, right half) are the pyramids, the tectospinal, vestibulospinal, and rubro-spinal tracts; and the spinal tract of the trigeminal nerve.

The ascending tracts are the medial lemniscus forming an anteroposterior L-shaped band lying next to the middle line; the spinothalamic, spinocerebellar and spinotectal tracts. At this level the dorsal spinocerebellar tract lies within the inferior cerebellar peduncle. The ventral spinocerebellar tract lies more anteriorly near the surface of the medulla. The spinothalamic tracts lie dorsolateral to the inferior olivary nucleus.

The medial longitudinal fasciculus lies dorsal to the medial lemniscus.

The connections of the cranial nerve nuclei of the medulla have been described in Chapter 9. The reticular formation is considered later in this Chapter. The connections of the gracile and cuneate nuclei are described on page 505. Connections of some other masses of grey matter to be seen in the medulla are considered below.

Connections of the Inferior Olivary Nucleus

The main afferents of the inferior olivary nucleus are from the cerebral cortex and from the spinal cord. The main efferents are to the cerebellar cortex and to the spinal cord. The nucleus may, therefore, be regarded as a relay station on the following pathways.

a. Cortico olivo cerebellar.
b. Cortico olivo spinal.
c. Spino olivo cerebellar.

Some details of olivocerebellar connections are considered on page 513.

Connections of Other Nuclei

The accessory olivary nuclei are connected to the cerebellum by parolivocerebellar fibres.

The arcuate nuclei are generally regarded as displaced pontine nuclei. Cortical fibres reach them through the pyramids. These are relayed to the cerebellum by fibres which follow two separate pathways. Some of them wind round the anterior and lateral aspect of the medulla as anterior external arcuate fibres to reach the inferior cerebellar peduncle of the opposite side. Other fibres pass dorsally through the substance of the medulla to reach the floor of the fourth ventricle. Here they run under the ependyma to the inferior cerebellar peduncle of the opposite side as fibres of the striae medullares. Fibres from the arcuate nuclei probably end in the flocculus of the cerebellum.

Like the arcuate nuclei, the ***pontobulbar body*** is made up of neurons that represent displaced pontine nuclei. Fibres arising in this body form the ***circumolivary bundle***. These fibres join those from the arcuate nuclei to reach the inferior cerebellar peduncle of the opposite side. Some of them possibly pass through the striae medullares.

THE PONS

Transverse sections through the upper and lower parts of the pons are illustrated in Figs. 16.8A and 16.8B. Some features common to both these levels have been already considered (Fig. 18.7). The subdivision of the pons into dorsal and ventral parts and its relationship to the superior, middle and inferior cerebellar peduncles have been noted. We have seen that the ventral part of the pons contains: (i) the pontine nuclei, (ii) vertically running corticospinal and corticopontine fibres, and (iii) transversely running fibres arising in the pontine nuclei and projecting to the opposite half of the cerebellum through the middle cerebellar peduncle.

The ***pontine nuclei*** (or ***nuclei pontis***) receive corticopontine fibres from the frontal, temporal, parietal and occipital lobes of the cerebrum. Their efferents form the transverse fibres of the pons. We have seen that most of these fibres cross to the opposite side, but some may end ipsilaterally.

The dorsal part of the pons is occupied, predominantly, by the reticular formation. Its posterior surface helps to form the floor of the fourth ventricle. This surface is lined by grey matter and is related to some cranial nerve nuclei. The dorsal part is bounded laterally by the inferior cerebellar peduncle in the lower part of the pons, and by the superior cerebellar peduncle in the upper part. The region adjoining the ventral part is occupied by important ascending tracts. The medial lemniscus occupies a transversely elongated oval area next to the middle line. Lateral to this are the trigeminal lemniscus and the spinal lemniscus (lateral spinothalamic tract). The fibres of the spinotectal tract run along with the spinal lemniscus, while those of the ventral spinothalamic tract lie within the medial lemniscus. Still more laterally, there is the lateral lemniscus. Ventral to these lemnisci there are conspicuous transversely running fibres that form the ***trapezoid body***. The ventral spinocerebellar tract lies ventromedial to the inferior cerebellar peduncle in the lower part of the pons (Fig. 16.8B). In the upper part of the pons it is seen within the superior cerebellar peduncle (Fig. 16.8A).

Descending tracts passing through the dorsal part of the pons are the tectospinal tract and the rubrospinal tract. The medial longitudinal fasciculus lies dorsally near the middle line.

We will now consider those features of the pons that are different in the upper and lower parts.

A section through the lower part of the pons (Fig. 16.8B) shows two cranial nerve nuclei that are closely related to the floor of the fourth ventricle. These are the abducent nucleus lying medially and the vestibular nuclei that lie laterally. At a deeper level in the lateral part of the reticular formation two additional nuclei are seen. These are the spinal nucleus of the trigeminal nerve (along with its tract) lying laterally, and the facial nucleus lying medially. The dorsal and ventral cochlear nuclei lie dorsal and ventral, respectively, to the inferior cerebellar peduncle.

The fibres arising from the facial nucleus follow an unusual course which has been described on page 247 (Fig. 9.59). We have seen that the abducent nucleus and the facial nerve fibres looping around it together form a surface elevation, the ***facial colliculus,*** in the floor of the fourth ventricle (Fig. 24.8).

The vestibular nuclei occupy the vestibular area in the lateral part of the floor of the fourth ventricle. These nuclei are to be seen in the lower part of the pons and in the upper part of the medulla (Figs. 16.6B, 16.8B). Other masses of grey matter to be seen in the lower part of the pons are the superior olivary complex (made up of several nuclei) which lies dorsomedial to the lateral lemniscus, and the nuclei of the trapezoid body which consist of scattered cells lying within this body.

A section through the upper part of the pons (Fig. 16.8A) shows that the dorsal part is bounded laterally by the superior cerebellar peduncles. Medial to the peduncle there is the main sensory nucleus of the trigeminal nerve, and further medially there is the motor nucleus of the same nerve. The superior olivary nucleus extends to this level, but is less prominent; while the lateral lemniscus forms a more conspicuous bundle. Some fibres of the trapezoid body can be seen ventral to the medial lemniscus.

The reticular formation of the pons is described later in this Chapter.

THE MIDBRAIN

Some features of the internal structure of the midbrain have been considered on page 476 (Fig. 18.8). The subdivision of the midbrain into the tectum, the tegmentum, the substantia nigra, and the crus cerebri (or basis pedunculi) has been noted. The superior and inferior colliculi, the red nucleus and the reticular formation have been identified.

A transverse section through the midbrain at the level of the inferior colliculus is shown in Fig. 16.9B and a section at the level of the superior colliculus in Fig. 16.9A. We will first consider those features that are common to both these levels.

The ***crus cerebri*** (or ***basis pedunculi***) consists of fibres descending from the cerebral cortex. Its medial one-sixth is occupied by corticopontine fibres descending from the frontal lobe; and the lateral one-sixth is occupied by similar fibres from the temporal, occipital and parietal lobes. The intermediate two-thirds of the crus cerebri are occupied by corticospinal and corticonuclear fibres. The fibres for the leg are most lateral and those for the head are most medial.

The ***substantia nigra*** lies immediately behind and medial to the basis pedunculi. It appears dark in unstained sections as neurons within it contain pigment (neuromelanin).

The midbrain is traversed by the cerebral aqueduct which is surrounded by central grey matter. Ventrally, the central grey matter is related to cranial nerve nuclei (oculomotor and trochlear). The region between the substantia nigra and the central grey matter is occupied by the reticular formation.

A section through the midbrain at the level of the inferior colliculus shows the following additional features (Fig. 16.9B).

The ***inferior colliculus*** is a large mass of grey matter lying in the tectum. It forms a cell station in the auditory pathway and is probably concerned with reflexes involving auditory stimuli. The ***trochlear nucleus*** lies in the ventral part of the central grey matter. Fibres arising in this nucleus follow an unusual course. They run dorsally and decussate (in the superior medullary velum) before emerging on the dorsal aspect of the brainstem. The ***mesencephalic nucleus of the trigeminal nerve*** lies in the lateral part of the central grey matter.

A compact bundle of fibres lies in the tegmentum dorsomedial to the substantia nigra. It consists of the medial lemniscus, the trigeminal lemniscus and the spinal lemniscus in that order from medial to lateral side. The medial lemniscus includes fibres of the ventral spinothalamic tract while the spinal lemniscus (made up mainly of the lateral spinothalamic tract) includes fibres of the spinotectal tract. More dorsally, the lateral lemniscus forms a bundle ventrolateral to the inferior colliculus (in which most of its fibres end). Important fibre bundles are also located near the middle line of the tegmentum. The medial longitudinal fasciculus lies ventral to the trochlear nucleus; and ventral to the fasciculus there is the tectospinal tract. The region ventral to the tectospinal tracts is occupied by decussating fibres of the superior cerebellar peduncle. These fibres have their origin in the dentate nucleus of the cerebellum. They cross the middle line in the lower part of the tegmentum. Some of these fibres end in the red nucleus while others ascend to the thalamus. The part of the tegmentum ventral to the decussation of the superior cerebellar peduncle is occupied by the rubrospinal tracts.

A section through the upper part of the midbrain (Fig. 16.9A) shows two large masses of grey matter not seen at lower levels. These are the ***superior colliculus*** in the tectum, and the ***red nucleus*** in the tegmentum. The superior colliculus is a centre concerned with visual reflexes. The red nucleus (so called because of a reddish colour in fresh material) lies in the anterior part of the tegmentum dorsomedial to the substantia nigra.

The ***oculomotor nucleus*** lies in relation to the ventral part of the central grey matter. The nuclei of the two sides lie close together forming a single complex. The ***Edinger Westphal nucleus*** (which supplies the sphincter pupillae and ciliaris muscle) forms part of the oculomotor complex. The oculomotor complex is related ventrally to the medial longitudinal fasciculus. Closely related to the cranial part of the superior colliculus there is a small collection of neurons that constitute the ***pretectal nucleus***. This nucleus is concerned with the pathway for the pupillary light reflex.

The bundle of ascending fibres consisting of the medial lemniscus, the trigeminal lemniscus and the spinal lemniscus lies more dorsally than at lower levels (because of the presence of the red nucleus). The lateral lemniscus is not seen at this level as its fibres end in the inferior colliculus. However, the ***inferior brachium*** that conveys auditory fibres to the medial geniculate body can be seen near the surface of the tegmentum.

The middle line region of the tegmentum shows two groups of decussating fibres. The ***dorsal tegmental decussation*** consists of fibres that have their origin in the superior colliculus and cross to the opposite side to descend as the tectospinal tract. The ***ventral tegmental decussation*** consists of fibres that originate in the red nucleus and decussate to form the rubrospinal tracts.

Connections of the Red Nucleus

The nucleus receives its main afferents from (i) the cerebral cortex, and (ii) the cerebellum (dentate, emboliform and globose nuclei). The main efferents are to the spinal cord through the rubrospinal tract, and also to motor cranial nerve nuclei. The red nucleus may, therefore, be considered as an integrating and relay centre on the following pathways: (a) cortico rubrospinal, (b) cortico rubro nuclear, and (c) cerebello rubro spinal.

Connections of the Inferior Colliculus

The inferior colliculus is an important relay centre in the acoustic (auditory) pathway. It receives fibres of the lateral lemniscus arising in the superior olivary complex. Each colliculus receives auditory impulses from both ears. These impulses are relayed to the medial geniculate body and from there to the acoustic area of the cerebral cortex.

Connections of the Superior Colliculus

The superior colliculus has a complex laminar structure, being made up of six (or more) layers. Its most important afferents are those that bring visual impulses from the retina. The major efferents are the tectospinal tract, and tectonuclear fibres to the nuclei of cranial nerves responsible for moving the eyes and head. The colliculus has, therefore, been regarded as a centre for reflex movements of the head and eyes in response to visual stimuli.

Connections of the Substantia Nigra

The main connections (both afferent and efferent) are with the striatum (i.e., caudate nucleus and putamen). Dopamine produced by neurons in the substantia nigra passes along their axons to the striatum. Dopamine is much reduced in patients with a disease called Parkinsonism in which there is a degeneration of the striatum.

RETICULAR FORMATION OF THE BRAINSTEM

The term reticular formation was originally used to designate areas of the central nervous system which were not occupied by well defined nuclei or fibre bundles, but consisted of a network of fibres within which scattered neurons were situated. Such areas are to be found at all levels in the nervous system. In the spinal cord there is an intermingling of grey and white matter on the lateral side of the neck of the dorsal grey column. This area is sometimes referred to as the reticular formation of the spinal cord. The reticular formation is, however, best defined in the brainstem where it is now recognized as an area of considerable importance. Some centres in the cerebrum and cerebellum are regarded by some authorities to be closely related, functionally, to this region.

The reticular formation extends throughout the length of the brainstem. In the medulla it occupies the region dorsal to the inferior olivary nucleus. In the pons it lies in the dorsal part, while in the midbrain it lies in the tegmentum.

Connections of the Reticular Formation

The reticular formation has numerous connections. Directly, or indirectly, it is connected to almost all parts of the nervous system. The pathways involved are both ascending and descending; crossed and uncrossed, somatic and visceral.

The reticular formation receives impulses from the motor and other areas of the cerebral cortex and relays them to the spinal cord through the medial and lateral reticulospinal tracts. It is also connected to the cerebellum and to the thalamus. Fibres passing from the reticular formation to the thalamus constitute the ascending reticular activating system (ARAS).

Functions of the Reticular Formation

Because of its diverse connections the reticular formation is believed to have a controlling or modifying influence on many functions. Some of them are as follows.

A. Somatomotor control

Through its direct connections with the spinal cord; and indirectly through the corpus striatum, the cerebral cortex and the cerebellum, the reticular formation has an influence on fine control of movements including those involved in postural adjustments, locomotion, skilled use of the hands, speech etc.

B. Somatosensory control

The reticular formation influences conduction through somatosensory pathways. Similar effects may also be exerted on visual and auditory pathways.

C. Visceral control

Physiological studies have shown that stimulation of certain areas in the reticular formation of the medulla has great influence on respiratory and cardiovascular function. These effects are mediated through connections between the reticular formation and autonomic centres in the brainstem and spinal cord, but the pathways concerned are not well defined.

D. Neuroendocrine control

Through its connections with the hypothalamus, the reticular formation influences activity of the adenohypophysis and of the neurohypophysis. A similar influence is also exerted on the pineal body.

E. Alertness

Through the ascending reticular activating system the reticular formation helps to maintain a state of alertness.

CHAPTER

21

Diencephalon and Basal Ganglia, Olfacatory Region and Limbic System

THE DIENCEPHALON

The diencephalon consists of the thalamus (or dorsal thalamus), the hypothalamus, the epithalamus, the subthalamus (or ventral thalamus), and the metathalamus. The third ventricle may be regarded as the cavity of the diencephalon.

THE THALAMUS

The thalamus (or dorsal thalamus) is a large mass of grey matter that lies immediately lateral to the third ventricle. It has two ends (or poles), anterior and posterior; and four surfaces, superior, inferior, medial and lateral.

The ***anterior end (or pole)*** lies just behind the interventricular foramen (Fig. 18.19). The ***posterior end (or pole)*** is called the pulvinar. It lies just above and lateral to the superior colliculus. The ***medial surface*** forms the greater part of the lateral wall of the third ventricle, and is lined by ependyma. The medial surfaces of the two thalami are usually interconnected by a mass of grey matter called the ***interthalamic connexus***. Inferiorly, the medial surface is separated from the hypothalamus by the ***hypothalamic sulcus***. This sulcus runs from the interventricular foramen to the aqueduct. The lateral surface of the thalamus is related to the internal capsule which separates it from the lentiform nucleus (Fig. 21.1). The ***superior (or dorsal) surface*** of the thalamus is related laterally to the caudate nucleus from which it is separated by a bundle of fibres called the ***stria terminalis***, and by the thalamostriate vein. The thalamus and the caudate nucleus together form the floor of the central part of the lateral ventricle. The medial part of the superior surface of the thalamus is, however, separated from the ventricle by the fornix, and by a fold of piamater called the ***tela choroidea***. At the junction of the medial and superior surfaces of the thalamus the ependyma of the third ventricle is reflected from the lateral wall to the roof. The line of reflection is marked by

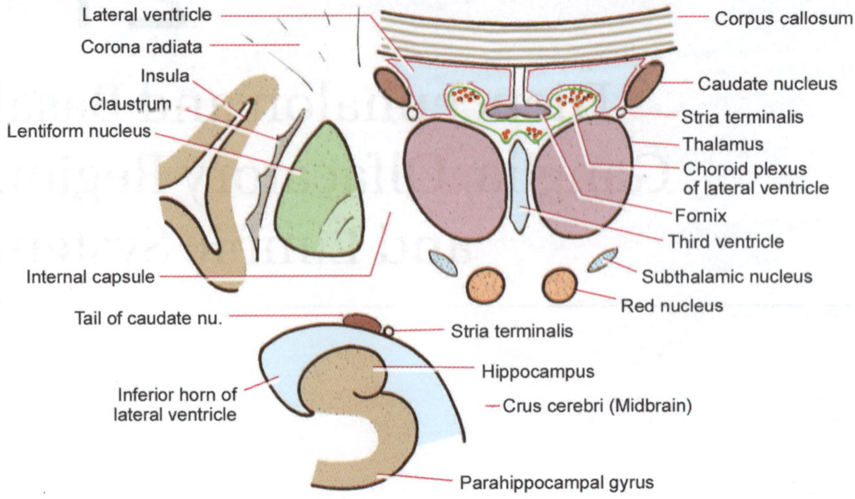

Fig. 21.1 Coronal section through the cerebrum to show structures related to the thalamus.

a line called the ***taenia thalami.*** Underlying it there is a narrow bundle of fibres called the ***stria medullaris thalami*** (not to be confused with the stria medullares present in the floor of the fourth ventricle). The ***inferior surface*** of the thalamus is related to the hypothalamus anteriorly (Fig. 18.19), and to the subthalamus posteriorly (Fig. 21.1). The subthalamus separates the thalamus from the tegmentum of the midbrain.

Internal Structure of the Thalamus

The thalamus consists mainly of grey matter. Its superior surface is covered by a thin layer of white matter called the ***stratum zonale;*** and its lateral surface by a similar layer called the ***external medullary lamina.***

The grey matter of the thalamus is subdivided into three main parts by a Y-shaped sheet of white matter which is called the ***internal medullary lamina*** (Fig. 21.2). This lamina is placed vertically. It divides the thalamus into a lateral part, a medial part, and an anterior part situated between the two limbs of the 'Y'.

A number of nuclei can be distinguished within each of these parts. Only the more important of these are listed below.

(a) Nuclei in the anterior part

A number of nuclei can be distinguished, but we shall refer to them collectively as the ***anterior nucleus.***[1]

(b) Nuclei in the medial part

The largest of these is the ***medial dorsal nucleus.***

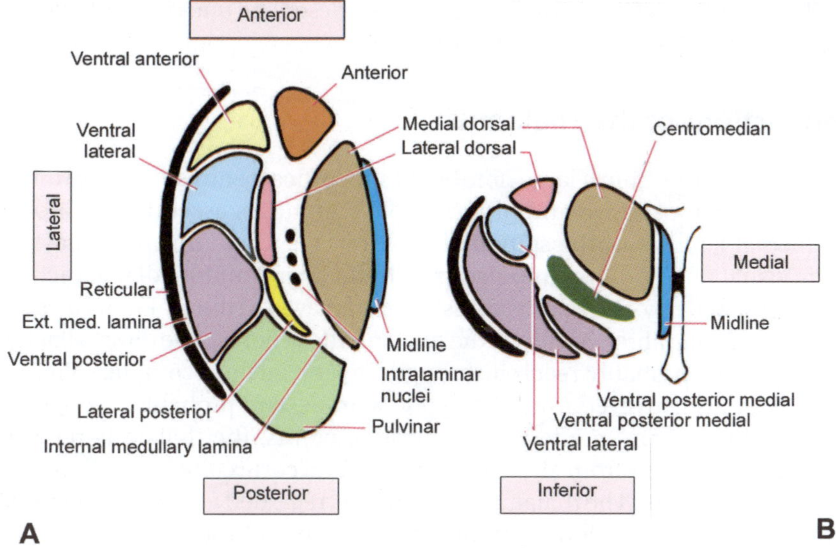

Fig. 21.2 Scheme to show the nuclei of the thalamus. A. Superior aspect. B. Coronal section.

(c) Nuclei in the lateral part

The nuclei in the lateral part can be subdivided into a ***ventral group*** and a ***lateral group.***

The ***nuclei in the ventral group*** are as follows (in anteroposterior order).

1. ***Ventral anterior nucleus.***
2. ***Ventral intermediate nucleus*** (also called the ***ventral lateral nucleus***).
3. ***Ventral posterior nucleus,*** which is further subdivided into a lateral part called the ***ventral posterolateral nucleus,*** and a medial part called the ***ventral posteromedial nucleus*** (Fig. 21.2B).

The ***nuclei of the lateral group*** are as follows (in anteroposterior order).

1. ***Lateral dorsal nucleus.***
2. ***Lateral posterior nucleus.***
3. ***Pulvinar.***

(d) In addition to the above the thalamus contains the following nuclei.

1. The ***intralaminar nuclei*** are embedded within the internal medullary lamina. The most important of these is the ***centromedian nucleus*** (Fig. 21.2B).
2. The ***midline nuclei*** consist of scattered cells that lie between the medial part of the thalamus and the ependyma of the third ventricle.
3. The ***reticular nucleus*** is made up of a thin layer of cells covering the lateral aspect of the thalamus. The cells of this nucleus are separated from the rest of the thalamus by the external medullary lamina. The reticular nucleus is related laterally to the internal capsule.

4. The ***medial and lateral geniculate bodies*** (described under metathalamus) are often included as part of the thalamus.

Connections of the Thalamus

Afferent impulses from a large number of subcortical centres converge on the thalamus. Exteroceptive and proprioceptive impulses ascend to it through the medial lemniscus, the spinothalamic tracts, and the trigeminothalamic tract. Visual and auditory impulses reach the lateral and medial geniculate bodies respectively. Sensations of taste are conveyed to the thalamus through solitariothalamic fibres. Although the thalamus does not receive direct olfactory impulses they probably reach it through the amygdaloid complex. Visceral information is conveyed from the hypothalamus, and probably through the reticular formation. In addition to these afferents, the thalamus receives profuse connections from all parts of the cerebral cortex, the cerebellum, and the corpus striatum. The thalamus is, therefore, regarded as a great integrating centre where information from all these sources is brought together. This information is projected to almost the whole of the cerebral cortex through profuse thalamocortical projections. These thalamocortical fibres form large bundles that are described as ***thalamic radiations*** or as ***thalamic peduncles***. These radiations are ***anterior*** (or ***frontal***), ***superior*** (or ***dorsal***), ***posterior*** (or ***caudal***), and ***ventral.*** Efferent projections from the thalamus also reach the corpus striatum, the hypothalamus, and the reticular formation. Besides its integrating function, the thalamus is believed to have some degree of ability to perceive exteroceptive sensations, specially pain.

Some further details are as follows.

The most important connections of the thalamus are those of the ***ventral posterior nucleus*** which receives the terminations of the major sensory pathways ascending from the spinal cord and brainstem. These include the medial lemniscus, the spinothalamic tracts, the trigeminal lemniscus and the solitariothalamic fibres carrying sensations of taste. All these sensations are carried to the sensory areas of the cerebral cortex (areas 3,2,1) by fibres passing through the posterior limb of the internal capsule (superior thalamic radiation).

Within the ventral posterior nucleus fibres from different parts of the body terminate in a definite sequence. The fibres from the lowest parts of the body end in the most lateral part of the nucleus. The medial lemniscus and spinothalamic tracts carrying sensations from the limbs and trunk end in the ventral posterolateral part; while the trigeminal fibres (from the head) end in the ventral posteromedial part, which also receives the fibres for taste.

THE HYPOTHALAMUS

The hypothalamus is a part of the diencephalon. As its name implies it lies below the thalamus. On the medial side, it forms the wall of the third ventricle below the level of the hypothalamic sulcus. Laterally, it is in contact with the internal capsule, and (in the posterior part) with the subthalamus. Posteriorly,

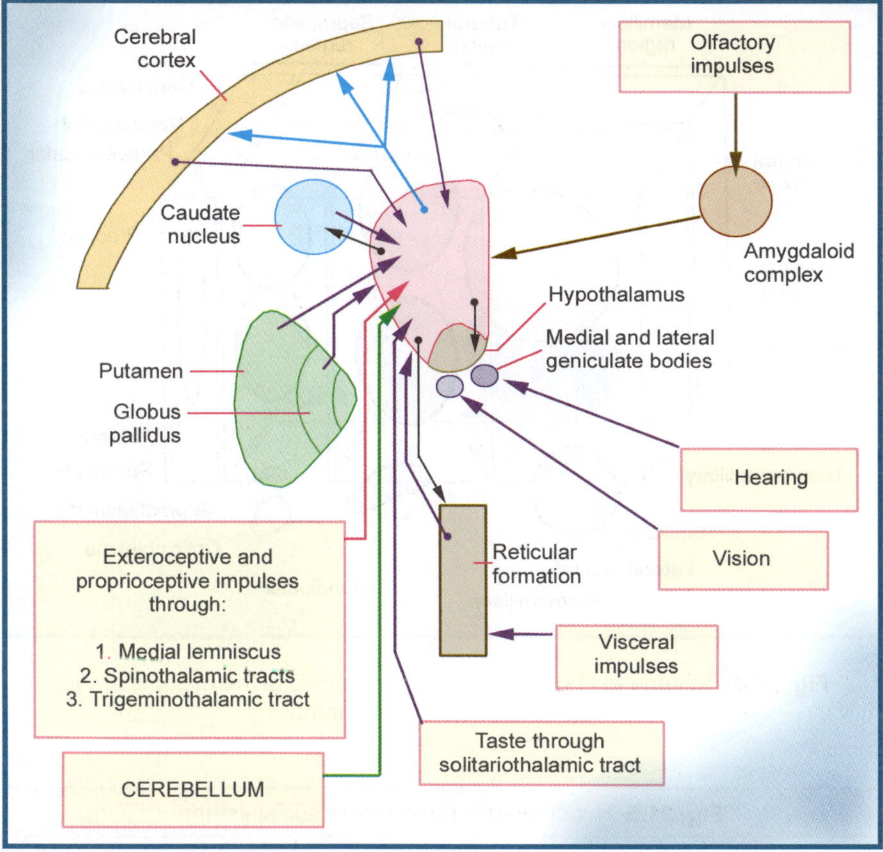

Fig. 21.3 Scheme to show the connections of the thalamus.

the hypothalamus merges with the subthalamus, and through it with the tegmentum of the midbrain. Anteriorly, it extends up to the lamina terminalis, and merges with certain olfactory structures in the region of the anterior perforated substance. Inferiorly, the hypothalamus is related to structures in the floor of the third ventricle. These are the tuber cinereum, the infundibulum, and the mamillary bodies, which are considered as parts of the hypothalamus.

Subdivisions of the Hypothalamus

For convenience of description the hypothalamus may be subdivided, roughly, into a number of regions (Figs. 21.4, 21.5). Some authorities divide it (from medial to lateral side) into three ***zones*** which are as follows.

a. ***Periventricular zone.***
b. ***Intermediate zone.***
c. ***Lateral zone.***

The periventricular and intermediate zones are often described collectively as the ***medial zone***. The column of the fornix lies between the medial and lateral zones. (The mamillothalamic tract also lies in this plane).

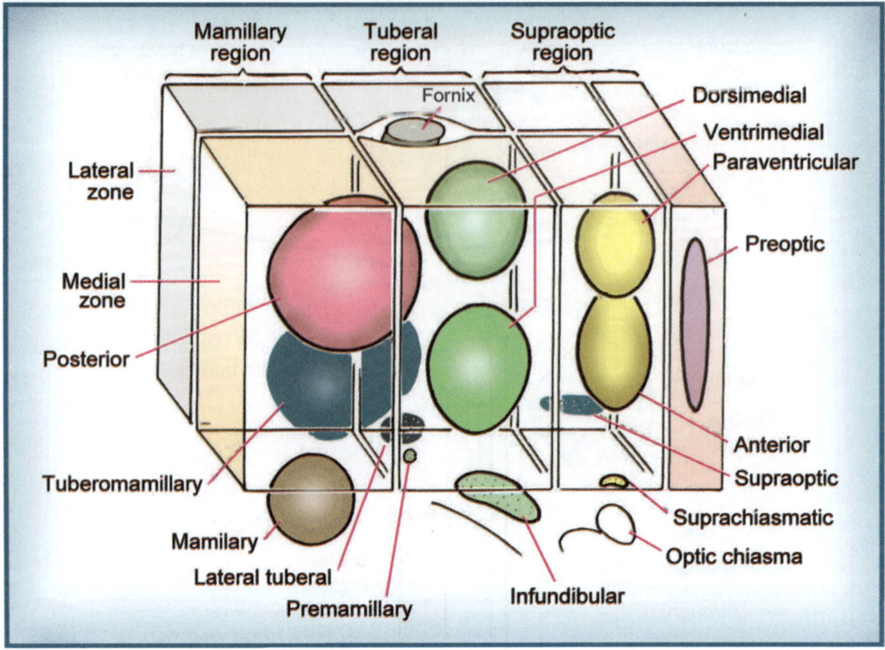

Fig. 21.4 Scheme to show the regions and zones of the hypothalamus, and the nuclei within them.

Fig. 21.5 Hypothalamic regions and nuclei in them.

	Medial zone (Periventricular and intermediate)	Lateral zone
	Preoptic nucleus	
Supraoptic region	Paraventricular nu. Periventricular cell groups Suprachiasmatic nu. Intermediate cell groups (= anterior nucleus ?)	Supraoptic nucleus*
Tuberal region	Dorsimedial nucleus Ventrimedial nucleus Arcuate (infundibular) nucleus Premamillary nucleus	Lateral tuberal nucleus
Mamillary or posterior region	Posterior nucleus (lies partly in tuberal region)	Tuberomamillary nucleus*
	Mamillary nuclei	

*From a functional point of view the supraoptic and tuberomamillary nuclei are grouped with the nuclei of the intermediate zone.

The hypothalamus is also subdivided anteroposteriorly into four ***regions***. These are as follows.

a. The ***preoptic region*** adjoins the lamina terminalis.
b. The ***supraoptic region*** lies above the optic chiasma.

c. The ***tuberal (or infundibulo-tuberal) region*** includes the infundibulum, the tuber cinereum and the region above it.
d. The ***mamillary region*** consists of the mamillary body and the region above it.

The preoptic region differs from the rest of the hypothalamus in being a derivative of the telen-cephalon. (The lamina terminalis also belongs to the telencephalon).

Hypothalamic Nuclei

The entire hypothalamus contains scattered neurons within which some aggre-gations can be recognised. These aggregations, termed the hypothalamic nuclei, are as follows (Figs. 21.4 to 21.6).

1. The ***preoptic nucleus*** extends through the periventricular, intermediate, and lateral zones of the preoptic part.
2. The ***mamillary nuclei*** lie within the mamillary body.
   The remaining nuclei of the hypothalamus lie either in the periventricular, intermediate, or lateral zones.
   Nuclei in the periventricular zone (Fig. 21.6).
3. The ***paraventricular nucleus,*** and
4. the ***suprachiasmatic nucleus,*** lie in the supraoptic region.
5. The ***infundibular nucleus*** lies in the tuberal region.
6. The ***posterior nucleus*** extends into both the tuberal and mamillary regions.
   Nuclei in the intermediate zone
7. The ***anterior nucleus*** occupies the supraoptic region.
8. The ***dorsimedial nucleus***, and
9. the ***ventrimedial nucleus*** lie in the tuberal part, which also contains small aggregations of cells that constitute
10. the ***premamillary nuclei.***
    Nuclei in the lateral zone
11. The lateral zone contains a diffuse collection of cells that extends through the supraoptic, tuberal and mamillary regions. These cells constitute the ***lateral nucleus.*** The lateral zone also contains the following nuclei.
12. The ***supraoptic nucleus*** lies in the supraoptic region.
13. The ***tuberomamillary nucleus*** extends into the tuberal and mamillary regions.
14. Small aggregations of neurons in the tuberal region constitute the ***lateral tuberal nuclei.***

Connections of the Hypothalamus

The hypothalamus is concerned with visceral function and is, therefore, connected to other areas having a similar function. These include the various parts of the limbic system, the reticular formation, and autonomic centres in the brainstem and spinal cord (Fig. 21.7).

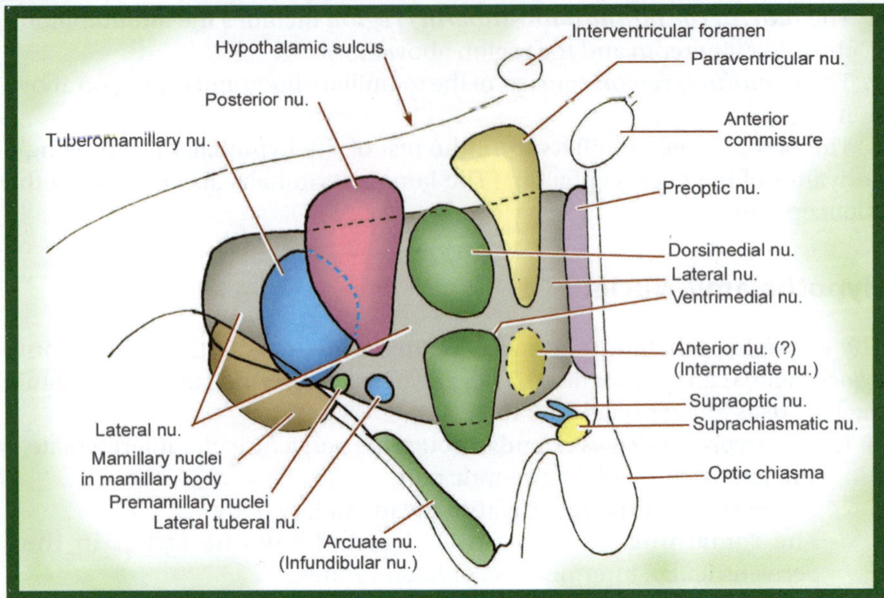

Fig. 21.6 Hypothalamic nuclei. Also see Figs. 21.4 and 21.5.

Afferent Connections

1. The hypothalamus receives visceral afferents (including those of taste) through the spinal cord and brainstem. The exact pathways are not known. They probably pass through the reticular formation and consist of several relays.

Many of these fibres pass through a bundle called the ***mamillary peduncle***. Other fibres pass through a bundle called the ***dorsal longitudinal fasciculus***. Fibres from the tegmentum of the midbrain also reach the hypothalamus through the ***medial forebrain bundle.***

2. The hypothalamus receives afferents from several centres connected to olfactory pathways, and to the limbic system.

These are the anterior perforated substance, the septal nuclei, the amygdaloid complex, the hippocampus and the piriform cortex. Many of these fibres reach the hypothalamus through the medial forebrain bundle. Fibres from the hippocampus travel through the fornix. Some fibres from the amygdaloid complex pass through the stria terminalis, and some through the medial forebrain bundle.

(3) The hypothalamus receives afferents from several parts of the cerebral cortex, and some from the cerebellum.

Efferent Connections

1. The hypothalamus sends fibres to autonomic centres in the brainstem and spinal cord.

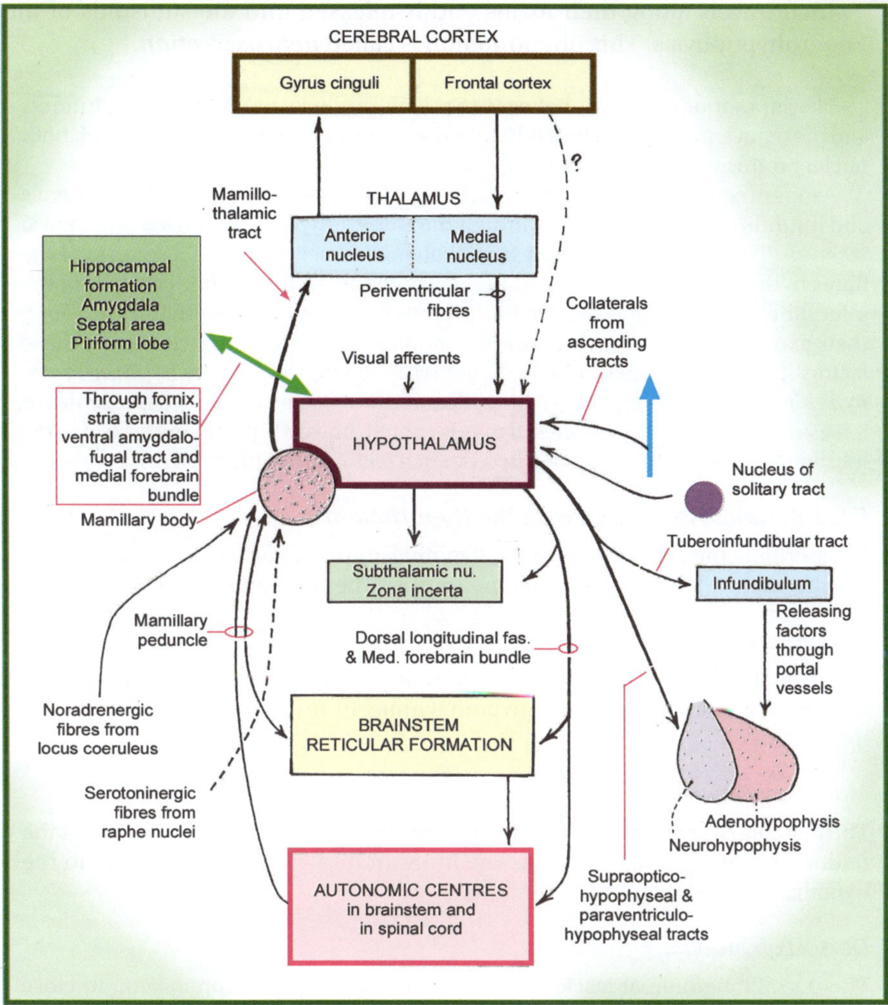

Fig. 21.7 Simplified scheme of the main connections of the hypothalamus.

It also sends fibres to the hippocampal formation, the septal nuclei, the amygdaloid complex, and the tegmentum of the midbrain, and autonomic centres in the brainstem and spinal cord. These fibres pass through the same bundles that convey afferent fibres from these centres.

2. Fibres from the mamillary body pass through the mamillothalamic tract to reach the anterior nucleus of the thalamus. New fibres arising here project to the gyrus cinguli.

3. The supraoptic, paraventricular and infundibular nuclei exert an important influence on the hypophysis cerebri. Fibres arising from the supraoptic and paraventricular nuclei reach the pars posterior (neurohypophysis) through the ***supraoptico-hypophyseal*** and ***paraventriculo hypophyseal*** tracts. The cells in these nuclei are peculiar in that they produce a secretion

which travels along their axons and is released into the sinusoids of the neurohypophysis. This phenomenon is called ***neurosecretion.***

The supraoptic nucleus is believed to mainly produce the antidiuretic hormone, and the paraventricular nucleus is believed to mainly produce oxytocin; though both nuclei produce both hormones.

Axons of cells in the infundibular (arcuate) nucleus end in the median eminence and infundibulum. They travel through the ***tubero-hypophyseal tract*** which also receives fibres from several other hypothalamic nuclei. The axon terminals of the fibres in these tracts are closely related to capillaries in the region. The cells of the infundibular nucleus are believed to produce ***releasing factors*** that travel along their axons and are released into the capillaries. These capillaries carry these factors into the pars anterior of the hypophysis cerebri through the ***hypothalamo-hypophyseal portal system***. In the pars anterior these factors are responsible for release of appropriate hormones. It may be noted, however, that in the case of some hormones their secretion is inhibited by such factors. (See Chapter 12).

Fibre Bundles Associated with the Hypothalamus

In describing the connections of the hypothalamus reference has been made to a number of fibre bundles not mentioned earlier. These are briefly described below.

Medial Forebrain Bundle

The medial forebrain bundle begins in the anterior olfactory areas. It runs caudally through the lateral zone of the hypothalamus, to reach the tegmentum of the midbrain.

Mamillary Peduncle

The mamillary peduncle is a bundle of fibres that connects the tegmentum of the midbrain to the mamillary body. The fibres in it carry visceral impulses to the hypothalamus (Fig. 21.7).

Dorsal Longitudinal Fasciculus

The dorsal longitudinal fasciculus runs vertically within the brainstem, in close relation to the central grey matter. It connects centres in the midbrain, pons, and the upper part of the medulla with the hypothalamus. .

Central Tegmental Tract

This is a bundle that travels from the region of the thalamus, and the basal ganglia, down to the medulla. The fibres in it establish connections with the thalamus, the basal ganglia, the red nucleus, the reticular formation and the inferior olivary complex.

Functions of the Hypothalamus

The hypothalamus plays an important role in the control of many functions that are vital for the survival of an animal. In exercising such control the hypothalamus acts in close co-ordination with higher centres including the limbic system and the prefrontal cortex, and with autonomic centres in the brainstem and spinal cord. The main functions attributed to the hypothalamus are as follows.

(1) Regulation of eating and drinking behaviour

The hypothalamus is responsible for feelings of hunger and of satiety, and this determines whether the animal will accept or refuse food. Stimulation of the lateral zone stimulates hunger while stimulation of the medial zone produces satiety. The lateral zone is also responsible for thirst and drinking.

(2) Regulation of sexual activity and reproduction

The hypothalamus controls sexual activity, both in the male and female. It also exerts an effect on gametogenesis, on ovarian and uterine cycles, and on the development of secondary sexual characters. These effects are produced by influencing the secretion of hormones by the hypophysis cerebri.

(3) Control of autonomic activity

The hypothalamus exerts an important influence on the activity of the autonomic nervous system, and thus has considerable effect on cardiovascular, respiratory and alimentary functions. Sympathetic activity is said to be controlled, predominantly, by caudal parts of the hypothalamus; and parasympathetic activity by cranial parts, but there is considerable overlap between the regions concerned.

(4) Emotional behaviour

The hypothalamus has an important influence on emotions like fear, anger and pleasure. Stimulation of some areas of the hypothalamus produces sensations of pleasure, while stimulation of other regions produces pain or other unpleasant effects.

(5) Control of endocrine activity

The influence of the hypothalamus in the production of hormones by the pars anterior of the hypophysis cerebri, and the elaboration of oxytocin and the antidiuretic hormone by the hypothalamus itself, have been described above. Through control of the adenohypophysis the hypothalamus indirectly influences the thyroid gland, the adrenal cortex, and the gonads.

(6) Temperature regulation

The hypothalamus acts as a thermostat to control body temperature. When body temperature rises or falls, appropriate mechanisms are brought into play to bring the temperature back to normal.

(7) Biological clock

Several functions of the body show a cyclic variation in activity, over the twenty four hours of a day. The most conspicuous of these is the cycle of sleep and waking. Such cycles (called ***circadian rhythms***) are believed to be controlled by the hypothalamus, which is said to function as a biological clock. The suprachiasmatic nucleus is believed to play an important role in this regard. Lesions of the hypothalamus disturb the sleep waking cycle.

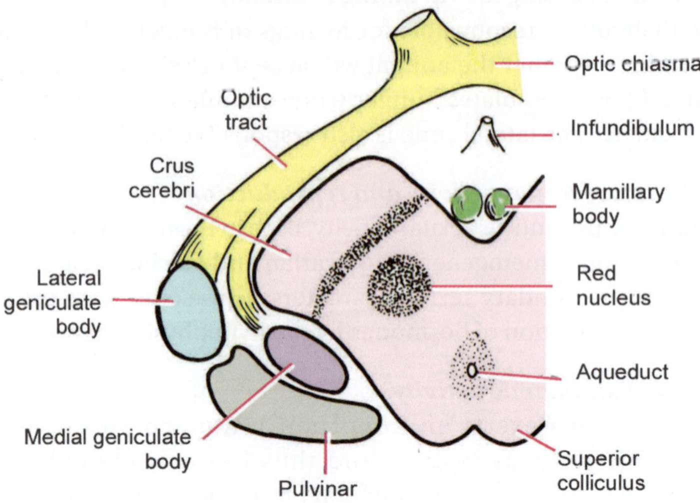

Fig. 21.8 Diagram to show the location of the medial and lateral geniculate bodies.

THE METATHALAMUS

The metathalamus is constituted by the medial and lateral geniculate bodies. These are small oval collections of grey matter situated below the posterior part of the thalamus, lateral to the colliculi of the midbrain (Fig. 21.8). Each mass of grey matter is bent on itself, hence the term 'geniculate'.

The Medial Geniculate Body

The medial geniculate body is a relay station on the auditory pathway. Several subdivisions of its grey matter have been described, but these will not be considered here. The medial geniculate body receives fibres of the lateral lemniscus either directly, or after relay in the inferior colliculus (Fig. 21.9). These fibres pass through the brachium of the inferior colliculus. Fibres arising in the medial geniculate body constitute the acoustic radiation. The acoustic radiation passes through the sublentiform part of the internal capsule to reach the acoustic areas of the cerebral cortex. Some other connections of the medial geniculate body are shown in Fig. 21.9. Each medial geniculate body receives impulses from the cochleae of both sides.

The Lateral Geniculate Body

The lateral geniculate body is a relay station on the visual pathway. It receives fibres from the retinae of both eyes (Fig. 21.10). Efferents arising in this body constitute the optic radiation which passes through the retrolentiform part of the internal capsule to reach the visual areas of the cerebral cortex.

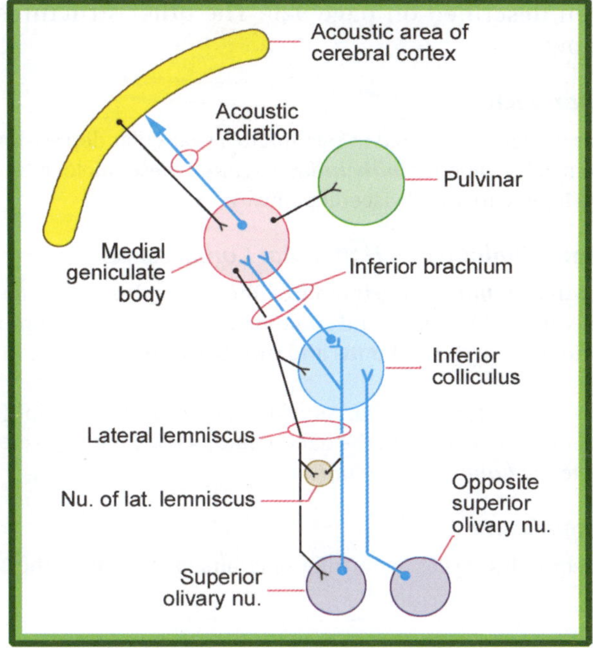

Fig. 21.9 Connections of the medial geniculate body.

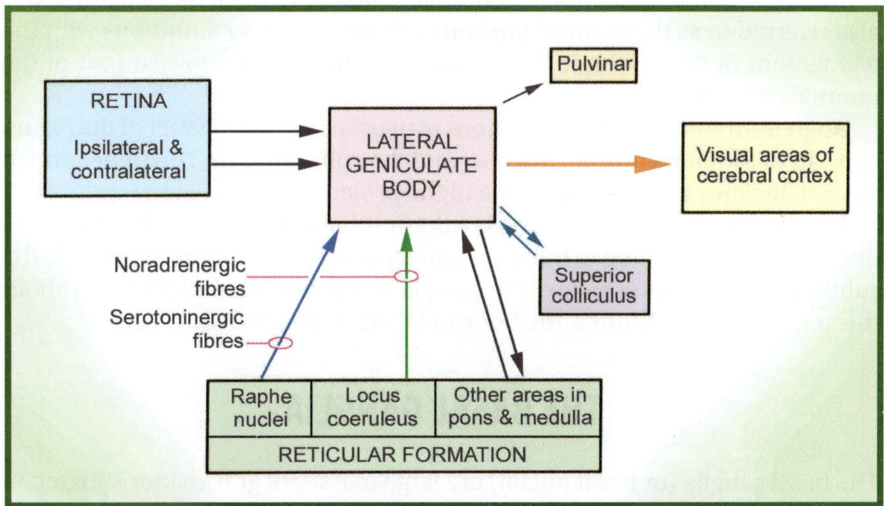

Fig. 21.10 Connections of the lateral geniculate body.

THE EPITHALAMUS

The epithalamus lies in relation to the posterior part of the roof of the third ventricle, and in the adjoining part of its lateral wall (Fig. 21.6A). It consists of the pineal gland, the habenular nuclei, and related structures. The pineal gland has been described on page 920. The other structures are briefly described below.

The Habenular Nuclei

The habenular nuclei are situated in relation to a triangular depression in the wall of the third ventricle called the ***habenular trigone***. These nuclei may be regarded as cell stations in olfactory and visceral pathways.

Stria Medullaris Thalami and Habenular Commissure

The ***stria medullaris thalami*** is a bundle of fibres lying deep to the taenia thalami (along the junction of the medial and superior surfaces of the thalamus). It begins near the anterior pole of the thalamus and runs backwards to reach the habenular region.

Some fibres of the stria medullaris thalami cross in the superior (or anterior) lamina of the pineal stalk to reach the habenular nuclei of the opposite side. These fibres constitute the ***habenular commissure.***

Posterior Commissure

The posterior commissure lies in the inferior lamina of the stalk of the pineal gland.

THE SUBTHALAMIC REGION

The part of the diencephalon that is called the subthalamus lies below the posterior part of the thalamus, behind and lateral to the hypothalamus. It is also referred to as the ***ventral thalamus***. Inferiorly, it is continuous with the tegmentum of the midbrain. Laterally, it is related to the lowest part of the internal capsule.

Apart from some small aggregations of neurons the grey matter of the region consists of the ***subthalamic nucleus*** and the ***zona incerta***. The upper end of the red nucleus, and the substantia nigra, project into the region.

Detailed studies of connections of the subthalamic nucleus show that this nucleus is closely related to the basal ganglia and some authorities include the subthalamic nucleus among these ganglia. For details of modern views about this region see the author's Textbook of HUMAN NEUROANATOMY.

THE BASAL GANGLIA

The basal ganglia (or basal nuclei) are large masses of grey matter situated in the cerebral hemispheres. They are derived from the telencephalon. The basal ganglia are as follows (Fig. 21.11).

a. ***Caudate nucleus.***
b. ***Lentiform nucleus***, which consists of two functionally distinct parts, the ***putamen*** and the ***globus pallidus***.
c. ***Amygdaloid nuclear complex.***
d. The ***claustrum*** is often included among the basal ganglia.

e. As stated above some authorities include the ***subthalamic nucleus*** amongst the basal ganglia.

Various other terms commonly used for some of the above nuclei are as follows. The caudate nucleus and the lentiform nucleus together constitute the ***corpus striatum.*** This consists of two functionally distinct parts. The caudate nucleus and the putamen form one unit called the ***striatum,*** while the globus pallidus forms the other unit, the ***pallidum.***

From an evolutionary point of view, the amygdaloid complex is the oldest of the basal ganglia and is, therefore, sometimes referred to as the ***archistriatum***. The globus pallidus constitutes the ***paleostriatum*** while the caudate nucleus and the putamen form the ***neostriatum.***

The Caudate Nucleus

The caudate nucleus is a C-shaped mass of grey matter (Fig. 21.11). It consists of a large head, a body and a thin tail. The nucleus is intimately related to the lateral ventricle. The head of the nucleus bulges into the anterior horn of the ventricle and forms the greater part of its floor (Fig. 24.3).

The body of the nucleus lies in the floor of the central part of the ventricle (Fig. 24.2); and the tail in the roof of the inferior horn (Fig. 24.4). The anterior part of the head of the caudate nucleus is fused, inferiorly, with the lentiform nucleus. In this situation the grey matter of these two nuclei is continuous with that of the anterior perforated substance. The anterior end of the tail of the caudate nucleus ends in relation to the amygdaloid complex. The body of the caudate nucleus is related medially to the thalamus, and laterally to the internal capsule which separates it from the lentiform nucleus (Fig. 21.12). Some other relationships of the caudate nucleus are shown in Fig. 21.1.

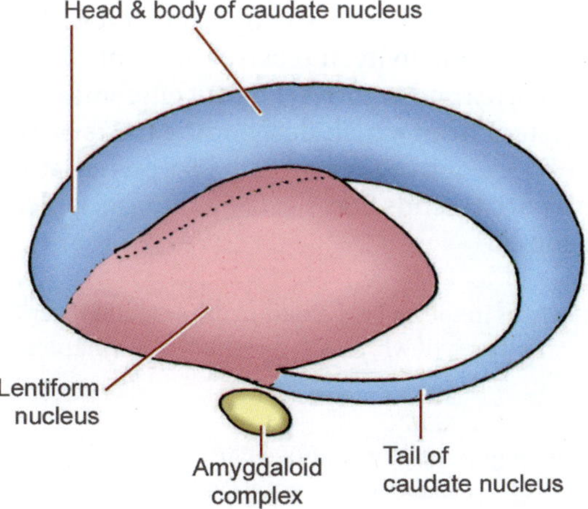

Fig. 21.11 The corpus striatum viewed from the lateral aspect.

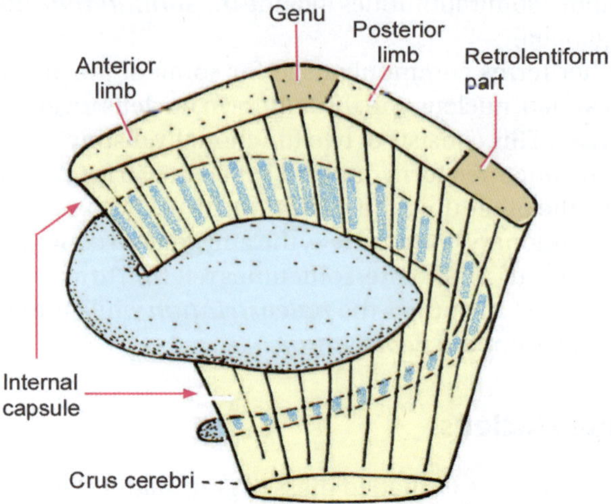

Fig. 21.12 Relationship of the corpus striatum to the internal capsule (viewed from the lateral side).

The Lentiform Nucleus

The lentiform nucleus lies lateral to the internal capsule. Laterally, it is separated from the claustrum by fibres of the external capsule. (Note that these capsules are so called because they appear, by naked eye, to form a covering for the lentiform nucleus). Superiorly, the lentiform nucleus is related to the corona radiata, and inferiorly to the sublentiform part of the internal capsule. Some other relationships are evident in Fig. 21.1. The lentiform nucleus appears triangular (or wedge shaped) in coronal section. It is divided, by a thin lamina of white matter, into a lateral part, the ***putamen;*** and a medial part, the ***globus pallidus.*** The globus pallidus is further subdivided into medial and lateral segments.

The corpus striatum is regarded as an important integrating centre. It plays an important role in motor activity. It receives afferents from various sources including the motor cortex and in turn sends out efferents to several important centres in the brainstem from which descending tracts arise (Fig. 19.3). The striatum constitutes the receiving centre of the corpus striatum, as most of the afferents end in this part. It sends fibres to the pallidum, which in turn projects fibres to various centres.

Degenerative changes in the corpus striatum are associated with a disease called ***Parkinsonism*** some features of which are considered in Chapter 26.

The Claustrum

This is a thin lamina of grey matter that lies lateral to the lentiform nucleus. It is separated from the latter by fibres of the external capsule. Laterally, it is separated by a thin layer of white matter from the cortex of the insula. Its connections are unknown.

The Amygdaloid Complex

This complex (also called the amygdaloid body, amygdala) lies in the temporal lobe of the cerebral hemisphere, close to the temporal pole. It lies deep to the uncus, and is related to the anterior end of the inferior horn of the lateral ventricle.

Before ending this section on the basal ganglia it may be mentioned that the clinician often uses the term basal ganglia in a wider sense than used here. The thalamus, the red nucleus, the substantia nigra and the subthalamic nuclei are included.

THE OLFACTORY REGION AND LIMBIC SYSTEM

THE OLFACTORY REGION

The peripheral end organ for smell is the ***olfactory mucosa*** that lines the upper and posterior parts of the nasal cavity. Nerve fibres arising in this mucosa collect to form about twenty bundles that together constitute an ***olfactory nerve.*** The bundles pass through foramina in the cribriform plate of the ethmoid bone to enter the cranial cavity where they terminate in the ***olfactory bulb*** (Figs. 21.13, 21.15).

The olfactory bulb is an elongated oval structure that lies just above the cribriform plate. It is continuous posteriorly with the ***olfactory tract*** through which it is connected to the base of the cerebral hemisphere. When traced posteriorly the olfactory tract divides into ***medial and lateral olfactory striae*** (Figs. 21.13, 21.14). The point of bifurcation is expanded and forms the ***olfactory trigone.*** An ***intermediate stria*** is sometimes present.

The olfactory striae are intimately related to a mass of grey matter called the ***anterior perforated substance***. The medial and lateral striae form the anteromedial and anterolateral boundaries of this substance. The intermediate stria extends into the anterior perforated substance and ends in a slight elevation (in the anterior part of the substance) called the ***olfactory tubercle***. Posterolaterally, the anterior perforated substance is related to the uncus (Fig. 21.13), while posteromedially it is bounded by a bundle of fibres called the ***diagonal band*** (of Broca) (Fig. 21.14).

The uncus is a part of the cerebral hemisphere that lies on the tentorial surface a little behind and medial to the temporal pole. It represents the anterior end of the ***parahippocampal gyrus*** and is separated from the temporal pole by the rhinal sulcus.

The anterior part of the parahippocampal gyrus, including the uncus, is referred to as the ***entorhinal area*** (area 28).

Some other areas present in the region are shown in Fig. 21.14. Their names may be noted, but further description is unnecessary.

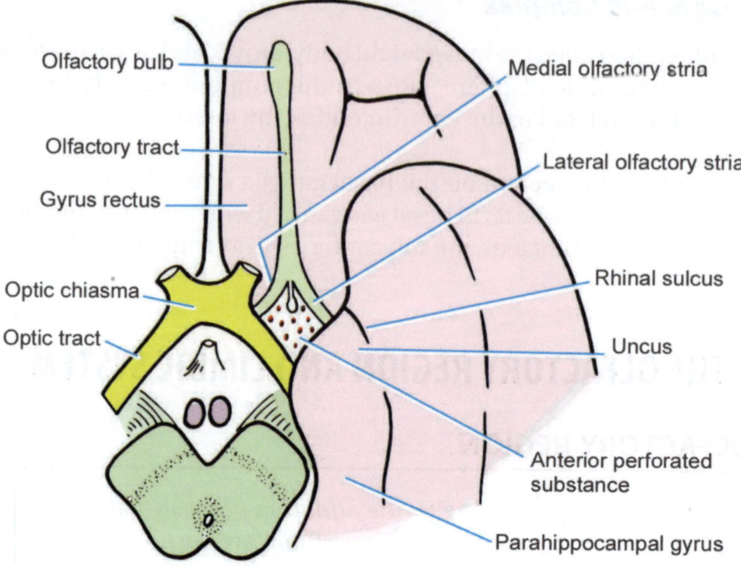

Fig. 21.13 Some structures related to the anterior part of the base of the brain.

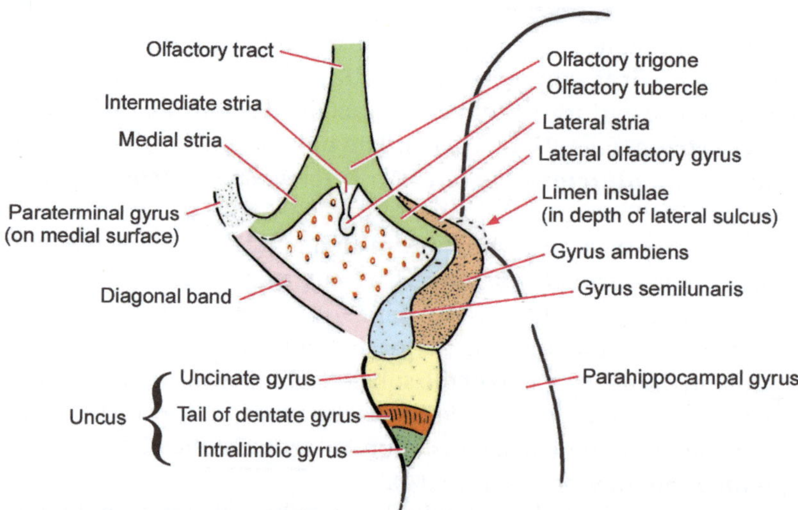

Fig. 21.14 Details of olfactory structures present in relation to the anterior perforated substance. Note the subdivisions of the uncus.

THE OLFACTORY PATHWAY

The fibres of the olfactory nerves are processes of ***olfactory receptor cells*** lying in the epithelium lining the olfactory mucosa (Fig. 21.15). These receptor cells are homologous to sensory neurons located in sensory ganglia. In other words,

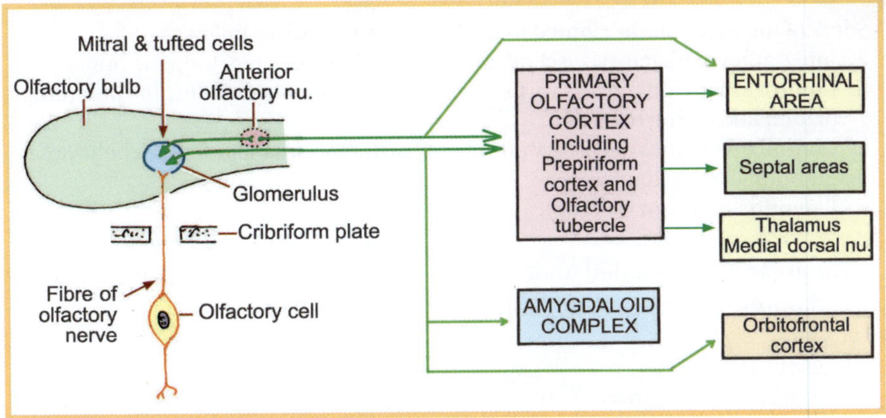

Fig. 21.15 Scheme to show the main features of the olfactory pathway.

the first order sensory neurons of the olfactory pathway are located within the olfactory epithelium itself.

Each receptor cell consists of a cell body and of two processes i.e., it is a bipolar cell. The peripheral process (dendrite) reaches the surface of the olfactory epithelium and ends in a small swelling. A number of cilia are attached to this swelling. The central process (axon) enters the submucosa, and forms one fibre of the olfactory nerve. The olfactory nerve fibres terminate in the olfactory bulb. Fibres arising in the olfactory bulb form the olfactory tract.

The fibres of the olfactory tract pass through the lateral olfactory stria to terminate in the anterior perforated substance and in some neighbouring areas that collectively constitute the ***primary olfactory cortex.*** Fibres arising in the primary cortex project to the entorhinal area. The entorhinal area is, therefore, called the ***secondary olfactory cortex.*** The sense of smell is believed to be perceived in both the primary and secondary olfactory cortex.

Some fibres of the olfactory tract, that pass through the medial stria, end in the anterior perforated substance. Others cross to the opposite side through the anterior commissure.

The primary olfactory cortex is connected to various other areas. In the past, many of these areas have been included under the term ***rhinencephalon*** or smell brain. It is now recognised, however, that although these areas might receive olfactory impulses their primary functions are not olfactory. Some of these areas and their connections are considered below as part of the limbic system.

THE LIMBIC SYSTEM

The term limbic system is applied to certain regions of the brain that are believed to play an important role in the control of visceral activity. Many of these areas have, in the past, been considered to have a predominantly olfactory function; but it is now realised that this is not so.

Some of the functions attributed to the limbic system are as follows.
a. Integration of olfactory, visceral, and somatic impulses reaching the brain.
b. Control of activities necessary for survival of the animal, including the procuring of food and eating behaviour.
c. Control of activities necessary for survival of the species including sex behaviour.
d. Emotional behaviour.
e. Retention of recent memory.

The areas to be included under the heading limbic system are not completely agreed upon. The most important of these are as follows.

1. Gyrus cinguli.
2. Entorhinal area (area 28), consisting of the anterior part of the parahippocampal gyrus, including the uncus.
3. Anterior perforated substance.
5. Prepiriform area consisting of the lateral olfactory gyrus and the gyrus ambiens (See Fig. 21.14).
6. Gyrus semilunaris (or periamygdaloid area) (Fig. 21.14).
7. Hippocampal formation including (a) the hippocampus, which is made up of the cornu ammonis and the dentate gyrus; and (b) the indusium griseum and smaller related structures.
8. Amygdaloid nuclear complex.
9. Septal region consisting of (a) the septal area (cortex); and (b) the septal nuclei (See below).
10. Olfactory nerves, bulb, tract, striae, trigone, tubercle; and the anterior olfactory nucleus.
11. Fornix, stria terminalis, stria medullaris thalami (or stria habenularis), diagonal band, and the anterior commissure.

The piriform lobe includes the prepiriform area, the entorhinal area, the lateral olfactory stria and the gyrus semilunaris.

In addition to the above, other regions that are included in the limbic system by some authorities are the hypothalamus and the reticular formation of the midbrain. The medial part of the thalamus, and the frontal cortex are closely related functionally to the limbic system.

Several of the above areas have been considered along with the olfactory pathway. The hypothalamus has already been considered. We shall now consider some other areas.

Amygdaloid Nuclear Complex

This region is also called the amygdaloid body or amygdala. It is situated near the temporal pole of the cerebral hemisphere in close relation to the anterior end of the inferior horn of the lateral ventricle. Superiorly, the complex is related to the anterior part of the lentiform nucleus. Inferiorly the complex is related to the gyrus semilunaris, the gyrus ambiens and the uncinate gyrus. Posteriorly, it becomes continuous with the tail of the caudate nucleus and with the stria terminalis (Fig. 21.11).

Stria Terminalis

This bundle of fibres is closely related to the inferior horn and central part of the lateral ventricle. It begins in the amygdaloid complex and runs backwards in the roof of the inferior horn. It then winds upwards and forwards to lie in the floor of the central part of the ventricle. Finally, it terminates near the interventricular foramen and anterior commissure by dividing into various smaller bundles. Throughout its course, it is closely related to the medial side of the caudate nucleus (Fig. 21.1). In the inferior horn it is related to the tail of this nucleus. In the central part of the ventricle it lies medial to the body of the caudate nucleus. Here the thalamus is medial to it.

Anterior Commissure

The anterior commissure is situated in the anterior wall of the third ventricle at the upper end of the lamina terminalis (Fig. 21.16).

When traced laterally, it divides into anterior and posterior bundles. Fibres passing through the commissure interconnect the regions of the two cerebral hemispheres concerned with the olfactory pathway.

Septal Region

This term is used to designate certain masses of grey matter that lie immediately anterior to the lamina terminalis and the anterior commissure (Fig. 21.16). The cerebral cortex of this region shows two small vertical sulci called the anterior and posterior ***parolfactory sulci.*** The region between the lamina terminalis and the posterior parolfactory sulcus is the ***paraterminal gyrus.*** The anterior part of this region which adjoins the posterior parolfactory sulcus is called the ***prehippocampal rudiment.*** The region between the anterior and posterior parolfactory sulci is the ***subcallosal area*** (or ***parolfactory gyrus***). The cortex of this region is referred to as the ***septal area*** in distinction to the ***septal nuclei*** which lie deep to the cortex.

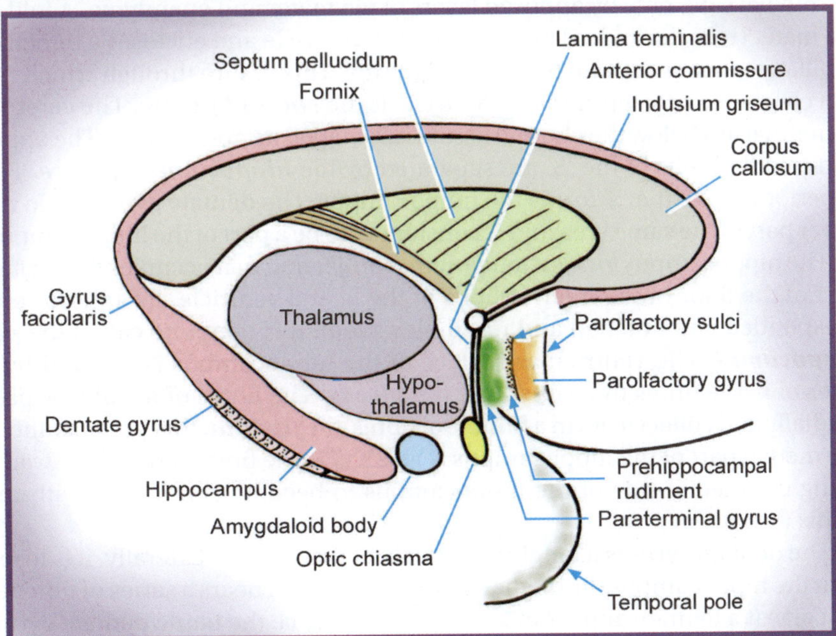

Fig. 21.16 The hippocampal formation and related structures. Note the positions of the parolfactory sulci and gyri.

Hippocampal Formation

In the human embryo, the hippocampal formation develops in relation to the medial surface of each cerebral hemisphere close to the choroid fissure of the lateral ventricle. It is at first approximately C-shaped in accordance with the outline of the body and inferior horn of the ventricle. The upper part of the formation is, however, separated from the ventricle because of the development of the corpus callosum between the two. For the same reason, this part of the formation remains underdeveloped and is represented by a thin layer of grey matter lining the upper surface of the corpus callosum. This layer is the ***indusium griseum.*** Within the indusium griseum are embedded two bundles of longitudinally running fibres called the ***medial and lateral longitudinal striae*** (on each side of the middle line). Posteriorly, the indusium griseum is continuous with a thin layer of grey matter related to the inferior aspect of the splenium of the corpus callosum. This grey matter is the ***splenial gyrus*** or ***gyrus faciolaris.*** The splenial gyrus runs forwards to become continuous with the ***dentate gyrus*** present in relation to the inferior horn of the lateral ventricle.

In the region of the inferior horn of the lateral ventricle, the developing hippocampus is pushed into the cavity of the ventricle because of the great development of the neighbouring neocortex. The hippocampal formation is best developed in this region and forms the ***hippocampus***: this term includes the dentate gyrus.

Several subdivisions of the region are described. These are shown in Fig. 21.17 which represents a coronal section through the inferior horn of the lateral ventricle. In this figure note that the cavity of the inferior horn is closed, on the medial side, only by apposed layers of pia mater and ependyma. A fold of pia mater (tela choroidea) projects into the ventricle and encloses a bunch of capillaries that constitute the choroid plexus. This fissure through which the tela choroidea projects into the ventricle is the ***choroid fissure.*** The cerebral cortex that lies below the choroid fissure is S-shaped in cross section. The upper and middle limbs of the 'S' are separated by the ***hippocampal fissure.*** The superior limb of the 'S' forms the hippocampus. The dentate gyrus lies in the lower part of the same area and is considered to be a part of the hippocampus.

The hippocampus forms a longitudinal projection that occupies the greater part of the floor of the inferior horn of the lateral ventricle. Its anterior end is expanded and notched and resembles a foot. It is therefore called the ***pes hippocampi.*** The ventricular surface of the hippocampus is covered by a layer of nerve fibres that constitute the ***alveus.*** The fibres of the alveus pass medially and collect to form a bundle of fibres, the ***fimbria,*** that projects above the medial part of the hippocampus (Fig. 21.17). The fimbria runs backwards along the medial side of the hippocampus to become continuous with the fornix (see below).

The dentate gyrus is a longitudinal strip of grey matter. Laterally, it is fused with the hippocampus. Its medial margin is free, and bears a series of notches that give it a dentate appearance (Fig. 21.17): hence the name dentate gyrus. When traced anteriorly the dentate gyrus runs medially across the inferior

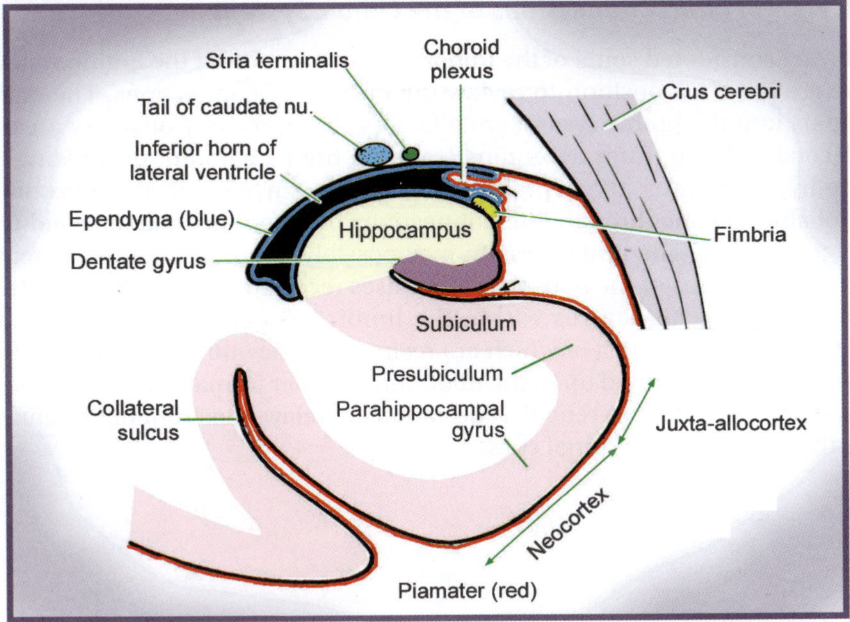

Fig. 21.17 Coronal section through the cerebral hemisphere in the region of the inferior horn of the lateral ventricle to show the hippocampus and related structures. C = choroid fissure. H = hippocampal fissure.

surface of the uncus. This part is called the ***tail of the dentate gyrus*** (Fig. 21.14). As stated above the posterior end of the dentate gyrus is continuous with the splenial gyrus (gyrus faciolaris) (Fig. 21.16). Because of its close relationship to the dentate gyrus the uncus is sometimes regarded as part of the hippocampal formation.

The Fornix

The fornix is a prominent bundle of fibres seen on the medial aspect of the cerebral hemisphere. It is made up, predominantly, of fibres arising in the hippocampus. The ***body*** of the fornix is suspended from the corpus callosum by the septum pellucidum (Figs. 21.1, 18.20) and comes into close relationship with the tela choroidea in the roof of the third ventricle. When traced posteriorly, the body of the fornix divides into two parts called ***crura.*** Each crus of the fornix becomes continuous with the fimbria of the corresponding side. The two crura are interconnected by fibres passing from one to the other. These crossing fibres constitute the ***hippocampal commissure*** or ***commissure of the fornix.*** The anterior end of the body of the fornix also divides into right and left halves called the ***columns*** of the fornix. Each column turns downwards just in front of the interventricular foramen and passes through the hypothalamus to reach the mamillary body.

Review of Main Connections of the Limbic System

Having considered some of the important components of the limbic system we are now in a position to review the major interconnections. The main inputs into the limbic system are olfactory (from primary olfactory areas); visceral through fibres ascending from the brainstem and terminating in the hypothalamus, the septal region and the amygdaloid complex; and probably somatic through interconnections between the thalamus and the hypothalamus. The limbic system may possibly be influenced by afferents from some areas of the neocortex. Impulses received from all these centres can spread to all centres within the limbic system through numerous interconnections, most of which are reciprocal. The output from the limbic system is concentrated upon the midbrain reticular formation. These inputs reaching the midbrain reticular formation are relayed to autonomic centres in the brainstem and spinal cord.

CHAPTER

22

Internal Capsule Commissures of the Brain

THE INTERNAL CAPSULE

A preliminary description of the internal capsule is given on page 497. This should be read before studying the details of the fibres passing through the capsule.

The fibres passing through the capsule may be ascending (to the cerebral cortex) or descending (from the cortex). The arrangement of fibres is easily remembered if it is realised that any group of fibres within the capsule takes ***the most direct path*** to its destination. Thus fibres to and from the anterior part of the frontal lobe pass through the anterior limb of the internal capsule. Those to and from the posterior part of the frontal lobe, and from the greater part of the parietal lobe, occupy the genu and posterior limb of the capsule. Fibres to and from the temporal lobe occupy the sublentiform part (Fig. 22.3), while those to and from the occipital lobe pass through the retrolentiform part. Some fibres from the lowest parts of the parietal lobe accompany the temporal fibres through the sublentiform part.

Ascending Fibres

These are predominantly ***thalamocortical fibres*** which go from the thalamus to all parts of the cerebral cortex (Figs. 22.1, 22.2B).

Fibres to the frontal lobe constitute the ***anterior thalamic radiation*** (or ***frontal thalamic peduncle***). They pass through the anterior limb of the internal capsule. The anterior thalamic radiation also carries fibres from the hypothalamus and limbic structures to the frontal lobe.

Fibres travelling from the ventral posterior nuclei of the thalamus to the somatosensory area (in the postcentral gyrus) constitute the ***superior thalamic radiation*** (or the ***superior, or dorsal, thalamic peduncle***). These fibres occupy the genu and posterior limb of the capsule. It should be noted that these fibres are third order sensory neurons responsible for conveying somesthetic sensations to the cerebral cortex. The superior thalamic radiation also contains some fibres that go from the thalamus to parts of the frontal and parietal lobes adjoining the postcentral gyrus.

Fibres from the thalamus to the occipital lobe constitute the ***posterior thalamic radiation*** (or the ***posterior, or caudal, thalamic peduncle***). This includes the ***optic radiation*** from the lateral geniculate body to the visual cortex. These radiations lie in the retrolentiform part of the internal capsule. The retrolentiform part also contains some fibres passing from the thalamus to the posterior part of the parietal lobe.

Fibres from the thalamus to the temporal lobe constitute the ***inferior thalamic radiation*** (or ***ventral thalamic peduncle).*** It includes the ***acoustic radiation*** from the medial geniculate body to the acoustic area of the cerebral cortex. These fibres pass through the sublentiform part of the internal capsule.

Descending Fibres

1. ***Corticospinal and corticonuclear fibres***

Corticonuclear fibres (for motor cranial nerve nuclei) pass through the genu of the internal capsule (Figs. 22.1, 22.2A).

Corticospinal fibres form several discrete bundles in the posterior limb. The fibres for the upper limb are most anterior, followed (in that order) by fibres for the trunk and lower limb.

2. ***Corticopontine fibres***

Frontopontine fibres are the most numerous. They pass through the anterior limb, genu, and posterior limb of the internal capsule.

Parietopontine fibres pass mainly through the retrolentiform part. Some fibres pass through the sublentiform part.

Temporopontine fibres pass through the sublentiform part (Fig. 22.3).

Occipitopontine fibres pass through the retrolentiform part.

3. ***Corticothalamic fibres***

These pass from various parts of the cerebral cortex to the thalamus. They form part of the thalamic radiations described above.

4. ***Fibres from Cerebral Cortex to Brainstem nuclei***

   a. ***Corticonuclear*** fibres to cranial nerve nuclei have been mentioned above.
   b. ***Corticorubral fibres*** pass through the posterior limb.
   c. ***Corticoreticular fibres*** pass through the genu and posterior limb.
   d. ***Occipitotectal fibres*** pass through the retrolentiform part.

5. ***Fibres of the subthalamic fasciculus***

These pass transversely through the posterior limb (intersecting the vertically running fibres). The fibres of this fasciculus connect the subthalamic nucleus to the globus pallidus

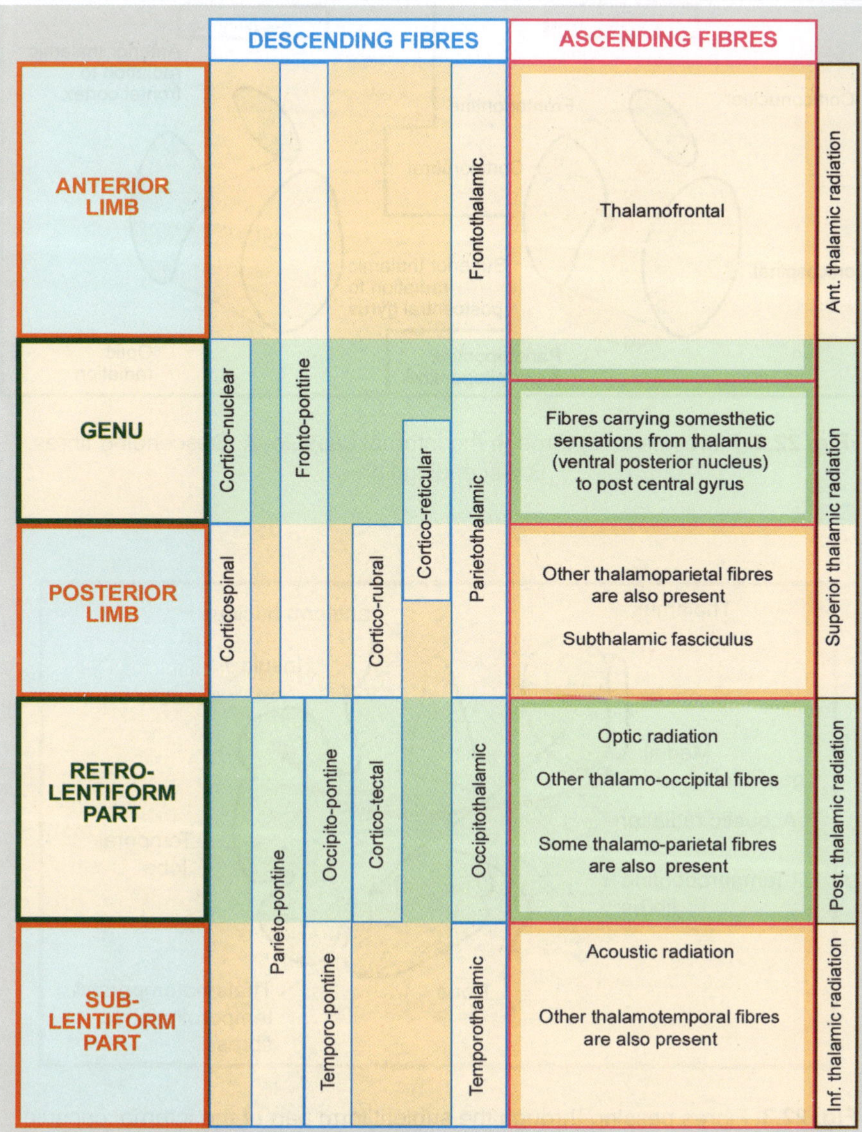

Fig. 22.1 Scheme to show the fibres passing through the internal capsule.

COMMISSURES OF THE BRAIN

The two halves of the brain and spinal cord are interconnected by numerous fibres that cross the middle line. In some situations such fibres form recognisable bundles that are called commissures. Strictly speaking commissural fibres are those that connect corresponding regions of the two sides. Many of the fibres passing through the so-called commissures do not fulfil this criterion as they connect different regions of the two sides. Such fibres are really association

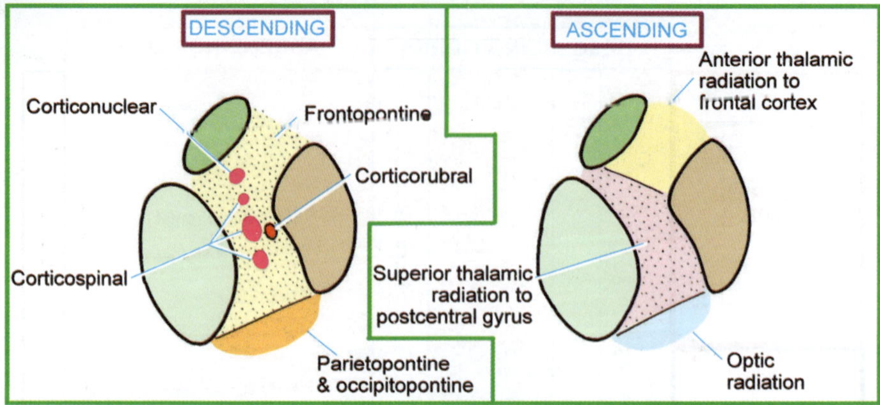

Fig. 22.2 Fibres passing through the internal capsule. A. Descending fibres. B. Ascending fibres.

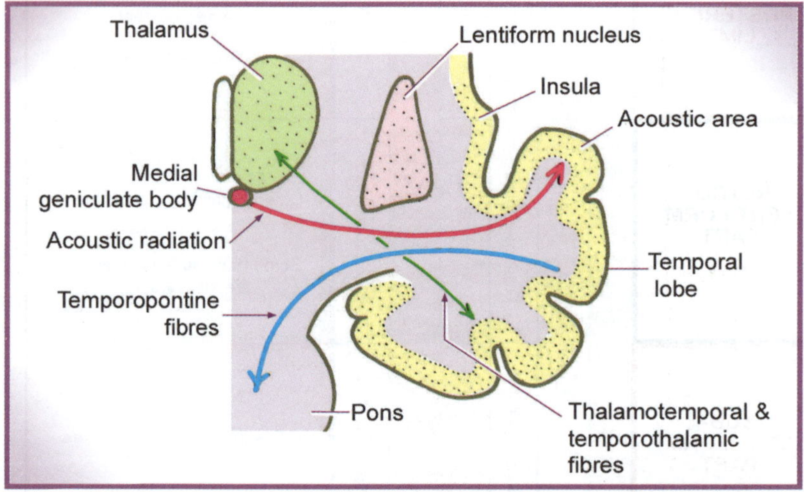

Fig. 22.3 Fibres passing through the sublentiform part of the internal capsule.

fibres. We have seen that several tracts passing through the spinal cord and brainstem cross from one side to the other. These crossings are ***decussations***, but collections of such fibres are sometimes loosely referred to as commissures e.g., the ventral white commissure of the spinal cord.

The Corpus Callosum

The corpus callosum is the largest commissure connecting the right and left cerebral hemispheres. It has been described on page 498.

The fibres passing through the corpus callosum are generally believed to interconnect corresponding regions of the entire neocortex of the right and left sides.

Other Commissures

Other commissures connecting the two cerebral hemispheres are the ***anterior commissure***, the ***posterior commissure***, the ***hippocampal commissure*** or commissure of the fornix and the ***habenular commissure***.

In close relationship to the optic chiasma a number of commissures carrying fibres not concerned with vision are described. These include the ***ventral supraoptic commissure*** (of Gudden), the ***dorsal supraoptic commissure*** (of Meynert) and the ***anterior hypothalamic commissure*** (of Ganser). The constitution of these commissures is controversial and will not be considered.

CHAPTER
23

Pathways for Special Senses

In this chapter we will consider the pathways responsible for perception of the special senses of vision, smell, taste, and hearing. In considering each pathway we have to consider (a) the peripheral organ concerned, (b) pathways through the cranial nerves, and (c) centres and pathways within the central nervous system.

VISUAL PATHWAY

1. The peripheral organ for sight is the eyeball. It has been described in Chapter 10.
2. We have seen that receptors for vision are the rods and cones located in the retina. It may be repeated here that the rods and cones are modified neurons. They give off central processes that synapse with peripheral processes of bipolar cells. The central processes of bipolar cells synapse with the dendrites of ganglion cells. Axons arising from ganglion cells form the fibres of the optic nerve.
   We may also recall that opposite the posterior pole of the eyeball the retina shows a ***central region*** about 6 mm in diameter. This region is responsible for sharp vision. In the centre of this region an area about 2 mm in diameter has a yellow colour and is called the ***macula lutea***. The fovea centralis is a depression in the centre of the macula and is 0.4 mm in diameter.
3. Visual impulses arising in the retina are carried to the brain through the optic nerve. The anatomy of the optic nerve and the main features of the visual pathway have been described in Chapter 9. We have seen that the optic nerves enter the cranial cavity through the optic canal and join each other to form the optic chiasma (Fig. 23.1). Many fibres of each optic nerve cross to the opposite side through the chiasma. The uncrossed fibres, along with those that have crossed over from the opposite side, form the optic tract. The optic tract terminates predominantly in the lateral geniculate body. Fresh fibres arising in the lateral geniculate body form the geniculocalcarine tract (or optic radiation) which ends in the visual areas of the cerebral cortex.

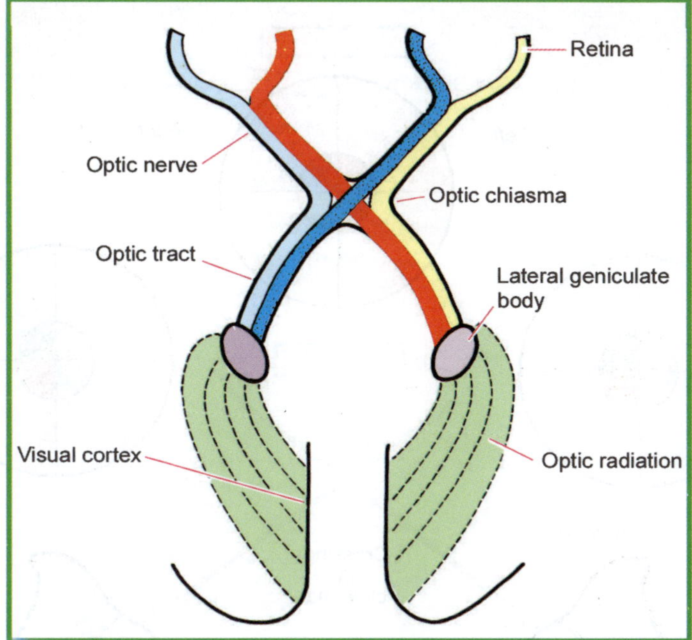

Fig. 23.1 The optic pathway. Note that the fibres from the medial (or nasal) half of each retina cross to the optic tract of the opposite side.

The Visual Field and Retinal Quadrants

When the head and eyes are maintained in a fixed position, and one eye is closed, the area seen by that eye constitutes the visual field for that eye. Now if the other eye is also opened the area seen is more or less the same as was seen with one eye. In other words the visual fields of the two eyes overlap to a very great extent. On either side, however, there is a small area seen only by the eye of that side. Although the two eyes view the same area, the relative position of objects within the area appears somewhat dissimilar to the two eyes as they view the object from slightly different angles. The difference though slight, is of considerable importance as it forms the basis for the perception of depth (***stereoscopic vision***).

For convenience of description, the visual field is divided into right and left halves. It may also be divided into upper and lower halves so that the visual field can be said to consist of four quadrants (Fig. 23.2). In a similar manner each retina can also be divided into quadrants. Images of objects in the field of vision are formed on the retina by the lens of the eyeball. As with any convex lens the image is inverted. If an object is placed in the ***right*** half of the field of vision its image is formed on the ***left*** half of the retina and ***vice versa.*** Unfortunately, instead of using the words right and left, the two halves of the retina are usually referred to as ***nasal*** (= medial) and ***temporal*** (= lateral) halves. This introduces a complication as the left half of the left eye is the temporal half, while in the

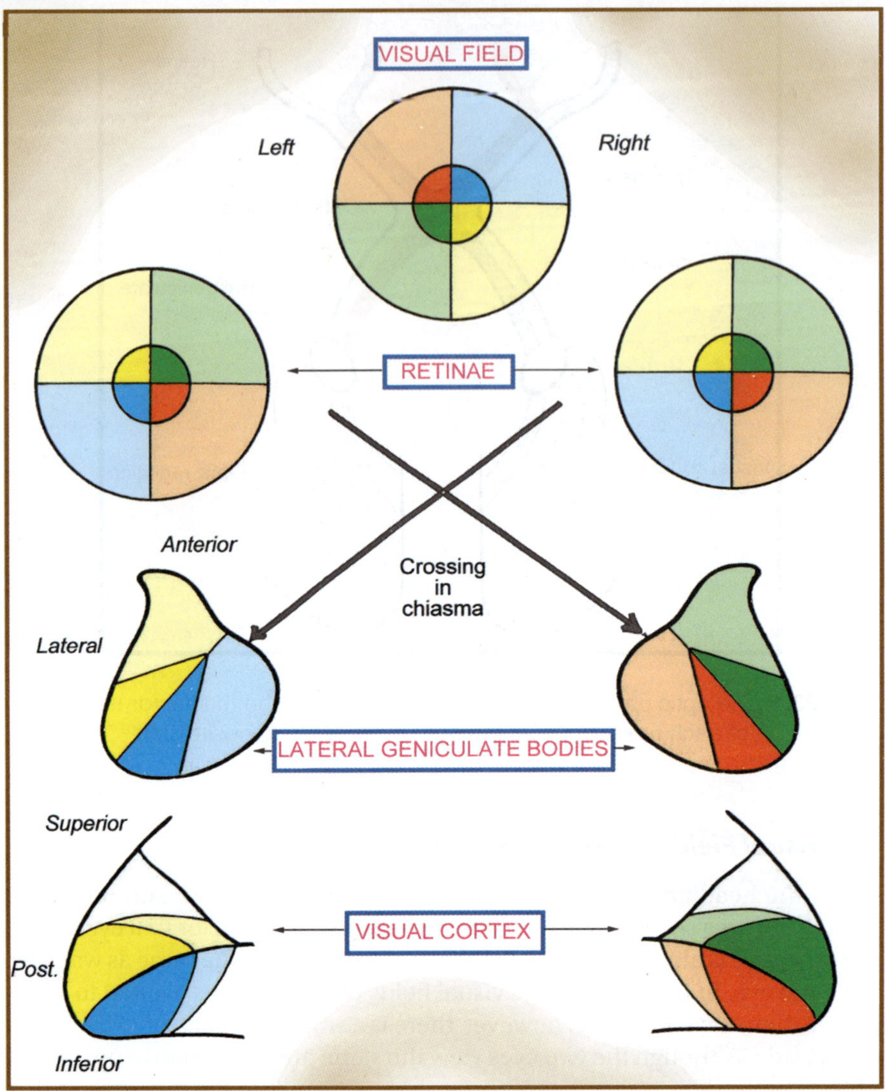

Fig. 23.2 Scheme to show the representation of the visual field in the retinae, the lateral geniculate bodies, and the visual cortex of the two sides. The retinal quadrants for the peripheral parts of the field of vision are shown in light colour, while the corresponding macular areas are shown in dark colour.

case of the right eye it is the nasal half. Thus the image of an object placed in the right half of the field of vision falls on the temporal half of the left retina, and on the nasal half of the right retina.

Optic Nerve, Optic Chiasma and Optic Tract

The optic nerve is made up of axons of the ganglion cells of the retina. These axons are at first unmyelinated. After passing through the sclera (in the region of the lamina cribrosa) each fibre acquires a myelin sheath. The fibres of the nerve arising from the four quadrants of the retina maintain the same relative position within the nerve. The fibres arising from the macula are numerous and form the ***papillomacular bundle***. Close to the eyeball, the macular fibres occupy the lateral part of the nerve, but by the time they reach the chiasma they lie in the central part of the nerve.

The fibres of the optic nerve arising in the nasal half of each retina enter the optic tract of the opposite side after crossing in the chiasma. Fibres from the temporal half of each retina enter the optic tract of the same side (Fig. 23.1). Thus the right optic tract comes to contain fibres from the right halves of both retinae, and the left tract from the left halves. In other words, all optic nerve fibres carrying impulses relating to the left half of the field of vision are brought together in the right optic tract and ***vice versa***. We have already noted that each optic tract carries these fibres to the lateral geniculate body of the corresponding side.

The Lateral Geniculate Body

Some aspects of the structure of the lateral geniculate body have been considered on page 536.

Sections through the lateral geniculate body show that its grey matter is split into six laminae. These layers are numbered one to six from ventral to dorsal side. Fibres from the eye of the same side end in laminae 2, 3, and 5; while those from the opposite eye end in laminae 1, 4, and 6. The macular fibres end in the central and posterior part of the lateral geniculate body, and this area is relatively large (Fig. 23.2). Fibres from the peripheral parts of the retina end in the anterior part of the lateral geniculate body. The upper half of the retina is represented laterally, and the lower half of the retina is represented medially. Specific points on the retina project to specific points in the lateral geniculate body. In turn, specific points of this body project to specific points in the visual cortex. In this way a point to point relationship is maintained between the retinae and the visual cortex.

Geniculocalcarine Tract and Visual Cortex

Fibres arising from cells of the lateral geniculate body constitute the ***geniculocalcarine tract*** *or* ***optic radiation.*** These fibres pass through the retrolentiform part of the internal capsule. The optic radiation ends in the visual areas of the cerebral cortex (areas 17, 18, 19) (Fig. 18.24).

The cortex of each hemisphere receives impulses from the retinal halves of the same side (i.e., from the opposite half of the field of vision). The upper quadrants of the retina are represented above the calcarine sulcus, and the lower quadrants below it (Fig. 23.2). The cortical area for the macula is larger than that for peripheral areas. It occupies the posterior part of the visual area. The cortical area for the peripheral part of the retina is situated anterior to the area for the macula.

Applied Anatomy of the Visual Pathway

Effects of injury to the visual pathway are considered on page 417. For relationship to an enlarged hypophysis cerebri see page 373.

PATHWAY FOR SMELL

The peripheral organ for smell is the olfactory mucosa, and the cranial nerve concerned is the olfactory nerve.

A complete description of olfactory pathways is given in Chapter 21.

PATHWAY FOR HEARING

The peripheral organ for hearing is the ear which is described in Chapter 10.

We have seen that sound waves travelling through air enter the external acoustic meatus and produce vibrations in the tympanic membrane. These vibrations are transmitted through the chain of ossicles present in the middle ear to reach the internal ear. Pressure waves set up in the perilymph reach the spiral organ (of Corti) present in intimate relationship to the cochlea. Hair cells present in the spiral organ convert these vibrations into nervous impulses.

The first neurons of the pathway of hearing are located in the spiral ganglion located in a bony tunnel running along the cochlea. These neurons are bipolar. Peripheral processes of neurons lying in this ganglion innervate the hair cells of the spiral organ. The central processes of the neurons form the cochlear nerve. The fibres of the cochlear nerve terminate in the dorsal and ventral cochlear nuclei (Figs. 9.72, 9.73, 16.8B, 23.3). The neurons in these nuclei are, therefore, second order neurons. Their axons pass medially in the dorsal part of the pons. Most of them cross to the opposite side, but some remain uncrossed (Fig. 23.3). The crossing fibres of the two sides form a conspicuous mass of fibres called the ***trapezoid body*** (Figs. 16.8 A, B).

The large majority of fibres from the cochlear nuclei terminate in the superior olivary complex (made up of a number of nuclei). Third order neurons arising in this complex form an important ascending bundle called the ***lateral lemniscus*** (Figs. 16.8 A, B, 16.9B). Some cochlear fibres that do not relay in the superior olivary nucleus join the lemniscus after relaying in scattered cells lying within the trapezoid body: these cells constitute the ***trapezoid nucleus (nucleus of the trapezoid body).*** Still other cochlear fibres relay in cells that lie within the lemniscus itself: these neurons form the ***nucleus of the lateral lemniscus.***

The fibres of the lateral lemniscus ascend to the midbrain and terminate in the inferior colliculus (Figs. 16.9B, 23.3). Fibres arising in the colliculus enter the inferior brachium to reach the medial geniculate body. Some fibres in the lemniscus reach this body without relay in the inferior colliculus. Fibres arising in the medial geniculate body form the ***acoustic radiation*** which ends in the acoustic area of the cerebral cortex. It may be stressed that each lateral lemniscus carries impulses arising in both the right and left cochleae.

The medial and lateral geniculate bodies are described in Chapter 21.

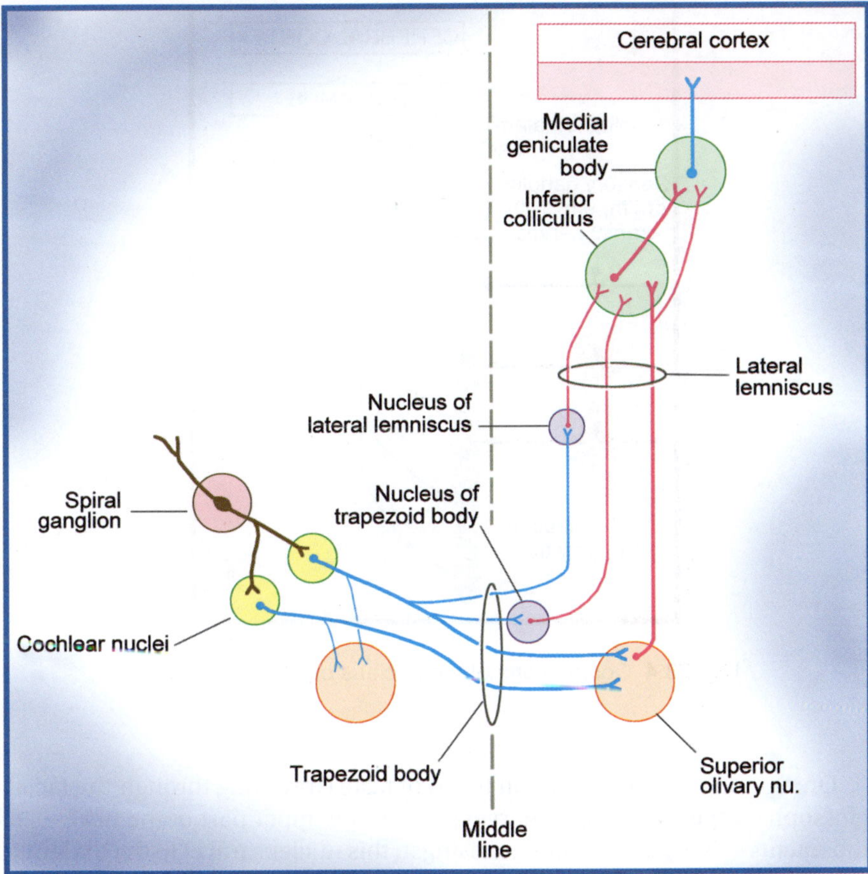

Fig. 23.3 Scheme to show the pathway for hearing.

PATHWAYS FOR TASTE

The end organs for taste are taste buds located mainly on the tongue. They are most numerous in relation to vallate papillae. Some taste buds are present in the mucosa of the soft palate, and of the epiglottis. Sensations of taste arising in the taste buds travel through a number of different pathways as follows.

1. Sensations of taste from the anterior two-thirds of the tongue (the part of the tongue lying anterior to the sulcus terminalis, but excluding the vallate papillae) travel through the lingual nerve, the chorda tympani and the facial nerve.
2. Sensations of taste from the posterior one third of the tongue (part of the tongue posterior to the sulcus terminalis, and including the vallate papillae) are carried by the glossopharyngeal nerve.
3. Taste fibres from the posteriormost part of the tongue (just in front of the epiglottis), and from taste buds on the epiglottis, are carried by the superior laryngeal branch of the vagus nerve.
4. The course of taste fibres from the soft palate is shown in Fig. 9.76.

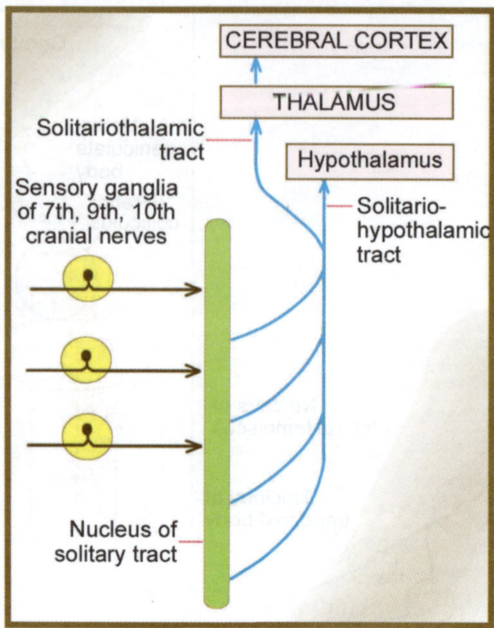

Fig. 23.4 Connections of the nucleus of the solitary tract.

On entering the brainstem all fibres of taste (travelling through the facial, glossopharyngeal and vagus nerves) end in the upper part of the nucleus of the tractus solitarius. New fibres arising in this nucleus travel to the thalamus through the solitario-thalamic tract (Fig. 23.4). The fibres reach the ventral posteromedial nucleus of the thalamus. From here they are relayed to the cerebral cortex (areas 3, 2, 1). The fibres form part of the superior thalamic radiation passing through the posterior limb of the internal capsule.

CHAPTER

24

The Ventricles of the Brain and Cerebrospinal Fluid

The interior of the brain contains a series of cavities (Fig. 24.1). The cerebrum contains a median cavity, the ***third ventricle***; and two ***lateral ventricles***, one in each hemisphere. Each lateral ventricle opens into the third ventricle through an ***interventricular foramen***. The third ventricle is continuous, caudally, with the ***cerebral aqueduct*** which traverses the midbrain and opens into the fourth ventricle. The ***fourth ventricle*** is situated dorsal to the pons and medulla, and ventral to the cerebellum. It communicates, inferiorly, with the ***central canal*** which traverses the lower part of the medulla and the spinal cord. The entire ventricular system is lined by an epithelial layer called the ***ependyma.***

THE LATERAL VENTRICLES

The lateral ventricles are two cavities, one situated within each cerebral hemisphere. Each ventricle consists of a central part which gives off three extensions called the anterior, posterior and inferior horns (Fig. 24.1).

The Central Part

The central part of the lateral ventricle is elongated anteroposteriorly. Anteriorly, it becomes continuous with the anterior horn, at the level of the interventricular foramen. Posteriorly, the central part reaches the splenium of the corpus callosum. The central part is triangular in cross section (Fig. 24.2). It has a roof, a floor, and a medial wall. The roof and floor meet on the lateral side.

The ***roof*** is formed by the trunk of the corpus callosum. The ***medial wall*** is formed by the septum pellucidum and by the body of the fornix. It is common to the two lateral ventricles. The ***floor*** is formed mainly by the superior surface of the thalamus (medially), and by the caudate nucleus (laterally). Between these two structures there are the stria terminalis (laterally) and the thalamostriate vein (medially).

From Fig. 24.2 it will be seen that there is a space between the fornix and the upper surface of the thalamus. This is the ***choroid fissure.*** A fold of pia

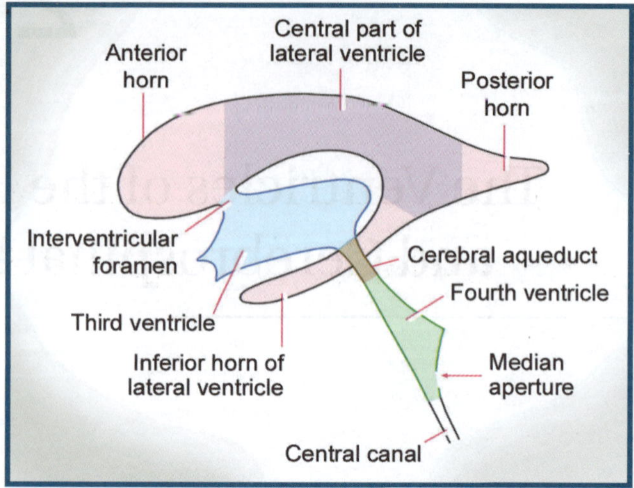

Fig. 24.1 The ventricular system of the brain. Lateral view.

mater, the ***tela choroidea***, invaginates into the ventricle through the fissure and covers part of the thalamus. The tela choroidea is common to the two lateral ventricles, and to the third ventricle. Within each lateral edge of the tela choroidea there are plexuses of blood vessels that constitute the ***choroid plexus*** (Figs. 24.2, 24.7). The tela choroidea and other structures forming the walls of the ventricle are lined by ependyma.

The Anterior Horn

The anterior horn of the lateral ventricle, lies anterior to its central part, the two being separated by an imaginary vertical line drawn at the level of the interventricular foramen (Fig. 24.1). This horn is triangular in section. It has a roof, a floor and a medial wall (Fig. 24.3). It is closed, anteriorly, by the genu and rostrum of the corpus callosum.

The ***roof*** is formed by the most anterior part of the trunk of the corpus callosum. The floor is formed mainly by the head of the caudate nucleus. A small part of the floor, near the middle line, is formed by the upper surface of the rostrum of the corpus callosum. The ***medial wall*** (common to the two sides) is formed by the septum pellucidum. It may be noted that the tela choroidea and the choroid plexus ***do not*** extend into the anterior horn.

The Posterior Horn

The posterior horn of the lateral ventricle extends backwards into the occipital lobe. It has a roof, a lateral wall, and a medial wall (Fig. 24.4). The ***roof*** and ***lateral wall*** are formed by the tapetum. The ***medial wall*** shows two elevations. The upper of these is the ***bulb of the posterior horn***, which is produced by fibres of the forceps major as they run backwards from the splenium of the

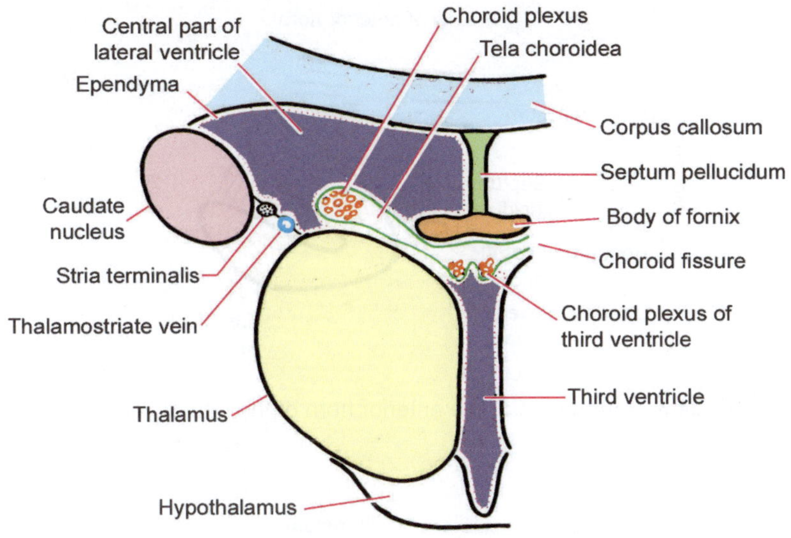

Fig. 24.2 Boundaries of the central part of the lateral ventricle and of the third ventricle. Note the relationship of the tela choroidea and choroid plexuses to these ventricles.

corpus callosum. The lower elevation is called the ***calcar avis***. It represents white matter 'pushed in' by formation of the calcarine sulcus.

The Inferior Horn

The inferior horn of the lateral ventricle begins at the posterior end of the central part. It runs downwards and forwards into the temporal lobe, its anterior end reaching close to the uncus. In considering the structures to be seen in the walls of the inferior horn it is useful to note that the anterior horn, the central part, and the inferior horn form one continuous C-shaped cavity. From Fig. 24.1 it will be obvious that the floor of the central part of the ventricle is continuous with the roof of the inferior horn. It is also useful to recall that the body of the fornix divides, posteriorly, into two crura which become continuous with the fimbria and hippocampus.

In the central part of the ventricle, the choroid fissure lies below the fornix. When traced into the inferior horn, the fissure lies ***above*** the fimbria and hippocampus. The choroid plexus extends into the inferior horn through the choroid fissure.

In cross section, the inferior horn is seen to have a narrow cavity (Fig. 24.5). The cavity is bounded above, and laterally, by the ***roof***; and below, and medially, by the ***floor.*** (Because of this orientation the lateral part of the roof is sometimes called the ***lateral wall,*** and the medial part of the floor is called the ***medial wall***).

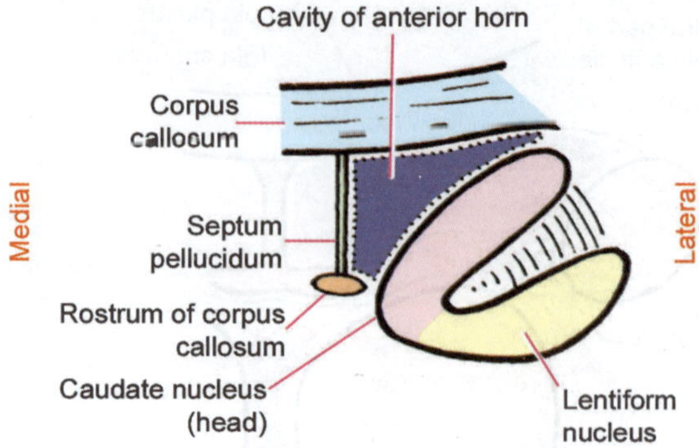

Fig. 24.3 Boundaries of the anterior horn of the lateral ventricle.

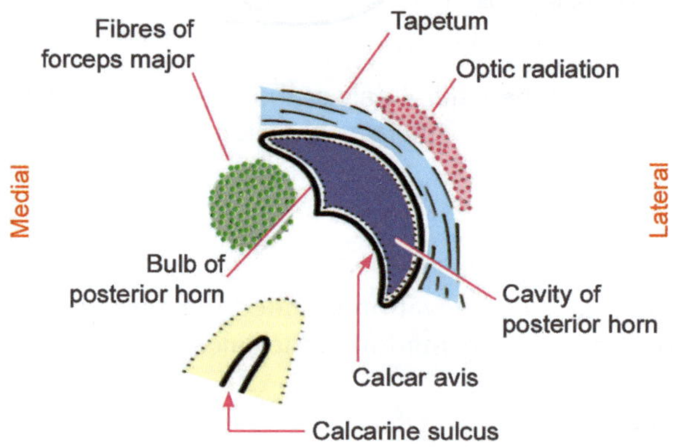

Fig. 24.4 Boundaries of the posterior horn of the lateral ventricle.

The lateral part of the roof (or lateral wall) is formed by fibres of the tapetum. The medial part of the roof is formed by the tail of the caudate nucleus (laterally) and the stria terminalis (medially). These structures are continued into the roof of the inferior horn from the floor of the central part. Anteriorly, the tail of the caudate nucleus and the stria terminalis end in relation to the amygdaloid complex, which lies in the most anterior part of the roof. The floor of the inferior horn is formed mainly by the hippocampus, along with the alveus and fimbria. In the lateral part of the floor there is an elevation, the ***collateral eminence***, produced by inward bulging of the white matter which lies deep to the collateral sulcus.

THE THIRD VENTRICLE

The third ventricle is the cavity of the diencephalon. It is a median cavity situated between the right and left thalami (Fig. 24.2). It communicates, on

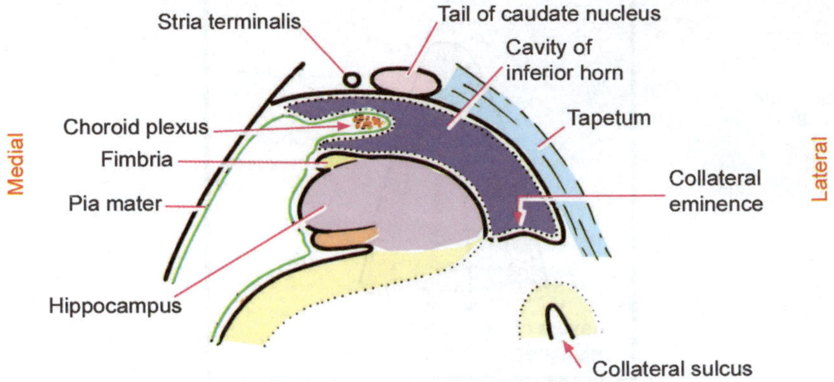

Fig. 24.5 Boundaries of the inferior horn of the lateral ventricle.

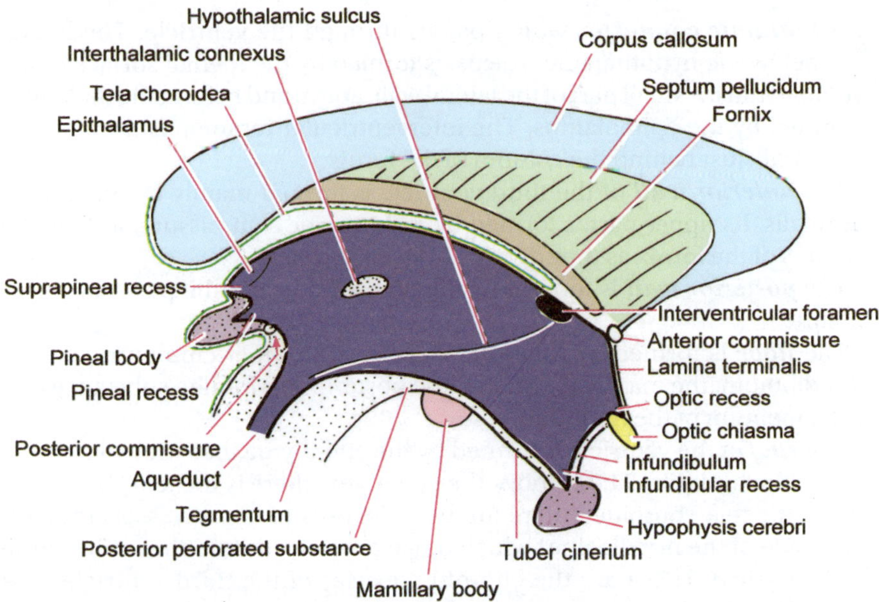

Fig. 24.6 Boundaries and recesses of the third ventricle. Note the mode of formation of the tela choroidea that lies in the roof of the ventricle.

either side, with the lateral ventricle through the interventricular foramen (Figs. 24.1, 24.6). Posteriorly, it continues into the cerebral aqueduct which connects it to the fourth ventricle. The ventricle has two lateral walls, an anterior wall, a posterior wall, a floor and a roof.

Each ***lateral wall*** is marked by the ***hypothalamic sulcus*** (Fig. 24.6) which follows a curved course from the interventricular foramen to the aqueduct. Above the sulcus, the wall is formed by the medial surface of the thalamus. The two thalami are usually connected by a band of grey matter called the

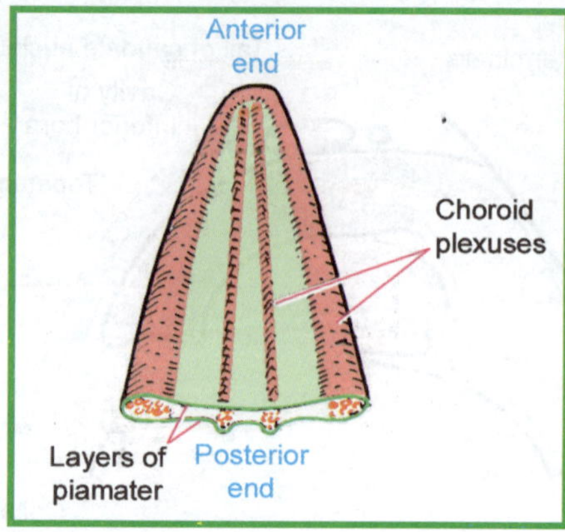

Fig. 24.7 Tela choroidea removed and viewed from above.

interthalamic connexus, which passes through the ventricle. The lateral wall, below the hypothalamic sulcus, is formed by the medial surface of the hypothalamus. A small part of the lateral wall, above and behind the thalamus, is formed by the epithalamus. The interventricular foramen is seen on the lateral wall, just behind the column of the fornix.

The ***anterior wall*** of the third ventricle is formed mainly by the lamina terminalis. Its upper part is formed by the anterior commissure, and by the columns of the fornix as they diverge from each other.

The ***posterior wall*** is formed by the pineal body and the posterior commissure.

The ***floor*** is formed by the optic chiasma, the tuber cinereum and the infundibulum, the mamillary bodies, the posterior perforated substance and the tegmentum of the midbrain.

The ***roof*** of the ventricle is formed by the ependyma that stretches across the two thalami (Fig. 24.2). Above the ependyma there is the tela choroidea. Within the tela choroidea there are two plexuses of blood vessels (one on either side of the middle line) which bulge downwards into the cavity of the third ventricle. These are the choroid plexuses of the third ventricle (See below) (Fig. 24.7).

The cavity of the third ventricle shows a number of prolongations or recesses (Fig. 24.6). The ***infundibular recess*** extends into the infundibulum. The ***optic recess*** lies just above the optic chiasma. The ***pineal recess*** lies between the superior and inferior laminae of the stalk of the pineal body. The ***suprapineal recess*** lies above the pineal body in relation to the epithalamus.

Tela Choroidea of the Third and Lateral Ventricles

The tela choroidea is a double layered fold of pia mater that occupies the interval between the splenium of the corpus callosum and fornix, above, and the two thalami below.

It is triangular in shape (Fig. 24.7). Its posterior end is broad and lies in the gap between the splenium (above) and the posterior part of the roof of the third ventricle (below) (Fig. 24.6). This gap is called the ***transverse fissure***. The anterior end (representing the apex of the triangle) lies near the right and left interventricular foramina. The median part of the tela choroidea lies on the roof of the third ventricle. Its right and left lateral edges project into the central parts of the corresponding lateral ventricles (Fig. 24.2). When traced posteriorly, the two layers of pia mater forming the tela choroidea separate. The upper layer curves upwards over the posterior aspect of the splenium. The lower layer turns downwards over the pineal body and tectum (Fig. 24.6).

Choroid Plexuses

The choroid plexuses are highly vascular structures that are responsible for the formation of cerebrospinal fluid.

The surface of each plexus is lined by a membrane formed by fusion of the ventricular ependyma with the pia mater of the tela choroidea. Deep to this membrane there is a plexus of blood vessels. Microscopic examination shows that the surface of the choroid plexus has numerous villous processes. Each process contains a plexus of capillaries that are connected to afferent and efferent vessels. Because of the presence of these processes the surface area of the choroid plexuses is considerable. It is further increased by the presence of microvilli (seen with the EM) present on the ependymal cells.

Four choroid plexuses are to be seen in relation to the tela choroidea of the third and lateral ventricles (Fig. 24.7). Two of these (one right and one left) lie along the corresponding lateral margins, and project into the central part of the corresponding lateral ventricle. Two other plexuses run parallel to each other, one on either side of the middle line. These are the choroid plexuses of the third ventricle. At each posterolateral angle of the tela choroidea the choroid plexus of the lateral ventricle continues into the inferior horn. The pial covering for this part of the plexus is provided by simple invagination of the pia, covering the medial aspect of the hemisphere, through the inferior part of the choroid fissure.

The tela choroidea and choroid plexuses of the fourth ventricle are considered later in this Chapter.

THE FOURTH VENTRICLE

For a proper understanding of the anatomy of the fourth ventricle, it is necessary that some features of the gross anatomy of the cerebellum and of related structures be clearly understood. Reference to Fig. 24.8 will show that the cerebellum is intimately related to the ventricle. The upper part of the ventricle is related to the ***superior medullary velum.*** When traced inferiorly (and posteriorly) the velum merges into the white matter of the cerebellum. The lower part of the ventricle is related to the nodule (Figs. 24.8, 24.9A). It will be recalled that the nodule forms the most anterior part of the inferior vermis. Immediately lateral to the nodule there is the tonsil of the cerebellum. If the tonsil is lifted away, we see that the nodule is continuous laterally with a membrane called the ***inferior medullary velum*** (Fig. 24.9B). Posteriorly, the inferior velum

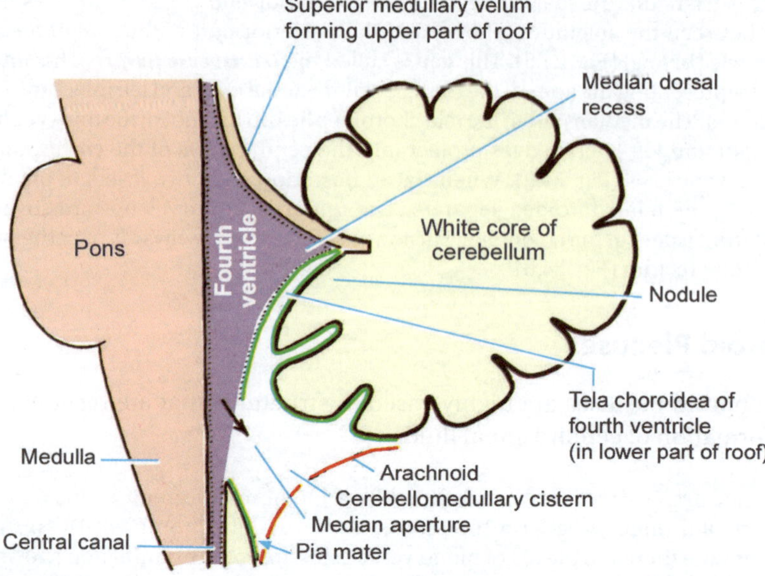

Fig. 24.8 Mid-sagittal section through the fourth ventricle and related structures. Note how the tela choroidea is formed. The piamater is shown in green.

merges into the white matter of the cerebellum. This is seen in Fig. 24.10 which is a sagittal section along the axis XY shown in Fig. 24.9B. The inferior medullary velum has a thickened free edge which connects the nodule to the flocculus. This edge is the peduncle of the flocculus. In the intact brain, this peduncle is very near the posterior surface of the medulla, and is separated from the inferior cerebellar peduncle only by a narrow interval. With these facts clearly recorded we may now consider the anatomy of the fourth ventricle.

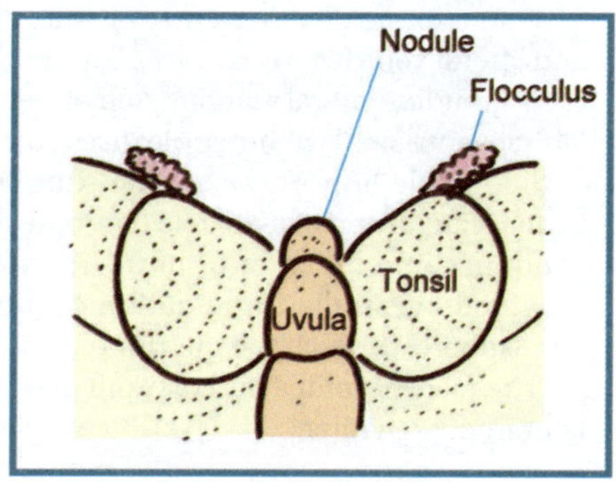

Fig. 24.9A Part of the inferior aspect of the cerebellum showing the nodule and some related structures.

The fourth ventricle is a space situated dorsal to the pons and to the upper part of the medulla; and ventral to the cerebellum. For descriptive purposes the ventricle may be considered as having a cavity, a floor, a roof and lateral walls.

The Cavity

The cavity of the ventricle is continuous, inferiorly, with the central canal; and, superiorly, with the cerebral aqueduct. It communicates with the subarachnoid space through three apertures, one median and two lateral (Figs. 24.8, 24.13A). A number of extensions from the main cavity are described (Fig. 24.11). The largest of these are two ***lateral recesses,*** one on either side. Each lateral recess passes laterally in the interval between the inferior cerebellar peduncle (ventrally), and the peduncle of the flocculus (dorsally) (Fig. 24.13A). The lateral extremity of the recess reaches the flocculus. At this extremity, the recess opens into the subarachnoid space as the ***lateral aperture.***

Another recess present in the middle line, is called the ***median dorsal recess.*** It extends into the white core of the cerebellum and lies just cranial to the nodule (Fig. 24.8, 24.11). Immediately lateral to the nodule, another recess projects dorsally, on either side, above the inferior medullary velum. This is the ***lateral dorsal recess*** (Figs. 24.10, 24.11).

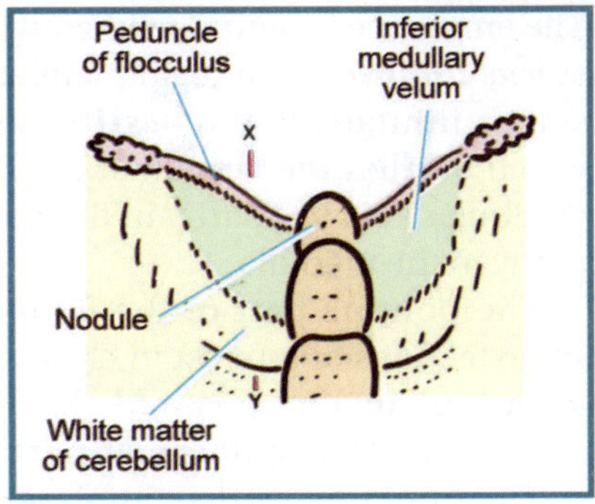

Fig. 24.9B Removal of the tonsil brings the inferior medullary velum into view. Note the peduncle of the flocculus connecting the nodule to the flocculus.

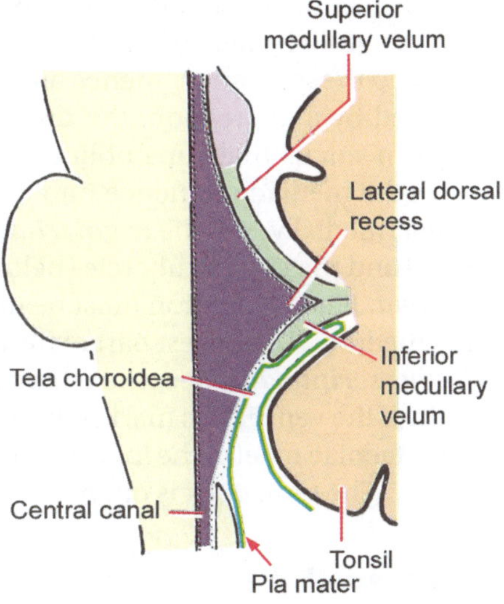

Fig. 24.10 Parasagittal section through the fourth ventricle a little to the nodule (along axis XY of Fig. 24.9B) to show the relationship of the inferior medullary velum to the roof of the ventricle. Note that the lateral dorsal recess lies just superior to the velum.

The Floor

Because of its shape, the floor of the fourth ventricle is often called the ***rhomboid fossa*** (Fig. 24.12). It is divisible into an upper triangular part formed by the posterior surface of the pons; a lower triangular part formed by the upper part of the posterior surface of the medulla; and an intermediate part at the junction of the medulla and pons. The intermediate part is prolonged laterally over the inferior cerebellar peduncle as the floor of the lateral recess. Its surface is marked by the presence of delicate bundles of transversely running fibres. These bundles are the ***striae medullares.***

The entire floor is divided into right and left halves by a ***median sulcus.*** Next to the middle line there is a longitudinal elevation called the ***median eminence.***

The eminence is bounded laterally by the ***sulcus limitans.*** The region lateral to the sulcus limitans is the ***vestibular area*** which overlies the vestibular nuclei. The vestibular area lies partly in the pons and partly in the medulla.

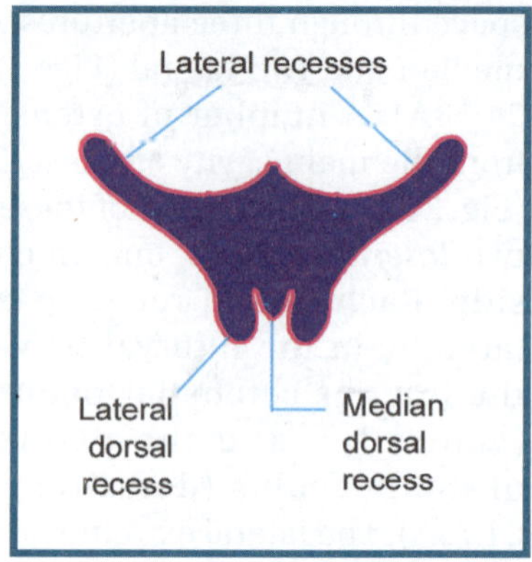

Fig. 24.11 Scheme of the cavity of the fourth ventricle to show its various recesses.

The pontine part of the floor shows some features of interest in close relation to the sulcus limitans and the median eminence. The uppermost part of the sulcus limitans overlies an area that is bluish in colour and is called the ***locus coeruleus.*** (Deep to the locus coeruleus there is the nucleus coeruleus which extends upwards into the tegmentum of the midbrain. It is regarded as part of the reticular formation). Somewhat lower down, the sulcus limitans is marked by a depression, the ***superior fovea.*** At this level the median eminence shows a swelling, the ***facial colliculus***.

The medullary part of the floor also shows some features of interest in relation to the median eminence and the sulcus limitans. The sulcus limitans is marked by a depression, the ***inferior fovea.*** Descending from the fovea, there is a sulcus that runs obliquely towards the middle line. This sulcus divides the median eminence into two triangles. These are the ***hypoglossal triangle***, medially; and the ***vagal triangle,*** laterally. Between the vagal triangle (above) and the gracile tubercle (below), there is a small area called the ***area postrema.*** Finally mention must be made of two terms often used in relation to the medulla. The lowest part of the floor of the fourth ventricle is called the ***calamus scriptorius,*** because of its resemblance to a nib. Each inferolateral margin of the ventricle is marked by a narrow white ridge or ***taenia.*** The right and left taeniae meet at the inferior angle of the floor to form a small fold called the ***obex.*** The term obex is often used to denote the inferior angle itself.

The Lateral Walls

The upper part of each lateral wall is formed by the superior cerebellar peduncle (Fig. 24.13B). The lower part is formed by the inferior cerebellar peduncle, and by the gracile and cuneate tubercles (Figs. 24.13 C, D).

The Roof

The roof of the fourth ventricle is tent-shaped and can be divided into upper and lower parts which meet at an apex (Figs. 24.8, 24.13A). The apex extends into the white core of the cerebellum. The upper part of the roof is formed by the superior cerebellar peduncles and the superior medullary velum (Figs. 24.13 A, B). The inferior part of the roof is devoid of nervous tissue in most of its extent. It is formed by a membrane consisting of ependyma and a double

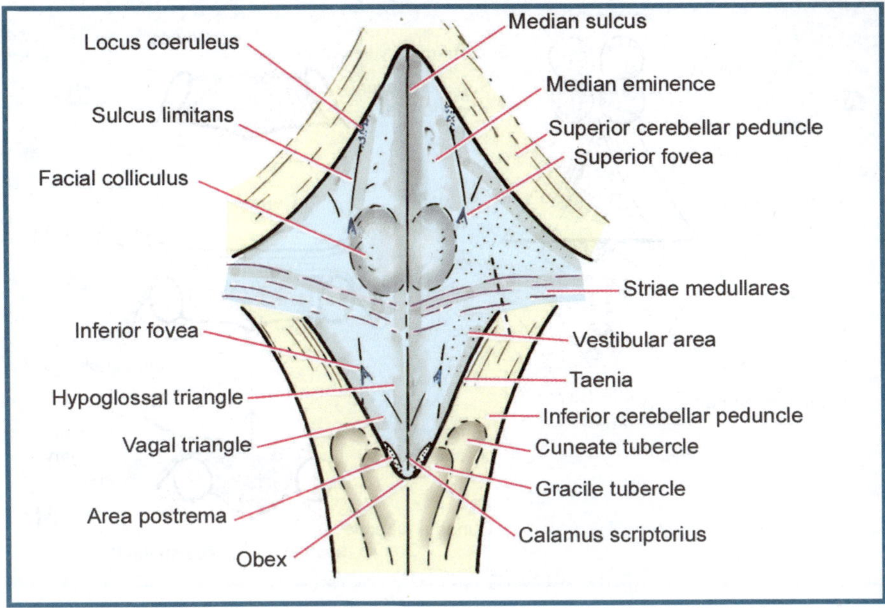

Fig. 24.12 Structures in the floor of the fourth ventricle.

fold of pia mater which constitutes the ***tela choroidea of the fourth ventricle*** (Fig. 24.13 A,C). Laterally, on each side, this membrane reaches and fuses with the inferior cerebellar peduncles. The lower part of the membrane has a large aperture in it. This is the ***median aperture*** of the fourth ventricle through which the ventricle communicates with the subarachnoid space in the region of the cerebello medullary cistern. In the region of the lateral recess, the membrane is prolonged laterally and helps to form the wall of the recess. The inferior medullary velum forms a small part of the roof in the region of the lateral dorsal recess (Fig. 24.10). It may be noted that some authors describe the entire membranous structure, forming the lower part of the roof of the fourth ventricle, as the inferior medullary velum. The nodule is intimately related to the roof of the ventricle in the region of the median dorsal recess.

As stated above the ***tela choroidea of the fourth ventricle*** is made up of two layers of pia mater. The superior (or dorsal) layer lines the inferior vermis. On reaching the nodule (and more laterally, the inferior medullary velum), it is reflected on itself to form the inferior (or ventral) layer (Fig. 24.8). When traced laterally the dorsal layer is continuous with the pia mater covering the cerebellar hemispheres, while the ventral layer is continuous with the pia mater lining the medulla (Fig. 24.13C).

The ***choroid plexuses of the fourth ventricle*** are similar in structure to those of the lateral and third ventricles. They lie within the folds of pia mater that form the tela choroidea, and project into the cavity of the ventricle from the lower part of the roof (Fig. 24.13C). Each plexus (right or left) consists of a vertical limb lying next to the midline, and a horizontal limb extending into the lateral recess.

The vertical limbs of the two plexuses lie side by side so that the whole structure is T-shaped. The lower ends of the vertical limbs reach the median aperture and project

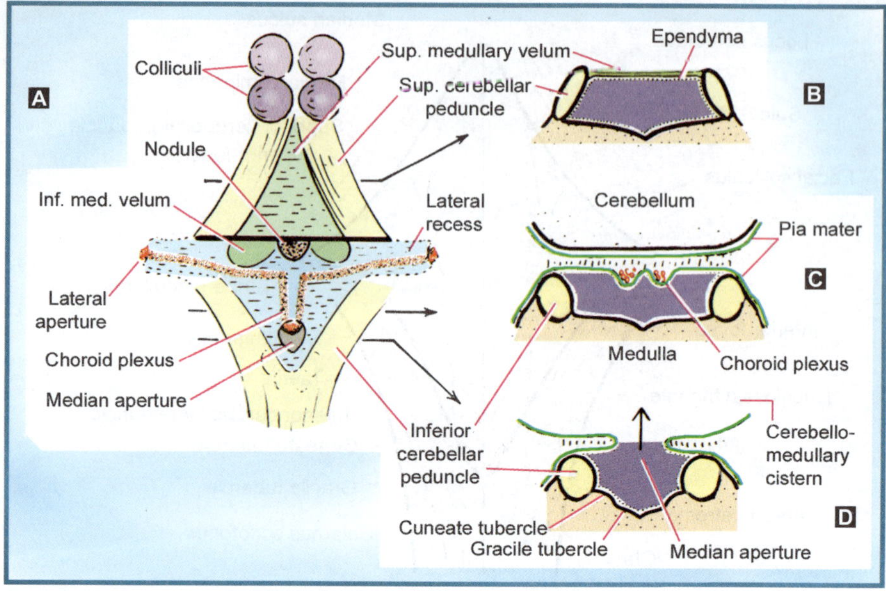

Fig. 24.13 Schemes to illustrate the formation of the roof of the fourth ventricle. The bold horizontal line in A represents the white core of the cerebellum. The part above this line represents the upper part of the roof, and the part below the line represents the lower part. B, C and D represent transverse sections across the ventricle at the levels indicated. In each figure the piamater is shown in pink.

into the subarachnoid space through it. The lateral ends of the horizontal limbs reach the lateral apertures, and can be seen on the surface of the brain, near the flocculus.

THE CEREBROSPINAL FLUID

The cerebrospinal fluid (CSF) fills the subarachnoid space. It also extends into the ventricles of the brain, and into the central canal of the spinal cord. The CSF provides a fluid cushion which protects the brain from injury. It probably also helps to carry nutrition to the brain, and to remove waste products.

CSF is formed by the choroid plexuses of the ventricles. The fluid formed in each lateral ventricle flows into the third ventricle through the interventricular foramen. From the third ventricle it passes through the aqueduct into the fourth ventricle. Here it passes through the median and lateral apertures in the roof of this ventricle to enter the part of the subarachnoid space which forms the cerebello medullary cistern. From here the fluid enters other parts of the subarachnoid space. In passing from the posterior cranial fossa into the upper (supratentorial) part of the cranial cavity the CSF traverses the narrow interval between the free margin of the tentorium cerebelli and the brain stem. It leaves the subarachnoid space by entering the venous sinuses through arachnoid villi.

The total volume of CSF is about 140 ml of which about 25 ml is in the ventricles. The CSF is constantly replaced.

The CSF consists of water in which are present sodium chloride, potassium, glucose and proteins. The proportion of these substances differ considerably in blood and CSF and hence it is believed that CSF is formed by an active secretory process, and not by passive filtration. The epithelium and other tissues of the choroid plexuses form an effective barrier between the blood and the CSF. This blood CSF barrier allows selective passage of substances from blood to CSF, but not in the reverse direction. The arachnoid villi provide a valvular mechanism for flow of CSF into blood without permitting back flow of blood into the CSF.

An abnormal increase in the quantity of CSF can lead to enlargement of the head in children. This condition is called ***hydrocephalus.***

Abnormal pressure of CSF leads to degeneration of brain tissue. Hydrocephalus may be caused by excessive production of CSF, by obstruction to its flow, or by impaired absorption through the arachnoid villi. It is classified as ***obstructive*** when there is obstruction to flow of CSF from the ventricular system to the subarachnoid space; or as ***communicating*** when such obstruction is not present. Obstruction is most likely to occur where CSF has to pass through narrow passages e.g., the interventricular foramina, the aqueduct, and the apertures of the fourth ventricle. In each of the above instances dilatation is confined to cavities proximal to the obstruction. Occasionally, meningitis may lead to obstruction of the narrow interval between the tentorium cerebelli and the brainstem. Meningitis may also lead to hydrocephalus by affecting the arachnoid villi, thus hampering the reabsorption of CSF.

Samples of CSF are often required for help in clinical diagnosis. They are obtained most easily by ***lumbar puncture.*** In this procedure a needle is introduced into the subarachnoid space through the interval between the third and fourth lumbar vertebrae.

Under exceptional circumstances CSF may be obtained by **cisternal puncture** in which a needle is passed into the cerebello medullary cistern.

Blood Brain Barrier

It has been observed that while some substances can pass from the blood into the brain with ease, others are prevented from doing so. This has given rise to the concept of a selective barrier between blood and the brain.

Anatomically, the structures that could constitute the barrier are as follows.

a. Capillary endothelium.
b. Basement membrane of the endothelium.
c. Closely applied to the vessels there are numerous processes of astrocytes. It has been estimated that these processes cover about eighty five percent of the capillary surface.

Some areas of the brain (and related structures) appear to be devoid of a blood brain barrier. These include the pineal body, the hypophysis cerebri, the choroid plexus and certain other regions.

Ventriculography

The ventricles of the brain can be studied in living subjects by taking radiographs after injecting a radio-opaque dye into the ventricular system. The procedure is called ventriculography (Fig. 16.12). Parts of the ventricles can also be seen using CT scans and magnetic resonance imaging.

CHAPTER

25

Blood Supply of the Brain

The nervous system is richly supplied with blood. Interruption of blood supply even for a short period can result in damage to nervous tissue. It is interesting to note that lymphatic vessels are not present in nervous tissue.

The blood supply of the spinal cord has been described on page 121. Here we will consider the blood supply of the brain.

ARTERIES THAT SUPPLY THE BRAIN

The arteries which supply the brain are derived from the internal carotid and vertebral arteries.

Internal Carotid Artery (Cerebral Part)

The internal carotid artery has been described on page 802. We have seen that the artery ascends up through the neck. After reaching the skull the artery follows a complicated course through the carotid canal, the foramen lacerum, and the cavernous sinus. Finally, it pierces the duramater forming the roof of the cavernous sinus, medial to the anterior clinoid process, and comes into relationship with the brain. The artery turns backwards to reach the anterior perforated substance of the brain, and terminates here by dividing into the ***anterior cerebral*** and ***posterior cerebral*** arteries. Other branches given off by the internal carotid artery in the intracranial part of its course are shown in Fig. 8.9. Two of these branches may be noted. These are the ***anterior choroidal artery***, and the ***posterior communicating artery*** which take part in supply of the brain. These branches are described briefly below. Further details will be mentioned when we take up the blood supply of different parts of the brain.

Anterior Cerebral Artery

We have seen that the anterior cerebral artery arises from the internal carotid artery below the anterior perforated substance, lateral to the optic chiasma (Figs. 25.1A, 25.2).

From here it runs forwards and medially crossing above the optic chiasma to reach the median longitudinal fissure. Here the arteries of the two sides lie close together and are united to each other by the ***anterior communicating artery***. The anterior cerebral artery now turns sharply to reach the medial surface of the cerebral hemisphere. Here it runs upwards to reach the genu of the corpus callosum (Fig. 25.1B). It winds round the front of the genu and then runs backwards just above the body of the corpus callosum, ending near its posterior part. The distribution of the artery is considered below, along with that of the middle cerebral and posterior cerebral arteries.

The anterior cerebral artery gives off a ***recurrent branch*** (also called the artery of Heubner). This branch runs backwards and laterally to enter the anterior perforated substance (Fig. 25.2).

Middle Cerebral Artery

After its origin from the internal carotid artery (just below the anterior perforated substance), the middle cerebral artery runs laterally on the inferior aspect of the cerebral hemisphere lying deep within the stem of the lateral sulcus (Fig. 25.1A). Reaching the superolateral surface of the hemisphere it runs backwards deep within the posterior ramus of the lateral sulcus (Fig. 25.1C). Along its course the artery gives off several branches to the brain. Their distribution is considered below along with that of the anterior and posterior cerebral arteries.

Posterior Communicating Artery

This artery arises from the internal carotid artery just before the termination of the latter (Fig. 25.2). The artery runs backwards crossing inferior to the optic tract, and ends by joining the posterior cerebral artery, thus helping to form an arterial circle in relation to the base of the brain (See below). It gives off some central branches that enter the cerebral hemisphere and supply part of the thalamus.

Anterior Choroidal Artery

This artery arises from the internal carotid artery near the termination of the latter. It runs backwards in relation to the uncus and the optic tract (Fig. 25.2). It ends in the choroid plexus in the inferior horn of the lateral ventricle. This artery also gives off branches to several parts of the brain including the internal capsule.

Vertebral Arteries

The vertebral artery has been described on page 178. We have seen that it is a branch of the subclavian artery. It ascends up the neck passing through foramina transversaria of the upper six cervical vertebrae, passes through the suboccipital region and enters the upper part of the vertebral canal. It then passes upwards to enter the cranial cavity through the foramen magnum, and comes to lie lateral to the lower part of the medulla oblongata. Continuing its ascent it gradually passes forwards and medially over the medulla and ends

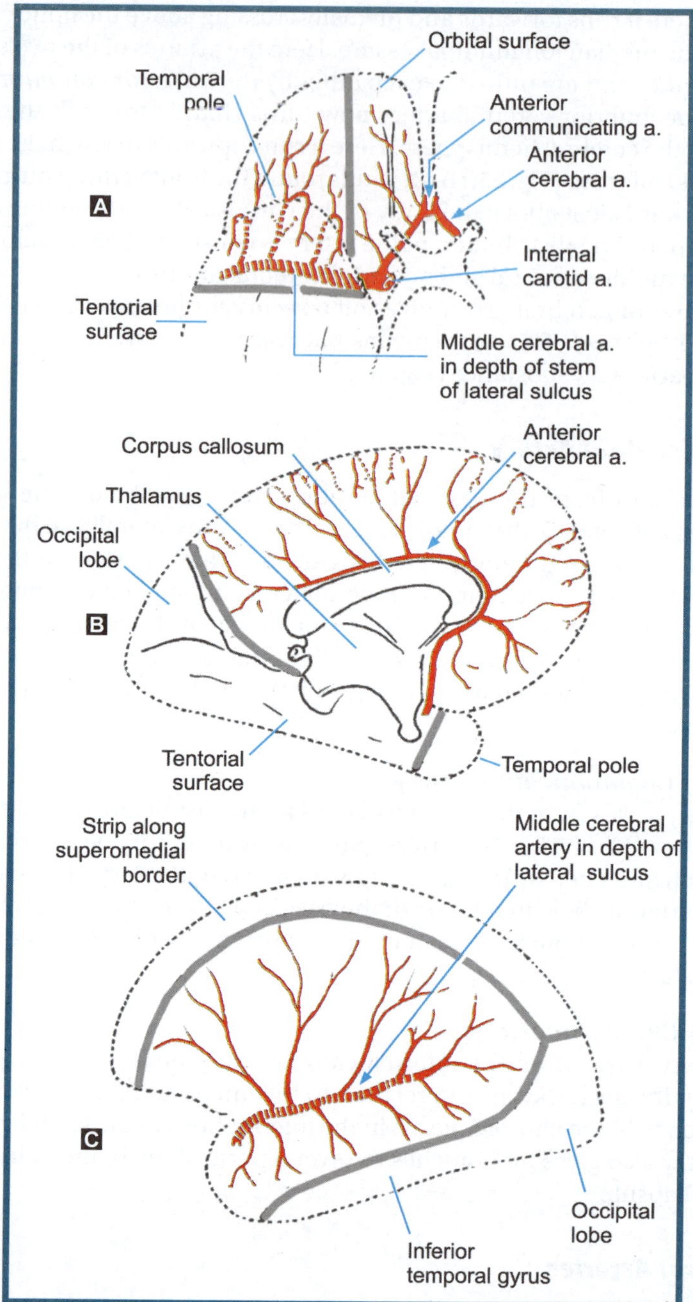

Fig. 25.1 A. Initial parts of the anterior and middle cerebral arteries (seen from below). B. Course of anterior cerebral artery (medial view). C. Course of middle cerebral artery (lateral view). The thick grey lines demarcate areas supplied.

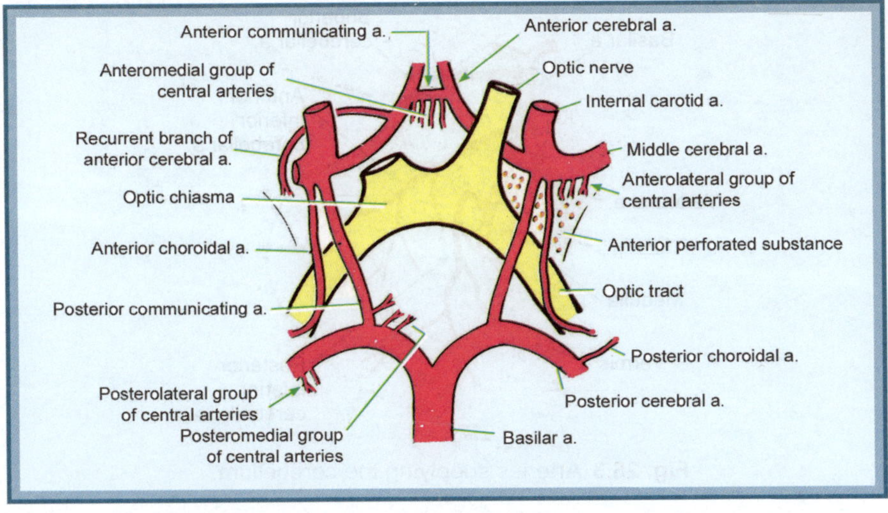

Fig. 25.2 The circulus arteriosus and related structures.

at the lower border of the pons by anastomosing with the opposite vertebral artery to form the basilar artery (Fig. 25.3).

The vertebral artery gives off several branches along its course. The branches that take part in supplying the brain are as follows.

1. ***Anterior and posterior spinal arteries***

These are described on page 179 (Fig. 8.37). They are meant for supply of the spinal cord, but they also give some branches to the medulla. See Fig. 25.12.

2. ***Posterior inferior cerebellar artery***

This is the largest branch of the vertebral artery. It first runs backwards in relation to the lateral aspect of the medulla, and then ramifies into branches over the posterior part of the inferior surface of the cerebellum (Fig. 25.3).

The Basilar Artery

The basilar artery is formed by the union of the right and left vertebral arteries at the lower border of the pons. It ascends in the middle line, ventral to the pons, and ends at its upper border by dividing into the right and left posterior cerebral arteries. The branches of the basilar artery are as follows (Fig. 25.4).

Posterior Cerebral Artery

The posterior cerebral artery is a terminal branch of the basilar artery. It passes backwards winding round the midbrain to reach the tentorial surface of the cerebral hemisphere (Fig. 25.5). Near its origin it is joined by the posterior communicating branch of the internal carotid artery. The posterior cerebral artery gives off cortical and central branches to the cerebral hemisphere. They are considered below along with those of the anterior and middle cerebral arteries.

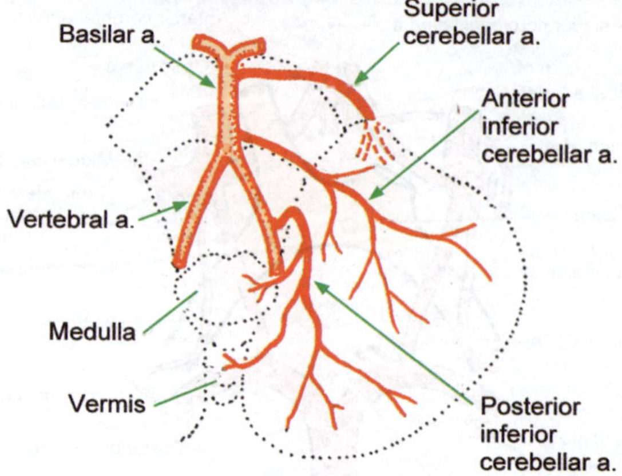

Fig. 25.3 Arteries supplying the cerebellum.

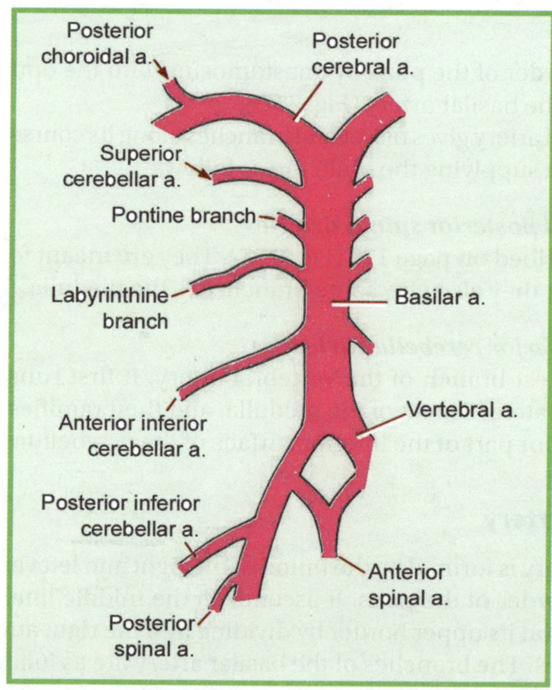

Fig. 25.4 Branches of the basilar artery. Some branches of the vertebral artery are also shown.

The ***posterior choroidal artery*** is a branch of the posterior cerebral artery (Fig. 25.2). It supplies the choroid plexuses of the lateral and third ventricles. It also supplies the lateral geniculate body.

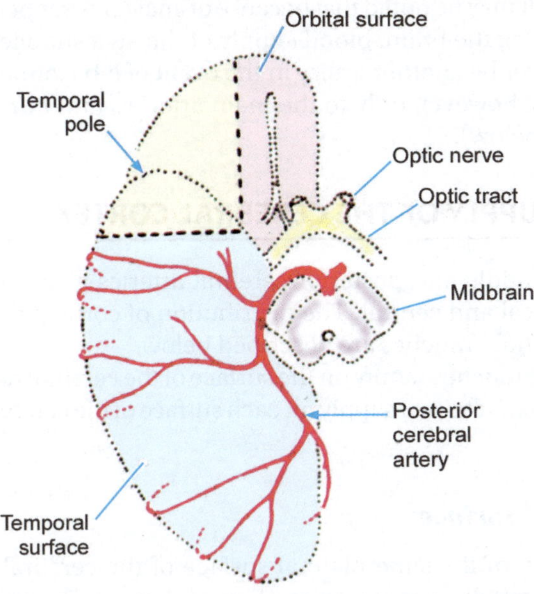

Fig. 25.5 Course and distribution of the posterior cerebral artery.

Superior Cerebellar Artery

This artery arises from the basilar artery just proximal to the termination of the latter. It winds round the midbrain to reach the superior surface of the cerebellum which it supplies (Fig. 25.3)

Anterior Inferior Cerebellar Artery

This artery arises from the basilar artery near its lower end. It runs backwards and laterally to reach the anterior part of the inferior surface of the cerebellum which it supplies (Fig. 25.3).

Other Branches of Basilar Artery

The basilar artery gives off some small ***pontine branches*** to the pons (Fig. 25.4). It also gives off the labyrinthine artery which accompanies the facial nerve into the internal acoustic meatus to reach the internal ear.

Circulus Arteriosus

From Fig. 25.2 we see that some of the arteries supplying the brain form an arterial circle that is present in relation to the base of the brain (in the region of the interpeduncular fossa). The anterior part of the circle is formed by the right and left anterior cerebral arteries, and the anterior communicating artery that unites them. On either side the ring is formed by the internal carotid artery and its posterior communicating branch. Posteriorly, the ring is completed by the bifurcation of the basilar artery into the right and left posterior cerebral arteries. We have already noted that the posterior communicating artery joins the posterior cerebral artery to complete the ring.

At this stage it may be noted that because of anastomoses between the major arteries supplying the brain, blood supply of the area supplied by one artery can be taken over by another artery in the event of it becoming blocked. This remark applies, however, only to the main arteries, and ***not*** to their smaller branches (see below).

ARTERIAL SUPPLY OF THE CEREBRAL CORTEX

The anterior, middle and posterior cerebral arteries give rise to two sets of branches, cortical and central. The distribution of cortical branches is given below. The central branches are described below.

The cortical branches ramify on the surface of the cerebral hemispheres and supply the cortex. Details of supply on each surface of the cerebral hemispheres are as follows.

Superolateral Surface

The greater part of the superolateral surface of the cerebral hemisphere is supplied by the middle cerebral artery (Figs. 16.1, 25.6). The areas ***not*** supplied by this artery are as follows.

a. A strip half to one inch wide along the superomedial border extending from the frontal pole to the parieto-occipital sulcus is supplied by the anterior cerebral artery.
b. The area belonging to the occipital lobe is supplied by the posterior cerebral artery.
c. The inferior temporal gyrus (excluding the part adjoining the temporal pole) is also supplied by the posterior cerebral artery.

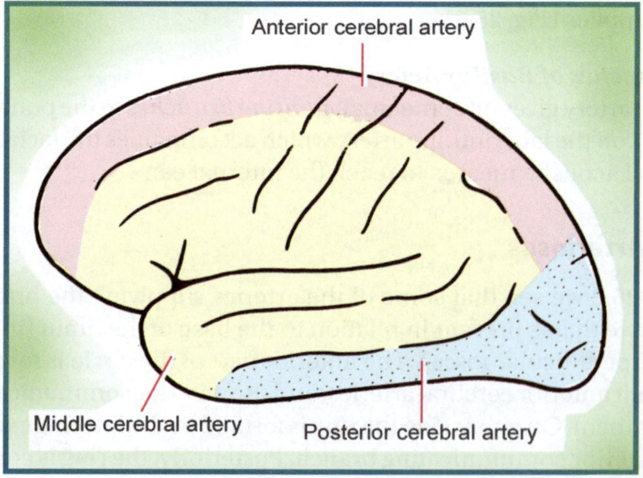

Fig. 25.6 Distribution of the anterior, posterior and middle cerebral arteries on the superolateral surface of the cerebral hemisphere.

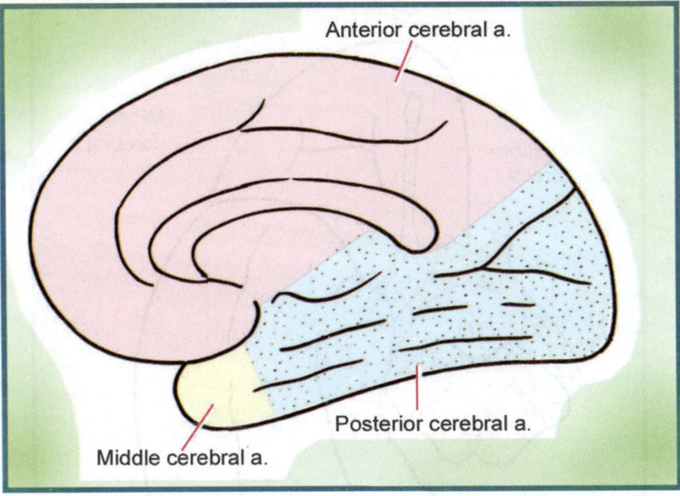

Fig. 25.7 Arteries supplying the medial surface of the cerebral hemisphere.

Medial Surface

The main artery supplying the medial surface is the anterior cerebral (Figs. 16.2, 25.7). The area of this surface belonging to the occipital lobe is supplied by the posterior cerebral artery.

Inferior Surface

The lateral part of the ***orbital surface*** is supplied by the middle cerebral artery, and the medial part by the anterior cerebral artery (Figs. 16.3A, 25.8).

The ***tentorial surface*** is supplied by the posterior cerebral artery. The temporal pole is, however, supplied by the middle cerebral artery (Figs. 16.3A, 25.8).

Additional Points of Interest

From the description given above it will be clear that the main somatic motor and sensory areas are supplied by the middle cerebral artery except in their uppermost parts (leg areas) which are supplied by the anterior cerebral. The acoustic area is supplied by the middle cerebral artery, and the visual area by the posterior cerebral.

The part of the visual area responsible for macular vision lies in the region where the territories of supply of the middle and posterior cerebral arteries meet. It may receive a supply from the middle cerebral artery, either directly, or through anastomoses with branches of the posterior cerebral artery. This is one explanation for the observation that macular vision is often spared in cases of thrombosis of the posterior cerebral artery. The phenomenon can also be explained by the observation that dye injected into the carotid system (for angiographic studies) often passes into the posterior cerebral artery through the posterior communicating artery (Fig. 16.13).

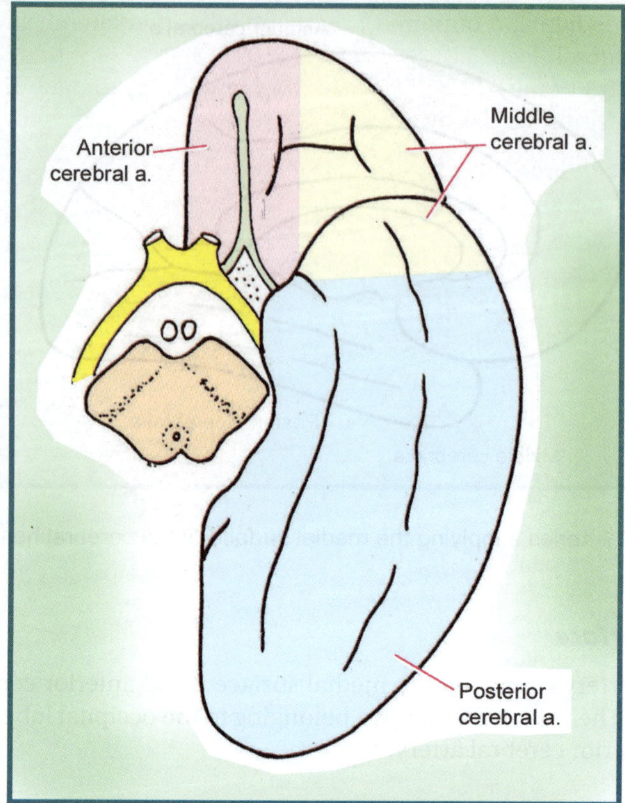

Fig. 25.8 Arteries supplying the orbital and tentorial surfaces of the cerebral hemisphere.

The cortical arteries give off branches that run perpendicularly into the substance of the cerebral hemisphere. Some of these are short and end within the grey matter of the cortex. Others are longer and penetrate into the subjacent white matter. While cortical branches may anastomose with each other on the surface of the brain, the perpendicular branches (both long and short) behave as terminal or end arteries. Each branch supplies a limited area of brain tissue, and does not anastomose with neighbouring arteries. As a result, blockage of such a branch leads to death (necrosis) of brain tissue in the region of supply.

ARTERIES SUPPLYING INTERIOR OF THE CEREBRAL HEMISPHERE

Central or Perforating Arteries

Structures in the interior of the cerebral hemisphere are supplied by central (or perforating) branches that arise from arteries lying in relation to the base of the brain. They consist of six main groups: anteromedial and posteromedial (which are median and unpaired); right and left anterolateral; and right and left posterolateral (Fig. 25.2).

The arteries of the ***anteromedial group*** arise from the anterior cerebral and anterior communicating arteries. They enter the most medial part of the anterior perforated substance. The arteries of the ***anterolateral group*** are the so called ***striate arteries***. They arise mainly from the middle cerebral artery. Some of them arise from the anterior cerebral artery. The anterolateral group of perforating arteries enter the anterior perforated substance and divide into two sets, medial and lateral. The ***medial striate arteries*** ascend through the lentiform nucleus. They supply this nucleus and also the caudate nucleus and the internal capsule. The ***lateral striate arteries*** ascend lateral to the lower part of the lentiform nucleus; they then turn medially and pass through the substance of the lentiform nucleus to reach the internal capsule and the caudate nucleus. One of these lateral striate arteries is usually larger than the others. It is called ***Charcot's artery***, or ***artery of cerebral haemorrhage***. The ***posteromedial group*** of central arteries arise from the posterior cerebral and posterior communicating arteries. They enter the interpeduncular region. The central branches of the ***posterolateral group*** arise from the posterior cerebral artery, as it winds around the cerebral peduncle.

Arterial Supply of Individual Structures

Internal Capsule

The main arteries supplying the internal capsule are the medial and lateral striate branches of the middle cerebral artery, the recurrent branch of the anterior cerebral, and the anterior choroidal artery. The internal capsule may also receive direct branches from the internal carotid artery, and branches from the posterior communicating artery (Fig. 25.9).

The ***upper parts*** of the anterior limb, the genu, and the posterior limb are supplied by striate branches of the middle cerebral artery. The ***lower parts*** of these regions are supplied as follows.

a. The lower part of the anterior limb is supplied by the recurrent branch of the anterior cerebral artery.
b. The lower part of the genu is supplied by direct branches from the internal carotid, and from the posterior communicating artery.
c. The lower part of the posterior limb is supplied by the anterior choroidal artery.

The entire ***retrolentiform part*** is supplied by the anterior choroidal artery. The ***sublentiform part*** is probably supplied by the anterior choroidal artery.

Thalamus

The thalamus is supplied mainly by perforating branches of the posterior cerebral artery (Fig. 25.10). The posteromedial group of branches (also called ***thalamo-perforating*** arteries) supply the medial and anterior part. The posterolateral group (also called ***thalamo-geniculate*** branches) supply the posterior and lateral parts of the thalamus. The thalamus also receives some branches from the posterior communicating, anterior choroidal, posterior choroidal, and middle cerebral arteries.

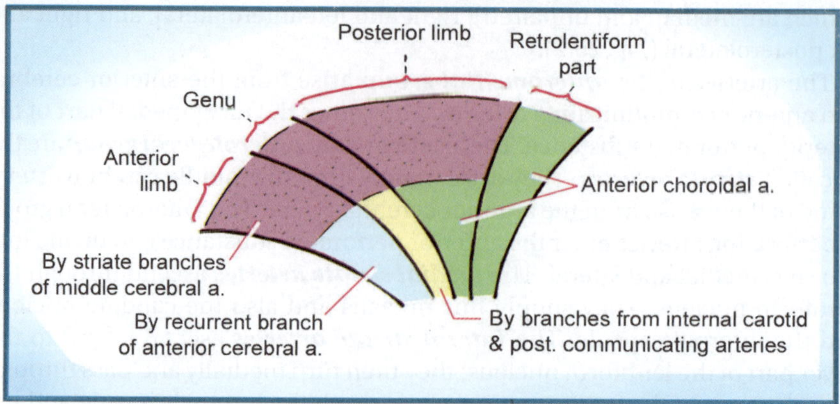

Fig. 25.9 Scheme to show the arterial supply of the internal capsule.

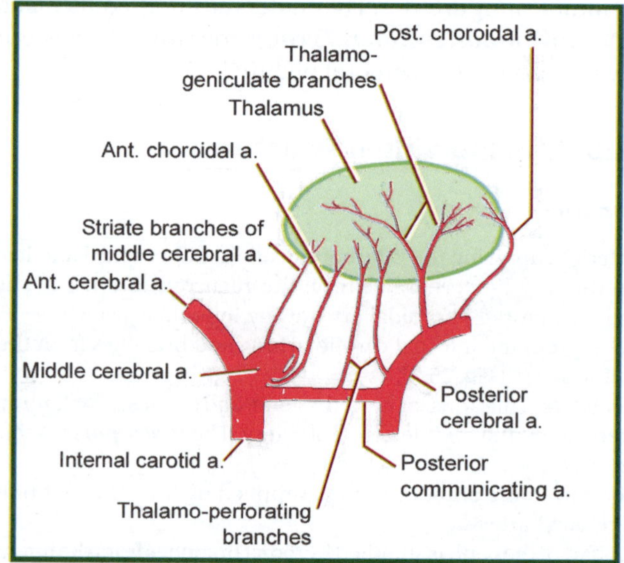

Fig. 25.10 Scheme to show the arteries supplying the thalamus.

Hypothalamus

The anterior part of the hypothalamus is supplied by central branches of the anteromedial group (arising from the anterior cerebral artery). The posterior part is supplied by central branches of the posteromedial group (arising from the posterior cerebral and posterior communicating arteries).

Corpus Striatum

The main arterial supply of the ***caudate nucleus*** and ***putamen*** is derived from the medial and lateral striate branches of the middle cerebral artery (Fig. 25.11).

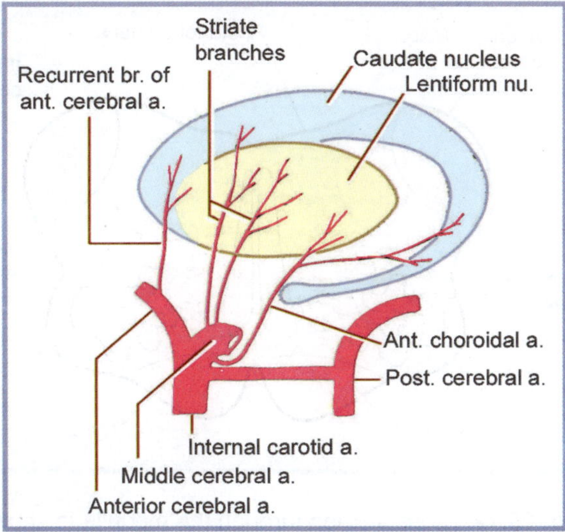

Fig. 25.11 Scheme to show the arteries supplying the corpus striatum.

In addition, their most anterior parts (including the head of the caudate nucleus) receive their blood supply through the recurrent branch of the anterior cerebral artery, and their posterior parts (including the tail of the caudate nucleus) through the anterior choroidal artery.

The main supply of the ***globus pallidus*** is from the anterior choroidal artery. Its lateral segment also receives blood through the striate arteries. The most medial part of the globus pallidus receives branches from the posterior communicating artery.

Arterial Supply of the Brainstem

Medulla

The medulla is supplied by various branches of the vertebral arteries. These are the anterior and posterior spinal arteries, the posterior inferior cerebellar artery, and small direct branches (Fig. 25.12).

The anterior spinal artery supplies a triangular area next to the middle line. This area includes the pyramid, the medial lemniscus, and the hypoglossal nucleus. The posterior spinal artery supplies a small area including the gracile and cuneate nuclei. The posterior inferior cerebellar artery supplies the retro-olivary region. This region contains several important structures including the spinothalamic tracts, the rubrospinal tract, the nucleus ambiguus, the dorsal vagal nucleus, and descending autonomic fibres. The posterior inferior cerebellar artery also supplies part of the inferior cerebellar peduncle. The rest of the medulla is supplied by direct bulbar branches of the vertebral arteries.

Thrombosis in an artery supplying the medulla produces symptoms depending upon the structures involved. Two characteristic syndromes are the ***medial medullary syndrome*** produced by thrombosis in the anterior spinal artery, and the ***lateral medullary syndrome*** produced by thrombosis in the posterior inferior cerebellar artery.

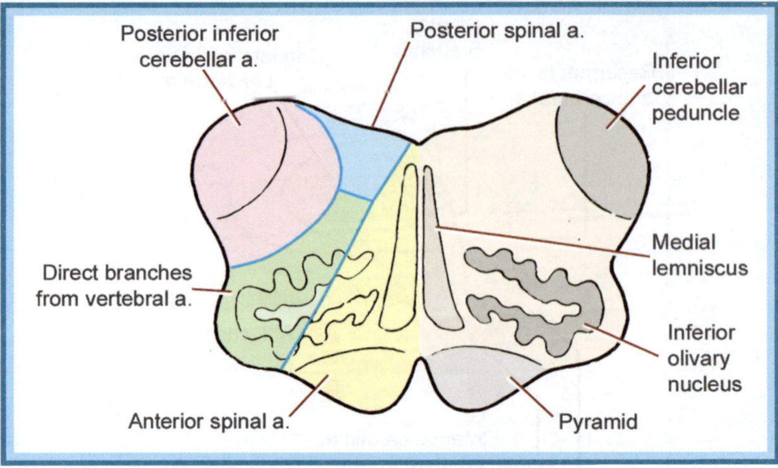

Fig. 25.12 Cross section through the medulla to show regions supplied by different arteries.

Pons

The pons is supplied by branches from the basilar artery.

The medial portion of the ventral part of the pons is supplied by ***paramedian branches.*** The lateral portion of the ventral part is supplied by ***short circumferential branches.*** The dorsal part of the pons is supplied by ***long circumferential branches.*** The dorsal part also receives branches from the anterior inferior cerebellar and superior cerebellar arteries. The paramedian branches of the basilar artery may extend into this region from the ventral part of the pons.

Midbrain

The midbrain is supplied mainly by branches of the basilar artery. These are the posterior cerebral and superior cerebellar arteries and direct branches from the basilar artery. Branches are also received from the posterior communicating and anterior choroidal arteries.

Branches arising from these vessels may either be ***paramedian,*** which supply parts near the midline; or ***circumferential*** which wind round the midbrain to supply lateral and dorsal parts. One of the latter arteries is called the ***quadrigeminal artery.*** It is the main source of blood to the colliculi.

Arteries Supplying the Cerebellum

The superior surface of the cerebellum is supplied by the ***superior cerebellar*** branches of the basilar artery (Fig. 25.3). The anterior part of the inferior surface is supplied by the ***anterior inferior cerebellar*** branches of the same artery.

The posterior part of the inferior surface is supplied by the ***posterior inferior cerebellar*** branch of the vertebral artery.

VENOUS DRAINAGE OF THE BRAIN

The veins draining the brain open into the dural venous sinuses (Fig. 25.13). These are the superior sagittal, inferior sagittal, straight, transverse, sigmoid, cavernous, sphenoparietal, petrosal and occipital sinuses. They have been

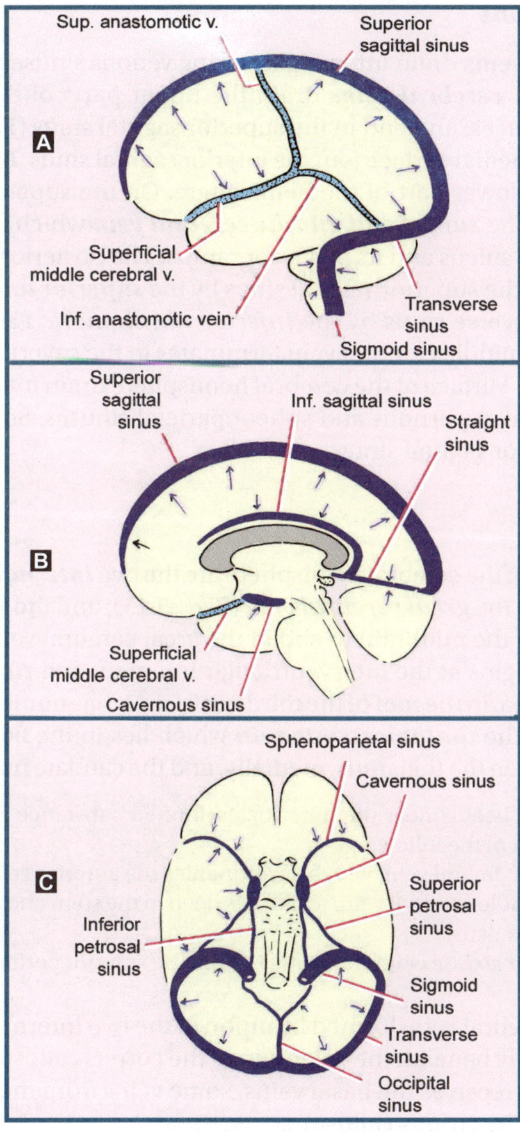

Fig. 25.13 Diagrams to show the position of the intracranial venous sinuses in relation to (A) lateral, (B) medial and (C) inferior aspects of the brain.

described in detail in Chapter 8. Ultimately, the blood from all these sinuses reaches the sigmoid sinus which becomes continuous with the internal jugular vein.

The venous drainage of individual parts of the brain is as follows.

Veins of the Cerebral Hemisphere

The veins of the cerebral hemisphere consist of two sets, superficial and deep.

Superficial Veins

The superficial veins drain into neighbouring venous sinuses.

The ***superior cerebral veins*** drain the upper parts of the superolateral and medial surfaces, and end in the superior sagittal sinus (Fig. 25.14). Some veins from the medial surface join the inferior sagittal sinus. ***Inferior cerebral veins*** drain the lower part of the hemisphere. On the superolateral surface, they drain into the ***superficial middle cerebral vein*** which lies superficially along the lateral sulcus and its posterior ramus. The posterior end of this vein is connected to the superior sagittal sinus by the ***superior anastomotic vein***; and to the transverse sinus by the ***inferior anastomotic vein*** (Fig. 25.13A). The superficial middle cerebral vein terminates in the cavernous sinus. Veins from the inferior surface of the cerebral hemisphere drain into the transverse, superior petrosal, cavernous and sphenoparietal sinuses. Some may ascend to join the inferior sagittal sinus.

Deep Veins

The deep veins of the cerebral hemisphere are the two ***internal cerebral veins***, that join to form the ***great cerebral vein*** (Fig. 25.15); and the two ***basal veins,*** that wind round the midbrain to end in the great cerebral vein. Each internal cerebral vein begins at the interventricular foramen, and runs backwards in the tela choroidea, in the roof of the third ventricle. It has numerous tributaries. One of these is the ***thalamostriate vein*** which lies in the floor of the lateral ventricle (between the thalamus, medially, and the caudate nucleus, laterally).

Each basal vein begins near the anterior perforated substance (Fig. 25.16). It is formed by union of the following.

a. The anterior cerebral vein, which accompanies the anterior cerebral artery.
b. The deep middle cerebral vein, which lies deep in the stem and posterior ramus of the lateral sulcus.
c. Some ***inferior striate veins*** that emerge from the anterior perforated substance.

The great cerebral vein, formed by union of the two internal cerebral veins, passes posteriorly beneath the splenium of the corpus callosum, to end in the straight sinus. It receives the basal veins, some veins from the occipital lobes, and some from the corpus callosum.

The deep cerebral veins described above are responsible for draining the thalamus, the hypothalamus, the corpus striatum, the internal capsule, the corpus callosum, the septum pellucidum, and the choroid plexuses.

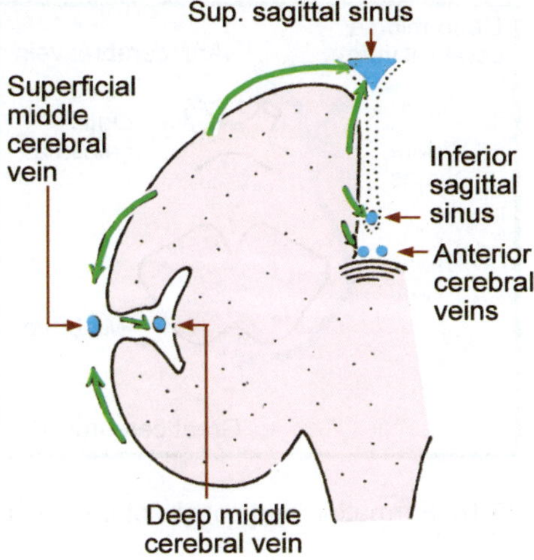

Fig. 25.14 Scheme to show venous drainage of the superolateral and medial surfaces of the cerebral hemisphere.

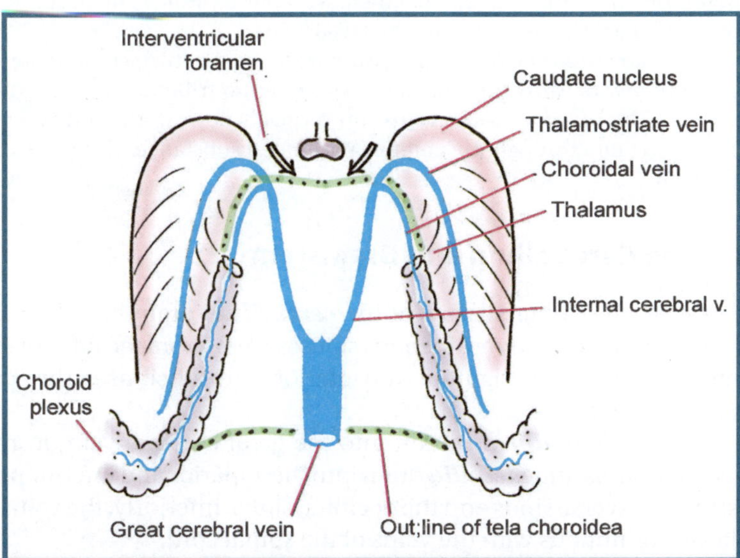

Fig. 25.15 Region of roof of third ventricle and floor of central part of lateral ventricle seen from above after removing the corpus callosum and parts above it. The deep veins are exposed.

Many tributaries of the internal cerebral veins extend beyond the corpus striatum into the white matter of the hemispheres. Here they establish communications with superficial veins. They can thus serve as alternative channels for draining parts of the cerebral cortex.

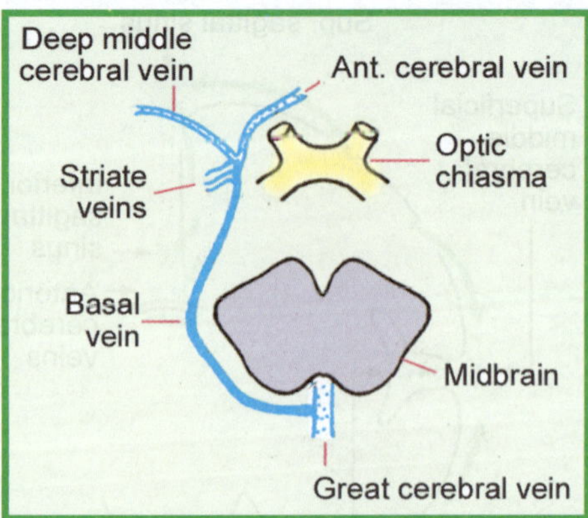

Fig. 25.16 Formation and course of the basal vein.

The upper part of the ***thalamus*** is drained by the tributaries of the internal cerebral vein (including the thalamostriate vein). The lower part of the thalamus, and the hypothalamus, are drained by veins that run downwards to end in a plexus of veins present in the interpeduncular fossa. This plexus drains into the cavernous and sphenoparietal sinuses, and into the basal veins.

The ***corpus striatum*** and ***internal capsule*** are drained by two sets of striate veins. The ***superior striate veins*** run dorsally and drain into tributaries of the internal cerebral vein. The ***inferior striate veins*** run vertically downwards and emerge on the base of the brain through the anterior perforated substance. Here they end in the basal vein.

Veins of the Cerebellum and Brainstem

The veins from the upper surface of the ***cerebellum*** drain into the straight, transverse, and superior petrosal venous sinuses. Veins from the inferior surface drain into the right and left sigmoid, and inferior petrosal, sinuses; the occipital sinus and the straight sinus.

The veins of the ***midbrain*** drain into the great cerebral vein or into the basal vein. The ***pons*** and ***medulla*** drain into the superior and inferior petrosal sinuses, the transverse sinus and the occipital sinus. Inferiorly, the veins of the medulla are continuous with the veins of the spinal cord.

CHAPTER

26

Some Clinical Correlations of the Central Nervous System

Some knowledge of anatomy is an essential prerequisite for the practice of any clinical discipline, but no where is this more true than in the diagnosis of neurological disorders. The localization of the areas of the nervous system involved in disease calls for a fairly thorough knowledge of the location of various masses of grey matter, and of the courses of various tracts. The purpose of this chapter is to provide some illustrations of how a knowledge of neuroanatomy can be of help in neurological diagnosis; and to introduce some terms that are commonly used in clinical practice.

Preliminary Remarks

Damage to nervous tissue can occur in various ways. Any part of the brain or spinal cord may be damaged by direct injury (***trauma***). Apart from other obvious causes such injury may occur during child birth. We have seen that if nervous tissue is deprived of blood even for a short period irreversible damage may result. Localized damage of this kind may occur if one of the arteries supplying the brain is blocked. This may occur by clotting of blood within the vessel (***thrombosis***). Such an event is more likely in older individuals in whom the arteries have undergone a degenerative change known as ***arteriosclerosis.*** A vessel can also be blocked by some extraneous material (e.g., clot, fat, air) reaching it from some other part of the body through the circulation. Such matter is called an ***embolus.*** Sometimes an artery may rupture, the blood leaking into brain tissue (***haemorrhage***) causing considerable damage. A haemorrhage in the brain is often fatal. Bleeding may be caused by rupture of small abnormal dilatations of arteries (***aneurysms***). Aneurysms may be congenital, or may be produced due to weakening of the arterial wall in the region. Another cause of brain damage is the presence of any abnormal mass within the cranial cavity. As the cranial cavity cannot expand such a mass inevitably presses on brain tissue. Such a ***space occupying lesion*** may be a tumour, a collection of pus, a collection of blood (in the epidural space) etc. Apart from producing general signs of increased intracranial tension, local effects are produced depending on the area involved. Nervous tissue may be affected by infections, both acute and chronic. An infection in the brain is referred to as ***encephalitis***; and that in the spinal cord is called ***myelitis.*** Defects in neural tissue may also be caused by ***maldevelopment*** (congenital anomalies), by ***degeneration*** in old age, and by various ***metabolic disorders.*** Finally, alterations in nervous function may occur in the absence of recognizable structural changes. These are called ***functional disorders.***

From the above it will be obvious that in some cases a neurological disorder will be of acute onset (as in trauma, vascular accidents, or acute infections). In such cases the patient may at first show signs indicative of widespread functional deficit quite out of proportion to the actual area involved. Deep unconsciousness (***coma***) is often present. In course of time, however, considerable recovery may take place, leaving residual defects dependent upon the area involved. In slowly developing diseases on the other hand, considerable structural damage may occur before symptoms become obvious. In the descriptions that follow we will deal only with signs and symptoms referable to the actual area of lesion.

DISORDERS OF MOTOR FUNCTION

Inability to move a part of the body is referred to as ***paralysis.*** This can be produced by interruption of motor pathways anywhere between the motor area of the cerebral cortex and the muscles themselves. We have seen that the pathway from cortex to muscle involves at least two neurons. The first of these is located in the cerebral cortex. Its axon terminates in the spinal cord or in motor cranial nerve nuclei in the brainstem. From a physiological and clinical point of view this neuron is referred to as the ***upper motor neuron***. The second neuron is located in the anterior grey column of the spinal cord (or in motor nuclei of the brainstem) and sends out an axon that travels through a peripheral nerve to innervate muscle. This neuron is referred to as the ***lower motor neuron.*** (For the present purpose we may ignore interneurons present in the pathway). When lower motor neurons are destroyed, or their continuity interrupted, the muscles supplied by them lose their tone (i.e., they become flaccid); and in course of time the muscles undergo atrophy. Changes in electrical responses of the muscles also take place. These alterations constitute the ***reaction of degeneration.*** In addition, because of interruption of the efferent part of reflex pathways tendon reflexes are abolished. Destruction or interruption of the upper motor neuron is not followed by any of these changes. On the other hand it is usually accompanied by an increase in muscle tone, and exaggeration of tendon reflexes. It is, therefore, possible to distinguish between an upper motor neuron paralysis (often called ***spastic paralysis***) and a lower motor neuron (or ***flaccid***) paralysis. Paralysis may be confined to one limb (***monoplegia***) or to both limbs on one side of the body (***hemiplegia***). Paralysis of both lower limbs is called ***paraplegia,*** and that of all four limbs is called ***quadriplegia.*** Paralysis of muscles supplied by one or more cranial nerves may occur in isolation, or in combination with hemiplegia. Destruction of a particular region often destroys lower motor neurons situated at that level resulting in a localized flaccid paralysis of muscles supplied from that level. This lesion may at the same time interrupt descending tracts (representing upper motor neurons) resulting in a spastic paralysis below the level of the lesion. The presence of a localized flaccid paralysis can thus serve as a pointer to the level of lesion.

It is also important to remember that the fibres of upper motor neurons meant for the limbs cross the midline in the lower part of the medulla (in the decussation of the pyramids); and those for the cranial nerves cross just above the level of their termination. A lesion above the level of crossing produces a paralysis in the opposite half of the body, and a lesion below this level produces a lesion on the same side.

Keeping the considerations discussed above in mind we may now consider the effects of lesions of the motor pathways at various levels.

1. Because of the large extent of the ***motor areas of the cerebral cortex*** lesions here produce a relatively localized paralysis e.g., a monoplegia.
2. A lesion in the ***internal capsule*** is capable of producing widespread paralysis on the opposite half of the body (hemiplegia) which may also involve the lower part of the face and the tongue. A lesion in the internal capsule is most likely to result from thrombosis or rupture of one of the arteries supplying the capsule. The artery most often involved is Charcot's artery of cerebral haemorrhage.
3. Lesions of corticospinal fibres at various levels in the ***brainstem***, above the level of the pyramidal decussation, can produce contra-lateral hemiplegia. If the lesion crosses the midline symptoms can be bilateral. Involvement of motor cranial nerve nuclei (or of fibres arising from them) may result in various combinations.

For example a lesion in the upper part of the midbrain can produce a paralysis of muscles supplied by the oculomotor nerve on the side of lesion, along with a hemiplegia on the opposite side (***Weber's syndrome***). A similar lesion in the pons, results in a paralysis of the lateral rectus muscle (abducent nerve) on the side of lesion with hemiplegia on the opposite side (***Raymond's syndrome***). Alternatively, facial paralysis of one side can be combined with contralateral hemiplegia (***Millard Gubler syndrome***). Various such combinations may result depending on the level of lesion.

4. Lesions affecting the lateral cortico-spinal tract in the spinal cord produce an upper motor neuron paralysis of muscles on the same side of the body. Lesions above the fifth cervical segment result in paralysis of both upper and lower extremities; while lesions below the first thoracic segment affect only the lower limbs. As in the brainstem, lesions in the spinal cord may be bilateral. Involvement of lower motor neurons at the level of lesion produces a flaccid paralysis of muscles supplied from that level, along with spastic paralysis below the level of injury. A knowledge of muscles supplied by individual spinal segments can thus help in locating the level of a lesion in the spinal cord.

In some diseases (e.g., ***poliomyelitis***) damage may be confined to lower motor neurons, and the resulting paralysis may be purely flaccid.

In the above description we have (for sake of simplicity) considered involvement of motor neurons in isolation. However, disease at any level can involve other structures resulting in sensory and other disturbances.

DISORDERS OF EQUILIBRIUM

We have seen that the maintenance of equilibrium, and of correct posture, is dependent on reflex arcs involving various centres including the spinal cord, the cerebellum, and the vestibular nuclei. Afferent impulses for these reflexes are carried by the posterior column tracts (fasciculus gracilis and fasciculus cuneatus), the spinocerebellar tracts, and others. Efferents reach the anterior horn cells through rubrospinal, vestibulospinal, and other 'extrapyramidal' tracts. Interruption of any of these pathways; or lesions in the cerebellum, the vestibular nuclei and other centres concerned; can result in various abnormalities involving maintenance of posture and coordination of movements.

Inability to maintain the equilibrium of the body, while standing, or while walking, is referred to as ***ataxia.*** This may occur as a result of the interruption of afferent proprioceptive pathways (***sensory ataxia***). Disease of the cerebellum itself, or of efferent pathways, results in more severe disability. Coordination of the activity of different groups of muscles is interfered with, leading to various defects.

The person is unable to stand with his feet close together: the body sways from side to side and the person may fall. While walking, the patient staggers and is unable to maintain progression in the desired direction. Lack of proprioceptive information can be compensated to a considerable extent by information received through the eyes. The defects mentioned are, therefore, much more pronounced with the eyes closed (***Romberg's sign***). Lack of coordination of muscles also interferes with purposeful movements (***asynergia***). Movements are jerky and lack precision. For example, the patient finds it difficult to touch his nose with a finger, or to move a finger along a line. There is difficulty in performing movements involving rapid alternating action of opposing groups of muscles (e.g., tapping one hand with the other; repeated pronation and supination of the forearm). This phenomenon is called ***dysdiadokokinesis.*** Incoordination of the muscles responsible for the articulation of words leads to characteristic speech defects (***dysarthria***). For the same reason, the eyes are unable to fix the gaze on an object for any length of time. Attempts to bring the gaze back to the same point result in repeated jerky movements of the eyes. This is called ***nystagmus.***

Apart from incoordination, cerebellar disease is characterized by diminished muscle tone (***hypotonia***). The muscles are soft, and tire easily (***asthenia***). Joints may lack stability (***flail joints***). Tendon reflexes may be diminished. Alternatively, tapping a tendon may result in oscillating movements of the part concerned, like a pendulum.

Abnormal Movements

Various kinds of abnormal movements are seen in neurological disorders involving the basal ganglia, the subthalamic nucleus and the cerebellum.

These may take the form of involuntary shaking (***tremor***) of the hands, head or other parts of the body, because of rapid alternating contraction of opposing groups of muscles. In some instances the tremor comes on when the patient tries to perform voluntary movement (***intention tremor***). Another type of abnormal movement consists of a slow twisting of a limb, or of the face or neck (***athetosis***). Sudden, jerky, shock-like movements involving any part of the body (***myoclonus***) may also occur. These can cause objects held in the hand to be thrown away (***hemiballism***). Sometimes different, complex, involuntary movements occur in succession, particularly in the distal parts of the limbs (***chorea***).

It has not been possible to precisely correlate specific abnormal movements with disease in specific regions of the basal ganglia and neighbouring structures. The movements are not a result of inactivity of the diseased centres but are, on the contrary, to be regarded as release phenomena, due to abolition of inhibitory influences. Hemiballism is known to be produced by lesions in the subthalamic nucleus. Intention tremor is seen in disorders of the cerebellum.

In many cases, abnormal movements are accompanied by rigidity of muscles, because of increased muscle tone. The increased tone is also a release phenomenon. One common syndrome characterized by rigidity and abnormal movements is called ***Parkinsonism*** or ***paralysis agitans*** (shaking palsy). It is characterized by marked rigidity which leads to a stooped posture, a slow shuffling gait, difficulty in speech, and a mask-like face. Characteristic involuntary 'pill-rolling' movements of the hands are seen. The condition is believed to be due to degenerative changes in the striatum and the substantia nigra.

SENSORY DISORDERS

Interruption of ascending pathways carrying various sensations results in loss of sensory perception (***anaesthesia***) over parts of the body concerned. In case of peripheral nerves the area of anaesthesia following injury is often much less than the area of distribution of the nerve. This is so because of considerable overlap in the areas supplied by different nerves. The area of skin supplied from one spinal segment is called a ***dermatome.*** Dermatomes for adjoining segments overlap, a given area of skin being innervated by two or more segments. In the case of spinal cord lesions, the level of disease can be inferred from the level of sensory loss. In this connection it must be remembered that the finer modalities of touch are carried by the posterior column tracts which are uncrossed. Crude touch, pain and temperature are carried by the spinothalamic tracts which are crossed. Thus a unilateral lesion in the spinal cord can result in loss of the power of tactile localization, tactile discrimination and of stereognosis on the side of lesion with loss of crude touch, pain and temperature on the opposite side. Because of a double pathway for touch, loss of sensations of pain and temperature is often more obvious than interference with touch. We have seen that, while crossing the midline, fibres of the spinothalamic tracts do not run horizontally. They ascend as they cross so that their path is oblique. The degree of obliquity is greater in the case of fibres carrying touch as compared to those carrying pain and temperature. Because of this there can be a difference of a few segments in the level at which (or below which) these sensations are lost when the crossing fibres are interrupted by a lesion. In a disease called ***syringomyelia***, the region of the spinal cord near the central canal undergoes degeneration with formation of cavities. Fibres of spinothalamic tracts crossing in this region are interrupted. Sensations of pain and temperature are lost over the part of the skin from which fibres are interrupted, but touch is retained as there is an additional pathway for it through the posterior column tracts. This phenomenon is called ***dissociated anaesthesia.***

Sensory disturbances can also result from lesions in the brainstem because of damage to the medial lemniscus or to the spinal and trigeminal lemnisci. Lesions of the thalamus can produce bizarre sensory disturbances. Lesions in the internal capsule can cause sensory loss in the entire opposite half of the body as thalamocortical fibres pass through this region. Pressure on sensory areas of the cerebral cortex can result in various abnormal sensations, or in anaesthesia over certain regions. Damage to pathways carrying special sensations of smell, vision and hearing can result in various defects.

Referred Pain

It sometimes happens that when one of the viscera is diseased pain is not felt in the region of the organ itself; but is felt in some part of the skin and body wall. This phenomenon is called ***referred pain.*** This pain is usually (but not always) referred to areas of skin supplied by the same spinal segments which innervate the viscus. Some classical examples of referred pain are as follows.

1. Pain arising in the diaphragm, or diaphragmatic pleura, is referred to the shoulder (C4).
2. Pain arising in the heart is referred to the lower cervical and upper thoracic segments. It is felt in the chest wall and along the medial side of the left arm. It may also be referred to the neck or jaw.
3. Referred pain from the stomach is felt in the epigastrium (T6 to T9); and that from the intestines is felt in the epigastrium and around the umbilicus (T7 to

T10). Pain from the ileocaecal region is felt in the right iliac region. Pain from the appendix is felt in the umbilical region.
4. Pain from the gall bladder is referred to the epigastrium. It may also be referred to the back just below the inferior angle of the right scapula.
5. Pain arising in the area of distribution of one division of the trigeminal nerve may be referred along other branches of the same division, or even along branches of other divisions.

SPINAL REFLEXES

We have seen that the nervous system is involved in various types of reflex activity. The basic pathways for such reflexes have been considered on page 462. Many of these reflexes can be demonstrated clinically, and constitute a valuable aid in establishing the integrity of various levels of the nervous system. Some of the reflexes that are used for this purpose are described below.

Myotatic or Stretch Reflexes

Sudden stretching of a muscle (by tapping its tendon) produces a reflex contraction of the muscle. The pathway for this reflex involves two neurons only. Stretching of the muscle stimulates proprioceptive nerve endings located in muscle spindles and other receptors. These impulses are carried to the spinal cord by neurons that synapse with motor neurons in the ventral grey columns (Fig. 17.2). Fibres arising from these motor neurons reach the muscle and produce contraction. Stretch reflexes are abolished if any part of the pathway for it (i.e., the reflex arc) is interrupted. Under certain conditions these reflexes may be exaggerated. From a clinical point of view it is important to know the level of the spinal cord at which each reflex is mediated. Some of the important stretch reflexes are described below. The spinal segments concerned are given in brackets.

1. The ***knee jerk*** or ***patellar tendon reflex*** consists of extension of the leg by contraction of the quadriceps when the ligamentum patellae is tapped (L2, L3, L4).
2. The ***ankle jerk*** or ***Achilles tendon reflex*** consists of plantar flexion of the foot on tapping the tendo calcaneus (L5, S1, S2).
3. The ***biceps tendon reflex*** consists of flexion of the forearm on tapping the biceps tendon (C5, C6).
4. The ***triceps tendon reflex*** consists of extension of the forearm on tapping the triceps tendon (C6, C7, C8).
5. The ***supinator jerk*** (or ***radial periosteal reflex***) consists of flexion of the forearm when the distal end of the radius is tapped (C7, C8). Note that the muscle responsible for this reflex is the brachioradialis, not the supinator. It is called the supinator jerk because the brachioradialis was at one time called the supinator longus.
6. The ***wrist tendon reflex*** consists of flexion of the fingers on percussion on wrist tendons (C8, T1).
7. The ***jaw*** or ***masseter reflex*** is a myotatic reflex mediated through the trigeminal nerve (and not through the spinal cord). To elicit this reflex the patient is asked to open the mouth slightly. The examiner places his index finger over the middle of the patients chin and taps it. This results in bilateral contraction of the masseter and temporalis muscles. Both afferent and efferent components of the reflex arc pass through the mandibular division of the trigeminal nerve, the nuclei concerned being located in the pons.

Superficial Reflexes

Stimulation of skin in certain regions of the body causes contraction of underlying muscles. This occurs reflexly, the reflex being mediated through the spinal cord. Some of these superficial reflexes are described below.

1. The ***abdominal reflexes*** consist of contraction of underlying muscles on stroking the skin of the abdomen in its upper (T6, 7), middle (T8, 9) and lower (T10 to T12) parts.
2. The ***cremasteric reflex*** consists of elevation of the scrotum on stroking the skin of the medial side of the thigh (T12 to L2).
3. The ***gluteal reflex*** consists of contraction of the glutei on stroking the overlying skin (L4 to S1).
4. The normal ***plantar reflex*** consists of plantar flexion of the toes on stroking the skin of the sole (L5 to S2). When there is an injury to the corticospinal system an abnormal response is obtained. There is extension (dorsiflexion) of the great toe and fanning out of other toes. This response is referred to as ***Babinski's sign.*** Such a response may also be seen in new born infants, and sometimes in sleeping or intoxicated adults.
5. The ***anal reflex*** consists of contraction of the external anal sphincter on stroking the perianal region (S4,5, coccygeal).

Other Important Spinal Levels

Movements of the head (through neck muscles) depend on segments C1 to C4; those of the diaphragm on segments C3 to C5; those of the upper extremity on segments C5 to T1; and those of the lower extremity on segments L1 to S2. Filling of the urinary bladder is mediated by segments T12 to L2, and evacuation by segments S3 to S5. Erection of the penis depends on segments S2 to S4, and ejaculation on segments L1 and L2 (smooth muscle), and also on S3 and S4 (striated muscle).

REFLEXES RELATED TO THE EYEBALL

Pupillary Reflexes

Light thrown on an eye causes the pupil of that eye to contract. This is called the ***direct pupillary light reflex.*** At the same time the pupil of the other eye also contracts. This is called the ***consensual light reflex.*** The pathway for the light reflex is shown in Fig. 26.1. Impulses from the retina (of the eye on which light is thrown) travel through the optic nerve, chiasma and optic tracts. Near the lateral geniculate body the fibres concerned pass into the midbrain and end in the pretectal nucleus. Axons arising from this nucleus reach the Edinger Westphal nuclei of both sides. Fibres arising in these nuclei supply the sphincter pupillae after relay in the ciliary ganglion. The consensual reflex may be explained by the following.

a. Fibres of each optic nerve enter both optic tracts as a result of partial crossing in the chiasma.
b. Fibres from each optic tract end in both pretectal nuclei.
c. Fibres from each pretectal nucleus reach the Edinger Westphal nuclei of both sides.

Constriction of the pupil also takes place when we look at a near object i.e., during accomodation. The pathway for this is different from that for the light reflex, and is believed to involve the visual cortex. In certain diseases (notably syphlitic infection) of the nervous system the pupillary light reflex may be abolished, but pupillary constriction in response to accomodation remains. This condition is called ***Argyll-Robertson-pupil.*** In such cases the lesion is believed to be in the pretectal area.

Corneal Reflex

If the cornea is touched with a small wisp of cotton this results in closing of both eyes. This is called the ***corneal reflex***. Impulses from the cornea travel along branches of the ophthalmic division of the trigeminal nerve to the sensory nuclei of this nerve. Secondary fibres establish connections with the motor nuclei of the facial nerve of both sides. Fibres arising in the facial nuclei, and reaching the muscles closing the palpebral aperture, complete the reflex arc. In the case of injury to the ophthalmic division of the trigeminal nerve, the corneal reflex cannot be elicited from that side, but a bilateral response is obtained by stimulating the cornea of the normal side. In facial paralysis the response is seen only on the normal side.

SOME INVESTIGATIVE PROCEDURES USED FOR NEUROLOGICAL DIAGNOSIS

In the preceding paragraphs we have briefly reviewed some of the manifestations of neurological disorders. These may be seen in various combinations. Diagnosis of the site, and nature, of disease depends on an analysis of the total picture presented by the patient. It is here that a knowledge of neuroanatomy becomes important. It is this knowledge that enables the physician to pinpoint the region, involvement of which could explain the various manifestations observed.

In some cases considerable help in localization of lesions and in diagnosis of their nature, may be obtained by the use of certain investigative procedures that are briefly mentioned below.

Lumbar Puncture

We have seen that a needle can be introduced into the subarachnoid space through the interval between the third and fourth lumbar vertebrae. This procedure, called lumbar puncture, is useful for several purposes.

a. The pressure of CSF can be estimated, roughly, by counting the rate at which drops flow out of the needle; or more accurately, by connecting the needle to a manometer.
b. Samples of CSF can be collected for examination. The important points to note about CSF are its colour, its cellular content, and its chemical composition (specially the protein and sugar content).
c. Lumbar puncture may be used for introducing air or radio-opaque dyes into the subarachnoid space for certain investigative procedures (see below). Drugs may also be injected for treatment.
d. Mention may be made here of a use of lumbar puncture, not related to neurological diagnosis. Anaesthetic drugs injected into the subarachnoid space act on the lower spinal nerve roots and render the lower part of the body insensitive to pain. This procedure, called ***spinal anaesthesia***, is frequently used for operations on the lower abdomen or on the lower extremities.

Radiological Procedures

1. Plain radiographs of the skull (Figs. 1.22, 1.23) may give evidence of disease when the skull bones are affected, or when there are areas of calcification.
2. Air injected into the subarachnoid space through lumbar puncture ascends in the spinal subarachnoid space to the cranial cavity. The air can be seen in radiographs. This procedure is called ***pneumoencephalography.*** The air injected

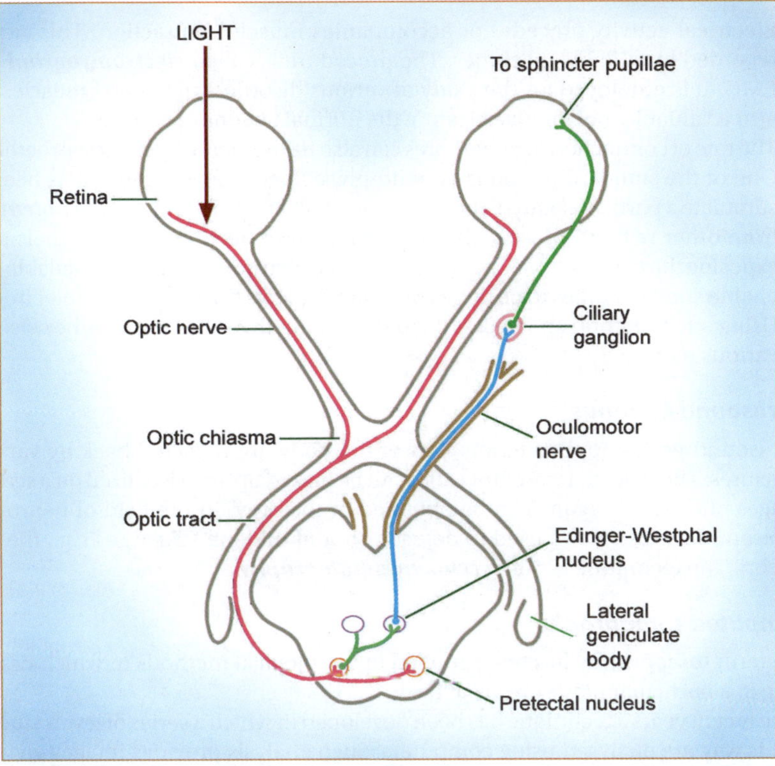

Fig. 26.1 Pathway for the light reflex. Note that all pathways shown are bilateral. Some of them are shown only on one side for sake of clarity.

may enter the ventricles. Their outlines can then be seen. (This procedure is no longer used and is of historical interest only).

3. The ventricles can be visualized by injecting radio-opaque dyes directly into the lateral ventricle (***ventriculography)*** (Figs. 16.12). Abnormal dilatations of the ventricular system (hydrocephalus) can be detected.
4. The vascular system of the brain can be visualized by injecting radio-opaque material into the common carotid or vertebral arteries (***Cerebral angiography).*** Radiographs taken immediately after the injection reveal the arterial pattern (Fig. 66.13). The capillary and venous patterns can be seen after brief intervals.
5. The spinal subarachnoid space can be visualized by injecting radio-opaque material (***myelography***).

Abnormal appearances seen with the procedures mentioned above help in determining the nature and location of tumours or other masses present in relation to the brain or spinal cord.

Electrophysiological Methods

1. Information about the functioning of the brain can be obtained by a study of the patterns of electrical activity within it. Electrodes are applied over the scalp at various points. These are connected to a machine which records the electrical potentials. The procedure is called ***electroencephalography*** or EEG).

2. Electrical activity precedes or accompanies muscle contraction. This can be recorded by suitable machines. The procedure is called ***electromyography*** or EMG. It is employed for the study of various disorders of skeletal muscle. It is also a valuable tool for investigating the normal actions of muscles.
3. The rate of conduction in nerve fibres can also be measured by electrical methods.
4. One of the standard methods of neurophysiological investigation has been to stimulate a particular part of the nervous system and to record ***evoked potentials*** from other regions. Most such experiments have been done on animals after exposing the regions concerned. Sophisticated instruments are now available that enable similar studies to be done in human subjects through surface electrodes. Using such methods it is possible to determine the integrity (or otherwise) of various pathways.

Ultrasound Methods

Ultrasound waves applied to any part of the body are reflected back by various structures. The reflected waves (or echo) can be picked up and visualized on a screen. Images of internal organs can be obtained in this way. In the field of neurology ultrasound waves can be used to detect a shift of midline structures e.g., the falx cerebri. The technique is called ***echoencephalography.***

Computed Tomography

The term ***tomography*** has been applied to radiological methods in which tissues lying in a particular plane are visualized.

In recent years a technique has been developed in which a series of levels studied in this way are analysed using computers. Such analysis provides images giving a remarkable degree of detail. The procedure is called ***computerized tomography*** or CT scan. The technique has revolutionized neurological diagnosis, and has rendered many older techniques obsolete. Tumours, areas of haemorrhage, and various other lesions can be identified with confidence.

Magnetic Resonance Imaging

It has been observed that if some radioactive materials are injected into the body, they induce a specific magnetic resonance in different tissues of the body. These differences can be recorded using sophisticated machines, and result in images of outstanding clarity (Fig. 66.14 to 66.6). The images are distinctly superior to those of CT scans but this technique is more expensive, and takes much more time to perform, than a CT scan.

Index

Page numbers followed by *f* refer to figure.

B

C

D

E

F

G

H

I

J

K

L

M

N

O

P

Q

R

S

T

U

V

W

X

Y

Z